T0198123

Imaging in
PEDIATRICS

MERROW | HARIHARAN

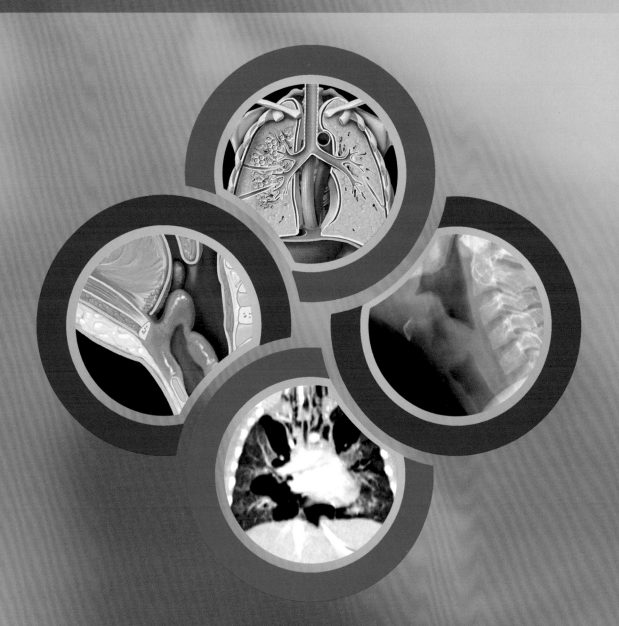

ELSEVIER

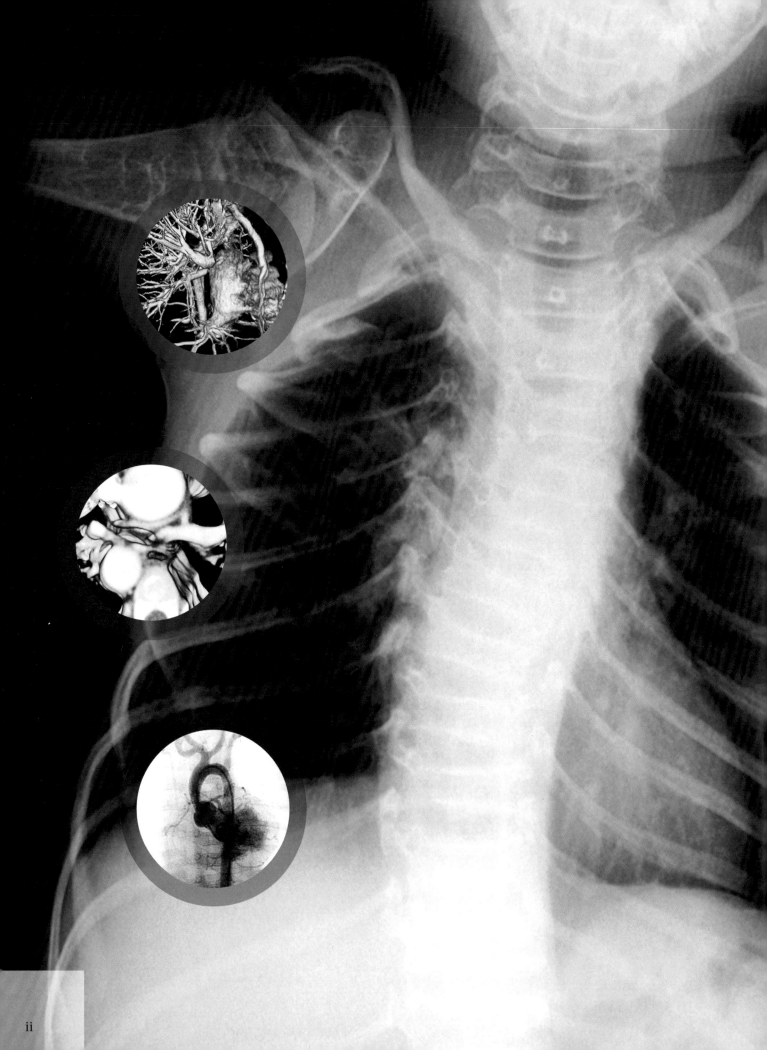

Imaging in
PEDIATRICS

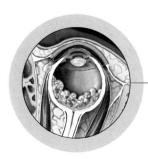

A. Carlson Merrow, Jr., MD, FAAP

Corning Benton Chair for Radiology Education
Cincinnati Children's Hospital Medical Center
Associate Professor of Clinical Radiology
University of Cincinnati College of Medicine
Cincinnati, Ohio

Selena Hariharan, MD, MHSA, FAAP

Division of Emergency Medicine
Cincinnati Children's Hospital Medical Center
Associate Professor of Pediatrics
University of Cincinnati College of Medicine
Cincinnati, Ohio

ELSEVIER

1600 John F. Kennedy Blvd.
Ste 1800
Philadelphia, PA 19103-2899

IMAGING IN PEDIATRICS

ISBN: 978-0-323-47778-9

Notices

Knowledge and best practice in this field are constantly changing. As new research and experience broaden our understanding, changes in research methods, professional practices, or medical treatment may become necessary.

Practitioners and researchers must always rely on their own experience and knowledge in evaluating and using any information, methods, compounds, or experiments described herein. In using such information or methods they should be mindful of their own safety and the safety of others, including parties for whom they have a professional responsibility.

With respect to any drug or pharmaceutical products identified, readers are advised to check the most current information provided (i) on procedures featured or (ii) by the manufacturer of each product to be administered, to verify the recommended dose or formula, the method and duration of administration, and contraindications. It is the responsibility of practitioners, relying on their own experience and knowledge of their patients, to make diagnoses, to determine dosages and the best treatment for each individual patient, and to take all appropriate safety precautions.

To the fullest extent of the law, neither the Publisher nor the authors, contributors, or editors, assume any liability for any injury and/or damage to persons or property as a matter of products liability, negligence or otherwise, or from any use or operation of any methods, products, instructions, or ideas contained in the material herein.

Publisher Cataloging-in-Publication Data

Names: Names: Merrow, A. Carlson, Jr. (Arnold Carlson) | Hariharan, Selena.
Title: Imaging in pediatrics / [edited by] A. Carlson Merrow, Jr. and Selena Hariharan.
Description: First edition. | Salt Lake City, UT : Elsevier, Inc., [2017] | Includes
  bibliographical references and index.
Identifiers: ISBN 978-0-323-47778-9
Subjects: LCSH: Pediatric diagnostic imaging--Handbooks, manuals, etc. | MESH: Diagnostic Imaging--methods--Atlases. | Child--
Atlases. | Infants--Atlases.
Classification: LCC RJ51.D5 I43 2017 | NLM WN 240 | DDC 618.9200754--dc23

International Standard Book Number: 978-0-323-47778-9

Cover Designer: Tom M. Olson, BA

Printed in Canada by Friesens, Altona, Manitoba, Canada

Last digit is the print number: 9 8 7 6 5 4 3 2 1

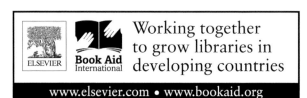

Dedications

To my family: Thank you for your patience, encouragement, and love.

To my colleagues: Thank you for your teaching, vision, wisdom, and support.

To my patients and their families: Thank you for your courage, trust, and endurance.

ACM

Thank you to my parents, P.R. and Brindha Hariharan, for always nurturing my dreams; to my children, Nikhil and Ami Hariharan, for reminding me that dreams can come true, both at work and at home; and to my husband, James Kalinowski, who supports my dreams so completely that he moved to a new city without any questions and laughs when people call him "Mr. Hariharan."

SH

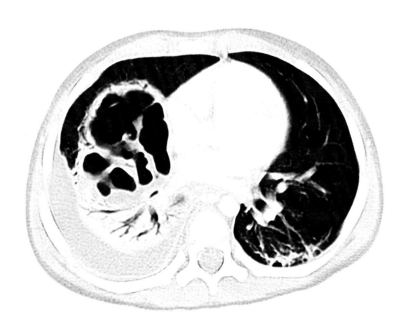

Contributing Authors

Christopher G. Anton, MD
Division Chief of Radiography
Cincinnati Children's Hospital Medical Center
Assistant Professor
Clinical Radiology and Pediatrics
Associate Radiology Residency
Program Director
University of Cincinnati College of Medicine
Cincinnati, Ohio

Michael R. Aquino, MD, MHSc
Staff Pediatric General Radiologist
The Hospital for Sick Children
Assistant Professor of Medical Imaging
University of Toronto
Toronto, Ontario, Canada

Hank Baskin, MD
Pediatric Imaging Section Chief
Primary Children's Hospital
Intermountain Healthcare
Adjunct Associate Professor of Radiology
University of Utah School of Medicine
Salt Lake City, Utah

Lane F. Donnelly, MD
Chief Quality Officer
Associate Radiologist-in-Chief
Texas Children's Hospital
Professor of Radiology
Baylor College of Medicine
Houston, Texas

Robert J. Fleck, Jr., MD
Section Chief of Cardiovascular Imaging
Cincinnati Children's Hospital Medical Center
Associate Professor of Clinical Radiology
University of Cincinnati College of Medicine
Cincinnati, Ohio

Blaise V. Jones, MD
Division Chief of Neuroradiology
Cincinnati Children's Hospital Medical Center
Professor of Clinical Radiology and Pediatrics
University of Cincinnati College of Medicine
Cincinnati, Ohio

Bernadette L. Koch, MD
Associate Chief of Radiology Academic Affairs
Cincinnati Children's Hospital Medical Center
Professor of Clinical Radiology and Pediatrics
University of Cincinnati College of Medicine
Cincinnati, Ohio

Nicholas A. Koontz, MD
Director of Fellowship Programs
Assistant Professor of Radiology
Department of Radiology and Imaging Sciences
Indiana University School of Medicine
Indianapolis, Indiana

Steven J. Kraus, MD
Division Chief of Fluoroscopy
Cincinnati Children's Hospital Medical Center
Associate Professor
Clinical Radiology and Pediatrics
University of Cincinnati College of Medicine
Cincinnati, Ohio

Luke L. Linscott, MD
Pediatric Neuroradiologist
Primary Children's Hospital
Intermountain Healthcare
Adjunct Assistant Professor of Radiology
University of Utah School of Medicine
Salt Lake City, Utah

B.J. Manaster, MD, PhD, FACR
Emeritus Professor
Department of Radiology
University of Utah School of Medicine
Salt Lake City, Utah

Prakash M. Masand, MD
Division Chief of Cardiovascular Imaging
Department of Radiology, Texas Children's Hospital
Assistant Professor of Clinical Radiology
Baylor College of Medicine
Houston, Texas

Arthur B. Meyers, MD
Nemours Children's Health System
Nemours Children's Hospital
Orlando, Florida

Ryan A. Moore, MD
Assistant Professor of Clinical Cardiology
Cincinnati Children's Hospital Medical Center
University of Cincinnati College of Medicine
Cincinnati, Ohio

Usha D. Nagaraj, MD
Neuroradiologist
Cincinnati Children's Hospital Medical Center
Assistant Professor
Clinical Radiology and Pediatrics
University of Cincinnati College of Medicine
Cincinnati, Ohio

Sara M. O'Hara, MD, FAAP
Division Chief of Ultrasound
Cincinnati Children's Hospital Medical Center
Professor of Clinical Radiology and Pediatrics
University of Cincinnati College of Medicine
Cincinnati, Ohio

Anne G. Osborn, MD, FACR
University Distinguished Professor
Professor of Radiology
William H. and Patricia W. Child Presidential Endowed Chair
in Radiology
University of Utah School of Medicine
Salt Lake City, Utah

Daniel J. Podberesky, MD
Radiologist-in-Chief
Nemours Children's Health System
Chair, Department of Radiology, Nemours Children's Hospital
Associate Professor of Radiology
University of Central Florida and
Florida State University Colleges of Medicine
Orlando, Florida

Mantosh S. Rattan, MD
Division Chief of Cardiac Imaging
Cincinnati Children's Hospital Medical Center
Assistant Professor of Clinical Radiology
University of Cincinnati College of Medicine
Cincinnati, Ohio

Randy R. Richardson, MD
Chairman of Radiology
St. Joseph's Hospital and Medical Center
Associate Dean
Professor of Radiology
Creighton University School of Medicine
Phoenix Regional Campus
Phoenix, Arizona

Ethan A. Smith, MD
Co-Director of Thoracoabdominal Imaging
Cincinnati Children's Hospital Medical Center
Associate Professor of Clinical Radiology
University of Cincinnati College of Medicine
Cincinnati, Ohio

Alexander J. Towbin, MD
Associate Chief of Radiology
Clinical Operations and Informatics
Neil D. Johnson Chair of Radiology Informatics
Cincinnati Children's Hospital Medical Center
Associate Professor
Clinical Radiology and Pediatrics
University of Cincinnati College of Medicine
Cincinnati, Ohio

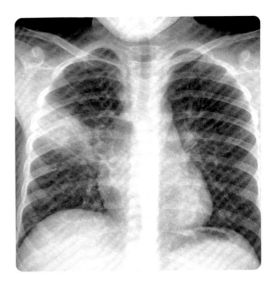

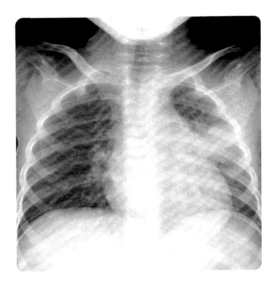

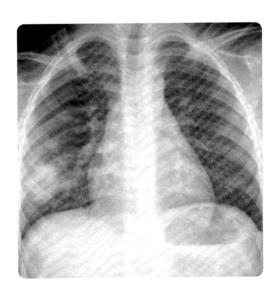

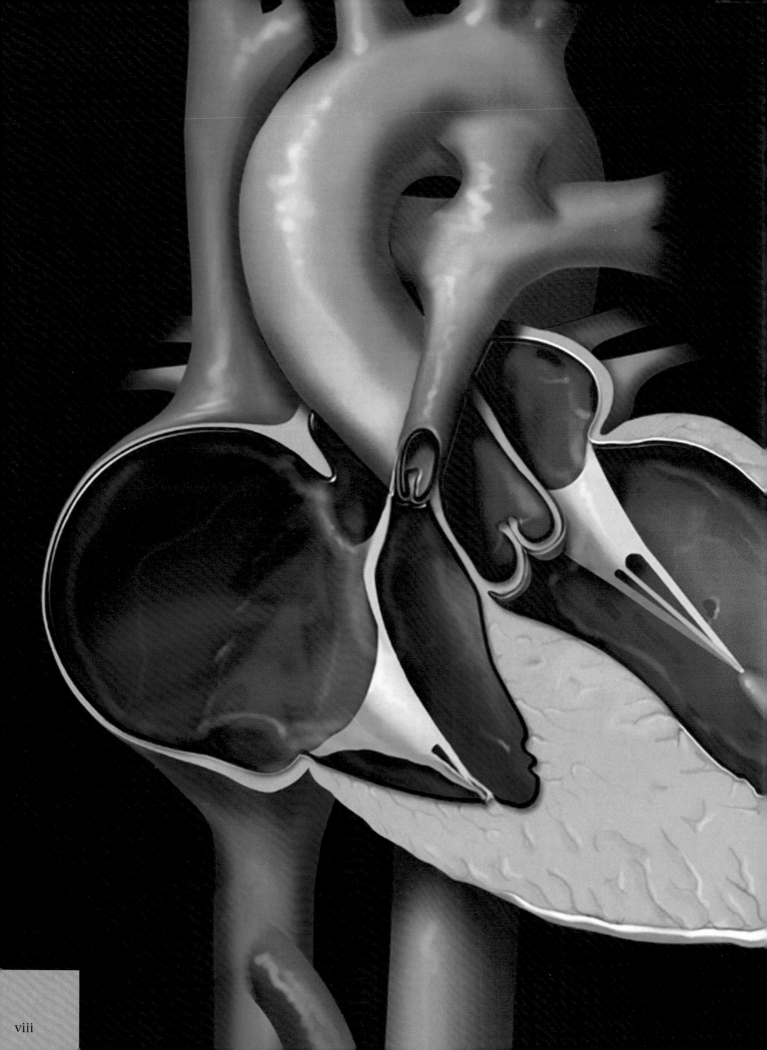

Foreword

In an era of rapid technological progress and virtually unlimited access to information, there are increasingly high expectations on pediatricians to coordinate efficient and accurate care for their patients. As a result, physicians may be anxious about choosing the best imaging modality to serve their patient, a decision that must include an evaluation of the accuracy, availability, risks, and costs of an ever-evolving array of diagnostic exams in relation to a specific diagnosis. *Imaging in Pediatrics* is designed to help answer the questions that not only lead up to choosing a radiologic study but also follow the exam, such as, "What does the radiologist mean by the wording in this report?" and "What can I as the pediatrician point out to the patient and family on these images?"

This work has been written and edited by a team of pediatric radiologists and pediatricians led by Drs. A. Carlson Merrow and Selena Hariharan from Cincinnati Children's Hospital Medical Center. Dr. Merrow is an associate professor of clinical radiology and holds the Corning Benton Chair for Radiology Education. He has received numerous teaching awards and has recently published a pediatric radiology text with online content that is used by the majority of radiology training programs in the USA. Dr. Hariharan is an associate professor of pediatrics and specializes in emergency medicine, which has provided her with a clear understanding of the clinical dilemmas and imaging conundrums faced by physicians who care for children. As a result, she is able to address the varied presentations of even common illnesses and ensures that the text is well suited for clinicians who are not radiology experts but are asked to incorporate imaging into their daily practice.

The text of *Imaging in Pediatrics* is an ideal marriage between practical information and visual examples. There are incredible images and illustrations that are highlighted by factual and easy-to-understand text. The chapters are grouped by physiologic systems with each chapter targeted to a suspected diagnosis and written with a bullet-point "Key Facts" style, creating a text that is easy to reference.

This book is ideally suited for anyone who is interested in becoming more proficient at understanding pediatric imaging in a primarily clinical setting. Physicians who use this volume will be able to intelligently discuss recommendations and results of imaging with the radiologist, clinical colleagues, and, most importantly, patients and families.

Karen Remley, MD, MBA, MPH, FAAP

Professor of Pediatrics
Eastern Virginia Medical School
Norfolk, Virginia

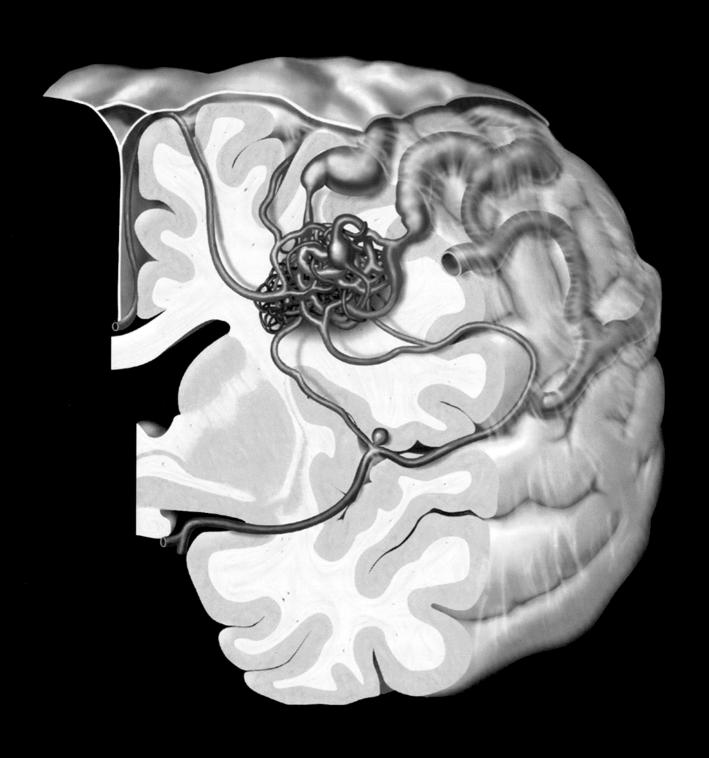

Preface

There is an ever-expanding world of resources available to the pediatrician for education and point-of-care reference, particularly in this era of nearly instantaneous access to data. We thank you for selecting this text that we believe offers a unique perspective on the clinical care of children by providing guidance through the increasingly complex landscape of available imaging tests. This book includes not only direction on when to employ imaging but also instruction on which studies to consider and how they should be ordered. This text will also lead you through the fundamentals of how these studies work as well as their advantages and disadvantages (including potential health risks). Common language employed by radiologists is explored, and numerous imaging examples are provided.

A quick glance through the book reveals that it is not a typical prose-filled reference. While you will find a few prose introductory chapters at the beginning of the book and leading each body section (which will help explain relevant imaging exams), the majority of the book utilizes a bullet point style to enable quick extraction of critical data from the text. Most of the chapters have only a "Key Facts" component (plus images), though we have chosen a number of important topics to expand for a more thorough discussion. Finally, please note that there is an abbreviation index to help guide you through the most common radiologic and anatomic notations.

Our ultimate hope is that this book will increase your comfort in the effective and efficient utilization of imaging in your practice, daily enhancing your care of children.

A. Carlson Merrow, Jr., MD, FAAP
Corning Benton Chair for Radiology Education
Cincinnati Children's Hospital Medical Center
Associate Professor of Clinical Radiology
University of Cincinnati College of Medicine
Cincinnati, Ohio

Selena Hariharan, MD, MHSA, FAAP
Division of Emergency Medicine
Cincinnati Children's Hospital Medical Center
Associate Professor of Pediatrics
University of Cincinnati College of Medicine
Cincinnati, Ohio

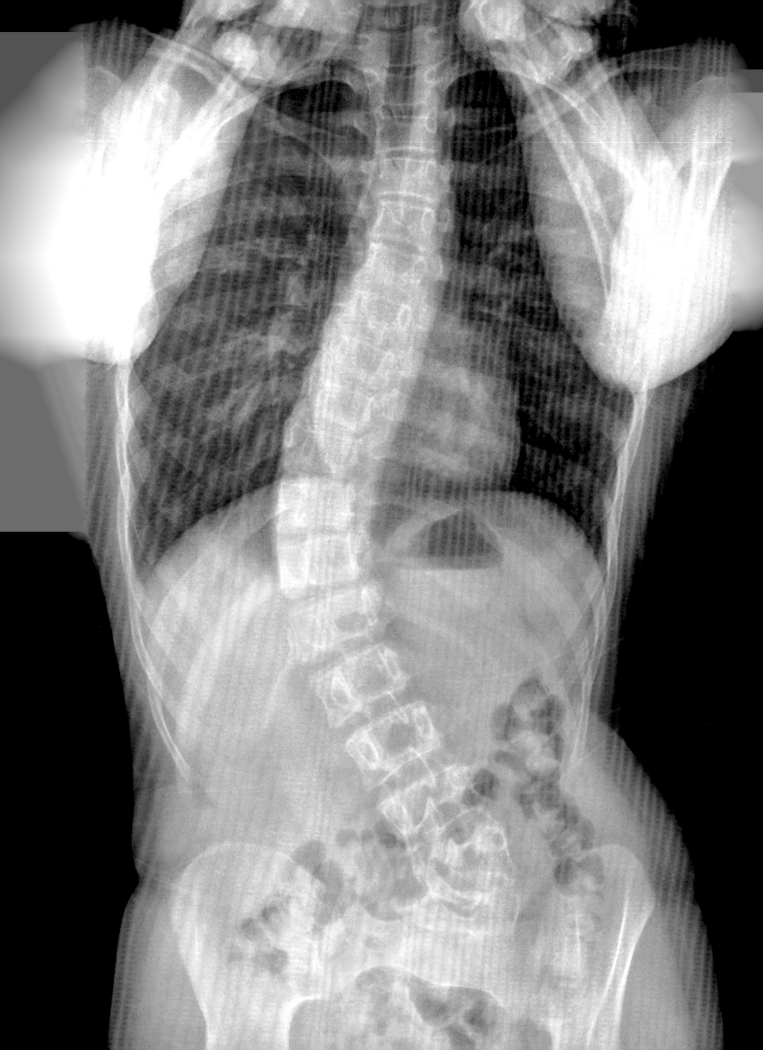

Acknowledgments

Text Editors

Arthur G. Gelsinger, MA
Terry W. Ferrell, MS
Lisa A. Gervais, BS
Karen E. Concannon, MA, PhD
Matt W. Hoecherl, BS
Megg Morin, BA

Image Editors

Jeffrey J. Marmorstone, BS
Lisa A. M. Steadman, BS

Medical Editors

Lauren C. Riney, DO
Caitlin Valentino, MD, MS

Illustrations

Laura C. Wissler, MA
Lane R. Bennion, MS
Richard Coombs, MS

Art Direction and Design

Tom M. Olson, BA
Laura C. Wissler, MA

Lead Editor

Nina I. Bennett, BA

Production Coordinators

Angela M. G. Terry, BA
Rebecca L. Bluth, BA
Emily C. Fassett, BA

ELSEVIER

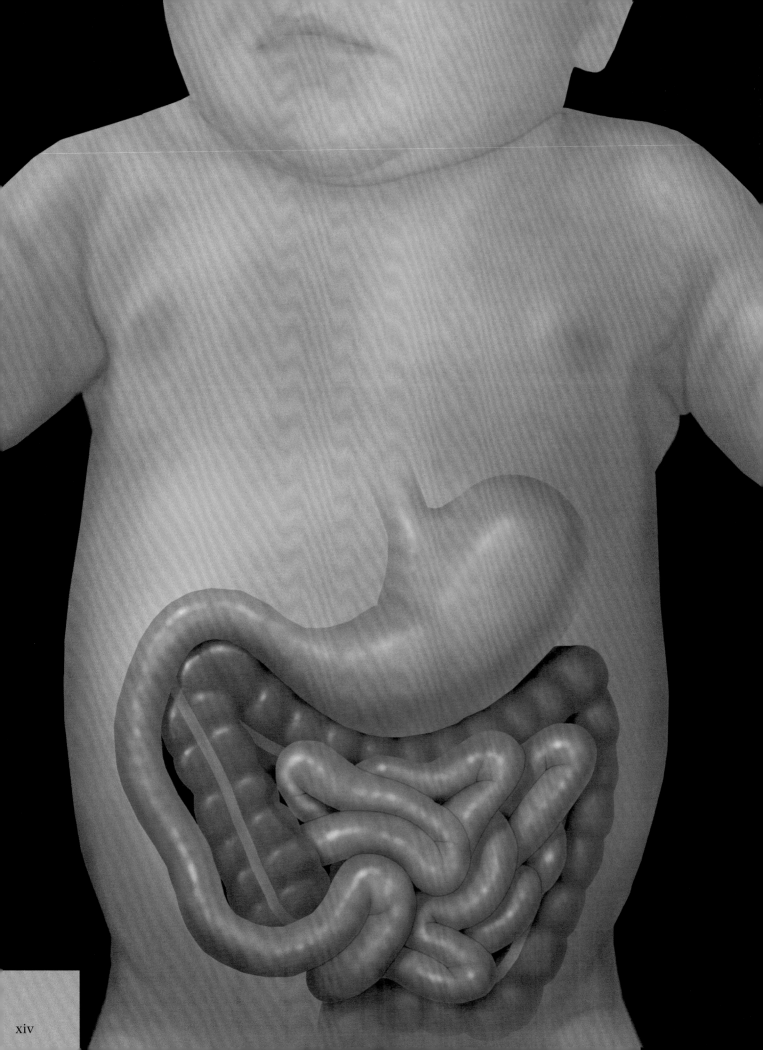

Sections

Section 1:
Airway

Section 2:
Chest

Section 3:
Cardiac

Section 4:
Gastrointestinal

Section 5:
Genitourinary

Section 6:
Musculoskeletal

Section 7:
Brain

Section 8:
Spine

Section 9:
Head and Neck

TABLE OF CONTENTS

TABLE OF CONTENTS

TABLE OF CONTENTS

TABLE OF CONTENTS

TABLE OF CONTENTS

TABLE OF CONTENTS

TABLE OF CONTENTS

Imaging in
PEDIATRICS

MERROW | HARIHARAN

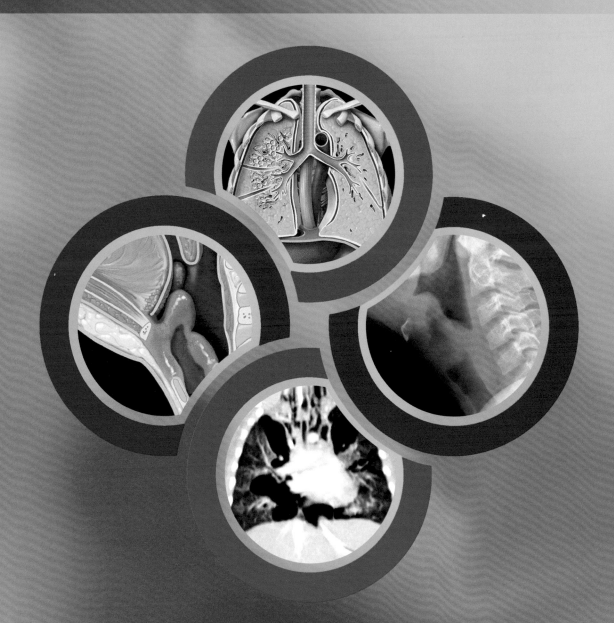

ELSEVIER

Introduction

There have been rapid technological advances in medical imaging over the last several decades, generally providing faster, more detailed, & readily available assessments of patients. Clinical work-ups have increasingly incorporated advanced imaging during these years, though not always in an effective or judicious manner. In addition to concerns of financial cost, apprehensions have been increasingly raised about the downsides of several imaging modalities (including the long-term effects of radiation, anesthesia, & contrast agents).

This chapter will serve as an overview of the various imaging modalities available in the work-up & treatment of pediatric patients, discussing basic techniques & terminology that can help the pediatrician better understand the studies they are ordering & the reports they are receiving. Basic applications of each modality will be covered here (though more thoroughly applied in the "Approach to..." chapters introducing each body section). We will also discuss some of the negatives associated with each modality, though the recognized & theorized health risks of these modalities will be covered in a separate chapter.

Radiography

Despite being the earliest discovered & medically adopted imaging technique, radiographs (the preferred term for "plain films" or "x-rays") remain the workhorse of radiologic imaging in the child (with the main exception being the head). They are widely used in the assessments of pediatric bone trauma, abdominal pain, & suspected lower respiratory tract infections, among many other indications. Radiographs remain the cheapest & most readily available imaging studies, though pediatric specific centers are most experienced with techniques to optimize not only the extraction of medical data from the study but also enhance the patient & family experience. Additionally, pediatric centers have been at the forefront of reducing the dose of ionizing radiation associated with these exams, which does require a balance with maintaining a diagnostically sufficient study.

In general, radiography uses a beam of x-rays coursing through the body to produce an image. The image generated will project as various shades of gray (from black to white) based on the density & thickness of the tissue being examined as well as the energy of the x-ray beam. The degree to which the x-ray beam is attenuated as it passes from the tube to the detector of the machine (with the patient in between these 2 components) determines how much of the detector is exposed to x-rays that then activate specific elements within the detector to create an image. Therefore, tissues such as the lung (which are filled with air) will attenuate relatively little of the x-ray beam on its way to the detector. In contrast, tissues such as bone will attenuate a much larger percentage of the x-ray beam, allowing relatively few x-rays to reach the detector. By convention, tissues of greater density (such as bone) will be displayed as relatively bright or white (radiopaque) while tissues of lesser density (such as lung) will be displayed as relatively dark or black (radiolucent). Classically, 5 main categories of density are recognized visually on radiographs (in order from least to most dense): Gas/air, fat, water (soft tissue), calcium, & metal.

Unlike the "cross-sectional" imaging modalities discussed below (i.e., computed tomography, magnetic resonance, ultrasound, & some nuclear medicine exams), where 2D images represent very thin slices of 3D patient anatomy, the 2D radiograph represents a single thick slice (or volume) of the entire patient where the 3D anatomy is all superimposed onto a single 2D image. Therefore, a particular point on the image likely represents the result of the x-ray beam passing through several different types of tissues. Structures will be most discrete when the interface of 2 tissues of differing densities (such as aerated lung vs. pneumonia) lies parallel to the x-ray beam. Overlapping structures (where 1 structure of interest lies deep to the other such that their interface is perpendicular to the x-ray beam) will be less apparent (e.g., a pneumonia hiding behind the heart). The loss of a normal interface can also represent pathology when 2 structures of similar density (such as the heart & pneumonia) lie directly adjacent to one another (obscuring the normal heart border). Because of this superimposition of structures & the need for visible interfaces of differing densities to increase the conspicuity of pathology, radiographs will be insensitive for some disease processes (such as a bowel obstruction that is fluid-filled rather than gas-filled) but highly sensitive for others (as with displaced fractures of bone).

Fluoroscopy

Whereas radiographs use a finite x-ray exposure to create a single image, fluoroscopy essentially creates real-time radiographic visualization of changing anatomy by continuous or pulsed x-ray beams. For decades, this technology has been used to study the gastrointestinal & urinary tracts when specific combinations of anatomic & physiologic information have been required. A fundamental example is the voiding cystourethrogram where key anatomy is only visualized during specific physiologic acts (e.g., voiding allows assessment of the urethra & can unmask previously occult vesicoureteral reflux).

As with many other radiologic studies, fluoroscopy frequently employs a relatively inert contrast agent to aid in viewing targeted anatomy. The interaction of these contrast agents with the x-ray beam (typically by increasing the density of the region of interest, thereby attenuating the x-ray beam) increases the conspicuity of the target organ in some way. For most pediatric fluoroscopic exams, this involves the introduction of the contrast agent into a hollow viscus (such as oral contrast into the stomach). The contrast is then allowed to propagate physiologically through the organ of interest (such as with bowel peristalsis) while images are intermittently obtained. A limitation of this type of imaging is that it does not directly visualize the tissue of interest. That is to say, as the contrast typically only outlines the mucosal surface of a viscus, it only allows inferences about the nature of the viscus wall & what is causing its distortion.

Computed Tomography (CT)

CT uses powerful rotating x-ray tubes & detectors, in conjunction with advanced computational processes, to rapidly generate high-quality 2D slices of the patient's anatomy. The differential attenuation of the x-ray beam by different patient tissues (based on electron density) produces varied shades of gray in the image. In CT, the different levels of image density are quantitatively measured in Hounsfield units (HU) that can help detect & characterize tissues & fluids on a basic level.

Various parameters set before & after the scan determine what information can be extracted from the acquired dataset. This applies to the orientation of the images displayed (in various 2D planes, 3D rotations, or time-resolved 4D reconstructions) as well as how the data is visually optimized (e.g., bone, soft tissue, or lung detail). That is to say, with appropriate acquisition & subsequent manipulation, some datasets will be able to generate images optimized to answer different questions than originally intended. For example, when a skull base fracture is detected on a trauma head CT, the same dataset can be used to create high-detail temporal bone images without a new scan.

Due to its ability to rapidly generate high-detail anatomic imaging of clinically urgent disease processes (now often on the order of seconds for a single body site), CT became widely used in emergency settings 10-15 years ago. This has tapered with increasing radiation concerns as well as the greater capacity & availability of other alternate modalities (such as ultrasound & MR). Clinical algorithms have also helped steer clinicians away from unnecessary scans.

The need for intravenous contrast varies by the body site & clinical questions at hand. Most urgent questions of head/brain pathology (such as hemorrhage, tumor, hydrocephalus, fractures, & sinusitis) will not require IV contrast for detection. However, complications of inflammatory processes will benefit from contrast administration. In contradistinction, most studies of the abdomen or pelvis will require IV contrast administration to increase the visibility of pathology against other fluid & soft tissue that may obscure the lesion on a noncontrast (nonenhanced) exam.

Modality Specific Terminology

High/hyper attenuation/density: Relatively bright or white.

Low/hypo attenuation/density: Relatively dark or black.

Enhancing: IV contrast is taken up by the lesion or organ of interest; this feature helps determine the vascularity of the lesion, increase its detectability, & provide clues to its origin.

Hyper- or hypoenhancing: Increased or decreased enhancement, respectively, of the site of interest relative to normal surrounding soft tissues.

Magnetic Resonance (MR)

Most clinical MR scanners generate images by manipulating magnetized hydrogen protons within a volume of tissue. Once aligned in a magnetic field, these protons are agitated with precisely timed radiofrequency energy pulses; as the protons return (or relax) to their baseline state of magnetization, a signal is emitted that is ultimately converted to an image. The hydrogen protons respond in different but predictable ways depending on their environment (i.e., protons bound to water behave differently than those bound to fat), which ultimately determines the imaging appearance of these tissues. The entire exam (which generally lasts 30-60 minutes) typically consists of 5-15 different pulse sequences designed to assess different properties of the tissues & reconstruct the data into specific orientations.

Modality Specific Terminology

Field strength: This is the strength of the main magnetic field in an MR scanner, typically ranging from 0.7-3.0 Tesla (T) for clinical applications. In general, the greater the field strength, the greater the capacity of the scanner to produce high-quality images quickly, though numerous parameters affect image quality & speed.

Spin-echo & gradient-echo: These are the 2 basic types of pulse sequences in MR. All other sequences are variations of these types & are designed to assess various properties of different tissues. The main vendors of MR machines have different names for each of their sequences (of which there are generally dozens per scanner). Unfortunately, this creates a vast lexicon that is ever changing.

T1, T2, & proton density: These are fundamental properties of tissues containing mobile hydrogen protons, & these properties are largely responsible for the appearance of tissue on MR images. Pulse sequences that emphasize tissue differences in T1 relaxation are called T1-weighted (T1W) & so on. Tissues with short T1 relaxation times (such as fat, melanin, & some proteins) produce high signal on T1W sequences, appearing "bright," whereas fluid will be relatively dark. Most fluids have a long T2 relaxation time & appear bright on T2W sequences. As most pathologies have increased fluid content, they will be bright on "fluid sensitive sequences" (T2W or certain types of inversion recovery sequences). However, the conspicuity of this abnormal signal depends on its contrast with the surrounding tissues. The visibility of a lesion can be increased by administering an IV contrast agent (which shortens T1 relaxation, generally making enhancing tissues brighter on T1W images) &/or applying fat saturation (a.k.a. fat suppression) to decrease the brightness of tissues surrounding the lesion. Techniques used to block the normally high signal of fat are particularly useful in identifying pathology in bone & soft tissues (where there is an abundance of macroscopic fat). Contrast is generally applied only when inflammation, infection, or tumors are suspected. Most cases of trauma do not benefit from IV contrast.

Fluid-attenuation inversion recovery (FLAIR): This sequence is used in the brain to eliminate the signal from CSF while maintaining the fluid signal of various pathologies. It is useful for highlighting parenchymal lesions that lie close to ventricles or sulci (like multiple sclerosis plaques, which are not as conspicuous on T2W sequences).

Short tau inversion recovery (STIR): This sequence is used to eliminate the signal from fat. It is particularly helpful in looking for edema of the bone marrow or soft tissues.

Diffusion-weighted imaging (DWI): This sequence displays the molecular motion or diffusion of water protons within tissue. It is most widely used to detect acute cerebral infarction as the cytoxic edema will be visible as early as 30 minutes after the insult, much sooner than on other types of sequences. However, restricted diffusion can also be seen in other processes like abscesses or highly cellular tumors, among others.

Gradient-echo sequence (GRE): There are numerous variations of this sequence to assess various tissue properties. Certain forms of the sequence are recognized for their ability to visualize cartilage, hemorrhage, or blood flow.

MR angiography (MRA) & venography (MRV): These sequences can be performed without or with IV contrast with advantages to each technique in specific scenarios. Contrast-enhanced techniques are generally faster than noncontrast versions & are less likely to suffer from artifacts.

Hyperintense/bright/high signal: Appearing more white than surrounding tissues.

Hypointense/dark/low signal: Appearing more black than surrounding tissues.

Ultrasound & Doppler

Sonography, or the interrogation of the tissues of the body with sound waves, is perhaps only 2nd to radiography in its importance in the imaging evaluation of children. That is largely due to its capacity to provide high spatial resolution cross-sectional imaging without requiring sedation, ionizing radiation, or an IV (for contrast). Additionally, these studies generally do not require absolute stillness or specific positioning. Furthermore, the body composition of most children, particularly infants, allows excellent visualization of soft tissues as compared to adults. This is largely because infants have an abundance of water-rich cartilage (which nicely transmits sound waves, unlike sound-reflective bone) & children in general have lower amounts of sound-attenuating fat than adults.

Despite its excellent spatial resolution in superficial tissues, the contrast resolution of ultrasound does not approach that of MR. However, the recent approval of ultrasound contrast in the USA will likely decrease this gap (though it will require an IV).

The Doppler modalities in ultrasound provide excellent characterization of blood flow within vessels, organs, & lesions. Arterial & venous signals are easily distinguished, & studies can be performed looking for occlusion, stenosis, & fistulas.

Modality Specific Terminology

Echogenicity: A visual representation of the degree of sound wave reflection from a tissue to the transducer/probe.

Hyperechoic/echogenic/increased echogenicity: The structure appears more bright or white on the image.

Hypoechoic/echolucent/decreased echogenicity: The structure appears more dark or black on the image.

Anechoic: Having relatively no reflection of sound waves (& thus appearing entirely black, as seen with simple fluid).

Color Doppler: A technique that is sensitive to the direction of vascular flow.

Power Doppler: A technique that is more sensitive for detecting vascular flow overall but lacks directionality.

Spectral/pulsed Doppler: A technique that characterizes the velocity of flow over time, demonstrating arterial & venous waveforms.

Nuclear Medicine

The basic idea of nuclear medicine is that a physiologically active compound (i.e., one processed by the body in a way that is of interest clinically) is coupled to a radioactive element & then introduced into the patient. External cameras then detect how that compound interacts with the body as radiation tagged to the compound is released through the patient's tissues. This differs from the previously discussed exams in which an external energy source is used to interrogate the patient's body.

Also, most of the previously discussed studies predominantly supply anatomic information. In nuclear medicine, studies have traditionally provided excellent physiologic information with relatively poor anatomic definition. SPECT imaging has enabled cross-sectional display of nuclear data to improve anatomic detail & has been employed in the spine & brain for many years. More recently, the additional fusion of SPECT images with CT (or even MR) has further increased the anatomic value of nuclear studies.

A final difference from traditional radiologic studies is that many nuclear medicine studies have served as a relatively quick way to screen large regions of the body for certain pathologies, though specificity for 1 disease is typically lacking. In contradistinction, MR has excelled at studying a single anatomic site in detail (with higher disease specificity) but has not (until recently) been capable of rapidly screening large segments of the body for pathology.

Many radiopharmaceuticals (radioisotope + physiologically active compound) have been designed, allowing the study of a wide range of processes related to the bones, brain, kidneys, hepatobiliary system, thyroid, blood cells, lungs, & gastric mucosa, among others. Each radiopharmaceutical has its own expected pattern of distribution throughout the body, which includes organs of physiologic uptake & excretion. Sites of pathologic concentration of the radiopharmaceutical are most commonly termed to have increased uptake (or are "hot"), though some pathologies (such as malignant thyroid nodules) are more likely to have decreased uptake (or be "cold" or "photopenic") relative to the expected uptake of the surrounding normal tissues.

A particular use of nuclear medicine that has rapidly expanded in the last 20 years is the oncologic use of positron emission tomography (PET). While many other applications have been introduced, it is the propensity of neoplasms to concentrate glucose (coupled to radioactive fluoride) that has seen PET imaging play a large role in the staging & follow-up of many malignancies. Another major area of PET use in pediatrics is in the study of epilepsy (where decreased metabolic activity may indicate a seizure focus). As with other radiotracers, PET agents show expected normal patterns of physiologic distribution in the body. Foci of disease will then show increased or decreased metabolic activity ("hypermetabolic" or "hypometabolic") relative to the physiologic uptake expected in that organ.

Interventional Radiology

Many invasive procedures can be performed with minimal percutaneous access using imaging guidance. These include the study & treatment of various blood vessel disorders & biliary abnormalities as well as tumor biopsies & abscess drainages, among others.

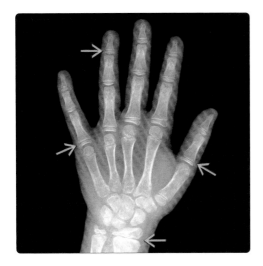

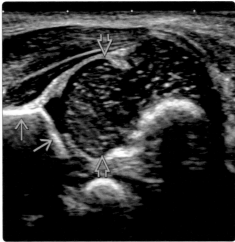

(Left) PA radiograph of the hand in a 7 year old after trauma shows no fracture or dislocation. Note the normal radiolucent cartilages of the primary growth plates ➡. (Right) Coronal hip ultrasound in a 14 day old with breech presentation but no hip click shows a normal configuration of the echogenic bony acetabular roof ➡ as well as a normal degree of coverage of the unossified femoral head ➡. Note how well the hypoechoic fluid-rich cartilage is visualized by ultrasound.

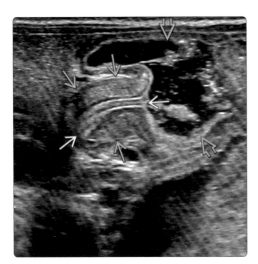

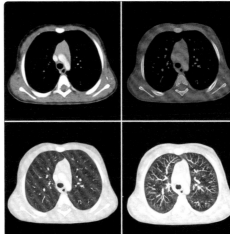

(Left) Oblique US in a 1 month old with vomiting shows abnormal thickening of the pyloric muscle ➡. The pyloric channel ➡ is abnormally elongated & failed to open during the exam, consistent with hypertrophic pyloric stenosis. Note the fluid distention of the stomach ➡. (Right) Axial CECT in a patient with neuroblastoma shows that a single CT dataset can be variably adjusted to highlight different anatomy. Clockwise from the top left, the image settings are: Mediastinal, bone, MIP (to improve nodule detection), & standard lung.

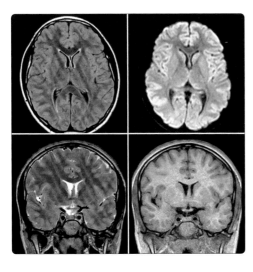

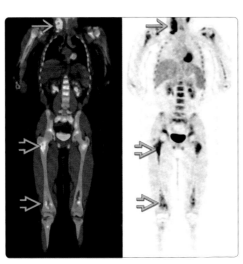

(Left) Normal MR images from a 14 year old show several types of sequences able to be obtained with MR, each providing different information. Clockwise from the top left are: Axial FLAIR, axial diffusion (DWI), coronal T1W, & coronal T2W images. (Right) Coronal fused PET/CT (left) & unfused PET (right) images in a teenager with a soft tissue rhabdomyosarcoma of the neck ➡ show extensive osseous metastases ➡.

Introduction

The parameters below often factor into imaging tests ordered to work-up pediatric diseases. In light of safety concerns associated with these elements, there are some situations where reasonable alternatives to the associated tests (including close clinical follow-up) should be employed as a substitute. However, the risks associated with these imaging facets do not mean that these exams should be avoided when the test is clinically justified for the well-being of the patient. If in doubt, such parameters should be discussed with the radiologist & other relevant specialists.

Contrast

Allergic reactions to contrast are uncommon with modern agents, & most true allergic reactions tend to be mild (such as hives). However, reactions are unpredictable & can be deadly, even in the patient with no prior history of allergies. Patients with a relevant allergy history are often premedicated with steroids, though there is no conclusive evidence that steroids are successful in preventing reactions. Patients with documented true allergic reactions to contrast should, if at all possible, avoid similar agents in the future.

Intravenous iodinated contrast agents (as used in CT) have traditionally been associated with nephrotoxicity & have been avoided in patients with impaired renal function. However, newer data suggests that this may not be true of modern contrast agents. Doubt has also been cast on the utility of preventative measures for avoiding renal injury by contrast, including IV hydration & oral Mucomyst. It should be noted that gadolinium-based contrast agents used in MR do not themselves cause renal injury.

The long-term deposition of dissociated gadolinium ions in patients receiving MR contrast has received much attention in the last decade. Patients with severe renal failure should not receive MR contrast as the retained gadolinium ion can deposit in the soft tissues & cause nephrogenic systemic fibrosis. More recently, individuals without renal impairment undergoing repeated contrast-enhanced MR scans have shown some accumulation of gadolinium in the brain, though the degree varies by the type of contrast agent; no clinical effects have been observed to date. This has led many centers to switch to the more stable macrocyclic forms of contrast, which are less likely to dissociate prior to clearance.

Radiation

The long-term effects of medical doses of ionizing radiation (which are employed with radiography, fluoroscopy, CT, & nuclear medicine) have raised significant concerns in recent years. The main issue at hand is an increased risk of latent cancer development in patients, particularly in children who are at higher risk of DNA damage & may undergo multiple studies during their lifetime. Most experts agree that the lifetime risk of developing a cancer from a single CT scan performed during childhood is low (ranging from < 0.1% to 0.4%), particularly compared to the baseline lifetime risk of developing a cancer in the USA otherwise (~ 40%). However, the risk in patients undergoing numerous scans is more difficult to predict. Whether or not the doses of multiple scans have a cumulative effect & how best to report & track patient radiation exposures remain controversial.

The ALARA (as low as reasonably achievable) principle guides radiologists to limit medical radiation exposure to that which is truly necessary to achieve a diagnostic quality exam. In the last 10 years, doses associated with medical imaging have notably decreased. Therefore, interpretation of any long-term risk data from studies of exposures 10-30 years ago may not be applicable to current practices.

Many of the developments in dose reduction are due to technical advances in equipment as well as adjustments in technique by medical physicists & radiologists. Additionally, clinical algorithms have been instituted in many centers to direct patients away from CT scanning if alternative work-up options are reasonable. Ultimately, it must be recognized that CT scans do save lives, & experts generally agree that the risks of not doing a medically justified study greatly outweigh the long-term risks of performing the exam.

Anesthesia

As motion can severely inhibit image quality, numerous techniques are employed by pediatric radiology departments to ensure stillness in young &/or uncooperative patients during radiologic exams. Distractions of various forms (including movies, toys, & child life specialists) can be invaluable in this setting. A component of physical restraint by the parents, technologists, & physicians may be required temporarily to appropriately position patients for relatively short exams (such as radiographs & CT). However, sedation or general anesthesia is often required for younger patients undergoing longer exams, especially MR. Concerns have recently been raised about the potential harmful effects of some anesthetic agents on the immature/developing nervous system, particularly in the setting of repeated administrations or even a single prolonged administration. While animal models have shown impaired neurodevelopment with some agents, there is conflicting data in humans, & the long-term effects remain under investigation.

Other Safety Issues

Patients may have implants that are incompatible with MR imaging, including most pacemakers, vagal nerve stimulators, & cochlear implants. The magnetic field may cause these devices to malfunction or heat up during scanning. Therefore, the specific details of implanted devices must be known before the patient will be allowed into the scan room. Retained metal fragments (such as from bullets or metal works) can also become mobile & injure the patient. While the MR technologists will thoroughly screen all patients before allowing them into the scanner, the pediatrician can facilitate this process by alerting the radiologist to such concerns.

Selected References

1. Davenport MS et al: The evidence for and against corticosteroid prophylaxis in at-risk patients. Radiol Clin North Am. 55(2):413-421, 2017
2. Ehrmann S et al: Contrast-associated acute kidney injury in the critically ill: systematic review and Bayesian meta-analysis. Intensive Care Med. ePub, 2017
3. World Health Organization: Communicating Radiation Risks in Paediatric Imaging. http://www.who.int/ionizing_radiation/pub_meet/radiation-risks-paediatric-imaging/en/. Published 2016. Accessed April 2017.
4. Davidson AJ et al: Neurodevelopmental outcome at 2 years of age after general anaesthesia and awake-regional anaesthesia in infancy (GAS): an international multicentre, randomised controlled trial. Lancet. 387(10015):239-50, 2016
5. Roberts DR et al: Pediatric patients demonstrate progressive T1-weighted hyperintensity in the dentate nucleus following multiple doses of gadolinium-based contrast agent. AJNR Am J Neuroradiol. 37(12):2340-2347, 2016
6. Nardone B et al: Pediatric nephrogenic systemic fibrosis is rarely reported: a RADAR report. Pediatr Radiol. 44(2):173-80, 2014
7. Brody AS et al: Radiation risk to children from computed tomography. Pediatrics. 120(3):677-82, 2007

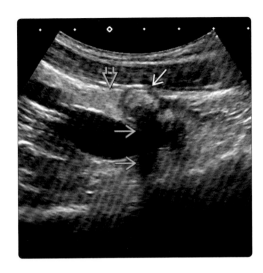

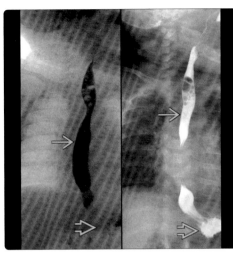

(Left) US shows a dilated noncompressible appendix ➡ with induration of the nearby fat ➥ & shadowing ➥ from an appendicolith. When performed with appropriate technique, US is very accurate in the diagnosis & exclusion of appendicitis, sparing the radiation of CT. (Right) Upper GI series shows contrast in the esophagus ➥ & stomach ➥. The noisier grayscale-inverted image on the left is a "last image hold" from fluoroscopy. The right image is a true radiograph that uses more radiation but yields higher detail.

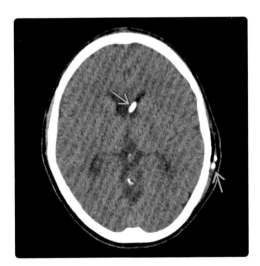

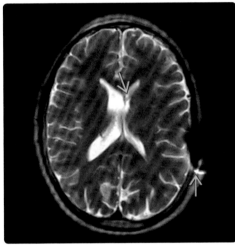

(Left) Axial NECT of the head in a teenager with shunted hydrocephalus shows normal ventricular size with metallic density from the shunt ➥. (Right) Axial SSFSE T2 MR (same patient) shows normal ventricular size & unchanged shunt position ➥. This sequence is much faster than a traditional T2WI, though brain detail is limited. In young patients with shunted hydrocephalus, this technique is usually adequate to assess for shunt malfunction without the radiation of CT or the anesthesia of a routine brain MR.

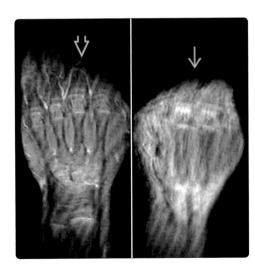

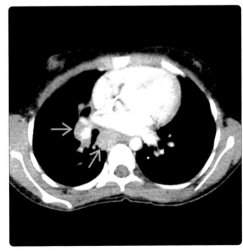

(Left) Coronal T1 C+ FS MR images of the right hand in an awake 5 year old show increasingly severe motion artifact on the repeat attempt ➥ of the first sequence ➥. Sedation/anesthesia is frequently required in this age range to achieve a diagnostic study. (Right) Axial CECT in a patient with ataxia-telangiectasia (AT) & fevers shows enlarged lymph nodes ➥, ultimately diagnosed as lymphoma. Patients with AT disorder are particularly sensitive to radiation, & CT must be avoided when possible.

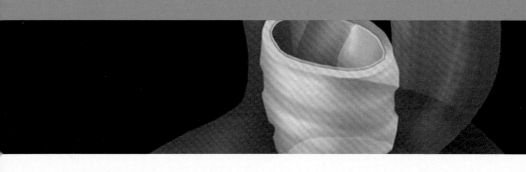

Introduction & Normals

Newborn Airway Obstruction

Infectious Causes of Airway Compromise

Obstructive Sleep Apnea

Extrinsic Vascular Compression of Airway

Miscellaneous Airway Obstructions

Introduction

Anatomically & functionally, the pediatric airway can be divided into upper & lower segments at the glottis (larynx) or large & small airways at the transition from the cartilage-containing bronchi proximally to the distal airways that lack supporting cartilage. The superimposed disease processes may be extrinsic or intrinsic, & they may manifest as acute or chronic airway compromise at a variety of ages. Broad categories of airway compromise include congenital airway obstructions (e.g., choanal atresia), acute infectious etiologies (e.g., croup, epiglottitis), noninfectious intrinsic & extrinsic obstructions (e.g., foreign bodies, vascular rings), & obstructive sleep apnea (e.g., tonsillar hypertrophy, glossoptosis). These general categories of disease are not always distinct, with some processes affecting multiple levels or presenting later in childhood despite an underlying congenital issue.

Imaging Modalities

Radiographs

Plain radiographs remain the imaging modality of choice for the initial evaluation of the pediatric airway. Two views (AP & lateral) are obtained to include the airway from the nasal passages & nasopharynx superiorly to the carina inferiorly. It is particularly important in young children to obtain the lateral view during inspiration & with the neck extended to prevent the simulation of pathology by normal tissue redundancy in these patients.

Airway radiographs are helpful in looking for ingested/inhaled foreign bodies (especially those that are radiopaque) & evaluating sites of midline pharyngeal or tracheal narrowing due to inflammation or extrinsic compression. Most extrinsic processes affecting the airway (such as peritonsillar abscesses & nodal conglomerations) will require further characterization with cross-sectional imaging.

Less acute indications for airway radiographs include infants with noisy breathing & older children with snoring (the latter of which could be obtained as a single lateral view of the upper airway).

Fluoroscopy

In the current era, fluoroscopy has a limited role in evaluating the pediatric airway. A commonly encountered circumstance is in the infant where a retropharyngeal space process is suspected clinically &/or radiographically. In this setting, the initial lateral radiograph will sometimes not be obtained with adequate extension &/or inspiration, making the retropharyngeal tissues appear abnormally thickened when they are not. Pulsed fluoroscopic visualization of such an airway during the respiratory cycle will demonstrate, in the lateral view, normal expansion & collapse of the retropharyngeal soft tissue in this age group (if there is no inflammatory change present).

Fluoroscopy may incidentally detect tracheomalacia or other sites of airway collapse in patients with obstructive sleep apnea, though it is not primarily used in the investigation of these entities.

Video swallowing studies (a.k.a. modified barium swallows) are frequently performed (in conjunction with speech pathologists) when aspiration or feeding difficulties are suspected. Another related study is the esophagram. While this exam is typically performed for dysphagia, it may have airway implications if there is a pattern of esophageal compression that suggests a vascular ring.

Computed Tomography

The applications of CT in evaluating the airway have become quite numerous. In the acute setting, CECT may be used to detail drainable abscesses of the retropharynx or peritonsillar tissues. In the setting of congenital or chronic airway anomalies, CT angiography can be used to look for vascular rings causing compression of the airway (typically during a pulmonary or otolaryngology work-up). Dynamic change in the airway caliber may also be assessed, creating 4D cine images of the airway lumen during the respiratory cycle. Given these applications & its rapid acquisition, CT has taken on a significant role in the work-up of complex airway anomalies.

Magnetic Resonance

While MR imaging has other applications in the neck, MR of the airway is typically limited to the evaluation of recurrent obstructive sleep apnea after tonsillectomy. Its strengths lie in its ability to distinguish the various soft tissue components contributing to intermittent airway obstructions, allowing observation of the supraglottic airway over numerous respiratory cycles & with the application of various interventions during the scan.

Ultrasound

Sonography is rarely used in the evaluation of the pediatric airway, primarily due to the artifacts associated with air. While palpable neck masses are well characterized by ultrasound, their depth of extension & exact relationship to the airway are much better visualized by CT or MR. Limited uses of airway ultrasound have been recently described, including the assessment of peritonsillar abscesses (using an intraoral probe), laryngeal motion (by otolaryngologists), & endotracheal tube position (during point of care ultrasound by the emergency or ICU physician).

Selected References

1. Berdan EA et al: Pediatric airway and esophageal foreign bodies. Surg Clin North Am. 97(1):85-91, 2017
2. Stagnaro N et al: Multimodality imaging of pediatric airways disease: indication and technique. Radiol Med. ePub, 2017
3. Ehsan Z et al: Pediatric obstructive sleep apnea. Otolaryngol Clin North Am. 49(6):1449-1464, 2016
4. Osman A et al: Role of upper airway ultrasound in airway management. J Intensive Care. 4:52, 2016
5. Richards AM: Pediatric respiratory emergencies. Emerg Med Clin North Am. 34(1):77-96, 2016
6. Salih AM et al: Airway foreign bodies: A critical review for a common pediatric emergency. World J Emerg Med. 7(1):5-12, 2016
7. Soyer T: The role bronchoscopy in the diagnosis of airway disease in children. J Thorac Dis. 8(11):3420-3426, 2016
8. Stafrace S et al: Essential ultrasound techniques of the pediatric airway. Paediatr Anaesth. 26(2):122-31, 2016
9. Vijayasekaran S et al: Airway disorders of the fetus and neonate: An overview. Semin Fetal Neonatal Med. 21(4):220-9, 2016
10. Bandarkar AN et al: Tonsil ultrasound: technical approach and spectrum of pediatric peritonsillar infections. Pediatr Radiol. ePub, 2015
11. Singhal M et al: Cardiovascular Causes of pediatric airway compression: a pictorial review. Curr Probl Diagn Radiol. 44(6):505-10, 2015

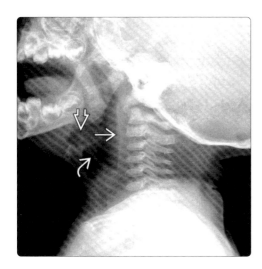

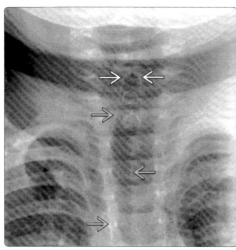

(Left) *Lateral radiograph of a normal airway shows a "thin" & well-defined epiglottis ➡. Note the normal retropharyngeal soft tissue width ➡ & thin aryepiglottic folds ➡.* (Right) *AP radiograph of a normal airway shows normal "shoulders" or lateral convexities ➡ of the glottis/subglottis, which differ from the vertically elongated "steeple" of croup. The tracheal air column ➡ is otherwise of uniform caliber from the glottis to the carina.*

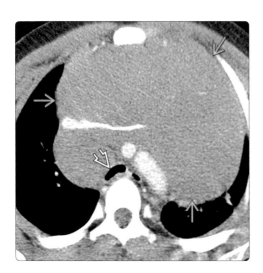

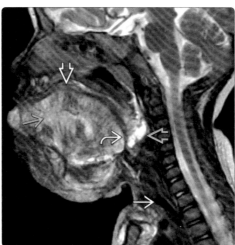

(Left) *Axial CECT in a child with lymphoma shows a large mediastinal mass ➡ posteriorly displacing & flattening the trachea ➡ (typical of extrinsic compression).* (Right) *Sagittal T2 MR in a 17 month old with an extensive facial lymphatic malformation shows marked infiltration & enlargement of the tongue ➡, floor of mouth tissues, & soft palate ➡ by the lesion, resulting in complete effacement of the oral cavity ➡, oropharynx ➡, & upper hypopharynx. A tracheostomy ➡ is partially visualized.*

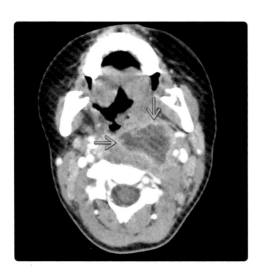

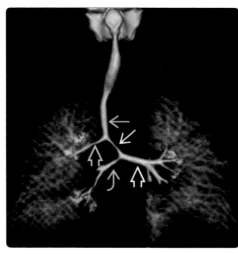

(Left) *Axial CECT in a 7 year old with fever & neck pain shows a rim-enhancing fluid collection ➡ of the deep neck soft tissues, typical of an abscess.* (Right) *Anterior view of a 3D NECT of the airways shows a round, narrow caliber distal trachea ➡, typical of complete cartilage rings. There is an isolated right upper lobe bronchus ➡ arising from the trachea & leaving a narrowed intermediate left bronchus ➡ that then gives rise to the left main bronchus ➡ & a right bridging bronchus ➡.*

Expiratory Buckling of Trachea

TERMINOLOGY

- Intermittent normal change in transverse & craniocaudal configuration of trachea in infants during expiration

IMAGING

- On AP view, trachea is normally straight vertically in older children & adults throughout respiratory cycle
- In infants, trachea is normally straight during inspiration but changes with expiration
  - Focal shortening, crinkle, bend, or curve at/above thoracic inlet without caliber change
  - Directed toward right in patients with left aortic arch
    - Buckling toward left suggests right aortic arch
  - Trachea becomes straight again with inspiration
- No need to repeat radiograph

TOP DIFFERENTIAL DIAGNOSES

- Croup: Symmetric narrowing of subglottic trachea in young child with characteristic "barky" cough

- Infantile hemangioma: Persistent asymmetric tracheal narrowing by intraluminal benign vascular neoplasm
  - Often associated with cutaneous infantile hemangioma in "beard" distribution
- Tracheomalacia: Abnormal dynamic tracheal collapse in anterior to posterior dimension (not transverse)
  - Static lateral view may show caliber narrowing; dynamic change confirms tracheomalacia rather than fixed stenosis or compression
- Compression by extrinsic mass or aberrant vessel
  - Persistent focal airway narrowing with deviation away from mass/vessel; mass may enlarge mediastinum

CLINICAL ISSUES

- Incidental finding on chest or airway radiographs if morphology & patient age correct
- Does not cause symptoms that lead to imaging

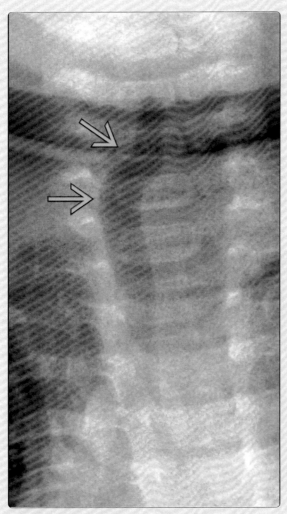

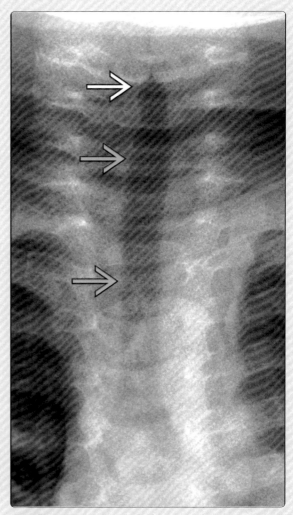

AP radiograph of the airway in an 8-month-old patient shows the typical configuration of expiratory tracheal buckling: The trachea at & just above the thoracic inlet demonstrates a focal bend toward the right ➡ but does not demonstrate narrowing.

AP radiograph in an 8-month-old patient during inspiration shows a trachea that is relatively straight vertically ➡. Also note the normal shouldering ➡ at the glottis.

Pseudothickening of Retropharyngeal Tissues

KEY FACTS

TERMINOLOGY

- Transient thickening of normal retropharyngeal soft tissues of infant on lateral airway radiograph
  - "Swelling" with expiration or poor extension
  - Resolution with inspiration & adequate extension
- Contributing factors to this appearance include
  - Relatively short necks of infants & young children, which lead to poor positioning for airway radiographs
  - Relatively long expiratory component of crying also challenges acquisition during maximal inspiration

IMAGING

- Generalized thickening/bulging of prevertebral soft tissues
  - ± retention of normal "step-off" at junction of hypopharynx & cervical esophagus
    - Persistent "step-off" favors pseudothickening over true retropharyngeal pathology
- Resolves on repeat lateral radiograph with improved inspiratory timing of exposure & ↑ neck extension

- Observation of dynamic airway changes under fluoroscopy can confirm intermittent thickening & resolution if radiographs unclear
  - Use "last image capture/image hold" for documentation

TOP DIFFERENTIAL DIAGNOSES

- Retropharyngeal cellulitis/abscess
  - Convex generalized bulging of prevertebral soft tissues persists despite inspiration & neck extension
  - Often lose normal "step-off" at hypopharyngeal-esophageal junction
- Cervical spine pathology
  - Trauma, inflammation/infection, or neoplasm → prevertebral soft tissue swelling
  - ± radiographically visible bony abnormality

CLINICAL ISSUES

- Uncommon in children > 2 years of age
- Unlike true pathology, pseudothickening does not cause characteristic signs/symptoms

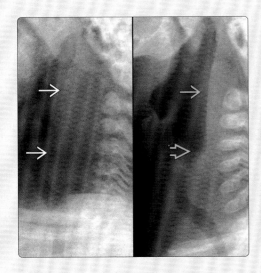
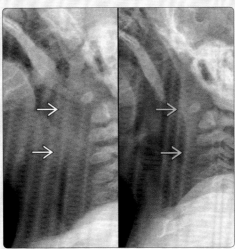

(Left) Lateral radiographs in an infant show pseudothickening of the prevertebral soft tissues initially ⮕ with resolution upon improved neck extension & inspiration ⮕. Note the normal "step-off" at the hypopharyngeal-esophageal junction ⮕ on the 2nd image. (Right) Lateral radiographs in a 4 month old show dynamic protrusion ⮕ & collapse ⮕ of the retropharyngeal tissues between expiration (left) & inspiration (right). The 2nd image confirms a normal thickness & morphology of the prevertebral tissues.

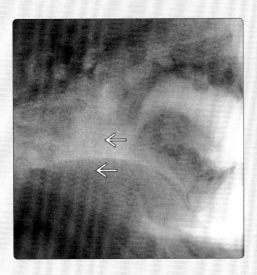
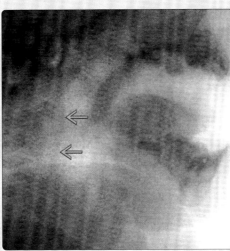

(Left) Lateral fluoroscopic "image hold" in an 11 month old with stridor & suggested retropharyngeal thickening on preceding radiographs (not shown) demonstrates bulging of the prevertebral soft tissues ⮕ during expiration. (Right) Lateral fluoroscopic "image hold" in the same patient during inspiration shows normal collapse of the prevertebral soft tissues ⮕, confirming pseudothickening on the initial image.

Congenital Nasal Pyriform Aperture Stenosis

TERMINOLOGY

- Congenital narrowing of anterior bony nasal passageway [pyriform aperture (PA)]

IMAGING

- Best tool: Bone CT in axial & coronal planes
  - Medial deviation of anterior maxillae with thickening & convergence of nasal processes
  - Triangle-shaped hard palate on axial images
  - Abnormal maxillary dentition: Solitary median maxillary central incisor (SMMCI) in 75%

TOP DIFFERENTIAL DIAGNOSES

- Nasolacrimal duct mucoceles
- Choanal stenosis/atresia

PATHOLOGY

- Congenital nasal pyriform aperture stenosis (CNPAS) without SMMCI: Almost always isolated
- SMMCI in 75% of CNPAS

- Associated with holoprosencephaly, pituitary-adrenal axis dysfunction, microcephaly, many other findings

CLINICAL ISSUES

- Respiratory distress in newborn/infant
  - Symptoms more pronounced with feeding
  - Breathing problems may be triggered by URI
  - Narrow nasal inlet on clinical exam
  - Nasogastric tube difficult to pass
- Congenital airway obstruction affects 1 in 5,000 infants
  - CNPAS much less common than choanal atresia
- Nasal cavity eventually grows; mild cases may improve
- Surgery for persistent respiratory difficulties & poor weight gain; PA width < 5.7 mm may predict surgical need

DIAGNOSTIC CHECKLIST

- Bone CT to confirm/characterize bony narrowing & identify dental/palatal abnormalities
- Brain MR if SMMCI to exclude midline brain anomalies

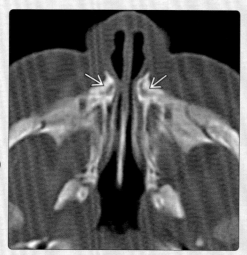

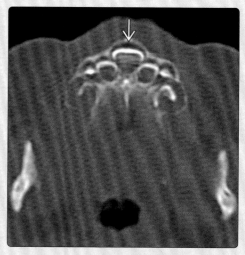

(Left) Axial bone CT in a newborn shows the typical features of congenital nasal pyriform aperture stenosis. There is overgrowth of the anterior maxillae ➡ causing marked narrowing of the pyriform aperture/nasal inlet. (Right) Axial bone CT at the level of the anterior maxilla in the same patient shows a solitary median maxillary central incisor (or megaincisor) ➡. This is a common associated finding in children with congenital pyriform aperture stenosis, ± midline intracranial abnormalities.

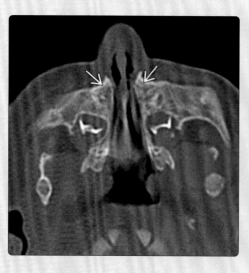

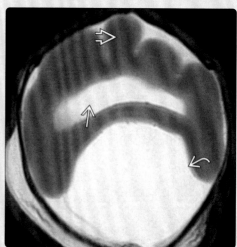

(Left) Axial bone CT in a newborn with respiratory distress shows thickening of the anterior & medial aspects of the maxillae ➡ causing pyriform aperture stenosis. This child did not have an associated solitary median maxillary central incisor or intracranial anomaly. (Right) Axial T2 brain MR necropsy image in a child with a solitary median maxillary incisor (not shown) reveals a monoventricle ➡, absence of frontal lobe cleavage ➡, & a large dorsal midline cyst ➡, findings that are all typical of alobar holoprosencephaly.

Nasolacrimal Duct Mucocele

TERMINOLOGY

- Synonym: Congenital dacryocystocele

IMAGING

- Well-defined, cystic medial canthal mass in continuity with enlarged nasolacrimal duct (NLD) in newborn
  - Unilateral or bilateral
- Little to no wall enhancement (unless infected) on CECT
- Coronal/sagittal reformatted images show continuity of proximal cyst (at lacrimal sac) with distal cyst (at inferior meatus) through dilated NLD

TOP DIFFERENTIAL DIAGNOSES

- Orbital dermoid & epidermoid: Lateral > medial canthus
- Acquired dacryocystocele: Uncommon in children

PATHOLOGY

- Tears & mucus accumulate in NLD with imperforate Hasner membrane (i.e., distal duct obstruction)

CLINICAL ISSUES

- Typically presents from 4 days to 10 weeks old
- Proximal cyst: Small, round, bluish, medial canthal mass identified at birth or shortly thereafter ± cellulitis (dacryocystitis)
- Distal cyst: Nasal airway obstruction with respiratory distress if bilateral (especially during feeding)
- Only 50% identified on prenatal MR ultimately have postnatal symptoms
- 90% of simple distal NLD obstructions resolve by 1 year of age
- Intervention recommended before infection occurs to prevent nasal airway obstruction, dacryocystitis, & permanent sequelae (such as nasolacrimal apparatus scarring, amblyopia, & permanent canthal asymmetry)
  - Daily manual massage ± prophylactic antibiotics
    - Manual massage inappropriate if NLD mucocele infected or causing airway obstruction
  - 10% require probing with irrigation ± silastic stent

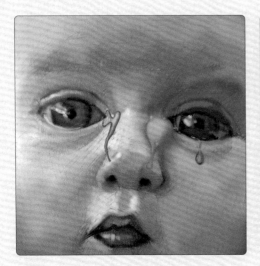

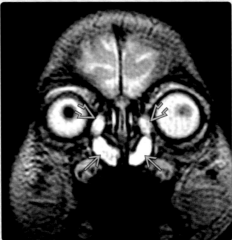

(Left) Graphic demonstrates a normal right nasolacrimal apparatus (in green). However, there is cystic dilation of the lacrimal sac on the left due to a distal obstruction at the membrane of Hasner. (Right) Coronal T2 MR in an infant shows hyperintense nasolacrimal duct mucoceles extending from the dilated lacrimal sacs proximally ➡ to the nasal passages inferiorly ➡.

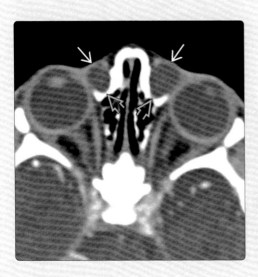

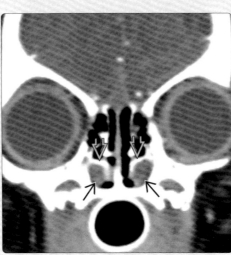

(Left) Axial CECT in a 4 day old with bluish bilateral medial orbital swelling & left purulent drainage shows bilateral lacrimal sac enlargement ➡. Also note the bilateral lacrimal sac fossae splaying ➡. (Right) Coronal CECT in the same patient demonstrates the typical locations of the distal intranasal components of nasolacrimal duct mucoceles ➡ inferior to the inferior turbinates ➡.

Choanal Atresia

TERMINOLOGY

- Congenital obstruction of posterior nasal aperture(s)
- Most common congenital abnormality of nasal cavity

IMAGING

- Unilateral or bilateral osseous narrowing of posterior nasal cavity
  - Thickening of vomer
  - Medial bowing of posterior maxilla(e)
- Obstruction completed by membrane or bony plate
  - Purely bony atresia in up to 30%
- ± air-fluid level in obstructed nasal cavity
- Bilateral in up to 25%
  - 75% of bilateral cases have other anomalies

TOP DIFFERENTIAL DIAGNOSES

- Choanal stenosis
- Pyriform aperture stenosis
- Nasolacrimal duct mucocele

CLINICAL ISSUES

- Typical presentations include
  - Bilateral choanal atresia: Significant respiratory distress in newborn (due to "obligate nasal breather" status); aggravated by feeding, relieved by crying
    - Grunting, snorting, low-pitched stridor
    - Inability to pass nasogastric tube through nasal cavity beyond 3-4 cm despite aerated lungs on chest radiograph
  - Unilateral choanal atresia: Chronic, purulent unilateral rhinorrhea with mild airway obstruction in older child
- Treatments
  - Establish oral airway immediately (to ensure breathing)
  - Membranous atresia may be perforated upon passage of nasogastric tube
  - Surgical treatment effective for alleviating respiratory symptoms
    - Postoperative scar & incomplete resection of atresia plate best evaluated with bone CT

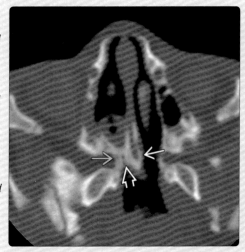
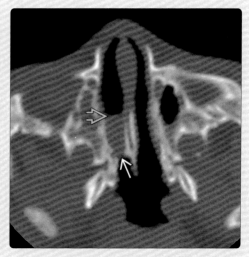

(Left) Axial NECT (in bone windows) through the upper choanae in a newborn shows a complete osseous right choanal obstruction ⇨ secondary to fusion of an enlarged vomer ⇨ to the thickened, medially positioned posterior maxilla ⇨. (Right) Axial NECT (in bone windows) in the same patient shows a component of membranous atresia ⇨ at the narrowed inferior aspect of the right choana. Note also the retained right nasal cavity secretions ⇨ secondary to choanal obstruction.

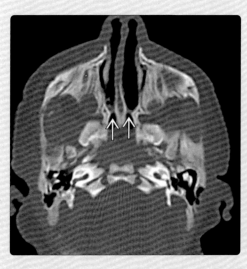
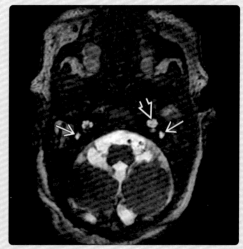

(Left) Axial bone CT in a child with CHARGE syndrome demonstrates bilateral choanal obstructions secondary to linear membranes ⇨ extending between the thickened vomer & each medially positioned posterior maxilla, typical of a mixed choanal atresia. (Right) Axial 3D SSFP MR in the same child shows typical inner ear anomalies of CHARGE syndrome, including small/dysplastic vestibules ⇨, absent semicircular canals, & left cochlear dysplasia ⇨.

Epiglottitis

TERMINOLOGY

- Airway obstruction secondary to inflammation of epiglottis & surrounding tissues; life threatening if untreated

IMAGING

- Diagnosis made clinically: Frontal & lateral radiographs only obtained in stable patients with questionable diagnosis
  - Child should be kept upright & comfortable
  - Patient may drool due to difficulty handling oral secretions: Should not be agitated or placed supine
- Lateral radiograph
  - Marked thickening of epiglottis
  - Thickening of aryepiglottic folds
    - Extend from epiglottis anterosuperiorly to arytenoid cartilages posteroinferiorly
    - Normally thin & convex inferiorly
    - May become thickened & convex superiorly
    - Swelling of these folds causes airway obstruction
- Frontal radiograph rarely helpful for this diagnosis

  - ± symmetric subglottic tracheal narrowing, similar to that seen in croup

CLINICAL ISSUES

- Marked ↓ in incidence in children since vaccine for *Haemophilus influenzae* introduced
  - Mean age in children has shifted from 3.5 to 14.6 years; now more common in adults than children
- High fever, sore throat, dysphonia, "hot potato voice," hoarseness, & drooling with abrupt onset of stridor (usually inspiratory), often associated with dysphagia
- Patients often toxic-appearing, anxious, & uncomfortable with ↑ respiratory distress when recumbent
  - May have characteristic "tripod position" (sitting up with neck extended & leaning forward with jaw thrust out to maximize laryngeal opening)
- Direct laryngoscopy & bronchoscopy with intubation performed in operating room with otolaryngology present
- Steroids & broad-spectrum IV antibiotics administered

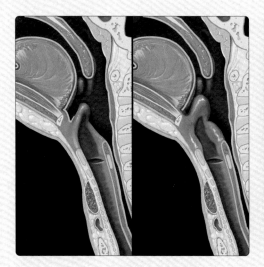

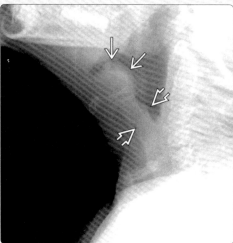

(Left) Sagittal graphics show epiglottitis (right) as compared with a normal epiglottis (left). The epiglottis & aryepiglottic folds are swollen & diffusely enlarged (right). (Right) Lateral radiograph in a young child shows marked thickening of the epiglottis ➡ & aryepiglottic folds ➡, typical of epiglottitis. The aryepiglottic folds are convex upward.

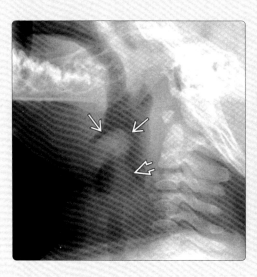

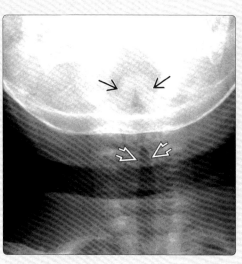

(Left) Lateral radiograph in an infant shows moderate to marked thickening of the epiglottis ➡ & the aryepiglottic folds ➡, typical of epiglottitis. (Right) AP radiograph of the same child shows thickening of the epiglottis & aryepiglottic folds ➡ seen through the skull base/foramen magnum. There is mild subglottic narrowing ➡ that can be seen in varying degrees with epiglottitis.

TERMINOLOGY

- Extranodal purulent fluid collection in retropharyngeal space (RPS)

IMAGING

- Lateral radiograph: Wide prevertebral distance with loss of normal contours at hypopharynx-esophagus interface
- CECT best tool for rapid characterization & evaluation of extent/complications
  - RPS distended by defined, ovoid, rim-enhancing low-density collection with convex anterior margin
  - Complications include airway compromise, jugular vein thrombosis/thrombophlebitis, mediastinal extension/mediastinitis, internal carotid artery pseudoaneurysm (rare, suggests methicillin-resistant *Staphylococcus aureus*)

TOP DIFFERENTIAL DIAGNOSES

- Pseudothickening of retropharyngeal soft tissues

- Retropharyngeal space edema
- Necrotic/suppurative adenopathy in RPS
- Lymphatic malformation

CLINICAL ISSUES

- Presentation: Dysphagia, sore throat, poor oral intake, dehydration, fever, chills, ↑ WBC & ESR; toxic-appearing child with marked neck pain & limited motion, especially extension
  - Most < 6 years old; increasing incidence in adults
- Etiology
  - Head & neck infection (pharyngitis, tonsillitis) seeds RPS lymph node → suppurative intranodal abscess → nodal rupture → RPS abscess
  - Pharyngeal penetration by foreign body
- Treatment: Early ENT consultation, IV antibiotics, airway management, fluid resuscitation

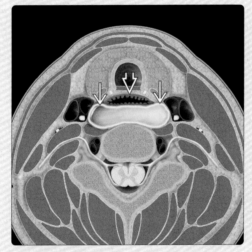
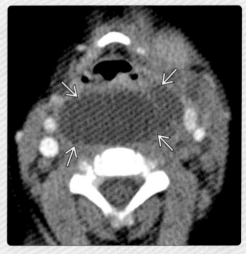

(Left) *Axial graphic illustrates the location & typical contour of a retropharyngeal space (RPS) abscess* ⇒ *displacing the cervical esophagus* ⇒ *anteriorly & flattening the prevertebral muscles.* (Right) *Axial CECT in a 10 month old with a 5-day history of febrile illness reveals a large, low-density, ovoid collection distending the RPS* ⇒ *with anterior displacement of the pharynx & splaying of the carotid sheaths. There is minimal enhancement of the collection wall.*

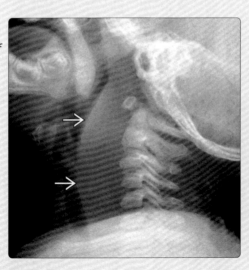
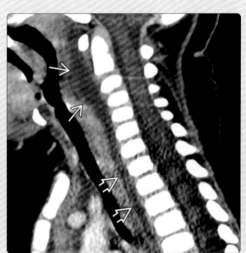

(Left) *Lateral radiograph in a 12-month-old boy with sepsis shows significant thickening of the prevertebral soft tissues* ⇒. *The normal step-off at the pharyngeal-esophageal junction has been effaced.* (Right) *Sagittal reformatted CECT in the same child clearly shows the cause of the prominent soft tissues to be a convex anterior RPS abscess* ⇒ *with extension of fluid into the posterior mediastinum* ⇒.

TERMINOLOGY

Definitions

- Retropharyngeal space (RPS): Midline space posterior to pharyngeal mucosa & cervical esophagus from skull base to T3 vertebral level in mediastinum
- RPS abscess: Extranodal purulent fluid collection in RPS

IMAGING

Radiographic Findings

- Lateral view critical
  - Normal prevertebral soft tissue thickness
    - C2 (at hypopharynx): ≤ 7 mm at any age
    - C6 (at cervical esophagus): ≤ 14 mm if < 15 years, ≤ 22 mm in adults
  - In children: Must perform lateral radiograph during inspiration & with neck extension
    - In infants, neck flexion & expiration often cause pseudothickening of prevertebral soft tissues
    - Lateral fluoroscopy can distinguish persistent true thickening vs. dynamic pseudothickening
- With RPS abscess, lateral view shows widened/thickened prevertebral soft tissues
  - Convex anterior bowing with loss of normal step-off at interface of hypopharynx & esophagus
  - Limited utility for defining extent of collection & differentiating cellulitis/phlegmon from abscess
  - RPS gas rare but diagnostic of abscess (if no trauma)

CT Findings

- CECT
  - Defined fluid collection with enhancing wall in RPS
    - In early stages, enhancement may be subtle
    - Thick enhancing wall suggests mature abscess

Imaging Recommendations

- Best imaging tool: CECT

DIFFERENTIAL DIAGNOSIS

Pseudothickening of Retropharyngeal Soft Tissues

- Common radiographic mimic of RPS pathology in infants
- Adequate extension & inspiration or fluoroscopy will confirm as transient finding

Retropharyngeal Space Edema

- Poorly defined, elongated, homogeneous fluid infiltration of prevertebral soft tissues without rim enhancement
  - Due to regional inflammation (e.g., pharyngitis) or venous/lymphatic obstruction
- Drainage not required

Suppurative Adenopathy in Retropharyngeal Space

- Centrally hypodense/necrotic lymph node in lateral RPS with adjacent cellulitis
- Suppuration of node may progress to extranodal RPS abscess with inadequate medical therapy

Lymphatic Malformation

- Uni- or multilocular, transspatial, cystic neck mass with thin, nonenhancing wall (unless infected)
- Typically involves anterior & lateral neck

PATHOLOGY

General Features

- Etiology
  - Head & neck infection (pharyngitis, tonsillitis) seeds RPS lymph node → suppurative intranodal abscess → nodal rupture → RPS abscess
    - Most common organisms: *Staphylococcus aureus*, *Haemophilus*, *Streptococcus*
  - Pharyngeal penetration by foreign body
    - Child running with object in mouth

CLINICAL ISSUES

Presentation

- Most common signs/symptoms
  - Dysphagia, sore throat, poor oral intake, dehydration
  - Septic patient: Fever, chills, elevated WBC & ESR
- Other signs/symptoms
  - Posterior pharyngeal wall edema or bulge; reactive cervical adenopathy
- Clinical profile
  - Toxic-appearing child with marked neck pain & limited movement, especially in extension
  - Uncommonly presents with stridor

Demographics

- Most often children < 6 years old

Natural History & Prognosis

- Prognosis generally excellent with early diagnosis & aggressive management
- Complications may result from infection spread
  - Narrowing of pharyngeal lumen → airway compromise
  - Inferior spread to mediastinum → mediastinitis
    - Up to 50% mortality (much less in infants)
  - Carotid space involvement
    - Jugular vein thrombosis or thrombophlebitis
    - Internal carotid artery (ICA) spasm; neurological sequelae infrequent
    - Rarely ICA pseudoaneurysm &/or rupture; described with MRSA infection
  - Grisel syndrome rare
    - Distension or loosening of atlantoaxial ligaments after head & neck inflammation → nontraumatic atlantoaxial subluxation

Treatment

- Early ENT consultation
- IV antibiotics, airway management, fluid resuscitation
- Surgical intervention (I&D) for significant or complex abscess, lack of improvement/worsening with IV antibiotics

SELECTED REFERENCES

1. Ho ML et al: The ABCs (airway, blood vessels, and compartments) of pediatric neck infections and masses. AJR Am J Roentgenol. 1-10, 2016
2. Novis SJ et al: Pediatric deep space neck infections in U.S. children, 2000-2009. Int J Pediatr Otorhinolaryngol. 78(5):832-6, 2014
3. Abdel-Haq N et al: Retropharyngeal abscess in children: the rising incidence of methicillin-resistant Staphylococcus aureus. Pediatr Infect Dis J. 31(7):696-9, 2012
4. Baker KA et al: Use of computed tomography in the emergency department for the diagnosis of pediatric peritonsillar abscess. Pediatr Emerg Care. 28(10):962-5, 2012

Croup

TERMINOLOGY

- Benign, self-limited viral inflammation of upper airway
- Symmetric subglottic edema results in stridor & characteristic "barky" cough

IMAGING

- Diagnosis usually clinical; radiographs used to exclude more serious causes of stridor
- Frontal view: Often more revealing than lateral view
  - Gradual symmetric tapering of subglottic trachea from inferior to superior
    - "Steeple," "pencil tip," or "inverted V" configuration
    - Loss of normal "shoulders" (focal lateral convexities) of subglottic trachea secondary to edema
- Lateral view: Best for excluding other diagnoses
  - Relatively mild narrowing of AP dimension
  - Haziness with loss of subglottic tracheal wall definition
  - ± hypopharyngeal overdistention

TOP DIFFERENTIAL DIAGNOSES

- Foreign body
- Infantile hemangioma
- Epiglottitis
- Iatrogenic subglottic stenosis
- Exudative tracheitis

CLINICAL ISSUES

- Acute clinical syndrome characterized by "barky" or "seal-like" ("croupy") cough, inspiratory stridor, hoarseness
  - Age range: 6 months to 3 years; peak age: 1 year
- ± prodrome of low-grade fever, mild cough, rhinorrhea
- Affected child usually well otherwise
- Most cases successfully treated with corticosteroids ± nebulized epinephrine with < 4 hours of observation
- Recurrent episodes or atypical age suggest alternate diagnosis

(Left) Lateral radiograph in a 9-month-old infant with stridor shows haziness of the subglottic airway ➡. Overdistention (ballooning) of the hypopharynx ➡ is noted. The epiglottis ➡ & aryepiglottic folds ➡ are normal. (Right) AP radiograph in the same patient shows symmetric narrowing of the subglottic trachea ➡, typical of croup. The loss of the normal abrupt subglottic/glottic shouldering plus gradual tapering of the subglottic airway lumen from inferior to superior is referred to as the steeple sign.

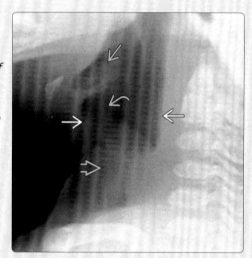
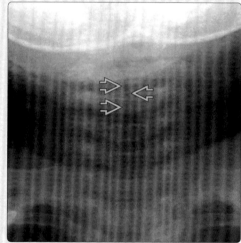

(Left) Endoscopic photograph shows a normal appearance of the subglottic airway. The subglottis is widely patent such that the mucosa is actually hidden beneath the vocal cords. (Right) Endoscopic photograph in a child with viral croup shows edematous subglottic mucosa ➡ that is visualized below the vocal cords. There is marked narrowing of the subglottic airway lumen, predominantly in the transverse dimension.

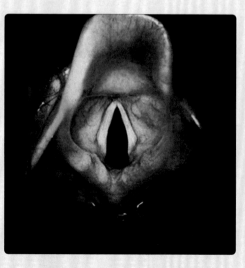
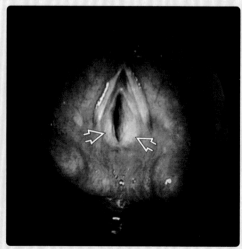

TERMINOLOGY

Definitions

- Croup: Self-limited viral inflammation of subglottic trachea causing stridor & characteristic cough
- Acute laryngotracheobronchitis: Croup + lower airway involvement
- Spasmodic croup: Recurrent episodes, typically without viral prodrome or fever
- Atypical croup: Recurrent episodes or croup outside expected age range

IMAGING

General Features

- Morphology of normal trachea: Uniform caliber from subglottis to carina
  - Normal "shoulders" at subglottis/glottis: Symmetric, focal convex/angular lateral margins of airway
  - Croup shows gradual tapering of subglottic trachea from inferior to superior

Radiographic Findings

- AP/frontal view
  - "Steeple," "pencil tip," or "inverted V" configuration of subglottic trachea
    - Loss of normal "shoulders" (lateral convexities) of subglottic trachea secondary to subglottic edema
    - Narrowing extends inferior to pyriform sinuses
- Lateral view
  - Mild narrowing of subglottic trachea in AP dimension
    - In contrast to moderate to marked narrowing of transverse dimension on frontal view
  - Haziness with poor definition of subglottic tracheal walls
  - ± hypopharyngeal overdistention
  - Normal epiglottis, aryepiglottic folds, retropharynx
  - No foreign body

Imaging Recommendations

- Best imaging tool
  - Diagnosis of croup primarily clinical, not imaging-based
    - Radiographs to exclude more serious causes of stridor
  - Frontal radiograph most useful view to confirm croup
  - Lateral radiograph helps exclude other diagnoses
- Protocol advice
  - Adequate neck extension + inspiration on lateral view
    - Decreases crowding of airway structures that may simulate disease in young child

PATHOLOGY

General Features

- Etiology
  - Benign, self-limited condition secondary to viral illness, most commonly parainfluenza viruses types 1-3
- Associated abnormalities
  - With atypical or spasmodic croup
    - 20-64% incidence of large airway lesions: Subglottic hemangioma, stenosis, laryngeal cleft or web, tracheomalacia, laryngomalacia, papillomatosis, or vocal cord paralysis

- Additional common disorders in this group: Gastroesophageal reflux, asthma, sleep-disordered breathing, allergies, chronic cough, prematurity

Staging, Grading, & Classification

- Clinical staging
  - Mild: Stridor at rest or when agitated
  - Moderate: Stridor + mild tachypnea, mild retractions
  - Severe: Stridor + respiratory distress, severe retractions, ± altered mental status

CLINICAL ISSUES

Presentation

- Most common signs/symptoms
  - "Barking" or seal-like ("croupy") cough, inspiratory stridor, hoarseness, respiratory distress
- Other signs/symptoms
  - ± prodrome of low-grade fever, mild cough, rhinorrhea
  - Usually well otherwise, able to manage secretions
  - More severe cases: Intercostal retractions, tachypnea, pallor, cyanosis, tachycardia, altered mental status
  - Symptoms worse at night or with agitation
  - May occur with other symptoms of lower respiratory tract infection (wheezing, cough, etc.)

Demographics

- Age range: 6 months to 3 years; peak: 1 year
  - If > 3 years, consider other acute causes of stridor
    - Mean age of atypical croup: 2.7-4.8 years
  - If < 6 months, consider predisposing abnormality

Natural History & Prognosis

- Benign, self-limited disease
- 75% of mild cases resolve within 3 days
- 11% of mild & 49% of moderate cases of croup worsen
- 53% of severe cases require endotracheal intubation
- Overall: 8% hospitalized, 1% admitted to intensive care unit
- 5% return to emergency department within 1 week
  - Consider other causes with recurrence, persistence

Treatment

- Most frequently managed supportively as outpatient
  - Mild croup: Systemic or nebulized corticosteroids, 2-hour observation
  - Moderate croup: Above + nebulized epinephrine, 4-hour observation
  - Severe croup: Above (can repeat epinephrine), admission to hospital
- Parents reassured, instructed to monitor for worsening
- Endoscopy/bronchoscopy rarely needed unless
  - Foreign body suspected
  - Exudative tracheitis suggested clinically/radiologically
  - Assistance required for intubation in severe croup

SELECTED REFERENCES

1. Darras KE et al: Imaging acute airway obstruction in infants and children. Radiographics. 35(7):2064-79, 2015
2. Delany DR et al: Role of direct laryngoscopy and bronchoscopy in recurrent croup. Otolaryngol Head Neck Surg. 152(1): 159-64, 2015
3. Johnson DW: Croup. BMJ Clin Evid. 2014, 2014
4. Petrocheilou A et al: Viral croup: diagnosis and a treatment algorithm. Pediatr Pulmonol. 49(5):421-9, 2014

Exudative Tracheitis

TERMINOLOGY

- Synonyms: Bacterial tracheitis, membranous or pseudomembranous croup, membranous laryngotracheobronchitis
  - Membranous croup: Confusing term overlapping much more common benign entity of viral croup
- Definition: Purulent infection of trachea
  - Results in thick, adherent, exudative plaques along tracheal walls that can slough, leading to airway obstruction
- Controversial disease
  - While many cases with significant morbidity & mortality have been confirmed, questions remain concerning overdiagnosis/overtreatment at certain centers

IMAGING

- Characteristic radiographic findings
  - Thin or thick linear or irregular soft tissue filling defects within airway (visualized pseudomembranes)
  - Loss of smooth well-defined parallel tracheal walls with nodular plaque-like irregularity
  - Hazy or indistinct tracheal air column
  - Symmetric or asymmetric subglottic narrowing in acutely ill child older than typically seen with viral croup

TOP DIFFERENTIAL DIAGNOSES

- Epiglottitis, croup, retropharyngeal abscess, foreign body

CLINICAL ISSUES

- Fever, cough, stridor, rapid onset (2-10 hours) of respiratory distress; often after viral prodrome
  - Favored to represent bacterial superinfection following compromise of respiratory mucosa by viral illness
    - Influenza A most common virus found; *Staphylococcus aureus* remains most common bacterial etiology
- Peak age: 3-8 years (older than classic viral croup)
- Aggressive treatment to prevent airway obstruction, death
  - Flexible laryngoscopy → rigid bronchoscopy + removal of pseudomembranes ± intubation; IV antibiotics ± steroids

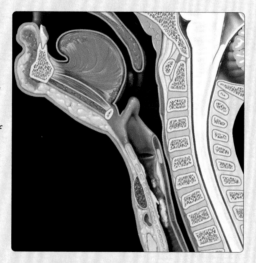

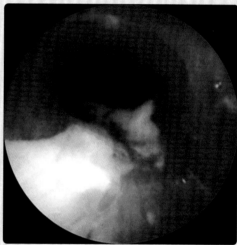

(Left) *Graphic shows inflammation of the trachea with the formation of inflammatory plaques & pseudomembranes along the tracheal walls. These plaques may detach from the tracheal wall & occlude the airway.* (Right) *Photograph from bronchoscopic visualization of the trachea in a child with bacterial tracheitis shows multiple purulent exudative plaques along the tracheal walls.*

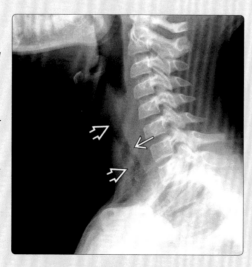

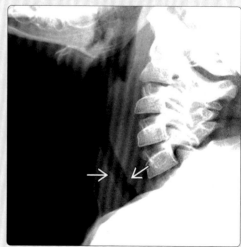

(Left) *Lateral airway radiograph shows multiple irregular intraluminal filling defects ➡ as well as tracheal wall irregularity ➡ & moderate luminal narrowing, consistent with exudative tracheitis.* (Right) *Lateral airway radiograph in a 5-year-old boy with fever, throat pain, & cough shows mild, generalized tracheal narrowing with subtle lobular & linear filling defects ➡, concerning for plaques/pseudomembranes. Exudative tracheitis was confirmed at laryngoscopy.*

TERMINOLOGY

- Adenoid tonsils (AT) lie along posterior wall of nasopharynx
- Enlargement may be chronic & idiopathic or acute/subacute with pathology (as from infection or neoplasm)
- Chronically enlarged AT can lead to obstructive sleep apnea (OSA) by obstructing posterior nasopharynx
- AT regrowth is common cause of recurrent/persistent OSA following palatine tonsillectomy & adenoidectomy (T&A)
  - Most MR sleep studies performed in this setting
  - Visualization of AT on such studies = recurrence

IMAGING

- Growth of normal adenoids without history of T&A
  - Absent at birth
  - Rarely visible radiographically prior to 6 months of life
  - Proliferate rapidly during infancy
  - Reach maximal size by 2-10 years of age
  - Progressively ↓ in size during 2nd decade of life
- Enlarged &/or recurrent AT

- Radiographs
  - Soft tissue fullness of nasopharyngeal posterior wall
    - \> 12-mm thickness
  - Encroachment on posterior nasopharyngeal airway
- MR imaging with cine sequences during respiratory cycle
  - T2 FS/STIR: High-signal AT tissue
    - V-shaped defect in midportion of anterior adenoid surface on axial images status post T&A
  - Cine: Intermittent collapse of posterior nasopharynx ± secondary collapse of retroglossal airway

CLINICAL ISSUES

- OSA in 3% of children, any age
  - OSA may manifest as snoring (± pauses, gasps), neurocognitive impairment, daytime sleepiness, pulmonary or systemic hypertension, failure to thrive
  - Treatment: Adenoidectomy; repeat for recurrence
- Pathologic causes of adenoid enlargement (acute to chronic, without OSA): Tonsillitis/pharyngitis > > neoplasm

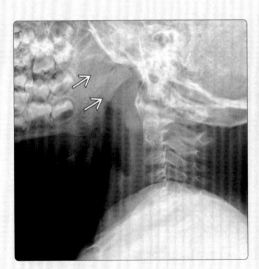

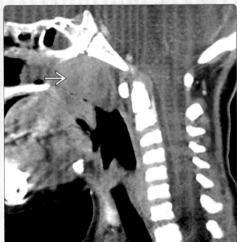

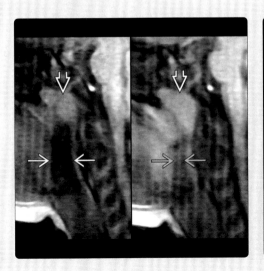

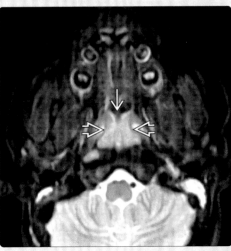

(Left) *Lateral radiograph in a 4 year old with fever & difficulty swallowing shows marked enlargement of the adenoid tonsils* ➡ *due to streptococcal pharyngitis.* **(Right)** *Sagittal midline CECT in the same patient shows marked enlargement of the adenoid tonsils* ➡ *with homogeneous enhancement. No abscess was identified in this patient with streptococcal pharyngitis.*

(Left) *Sagittal MR cine images during expiration (left) & inspiration (right) in a patient with obstructive sleep apnea show enlarged adenoid tonsils* ➡ *with effacement of the nasopharynx. The retroglossal airway is patent during expiration* ➡ *but collapses during inspiration* ➡ *due to the negative pressure generated by the more cephalad obstruction.* **(Right)** *Axial STIR MR in the same patient after adenoidectomy shows recurrent adenoid tonsils* ➡. *Note the anterior midline defect* ➡, *a typical postoperative appearance.*

Enlarged Palatine Tonsils

TERMINOLOGY

- Palatine tonsils: Paired, discrete masses of lymphoid tissue on either side of oropharynx
- Enlargement may be chronic & idiopathic or acute/subacute (as from infection or neoplasm)
  - Chronic may lead to obstructive sleep apnea (OSA)

IMAGING

- Clinical evaluation based on
  - Local & systemic symptoms
  - Size, asymmetry, & discoloration of palatine tonsils + presence of cervical adenopathy
    - No clear size measurements established on imaging
    - Enlargement determined by clinically visible percentage of oropharynx occupied by palatine tonsils
- Lateral airway radiograph obtained to evaluate upper airway pathologies other than palatine tonsils
  - Palatine tonsils appear as well-circumscribed soft tissue mass superimposed over mandibular angle

- CECT for acute presentations suggesting drainable abscess
  - Symmetric, homogeneously enhancing paired palatine tonsils show variable degrees of airway effacement
  - Asymmetry & heterogeneous enhancement may indicate pathology (e.g., abscess, necrotic tumor)
- MR sleep studies typically reserved for
  - Recurrent OSA despite previous surgery
  - Complex syndromes with multilevel obstruction

CLINICAL ISSUES

- Tonsillitis/pharyngitis: Fever, odynophagia, tonsillar erythema & exudate, preceding viral prodrome, tender cervical adenopathy
- Neoplasm (lymphoma): Tonsillar asymmetry, dysphagia, mucosal color alteration, snoring, recurrent tonsillitis, cervical adenopathy
- OSA: Chronic snoring (± pauses, gasps), neurocognitive impairment, daytime sleepiness, pulmonary or systemic hypertension, failure to thrive

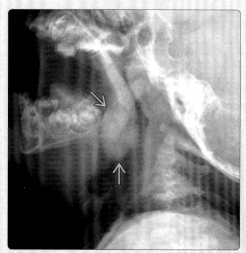
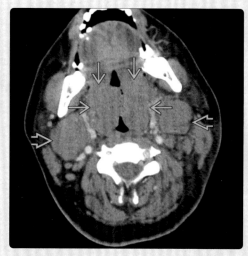

(Left) *Lateral airway radiograph in a 1-year-old child with drooling & decreased oral intake due to pharyngitis shows markedly enlarged palatine tonsils* ➡ *outlined by air.* (Right) *Axial CECT in a 17-year-old girl with cervical adenopathy* ➡ *due to Epstein-Barr virus shows marked symmetric enlargement of homogeneously enhancing "kissing" palatine tonsils* ➡ *that efface much of the oropharynx.*

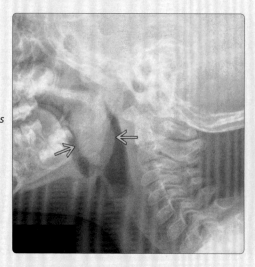
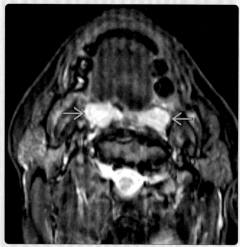

(Left) *Lateral radiograph of the neck in a 2-year-old child with snoring shows marked enlargement of the palatine tonsils* ➡. (Right) *Axial STIR MR shows paired palatine tonsils* ➡ *as symmetric, well-defined, fairly homogeneous high signal intensity structures in the palatine fossae.*

KEY FACTS

TERMINOLOGY

- Chronic idiopathic enlargement of lingual tonsils (lymphoid tissue at base of tongue) contributing to obstruction of retroglossal airway

IMAGING

- AP & lateral radiographs initially obtained in child with suspected upper airway pathology
  - Lingual tonsils best seen on lateral view
    - Round or lobulated mass protruding posteriorly from tongue base into vallecula & oropharyngeal/hypopharyngeal airway
    - Markedly enlarged if AP diameter ≥ 10 mm
- MR sleep study for recurrent/complex obstructive sleep apnea (OSA)
  - High T2 FS/STIR signal round, lobulated, or dumbbell-shaped mass protruding posteriorly from tongue base & filling retroglossal airway
    - Normally separate left & right lingual tonsils

TOP DIFFERENTIAL DIAGNOSES

- Other causes of OSA
- Lingual tonsil hypertrophy from infection or neoplasm
- Other vallecular masses

CLINICAL ISSUES

- OSA presentations: Snoring, poor rest, daytime fatigue
- Enlargement of lingual tonsils occurs most commonly
  - After previous palatine tonsillectomy & adenoidectomy
  - In children with Down syndrome (trisomy 21)
  - In obese children
  - With other systemic processes (e.g., Epstein-Barr virus infection, lymphoma) causing enlargement of lymphoid tissue
- If lingual tonsils causative of recurrent OSA, lingual tonsillectomy usually curative

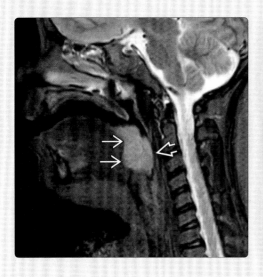

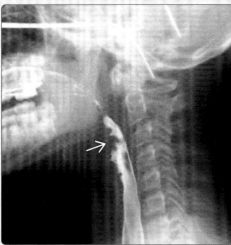

(Left) Lateral airway radiograph in an 11 year old with snoring shows round, mildly lobulated soft tissue ➡ at the tongue base filling the vallecula consistent with lingual tonsil enlargement. Note the concurrent enlargement of the adenoids ⮑. (Right) Lateral esophagram in a child with Down syndrome shows a fungiform filling defect ➡ of the barium column at the posterior aspect of the tongue consistent with enlarged lingual tonsils.

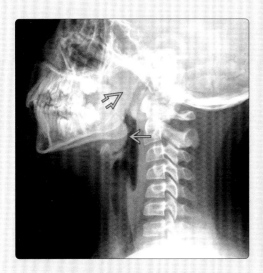

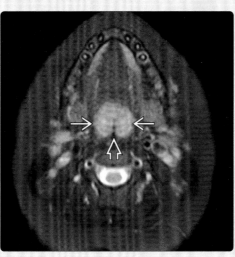

(Left) Sagittal STIR MR in a child with Down syndrome & other causes of obstructive sleep apnea (OSA) shows enlarged lingual tonsils ➡ as a high-signal mass at the base of the tongue. Note the filling & obstruction of the retroglossal airway ⮑. (Right) Axial T2 FS MR in a child with Down syndrome & OSA shows enlarged lingual tonsils ➡ as a high-signal mass at the base of the tongue. The enlarged lingual tonsils fill much of the retroglossal airway, leaving only a tiny patent lumen ⮑.

TERMINOLOGY

- Abnormal posterior motion of tongue during sleep leading to obstructive sleep apnea (OSA)
- Typically associated with underlying hypotonia, macroglossia, &/or micrognathia
- Glossoptosis very rare in otherwise healthy children

IMAGING

- MR sleep study evaluates airway motion & anatomic abnormalities during real-time respiratory cycle
- Indications for dynamic MR sleep imaging
  - Persistent OSA despite previous tonsillectomy & adenoidectomy (T&A) or other airway surgery
  - Complex OSA with predisposition to obstruction at multiple sites (e.g., Down syndrome)
  - Evaluation of OSA prior to any complex airway surgery
  - OSA & severe obesity
- Characteristic findings of glossoptosis
  - Tongue "falls" posteriorly → posterior border of tongue abuts posterior wall of pharynx → obstruction of retroglossal airway during inspiration
    - Can also abut & displace velum (soft palate) → obstruction of posterior nasopharynx
  - Stationary posterior & lateral walls of hypopharynx
    - In contrast to hypopharyngeal collapse
  - ± macroglossia & fatty infiltration of tongue

PATHOLOGY

- OSA difficult to manage in Down syndrome: Multiple anatomic abnormalities + ↓ muscle tone
  - Findings in Down syndrome & persistent OSA after T&A: Glossoptosis (63%), recurrent & enlarged adenoid tonsils (63%), enlarged lingual tonsils (30%), macroglossia (74%)

CLINICAL ISSUES

- Treatment: Initially conservative with positive pressure ventilation (CPAP or BIPAP); may require procedures to ↓ tongue bulk &/or reposition tongue

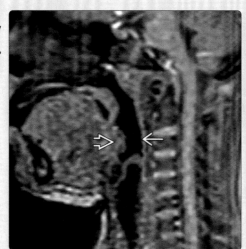
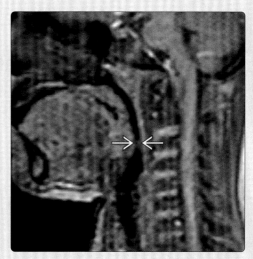

(Left) *Sagittal cine MR obtained during the expiratory phase of the respiratory cycle in a child with Down syndrome shows the retroglossal airway* ⟹ *to be patent despite the large posteriorly positioned tongue. The lingual tonsils* ⟹ *are also enlarged.* (Right) *Sagittal cine MR in the same patient, obtained during inspiration, shows the posterior aspect of the tongue & lingual tonsils to have moved posteriorly, nearly obstructing the retroglossal airway* ⟹.

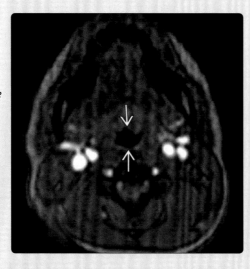
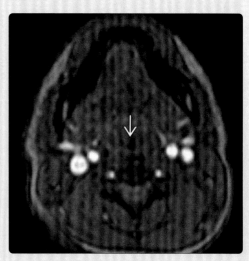

(Left) *Axial cine MR obtained during expiration shows the retroglossal airway* ⟹ *to be patent.* (Right) *Axial cine MR in the same patient, obtained during inspiration, shows the posterior aspect of the tongue & lingual tonsils to have moved posteriorly, nearly completely obstructing the retroglossal airway* ⟹.

Double Aortic Arch

KEY FACTS

TERMINOLOGY

- Congenital aortic arch anomaly related to persistence of both left & right 4th aortic arches

IMAGING

- Chest radiography often suggestive of diagnosis
  - Bilateral tracheal indentations & mid tracheal narrowing
  - Right arch indentation commonly higher & more substantial than left ("right dominant")
- Esophagram shows characteristic bilateral & posterior indentations
- Cross-sectional imaging (CTA/MR) for definitive diagnosis & characterization
  - Left & right arches arise from ascending aorta, encircle trachea & esophagus, & join to form descending aorta
  - Each arch gives rise to 1 ventral carotid & 1 dorsal subclavian artery (4 artery sign on axial slice)
  - Right arch commonly larger, more superior, & more posterior extending than left (70% of cases)

- Left descending aorta in these cases

PATHOLOGY

- Typically isolated; congenital intracardiac disease in 20%
- Dominant right arch, left descending aorta: 70-75%
- Dominant left arch, right descending aorta: 15-20%
- Arches equal in size: 5-10%
- Smaller of 2 arches may be partially atretic

CLINICAL ISSUES

- Most common symptomatic vascular ring (55%)
- Typically presents < 3 years of age (often immediately after birth) with stridor, wheezing, choking that worsens with feeding, apneic attacks, noisy breathing, "seal bark" cough
- Surgery: Left (usually) thoracotomy with division of smaller arch, atretic segment, & ligamentum arteriosum with mobilization of trachea & esophagus
  - Up to 11% require 2nd operation to relieve persistent airway symptoms (most commonly stridor)

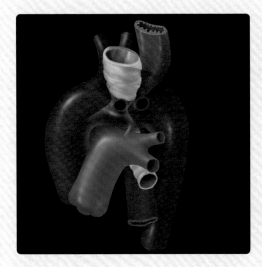
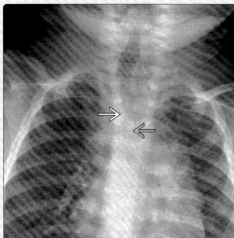

(Left) Oblique graphic shows a double aortic arch anomaly with a complete vascular ring encircling & compressing the trachea & esophagus. (Right) AP radiograph of a 2 month old with biphasic stridor shows impressions on the trachea from both the right & left, with the right impression ➡ being higher than the left ➡. Radiography can be highly suggestive of a double aortic arch, though the airway morphology is often overlooked.

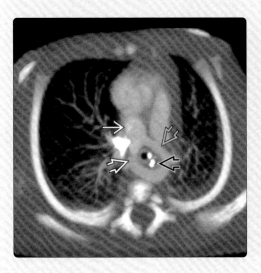
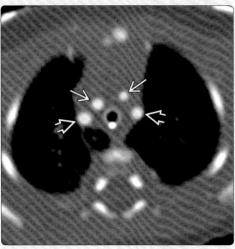

(Left) Axial CTA MIP image shows the ascending aorta ➡ dividing into the right ➡ & left ➡ arches, which extend along either side of the trachea. The right arch is dominant, as is typically seen. Both arches converge to form the descending aorta to the left of the thoracic spine. The trachea & esophagus ➡ are both surrounded & compressed by the arches. (Right) Axial CTA just above both aortic arches shows separate ostia of both carotid ➡ & subclavian ➡ arteries (the 4 artery sign), typical of a double aortic arch.

TERMINOLOGY

- Left pulmonary artery (LPA) sling: Left branch pulmonary artery originates from posterior aspect of proximal right branch pulmonary artery, coursing around right & posterior distal tracheal walls as it passes leftward between trachea & esophagus

IMAGING

- Only vascular ring (essentially) to course between trachea & esophagus
  - Compresses posterior trachea & anterior esophagus
  - Lateral chest radiograph: Round opacity between distal trachea & esophagus
  - Lateral esophagram: Anterior indentation on esophagus
- Often causes asymmetric lung inflation
- Multidetector CT angiography preferred over MR to confirm diagnosis & delineate anatomy prior to surgery
  - Rapid acquisition of CTA avoids intubation
  - Exquisite 3D reconstructions of airway & vessels

PATHOLOGY

- Compression of distal trachea, carina, & main bronchi by sling, resulting in asymmetric inflation of lungs
  - Obstructive hyperinflation > atelectasis
- ± tracheobronchomalacia, intrinsic airway narrowing (by complete cartilage rings), &/or branching anomalies
- ± associated pulmonary, cardiac, & GI anomalies

CLINICAL ISSUES

- Typically presents in neonatal period
  - Severe stridor, cough, apneic spells, hypoxia, ventilator dependency
- Surgical repair
  - Division of LPA from its anomalous origin with implantation to its normal origin (main pulmonary artery)
  - Tracheobronchial reconstruction required for complete cartilaginous rings or other associated tracheobronchial malformations

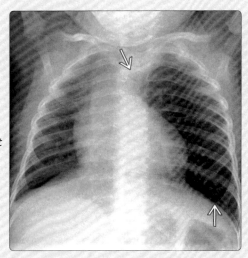
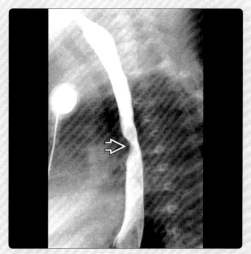

(Left) AP radiograph in a patient with a left pulmonary artery sling (LPAS) shows asymmetric hyperinflation of the left lung ➡ with rightward mediastinal shift. There is an inapparent (poorly visualized) distal trachea. (Right) Lateral esophagram shows an anterior impression ➡ on the esophageal contrast column from the aberrant LPAS, a classic finding on fluoroscopy.

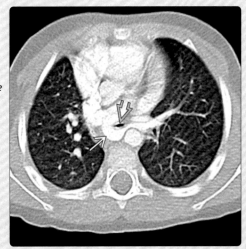
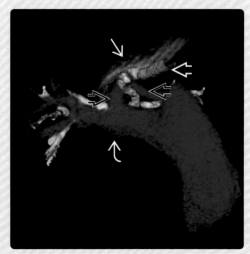

(Left) Axial CTA (in lung windows) shows an aberrant left pulmonary artery ➡ coursing posterior to the airway. Note the distal tracheal narrowing ➡ in this child with associated complete tracheal rings. Also note the mild hyperinflation of the left lung compared to the right. (Right) Anterior 3D CTA surface rendering shows an aberrant LPAS ➡ originating from the right pulmonary artery ➡ & coursing between the esophagus ➡ & trachea ➡.

IMAGING

- AP radiograph: Right aortic arch (RAA) deviates trachea to left
- Lateral radiograph: Anterior tracheal bowing due to retroesophageal aberrant left subclavian artery (ALSCA) arising from Kommerell diverticulum
- Esophagram: Posterior indentation by aberrant vessel
- CTA or MRA with 3D reconstructions now preferred modality for diagnosis prior to surgical intervention

TOP DIFFERENTIAL DIAGNOSES

- Right aortic arch with mirror image branching
  - High association with cyanotic congenital heart disease, such as tetralogy of Fallot & truncus arteriosus
- Double aortic arch with atretic left arch
  - Inferior tenting of left common carotid artery & 4-pronged branching pattern of arches at thoracic inlet
- Left aortic arch with aberrant right subclavian artery

- Typically isolated & incidental abnormality (without airway compression)

PATHOLOGY

- Related to embryologic persistence of right 4th aortic arch
- Left ductus persists as ligamentum arteriosum, which completes vascular ring
- Right arch often found in 22q11 deletion patients

CLINICAL ISSUES

- Symptoms of stridor, apnea, cyanosis, recurrent respiratory infection, or chronic cough; can be incidental finding on esophagram
- RAA-ALSCA with constricting (symptomatic) left ligamentum arteriosum treated with division of ligamentum via left thoracotomy
  - Prognosis generally good after division of vascular ring
  - Symptoms may persist from tracheomalacia & residual stenosis after vascular ring repair

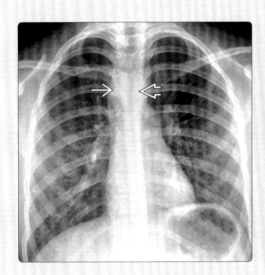

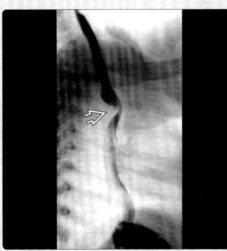

(Left) PA radiograph of the chest shows a right aortic arch ➡ causing an impression on the right side of the trachea & displacing the trachea to the left ➡. This is an initial clue to diagnosing a right aortic arch with aberrant left subclavian artery (RAA-ALSCA) & is often overlooked. (Right) Lateral esophagram in an infant shows a large posterior indentation ➡ on the esophagus due to a RAA-ALSCA with a diverticulum of Kommerell.

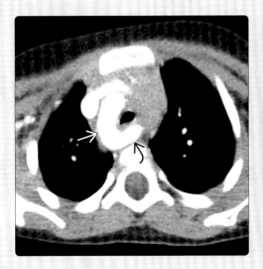

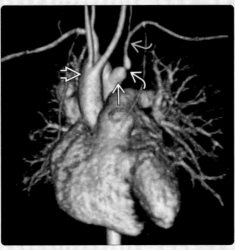

(Left) Axial CECT shows an RAA ➡ with an ALSCA ➡ arising from the dorsal aorta & coursing posterior to the trachea. This RAA, in concert with a tight left ligamentum arteriosum (that is usually not visible), creates a complete vascular ring. (Right) 3D volume-rendered CTA (anterior projection) shows an RAA ➡ with an ALSCA ➡ originating from a diverticulum of Kommerell ➡. There is stenosis ➡ at the origin of the ALSCA from the diverticulum.

Infantile Hemangioma, Airway

TERMINOLOGY

- Benign vascular neoplasm of capillaries in infant
- Can arise in many locations; airway occurrence potentially life threatening

IMAGING

- Asymmetric subglottic tracheal narrowing in young child
  - May be transglottic, rarely distal
- Avidly enhancing submucosal mass on CT/MR
  - Unilateral > bilateral or circumferential

TOP DIFFERENTIAL DIAGNOSES

- Congenital or iatrogenic subglottic tracheal stenosis
- Croup
- Tracheomalacia
- Papillomatosis

PATHOLOGY

- Predictable life cycle of infantile hemangioma

- Proliferative phase: Appears days-weeks after birth & grows rapidly for ~ 4-12 months
  - Involuting phase: Slow gradual regression over years
  - Involuted phase: Static minimal residua of lesion
- May occur with PHACES association
  - **P**osterior fossa brain malformations, **h**emangiomas of face, **a**rterial anomalies, **c**ardiac anomalies, **e**ye abnormalities, **s**ternal clefts or **s**upraumbilical raphe

CLINICAL ISSUES

- Inspiratory stridor, hoarseness, or abnormal cry < 6 months of age; often progressive as lesion proliferates
- Cutaneous hemangiomas in 50%
  - Classically in "beard" distribution
- Treatment
  - Most common: Conservative monitoring or propranolol
  - Others: Corticosteroids, laser therapy, surgical excision
  - Combination of therapies used in 75% of children

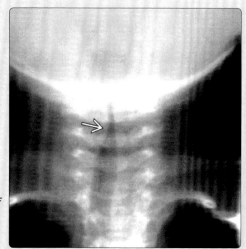

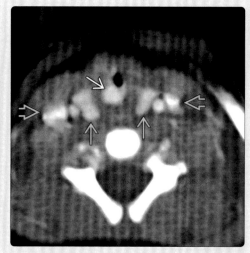

(Left) AP radiograph shows asymmetric subglottic tracheal narrowing ➡ in a 2-week-old infant presenting with stridor. Asymmetric narrowing is always concerning for a hemangioma, as opposed to the symmetric subglottic narrowing that is typical of croup. (Right) Axial CECT in the same patient shows a well-defined, avidly enhancing infantile hemangioma ➡ along the posterior aspect of the subglottic airway. The lobes of the thyroid ➡ & adjacent cervical vessels ➡ are noted for reference.

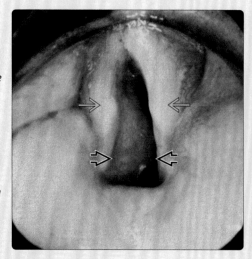

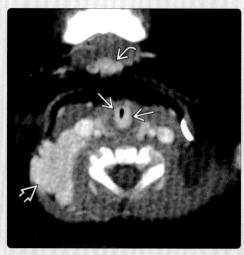

(Left) Endoscopic photograph above the vocal folds ➡ demonstrates a bulging red mass ➡ protruding into & narrowing the subglottic trachea, typical of an infantile hemangioma. (Right) Axial CECT in an 11-week-old girl demonstrates a circumferential, well-defined subglottic infantile hemangioma ➡. Note the additional posterior cervical space ➡ & submental ➡ infantile hemangiomas, which should raise suspicion for PHACES association.

Tracheobronchomalacia

TERMINOLOGY

- Excessive expiratory collapse of trachea &/or bronchi due to weakness of airway wall/supporting cartilage
  - May be purely intrinsic or in association with longstanding extrinsic compression

IMAGING

- Dynamic 4D CT (real-time model of airway during respiration) vs. static inspiratory & expiratory CT scans
  - 3D & multiplanar reconstructions of airway helpful
  - IV contrast useful to look for contributory adjacent mass or aberrant vessel
- > 50% ↓ in cross-sectional area of tracheal &/or bronchial lumen during expiration or coughing
  - Correlates well with bronchoscopy (which remains gold standard for diagnosis)
  - Relatively underdiagnosed as imaging is routinely performed only at end inspiration
- ↑ frequency & severity of air-trapping

TOP DIFFERENTIAL DIAGNOSES

- Difficult to control asthma
- Foreign body aspiration
- Extrinsic compression
- Complete tracheal rings

PATHOLOGY

- Primary (congenital): Impaired cartilage maturation
- Secondary (acquired): Otherwise normal cartilage degenerates following infection, chronic inflammation, intubation, trauma, or longstanding extrinsic compression

CLINICAL ISSUES

- Presentations: Expiratory stridor, dyspnea, cough, sputum production, ALTE/BRUE
- Conservative therapy in mild cases (may improve with age)
- Continuous positive airway pressure (CPAP) if moderate
- If necessary, procedures include aortopexy, anterior tracheal suspension, or rarely stenting

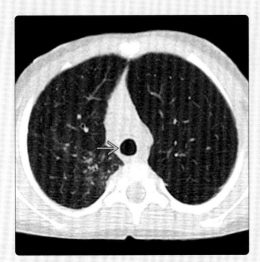
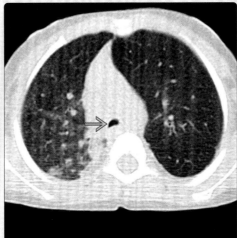

(Left) Inspiratory axial HRCT shows a normal, nearly rounded appearance of the trachea ➡. The posterior aspect is often nearly flat as it lacks supportive cartilage. The caliber of the trachea should be uniform from the glottis to the carina & relatively unchanging between inspiration & expiration. (Right) Expiratory axial HRCT in the same patient shows marked narrowing of the trachea ➡, a substantial change from the inspiratory image that is consistent with tracheomalacia.

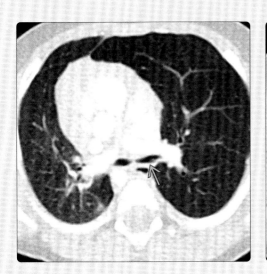
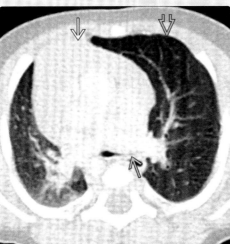

(Left) Inspiratory axial HRCT with contrast shows a patent left main bronchus ➡. (Right) Expiratory axial HRCT in the same patient shows interval collapse of the left main bronchus ➡, consistent with bronchomalacia. No adjacent mass or abnormal vessel was noted on soft tissue windows (not shown). Note the air-trapping of the left lung ➡ & the L → R mediastinal shift ➡.

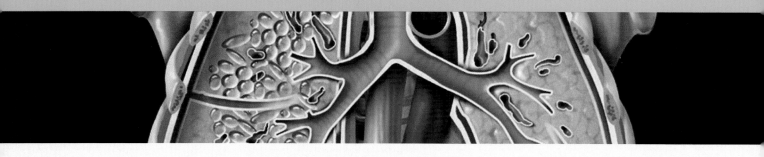

SECTION 2
Chest

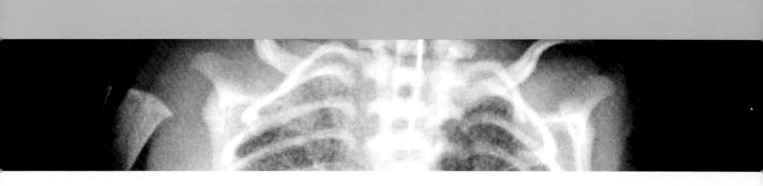

Mediastinal Masses

Trauma

Miscellaneous

Imaging Modalities

Radiography

Imaging investigation of most thoracic symptoms (whether suggestive of pulmonary, cardiovascular, gastrointestinal, or chest wall origin) almost always begins with chest radiographs. In patients who are clinically stable & capable of following directions, the preferred technique is upright frontal (PA) & lateral views of the chest with full inspiration. However, supine (AP) views will typically be employed in patients who are unstable or are otherwise not able to support themselves upright. It is important to note how the image was obtained as this can cause problems with interpretation. One pitfall is that the lungs will typically be hypoinflated in supine patients, which can accentuate lung opacity (thereby mimicking disease such as edema or pneumonia) & create the appearance of an enlarged heart. Additionally, gas collections (such as pneumothorax & free peritoneal air) will accumulate anteriorly in the supine patient (rather than superiorly on an upright view). This change in the position of gas can help determine the position of the patient on the study at hand (though this is often indicated on the image by an arrow or note by the technologist): Gas in the stomach will outline the gastric fundus on an upright view but will outline the anterior body or antrum on a supine cross-table lateral view.

Additional views are rarely needed but do arise in specific circumstances. Oblique views of the ribs are sometimes requested to look for bone pathology. Such views have shown to increase rib fracture detection in the infant with suspected nonaccidental trauma. However, their utility in the older child with accidental trauma or chest wall pain is questionable (as the routinely obtained 2 views will typically suffice for clinical significance).

If a bronchial foreign body is suspected, bilateral decubitus views or inspiratory/expiratory views may be requested to look for unilateral air-trapping that suggests airway obstruction with a 1-way valve mechanism. However, the sensitivity & specificity of these techniques are limited, & these studies may be bypassed for CT or bronchoscopy depending on the level of clinical suspicion.

Fluoroscopy

Fluoroscopic imaging of the chest is rarely employed. One such circumstance is the patient with possible hemidiaphragm paralysis. Diaphragmatic excursion is easily observed during the respiratory cycle with limited radiation required to determine whether or not the diaphragm moves in an expected manner.

Ultrasound

Virtually any palpable mass can be interrogated successfully with ultrasound. It is particularly helpful for soft or compressible lesions, while very hard lesions (that may be calcified or of bony origin) may benefit 1st from radiography. If the mass is painful, further cross-sectional imaging is often required.

Ultrasound is excellent at detecting & characterizing pleural effusions. This can be particularly helpful in the patient with complex loculated collections associated with pneumonias as septations that may require more aggressive therapy will often not be visualized on CECT.

While not widely used, there has been increasing interest in the capability of ultrasound to detect pneumonia, pneumothorax, & pulmonary edema, particularly in the emergency department. Ultrasound will likely see an enhanced role in these diagnoses over the upcoming years.

Computed Tomography

CT has many uses in the chest, though they are generally driven by specific clinical scenarios that started with a chest radiograph. It should be recognized that the terms "spiral/helical CT" & "high-resolution chest CT" are now antiquated & based on techniques that were at one time advanced & required choosing one method over another. In the current era, most CT scanners are so powerful that using a helical or volume acquisition of data (which is now routine) allows reconstruction of the data in innumerable ways, both in visualized formats (e.g., 2D planes of any orientation or various 3D reconstructions) & types of tissue displayed (i.e., settings idealized for lung, vessels, mediastinal tissues, & bones). Therefore, simply ordering a "chest CT" with a clear clinical indication (including signs/symptoms & concerns) will allow the radiologist to determine exactly how the study should be performed & what data should be extracted from it. The main question remaining in ordering the exam is whether or not IV contrast is needed. Most indications targeted at the lung parenchyma (such as the detection of lung nodules in a patient with cancer or characterization of interstitial disease) do not require IV contrast. Most other questions will require contrast, including assessments of the vasculature (such as pulmonary emboli, arterial injuries, & vascular rings), mediastinal or hilar masses, & complicated pneumonias. Other techniques (including adding expiratory images to look for air-trapping) are usually driven by subspecialists.

Magnetic Resonance

Currently, CT provides much better evaluation of the lung parenchyma than MR. However, new ultrafast MR techniques show promise & may soon have a role in evaluating pediatric lung disease. The role of MR in the chest has largely been to evaluate soft tissue masses, particularly those near the spine that may be affecting the neural elements. MR also can be used to evaluate the vasculature of the chest. Beyond cardiac & aortic applications, it can be used in the evaluation of suspected chronic or dynamic venous occlusion (such as with thoracic outlet syndrome).

Nuclear Medicine

Currently, most nuclear chest imaging is limited to PET for staging & follow-up of lymphoma or other malignancies. The chest may also be imaged with the entire body in the setting of other malignancies, such as neuroblastoma (MIBG scan) or thyroid cancer (iodine scan). Due to the availability & accuracy of CECT for the diagnosis of pulmonary embolism, nuclear V/Q scans are rarely used now.

Selected References

1. ACR Appropriateness Criteria: Fever Without Source or Unknown Origin—Child. https://acsearch.acr.org/docs/69438/Narrative/. Published 1999. Reviewed 2015. Accessed April 14, 2017
2. Pereda MA et al: Lung ultrasound for the diagnosis of pneumonia in children: a meta-analysis. Pediatrics. 135(4):714-22, 2015
3. Thacker PG et al: Imaging evaluation of mediastinal masses in children and adults: practical diagnostic approach based on a new classification system. J Thorac Imaging. 30(4):247-67, 2015
4. Trinavarat P et al: Potential of ultrasound in the pediatric chest. Eur J Radiol. 83(9):1507-18, 2014
5. Manson DE: MR imaging of the chest in children. Acta Radiol. 54(9):1075-85, 2013
6. Frush DP: Radiation, thoracic imaging, and children: radiation safety. Radiol Clin North Am. 49(5):1053-69, 2011
7. Moore MA et al: Chest trauma in children: current imaging guidelines and techniques. Radiol Clin North Am. 49(5):949-68, 2011

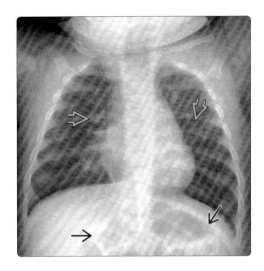

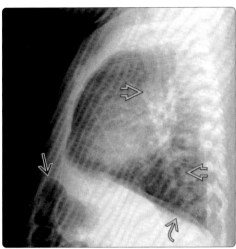

(Left) *Frontal radiograph in a 5 month old with cough & fever shows symmetric hyperinflation of the lungs with increased peribronchial thickening ⊟, typical of bronchiolitis. Gaseous distention of bowel in the upper abdomen ⊟ is due to air swallowing, & its location suggests a supine position.* (Right) *Lateral radiograph in the same patient shows lung hyperinflation with depression of the hemidiaphragms ⊟ & peribronchial thickening ⊟. The anterior location of the bowel gas ⊟ confirms a supine position of the patient.*

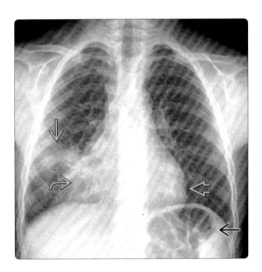

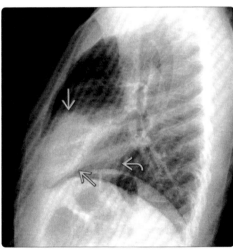

(Left) *Frontal radiograph in a 5 year old with fever & cough shows a poorly defined opacity ⊟ obscuring the right heart border ⊟, consistent with a right middle lobe (RML) pneumonia. Note that the left heart border is well seen ⊟ because the lingula is clear. There is gas ⊟ in the stomach & colon just under the left hemidiaphragm, confirming an upright patient position.* (Right) *Lateral radiograph in the same patient confirms a pneumonia of the RML ⊟. The portion of the heart that is not overlapped by the pneumonia is less dense ⊟.*

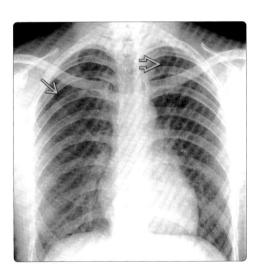

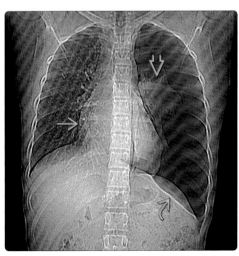

(Left) *Frontal radiograph in a 17 year old with difficulty breathing shows a small to moderate right apical pneumothorax that is visualized by the interface ⊟ of the right upper lobe & pleural gas. Note the lack of lung markings superiorly, unlike the left apex ⊟.* (Right) *Scout image from an NECT in a teenager with tuberous sclerosis shows a large left tension pneumothorax with rightward mediastinal shift ⊟ & depression of the left hemidiaphragm ⊟. The left lung is completely collapsed ⊟.*

(Left) *Frontal radiograph in a 1 year old with fever & cough shows a poorly defined opacity* ➡ *in the medial left lower lobe (LLL) partially obscuring the left hemidiaphragm. No adjacent bony abnormality is seen.* (Right) *Lateral radiograph in the same child shows the LLL pneumonia* ➡. *Most of the left hemidiaphragm is obscured on this view by the adjacent consolidated lung (unlike the right side* ➡). *Note the position of the air-fluid level in the stomach* ➡ *on this image, typical of a supine view.*

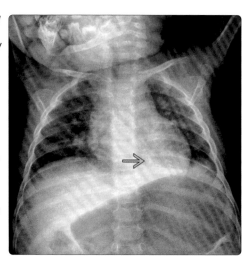
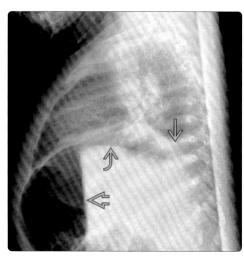

(Left) *Frontal radiograph in a 7 year old with cough & decreased breath sounds shows a dense retrocardiac LLL pneumonia* ➡ *obscuring the left hemidiaphragm. The ascending crescentic opacities laterally* ➡ *are due to a parapneumonic effusion on this upright view.* (Right) *Longitudinal ultrasound of the chest in a 15 year old with tachypnea shows a complex hypoechoic right pleural effusion* ➡ *with numerous echogenic septations* ➡. *Note the adjacent consolidated echogenic lung* ➡ *& hypoechoic liver* ➡.

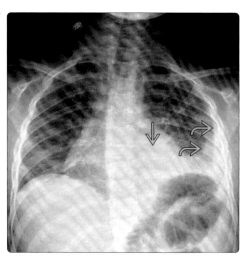
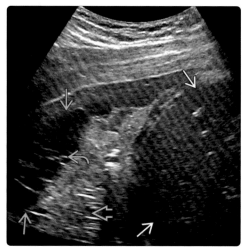

(Left) *Frontal radiograph of a 5 year old with cough & fever shows a round right perihilar opacity* ➡ *with air bronchograms. There is no bony abnormality. The appearance, symptoms, & age are typical for a round pneumonia.* (Right) *Axial CECT in a 2 year old with wheezing shows a heterogeneous mass* ➡ *filling & expanding the right hemithorax. The mass proved to be a pleuropulmonary blastoma.*

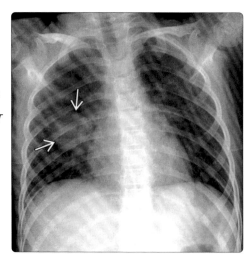
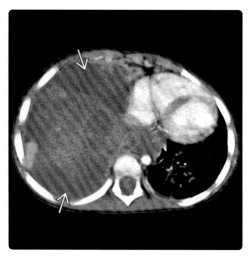

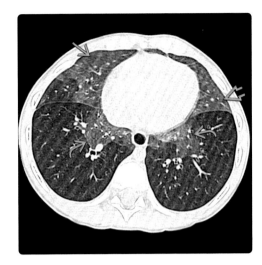

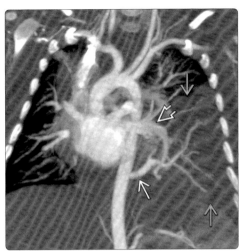

(Left) *Axial lung CT in a 13 month old with dyspnea, crackles, & failure to thrive shows a characteristic distribution of ground-glass opacities in the middle lobe ⊟, lingula ⊟, & paramediastinal lower lobes ⊟, typical of neuroendocrine cell hyperplasia of infancy.*
(Right) *Coronal chest CTA MIP image in a 2 month old with a prenatally diagnosed congenital lung lesion shows both the systemic arterial supply ⊟ & the pulmonary venous drainage ⊟ of a large bronchopulmonary sequestration ⊟.*

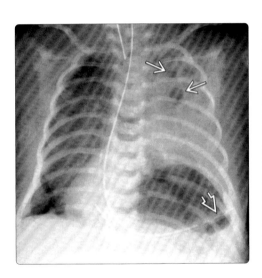

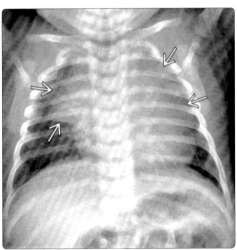

(Left) *Frontal radiograph of a neonate with a left congenital diaphragmatic hernia shows several gas-containing bowel loops ⊟ in the left upper hemithorax. The stomach is also in the chest, as confirmed by the nasogastric tube ⊟.*
(Right) *Frontal radiograph of a 1 month old shows a large but normal thymus ⊟ that could be mistaken for a mediastinal mass. The shape, mild undulation, location, lack of mass effect, & age are typical for thymus. If uncertain, ultrasound can confirm normal thymic tissue.*

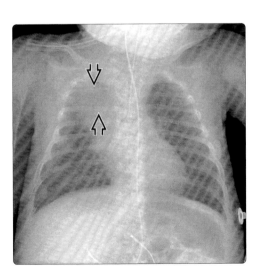

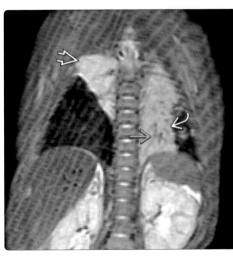

(Left) *Frontal radiograph in a 3 week old with respiratory distress shows a right upper lobe opacity that could easily be mistaken for atelectasis. However, there is splaying of the adjacent ribs ⊟, a finding that strongly suggests a paraspinal neuroblastoma.*
(Right) *Coronal STIR MR in the same patient shows a right apical paraspinal neuroblastoma ⊟. There is also atelectasis of much of the LLL ⊟. Note the dark, air-filled branching bronchi ⊟ within the atelectatic lung that are not visible in the solid tumor.*

TERMINOLOGY

- Normal organ of anterior superior mediastinum involved in production of T cells
  o Appears prominent in many young children

IMAGING

- Normal thymus variable in size but ↓ with age
  o Moderate to large on chest x-ray up to 5 years of age
  o ↓ in relative size by end of 1st decade
  o No "mass" should be present in 2nd decade
- Normal thymus variable in contour
  o Smooth curvilinear borders ± undulation with ribs
- Normal thymus variable in shape & symmetry
  o Bilobed with convex margins in young children vs. concave margins in older children
  o Sail sign: Lateral triangular extension (right > left)
- Homogeneous consistency without Ca²⁺ or cysts
  o Slightly lucent: Vessels seen through thymus
- No mass effect on adjacent structures

- Normal variant locations: Cervical & retrocaval extensions
  o Can be confused with lymphadenopathy or mass
  o Keys to diagnosing normal variant thymic extensions
    – Continuous with & similar imaging appearance (on US, CT, MR) to normally located thymus
      □ Ultrasound best tool for confirmation in children
- Aberrant, ectopic thymic tissue may occur in inferior lateral neck or thyroid, ± thymic tissue in normal location
- Thymic rebound: Volume can ↓ by > 40% with chemotherapy & other stresses
  o Volume ↑ or rebounds to original (or larger) size upon stress cessation, potentially mimicking recurrent mass
- Absent thymic visualization on lateral neonatal chest radiograph occurs with ectopia, DiGeorge syndrome, severe combined immunodeficiency, or prior sternotomy for congenital heart disease

CLINICAL ISSUES

- Prominent but normal thymus should be asymptomatic

(Left) AP chest radiograph in a 6-month-old girl shows a normal prominent thymus ⇨ with a triangular configuration extending into the right hemithorax (sail sign). The normal thymus is lucent & "soft" with undulations at the ribs & intercostal spaces ⇨. (Right) AP chest radiograph in a neonate shows prominence of the superior mediastinum ⇨ about the trachea ⇨. This appearance of smooth convex margins with no tracheal compression is consistent with a normal thymus in a patient of this age.

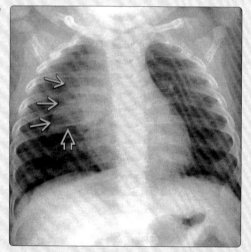
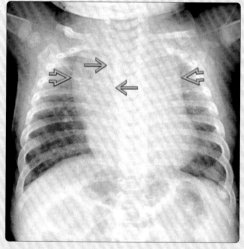

(Left) Longitudinal grayscale (left) & color Doppler (right) US in a 2 day old show a normal thymus ⇨. Punctate & linear (dot-dash pattern) echogenic foci ⇨ are present throughout the hypoechoic parenchyma with no increased vascularity. The great vessels are posteroinferior ⇨ to the thymus. (Right) Axial chest CECT images are shown in 2 boys of different ages. In the 2 year old, the normal thymus is prominent with convex borders ⇨. In the 17 year old, the normal thymus is small & relatively triangular in shape with concave borders ⇨.

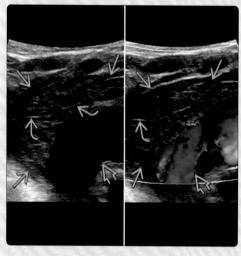
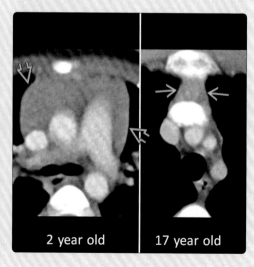

2 year old   17 year old

Palpable Normal Variants of Chest Wall

KEY FACTS

TERMINOLOGY

- Commonly occurring normal variations of anterior chest wall that may be mistaken for pathology
- Typically isolated variant morphologies of costal cartilages, ribs, &/or sternum
  - Prominent asymmetric convexity or thickness of costal cartilage; may be isolated or due to bifid rib
  - Tilted sternum

IMAGING

- Ultrasound best initial study for palpable mass unless bony abnormality primarily suspected
- Radiographs best for initial bone evaluation
  - May show bifid rib or bony sternal anomaly
  - Purely cartilaginous variants will not be seen
  - Help exclude other significant processes
    - Scoliosis, bone destruction by malignancy

TOP DIFFERENTIAL DIAGNOSES

- Vascular anomaly
- Soft tissue or bone sarcoma
- Osteochondroma
- Pectus excavatum or pectus carinatum
- Scoliosis

CLINICAL ISSUES

- Asymptomatic palpable "mass" detected by patient, parent, or clinician; usually painless
  - History often erroneously suggests finding as newly or rapidly developed
  - Recent trauma to region may bring palpable abnormality to attention
- Typically isolated finding of little consequence
  - ~ 33% of children imaged for other causes have minor variations in chest wall configuration
  - Isolated bifid rib in 0.15-3.4% of population

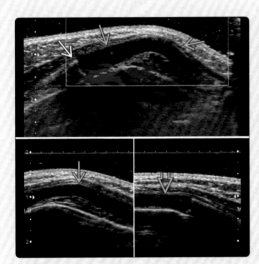

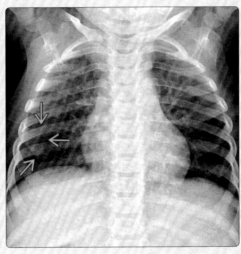

(Left) Transverse color Doppler (top) & grayscale (bottom) ultrasounds of a 2 year old with an asymptomatic palpable abnormality of the right chest wall show an avascular, nearly anechoic anteriorly protuberant costal cartilage ➡ that is continuous with the bony anterior rib ➡. The normal comparison left side is shown at the same level ➡. (Right) AP chest radiograph in the same 2 year old shows a bifid configuration of the right 5th rib ➡ at this same level, a normal variant.

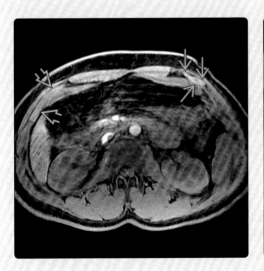

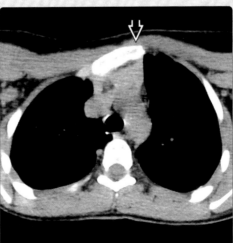

(Left) Axial T1 GRE FS MR in a teenager with a left lower anterior chest wall palpable abnormality shows focal protuberance & undulation of a costal cartilage on the left ➡, a normal variant. The normal right side is noted for comparison ➡. (Right) Axial NECT in a patient with a palpable "mass" shows tilting of the sternum with the left margin ➡ being more anterior in location as compared to the right.

Congenital Pulmonary Airway Malformation

TERMINOLOGY

- Heterogeneous group of cystic & noncystic lung lesions resulting from early airway maldevelopment
- CPAM term now recommended over CCAM, as lesions may not be cystic or adenomatoid

IMAGING

- Multicystic lung mass with variable amounts of air & fluid; no Ca^{2+} or rib abnormalities
- By imaging, categorized into large cyst, small cyst, & microcystic/solid subtypes; lesions often mixed
- Radiograph remains initial postnatal study
  - Prenatally detected lesion may be radiographically occult in asymptomatic patient due to recognized phenomenon of partial or complete in utero regression
- CTA for evaluation of residual lesion & surgical planning
  - Identification of systemic feeding artery of "hybrid lesion" [combined CPAM & bronchopulmonary sequestration (BPS)] critical

TOP DIFFERENTIAL DIAGNOSES

- BPS
- Congenital diaphragmatic hernia
- Bronchogenic cyst
- Pleuropulmonary blastoma
- Congenital lobar overinflation

CLINICAL ISSUES

- Overall survival > 95%
- ~ 25% with respiratory distress at birth
  - Depends on size of lesion, mediastinal shift, hydrops
  - ~ 13% require neonatal respiratory support: Be prepared if attending delivery
- All symptomatic CPAMs resected
- Asymptomatic lesions: Expectant vs. elective resection
  - Primary risk: Recurrent infections
  - Less common: Malignant degeneration

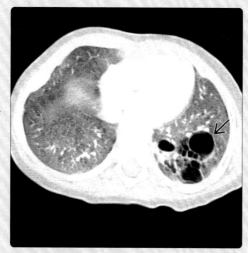
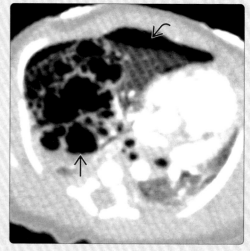

(Left) Axial chest CTA of a newborn (in lung windows) shows a multicystic lesion ➡ in the left lower lobe. The cysts are of varying size, typical of a congenital pulmonary airway malformation (CPAM). (Right) Axial CTA of a newborn shows a large right lower lobe, predominately macrocystic CPAM. Note the air-fluid level ➡ in one of the cysts as well as the accompanying pneumothorax ➡.

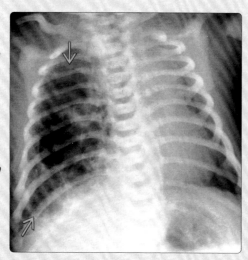
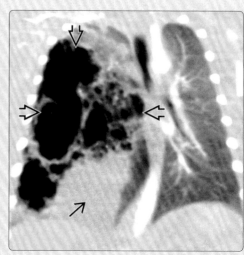

(Left) Frontal newborn chest radiograph shows a large multiseptated cystic lesion ➡ in the right lower lobe causing right to left mediastinal shift. (Right) Coronal CTA of the same patient shows that, in addition to the large multiseptated macrocystic lesion ➡, there are solid components in the right lower lobe ➡. This was found to be a mixed type 1 & 3 CPAM upon surgical resection.

Bronchopulmonary Sequestration

TERMINOLOGY

- Congenital focus of abnormal lung that does not connect to bronchial tree or pulmonary arteries
- Divided into intralobar (75%) & extralobar (25%) types
  - Intralobar shares pleural investment with normal lung & usually has pulmonary venous drainage
  - Extralobar has separate pleural investment from lung & usually has systemic venous drainage

IMAGING

- Lower lobe (left > right) opacity persisting over time
  - Mass may occur in mediastinum or in/below diaphragm
- Systemic arterial supply characteristic
  - Identification important for diagnosis, surgical planning
    - Postnatal CTA recommended for all congenital lung lesions (even with 3rd-trimester regression)
  - Arterial supply may be subdiaphragmatic in origin even if lesion supradiaphragmatic
    - Chest CTA must cover through celiac axis

PATHOLOGY

- Abnormal dysplastic lung tissue lacking normal/functional tracheobronchial connection
- Often occurs as "hybrid lesion" with congenital pulmonary airway malformation (CPAM)

CLINICAL ISSUES

- Intralobar typically presents as isolated anomaly in older children/adults with recurrent pneumonias
  - Incidental in 15%
- Extralobar typically detected in prenatal/neonatal period, often with additional congenital anomalies (65%)
  - May be asymptomatic postnatally
  - Rarely becomes infected
  - May cause neonatal respiratory distress from mass effect or adjacent pulmonary hypoplasia
  - May torse & infarct, causing chest/abdominal pain
- Symptomatic lesions resected; management of asymptomatic lesions controversial

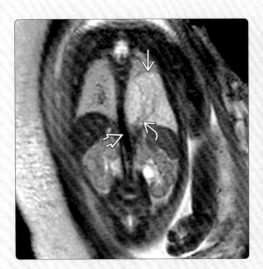

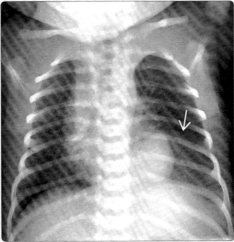

(Left) Coronal T2 SSFSE MR of a 31-week gestation fetus shows a large, homogeneously hyperintense left lower lobe mass ➡ displacing the left upper lobe & aorta ➡. Vascular flow voids ➡ are seen extending into the mass from the aorta. (Right) AP radiograph of the same patient 5 days after birth shows mild decreased size of the left lower lobe mass ➡.

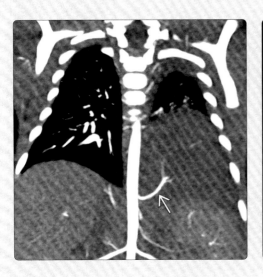

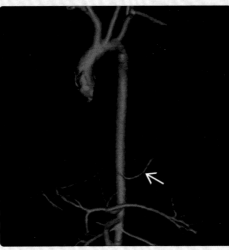

(Left) Coronal CT angiogram of the same patient 11 days later shows an arterial feeding vessel ➡ extending into the solid mass from the upper abdominal aorta, confirming systemic arterial supply in a bronchopulmonary sequestration (BPS). Upon resection, the mass contained components of both BPS & a congenital pulmonary airway malformation, consistent with a "hybrid lesion." (Right) 3D coronal oblique reconstruction from the same CT angiogram shows the feeding vessel ➡ relationship to other upper abdominal arterial origins.

Bronchogenic Cyst

TERMINOLOGY

- Congenital mass in family of foregut duplication cysts

IMAGING

- Mediastinal location (usually middle) > > lung (medial 1/3 of lower lobes) > neck, abdomen, heart, subcutaneous tissues
- Well-defined, round to ovoid, unilocular, thin-walled fluid-filled cyst with smooth margins
- Radiography: Often subtle, depending on size & location
  - Compression of adjacent bronchus may lead to hyperinflation or atelectasis
- CECT: Variable attenuation due to protein, hemorrhage, or (rarely) calcium; minimal enhancement of thin wall
- MR: Variable signal in cyst
  - MR provides more comprehensive evaluation of lesion to exclude other diagnoses & determine full extent
  - Lung parenchyma & airways better seen on CT
- UGI: Incidental extrinsic mass compressing/distorting contrast-filled esophagus

- US: Hypoechoic mass with posterior acoustic enhancement
  - Limited utility as cyst often surrounded by air-filled lung (impairing sound wave transmission)

TOP DIFFERENTIAL DIAGNOSES

- Round pneumonia
- Bronchopulmonary sequestration
- Congenital pulmonary airway malformation
- Lymphatic malformation
- Neuroblastoma/other malignancy

CLINICAL ISSUES

- Common presentations
  - In infants: Respiratory distress (airway compression)
  - In older children: Chest pain, dysphagia, vomiting, recurrent infections
  - May be asymptomatic in older children & adults
  - Cervical & subcutaneous lesions palpable
- Definitive treatment: Surgical resection

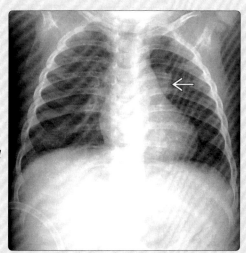

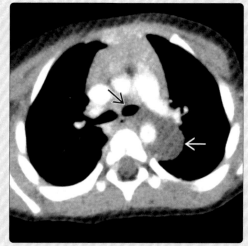

(Left) Chest radiograph of a 14-month-old boy reveals an ovoid left perihilar mass ➡. (Right) Axial CECT of the same patient shows a well-circumscribed, homogeneous, fluid-attenuation mass ➡ partially encasing the aorta. This bronchogenic cyst extends posteriorly from the margin of the left main bronchus to the left paraspinal region. There is mild mass effect on the left main bronchus ➡ without significant narrowing.

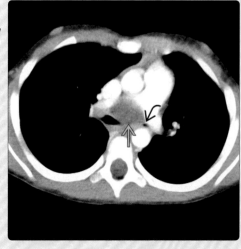

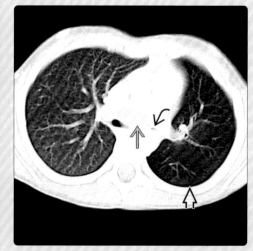

(Left) Axial CECT of a 5-year-old girl with recurrent left lower lobe pneumonia shows a 2-cm, well-circumscribed, fluid-attenuation mass ➡ in a subcarinal location. There is marked narrowing of the left main bronchus ➡. (Right) Axial lung window image from the same CECT shows diffuse hyperlucency of the left lung ➡, indicating postobstructive air-trapping due to extrinsic compression of the left main bronchus ➡ by the bronchogenic cyst ➡ (with the cyst being poorly visualized on this setting).

Congenital Lobar Overinflation

KEY FACTS

TERMINOLOGY

- Congenital abnormality of lower airways that results in progressive overexpansion of pulmonary lobe
- Synonyms: Congenital lobar emphysema, congenital lobar hyperinflation, infantile lobar emphysema

IMAGING

- Hyperlucent & hyperexpanded lobe in neonate
  - Lobar predilection: Left upper lobe > right middle lobe > right upper lobe > > lower lobes
  - Persistent hyperinflation in ipsilateral decubitus position
  - Mass effect on adjacent lung + mediastinal shift
- Diagnosis typically made by chest radiography
- CTA to confirm diagnosis/exclude other lesions, elucidate cause, define extent of disease

TOP DIFFERENTIAL DIAGNOSES

- Pneumothorax, congenital pulmonary airway malformation, bronchial atresia

PATHOLOGY

- Cause found in ~ 50% of cases
  - Wall abnormality, lumen obstruction, extrinsic compression

CLINICAL ISSUES

- Majority become symptomatic in neonatal period & infancy
  - 50% in first 4 weeks; 75% in first 6 months
- Presentations include: Respiratory distress in neonatal period, asymmetry of movement of chest with respiration, use of accessory muscles of respiration, breath sounds ↓ on affected side, hyperresonant hemithorax
  - Respiratory distress may be progressive & fatal
- Associated with cardiac anomalies (~ 15%), renal, GI, & MSK abnormalities
- Treatment: Bronchoscopy to exclude endobronchial lesion, surgical lobectomy

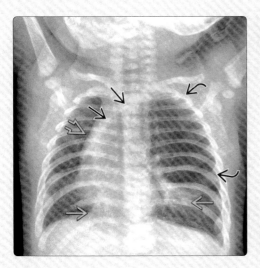
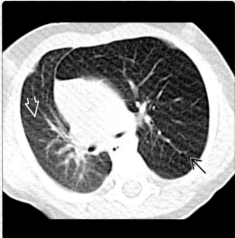

(Left) Frontal radiograph of an infant with chronic wheezing shows an abnormally lucent left upper lobe ➡ that is so hyperexpanded it herniates across the midline ➡. Note the mass effect causing mediastinal shift ➡ & lower lobe atelectasis ➡. (Right) Axial NECT from the same patient with congenital lobar overinflation (CLO) reveals smaller vessels in the affected hyperexpanded & hyperlucent left upper lobe ➡ with compressive atelectasis in the right lung ➡.

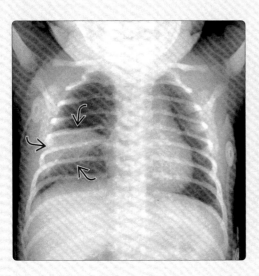
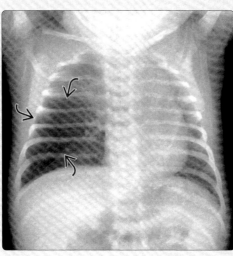

(Left) Chest radiograph obtained in the 1st few hours of life demonstrates segmental airspace opacification of the right middle lobe ➡. The opacity reflects retained fetal fluid filling alveoli in the affected segment. (Right) A follow-up radiograph in the same patient the next day shows that the same segment is now gas-filled, lucent, & hyperexpanded ➡. The retained fetal fluid has been resorbed with the findings now reflecting air-trapping in this case of CLO.

TERMINOLOGY

- Atresia: Congenital occlusion of lumen
- Fistula: Anomalous connection between 2 lumens

IMAGING

- 5 major anatomic variations of esophageal atresia-tracheoesophageal fistula (EA-TEF)
- Fistula level variable depending on type of EA-TEF
  - Most commonly above/near carina
- Atretic segments variable in length
  - Gap often long in EA without TEF
- Radiographs
  - Air-distended upper esophageal pouch
  - Enteric tube tip near thoracic inlet in pouch
  - EA with TEF: Gas in stomach & bowel
  - EA without TEF: Gasless stomach & bowel
- Limited indications for preoperative esophagram (except isolated TEF)
- Postoperative esophagram

  - Esophageal anastomotic leak, anastomotic stricture, recurrent/additional TEF, esophageal dysmotility, gastroesophageal reflux

TOP DIFFERENTIAL DIAGNOSES

- Tube malposition
- Laryngotracheal cleft
- Esophageal strictures of various etiologies

CLINICAL ISSUES

- Presentation: Excessive oral secretions, cyanosis, choking, coughing during feeding, recurrent pneumonia; nasogastric tube fails to reach stomach
  - 47-75% have associated anomalies
- Treatment: Bronchoscopy, esophagoscopy to visualize fistula(s) + extrapleural ligation of fistula + anastomosis of esophageal segments; may require staged surgeries
- Postsurgical survival: 75-95% (depends on associated cardiac anomalies, birth weight)

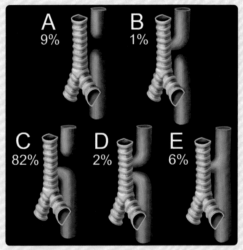
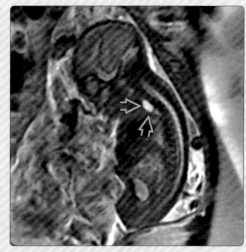

(Left) *Graphic shows the Gross classification of esophageal atresia with tracheoesophageal fistula (EA-TEF), including the isolated TEF without EA (H-type fistula, type E) & the isolated EA without TEF (type A).* (Right) *Sagittal T2 SSFSE MR of a 26-week gestation fetus imaged for polyhydramnios shows a collection of fluid in the region of the upper esophagus ➡ that is suggestive of an atretic esophageal pouch, which was confirmed during surgery in the newborn period.*

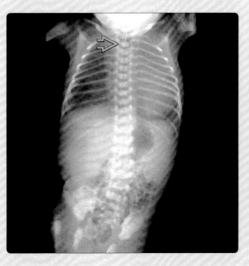
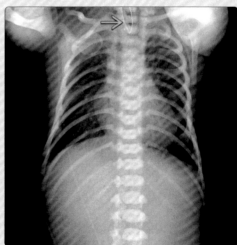

(Left) *AP radiograph of a premature newborn boy with a history of not handling secretions shows a nasogastric tube (NGT) tip ➡ overlying the thoracic inlet due to EA. The bowel gas confirms the presence of a distal TEF. The cardiomegaly suggests congenital heart disease.* (Right) *AP chest radiograph in a newborn shows an NGT coiled at the thoracic inlet ➡, suggesting EA. Note the lack of gas in the upper abdomen, which is typical of EA without a distal TEF.*

TERMINOLOGY

Definitions

- Esophageal atresia (EA): Congenital occlusion of upper esophagus
- Tracheoesophageal fistula (TEF): Single (less commonly multiple) anomalous congenital connection(s) from esophagus to trachea

IMAGING

Radiographic Findings

- Intermittently air-distended upper esophageal pouch
- Nasogastric tube (NGT) tip in esophageal pouch near thoracic inlet
- Gas in stomach & bowel: EA with TEF
- Gasless stomach & bowel: EA without TEF
- Displaced, bowed, narrowed trachea due to dilated esophageal pouch & tracheomalacia
- Signs of other congenital anomalies
  - Cardiomegaly, abnormal pulmonary vascularity, vertebral anomalies, dilated bowel

Fluoroscopic Findings

- Rarely needed for diagnosis of EA
  - Can inject air into NGT to confirm blind-ending pouch
- Contrast esophagram useful preoperatively for
  - H-type TEF without EA (clinical & radiographic diagnosis less clear in this type)
  - EA without TEF (often has long esophageal gap)
    - Often 2-stage repair if long gap
    - Preoperative measurement of gap
      - □ Surgical bougie into upper pouch ± contrast
      - □ Surgical bougie into lower pouch ± contrast via gastrostomy
      - □ Measure gap prior to 2nd surgery

Imaging Recommendations

- Best imaging tool
  - Radiographs ± air injection of NGT for EA
  - Esophagram for suspected isolated TEF or postoperative complication

DIFFERENTIAL DIAGNOSIS

Tube Malposition

- Traumatic pharyngeal perforation by NGT

Laryngotracheal Cleft

- High fistulous connection, variable length

Chronic Respiratory Issues (Mimicking H-Type TEF)

- Gastroesophageal reflux (GER) with aspiration, bronchial foreign body, cystic fibrosis, congenital lung lesion

Esophageal Strictures

- Caustic injury, eosinophilic esophagitis, prior foreign body, epidermolysis bullosa, mediastinal radiation

Extrinsic Esophageal Compression

- Vascular rings or mediastinal masses

PATHOLOGY

General Features

- 47-75% have additional anomalies
  - 10-20% have VACTERL (vertebral, anal, cardiac, tracheoesophageal, renal, limb anomalies) association

Staging, Grading, & Classification

- Most widely cited surgical classification (Gross)
  - Type A: EA with no TEF (7-9%)
  - Type B: EA with proximal TEF (1%)
  - Type C: EA with distal TEF (82-86%)
  - Type D: EA with proximal & distal TEF (2%)
  - Type E: Isolated (H-type) TEF (no EA) (4-6%)

CLINICAL ISSUES

Presentation

- Most common signs/symptoms
  - Excessive oral secretions, cyanosis, choking, coughing during 1st attempts at feeding
- Other signs/symptoms
  - NGT fails to reach stomach
  - Recurrent pneumonia, dysphagia (H-type TEF)

Natural History & Prognosis

- Postoperative survival: 75-95% (depends on associated cardiac anomalies, birth weight)

Treatment

- Bronchoscopy, esophagoscopy to visualize fistula(s) + extrapleural ligation of fistula + anastomosis of esophageal segments
  - If EA without TEF, esophageal ends often far apart
    - 1st surgery: Place gastrostomy tube
    - 2nd surgery: Connect esophagus after growth
    - Ultralong gap requires conduit
      - □ Colonic interposition vs. gastric pull-up/tube
    - Foker procedure: Actively stretches esophagus over time → primary anastomosis
- Early postsurgical complications
  - Anastomotic leak (up to 15%; most small leaks resolve spontaneously)
  - Additional TEF not seen initially
- Longer term postsurgical issues
  - Anastomotic stricture (18-50%)
    - ↑ with ↑ EA gap length, anastomotic tension, GER
    - Treated with repeated balloon or bougie dilations
  - Recurrent TEF (up to 10% of cases)
  - Esophageal dysmotility (nearly 100%)
  - GER; esophagitis (51%), Barrett esophagus (6%)
    - Surgical treatment (Nissen) if medical therapy fails
  - Respiratory infections
  - Tracheomalacia (10-20%)

SELECTED REFERENCES

1. Teague WJ et al: Surgical management of oesophageal atresia. Paediatr Respir Rev. 19:10-5, 2016
2. Smith N: Oesophageal atresia and tracheo-oesophageal fistula. Early Hum Dev. 90(12):947-50, 2014
3. Zani A et al: International survey on the management of esophageal atresia. Eur J Pediatr Surg. 24(1):3-8, 2014

Congenital Diaphragmatic Hernia

TERMINOLOGY

- Herniation of abdominal contents into chest via congenital defect in diaphragm, most commonly posterior (Bochdalek)
- Side of congenital diaphragmatic hernia (CDH): Left 85%, right 13%, bilateral 2%

IMAGING

- Best clue: Bubbly, round, or tubular, relatively uniform air-filled lucencies in hemithorax displacing mediastinum
- Intrathoracic herniated contents may include stomach, small & large bowel, liver, gallbladder, spleen
  - Results in paucity of bowel gas in abdomen
- Support devices distorted in relatively specific ways
  - Nasogastric tube due to stomach herniation
  - Umbilical venous catheter due to liver herniation
- Postnatal chest imaging of CDH beyond radiography typically unnecessary

CLINICAL ISSUES

- Presentation: Most detected prenatally or at birth; delayed presentation uncommon
  - Respiratory distress at birth in majority
  - Presence of intrathoracic bowel sounds
  - Absence of ipsilateral breath sounds
  - Scaphoid abdomen
- Treatment: Immediate initiation of supportive postnatal care until patient can tolerate surgical repair (primary vs. patch)
- Prognosis most related to severity of pulmonary hypoplasia, pulmonary arterial hypertension, congenital heart disease, & other anomalies
  - Survival ↑ if diagnosis known prenatally & patient delivers at high-volume center
  - Long-term morbidity: Impaired lung function + recurrent respiratory infections, neurocognitive & language delays, failure to thrive, chest wall deformities, scoliosis

(Left) Graphic shows a large posterior defect in the left hemidiaphragm with partial herniation of the stomach & bowel into the left hemithorax. There is rightward mediastinal shift with compression & hypoplasia of both the ipsilateral & contralateral lungs. (Right) Coronal SSFSE T2 MR of a 32-week gestation fetus shows herniated bowel loops ➡ filling the left hemithorax. The hypoplastic right lung ➡ overlies the aorta ➡ & herniated stomach ➡, which are shifted into the right hemithorax.

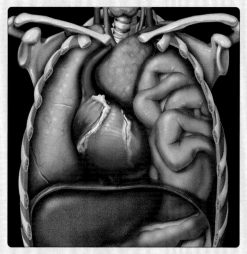 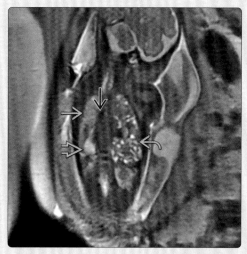

(Left) Sagittal T1 MR in the same fetus shows a herniated left hepatic lobe ➡ separated from the remaining intraabdominal right hepatic lobe ➡ by residual anterior diaphragm ➡. Note the herniated stomach ➡ & meconium-containing bowel ➡. (Right) AP chest radiograph of the same patient after delivery shows gas-filled bowel ➡ in the left hemithorax. The herniated stomach has an organoaxial rotation ➡ & overlies the herniated left hepatic lobe. Note the arterial ➡ & venous ➡ ECMO cannulae.

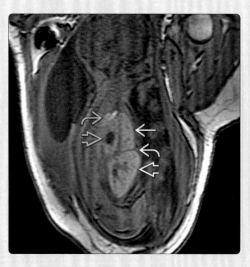 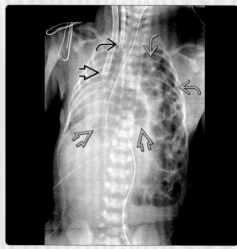

TERMINOLOGY

Definitions

- Herniation of abdominal contents into chest via developmental defect in diaphragm
  - Bochdalek hernia (70-95%): Posterior
  - Morgagni hernia (2-28%): Anterior
  - Central tendon hernia (2-7%)

IMAGING

General Features

- Best diagnostic clue
  - Bubbly, round, & tubular lucencies in neonatal hemithorax with contralateral mediastinal shift
- Location: Left 85%, right 13%, bilateral 2%
- Morphology: Degrees of diaphragmatic deficiency & herniated contents variable; may contain stomach, small & large bowel, liver, gallbladder, spleen

Radiographic Findings

- Depend on hernia contents & amount of air in bowel
  - Uniform soft tissue density of herniated solid organs
  - Herniated bowel may appear solid prior to progression of swallowed air
    - Upon air entering bowel, loops appear relatively uniform in size with round & tubular morphologies
      - Degree of gaseous distention changes day to day
    - Herniated gas-filled stomach larger than bowel & often abnormally rotated
- Mediastinal shift away from hernia
- Low lung volumes from hypoplasia
  - Ipsilateral lung more severe than contralateral
- Abnormal positions of support lines & tubes
- ↓ intraabdominal bowel gas
- Postoperative appearance
  - Resolution of herniated contents
  - Pleural fluid in 28%, eventually resolves
  - Ex vacuo negative pressure pneumothorax: Hypoplastic lung does not fill space initially but gradually expands
  - Repaired hemidiaphragm may be angular or sloped

Imaging Recommendations

- Best imaging tool
  - Prenatal US & MR: Diagnostic & prognostic information
  - Postnatal radiograph: Lung expansion, support devices

DIFFERENTIAL DIAGNOSIS

Congenital Pulmonary Airway Malformation

- Macrocystic type appears as multicystic, air-containing mass
  - Cysts typically not uniform in size
  - After gas replaces fluid in cysts (in 1st few days after birth), congenital pulmonary airway malformation appearance typically static

Diaphragmatic Eventration

- Focal muscle aplasia of diaphragm without free protrusion of bowel into thorax; contents contained by sac of peritoneum, diaphragm tendon, & parietal pleura

Congenital Lobar Overinflation

- Progressive overdistention of single lobe (rarely lower)

Bronchopulmonary Sequestration

- Solid mass near diaphragm with systemic arterial supply

PATHOLOGY

General Features

- Etiology
  - Underlying cause of defective diaphragm development unknown in ~ 70-80%
    - Various chromosomal anomalies (2-35%): Trisomy 18 most common (2-5%); Down syndrome (trisomy 21) most likely to have Morgagni type
    - Known specific genetic mutations (< 10%)
- Associated abnormalities
  - Isolated in ~ 50%; cardiac malformations in 20-40%

CLINICAL ISSUES

Presentation

- Most common signs/symptoms
  - Diagnosis known prenatally in 60-80%
  - Respiratory distress at birth
- Other signs/symptoms
  - Presence of intrathoracic bowel sounds
  - Absence of ipsilateral breath sounds
  - Scaphoid abdomen
  - < 3% present after 30 days (100% survival)
    - Gastrointestinal symptoms more likely

Natural History & Prognosis

- Prognosis related to severity of pulmonary hypoplasia, pulmonary hypertension, & other anomalies
- Mortality rates variable: 10-68%
  - ↑ survival reported at high-volume centers
- Long-term morbidity: Impaired lung function + recurrent respiratory infections, neurocognitive & language delays, failure to thrive, chest wall deformities, scoliosis

Treatment

- Varying degrees of supportive care required until definitive surgery able to be tolerated
  - Ventilation/oxygenation: Immediate intubation ± ECMO
  - Pulmonary hypertension: Inhaled nitric oxide or IV sildenafil
- Surgery: Primary closure of small defects vs. patch repair for larger; timing debated
  - Complications include chylothorax, abdominal compartment syndrome, recurrent hernia, malrotation
- Fetal tracheal occlusion therapy: Temporary balloon occlusion of trachea in utero stimulates lung growth
  - Still under study at limited centers

SELECTED REFERENCES

1. Puligandla PS et al: Management of congenital diaphragmatic hernia: a systematic review from the APSA outcomes and evidence based practice committee. J Pediatr Surg. 50(11):1958-70, 2015
2. Danzer E et al: Controversies in the management of severe congenital diaphragmatic hernia. Semin Fetal Neonatal Med. 19(6):376-84, 2014
3. Harting MT et al: The congenital diaphragmatic hernia study group registry update. Semin Fetal Neonatal Med. 19(6):370-5, 2014
4. Leeuwen L et al: Congenital diaphragmatic hernia. J Paediatr Child Health. 50(9):667-73, 2014
5. Slavotinek AM: The genetics of common disorders - congenital diaphragmatic hernia. Eur J Med Genet. 57(8):418-23, 2014

Surfactant Deficiency Disease

TERMINOLOGY

- Surfactant deficiency disease (SDD) favored term
  - a.k.a. respiratory distress syndrome & hyaline membrane disease (archaic)
- Common lung disease occurring in premature infants due to lack of surfactant
- Microatelectasis & abnormal pulmonary compliance are hallmarks of disease

IMAGING

- Premature infants < 32-week gestation at risk
- Initial findings are low lung volumes & diffuse granular opacities
- Signs of tension (lung collapse, mediastinal shift) less likely if pneumothorax develops (due to ↓ lung compliance)
- High incidence of patent ductus arteriosus, leading to pulmonary edema ("whiteout" of lungs with cardiomegaly)
- Bronchopulmonary dysplasia (BPD) eventually occurs in 17-55% of premature infants

PATHOLOGY

- Surfactant normally coats alveoli & ↓ surface tension, allowing alveoli to stay open
  - Prematurity-related SDD: Immature type II pneumocytes cannot produce sufficient surfactant
  - Secondary SDD: Surfactant deactivation from meconium aspiration or infection
  - Primary SDD: Dysfunctional surfactant due to abnormalities of 1 of several gene products

CLINICAL ISSUES

- Respiratory distress, usually with history of prematurity
- Acute complications: Alveolar rupture with barotrauma (pneumothorax, pneumomediastinum, PIE)
- Chronic complications: BPD, ↑ incidence of sudden death
- Treatment
  - Prenatal prevention (delay delivery, maternal steroids)
  - Surfactant administration
  - Mechanical ventilation + positive end-expiratory pressure

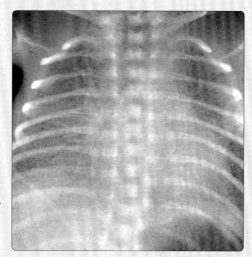
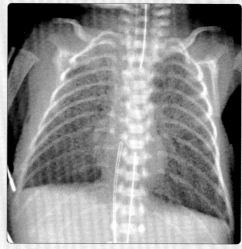

(Left) AP radiograph of the chest in a premature patient with surfactant deficiency disease (SDD) shows pulmonary hypoventilation & granular densities bilaterally. (Right) AP radiograph of the chest in a premature neonate shows diffuse granular opacities with marked hyperinflation of the lungs. Although classically lung volumes are decreased in patients with SDD, artificial ventilation can make them hyperinflated, especially after surfactant administration.

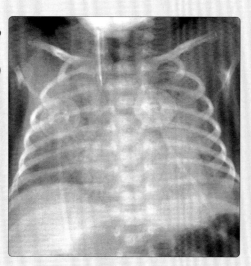
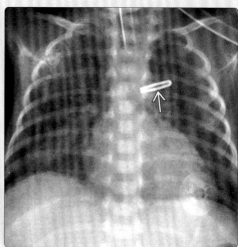

(Left) AP radiograph of the chest in a 1 week old with SDD shows diffuse opacification of the lungs. This neonate's patent ductus arteriosus (PDA) had recently reversed direction due to decreasing pulmonary vascular resistance & was now causing pulmonary edema. (Right) AP radiograph of the chest in the same patient shows increased aeration of the lungs after PDA ligation (with a surgical clip ➡ now in place).

Surfactant Deficiency Disease

TERMINOLOGY

Synonyms
- Surfactant deficiency disease (SDD) = lung disease of prematurity, respiratory distress syndrome, hyaline membrane disease (archaic)

Definitions
- Prematurity-related SDD (most common usage)
  - Surfactant deficiency in premature newborns
  - Lungs begin producing surfactant at ~ 24-week gestational age (GA); adequate amounts are usually present by 36-week GA
  - Lack of sufficient surfactant causes diffuse microatelectasis & abnormal pulmonary compliance
- Secondary SDD (less common usage)
  - Meconium aspiration or pneumonia can cause surfactant deactivation
  - Results are similar to those seen in prematurity but are usually heterogeneous & superimposed on other findings
- Primary SDD (least common usage)
  - Abnormal gene products adversely affect composition &/or function of surfactant
    - Surfactant protein-B, surfactant protein-C, ABCA3, & TTF-1 deficiencies
  - Often termed "surfactant dysfunction disorders"

IMAGING

Radiographic Findings
- Initial features
  - Low lung volumes secondary to microcollapse of innumerable alveoli
  - Diffuse granular opacities represent collapsed alveoli interspersed with open alveoli (microatelectasis)
  - Air bronchograms demonstrate patent bronchi in abnormal lungs
  - Pleural effusions very uncommon
  - Potential acute complications include pulmonary interstitial emphysema (PIE), pneumomediastinum, pneumothorax, pneumonia, pulmonary hemorrhage
- Features after surfactant administration
  - Clearing of granular opacities & ↑ lung volumes
  - May have asymmetric or partial response
- Findings after several days
  - Intubation & ventilatory support change appearance
  - High incidence of patent ductus arteriosus (PDA), which may cause pulmonary edema ("whiteout" of lungs with cardiomegaly) upon ↓ of pulmonary vascular resistance
- Bronchopulmonary dysplasia (BPD) develops in 17-55% of premature infants
  - Chronic lung disease characterized by coarse interstitial opacities with focal areas of atelectasis & hyperinflation vs. diffuse hyperinflation

DIFFERENTIAL DIAGNOSIS

Congenital Heart Disease
- Echocardiography gold standard for diagnosis
- PDA more common with prematurity

Group B Streptococcal Pneumonia
- Very common in neonates, especially premature
- Pleural effusion common (67%): Only imaging finding that helps differentiate from SDD

Meconium Aspiration Syndrome
- Term infants with meconium staining at delivery
- Rope-like densities radiating from hila
- Usually high lung volumes

PATHOLOGY

General Features
- Surfactant normally coats alveoli & ↓ surface tension, allowing alveoli to stay open & improving lung compliance
- Immature type II pneumocytes cannot produce surfactant → alveolar atelectasis

CLINICAL ISSUES

Presentation
- Most common signs/symptoms
  - Respiratory distress with history of prematurity

Demographics
- 50% of premature infants will have SDD
  - Infants < 27-week GA have ↑ sequelae

Natural History & Prognosis
- Acute complications & associations
  - Alveolar rupture with pneumothorax, pneumomediastinum, PIE
  - Sepsis & pulmonary infections
  - PDA with shunting & wide pulse pressures
  - Pulmonary hemorrhage
- Chronic complications
  - BPD defined as ≥ 28-days oxygen (O_2) dependence in premature infant
    - O_2 challenge at 36-week postmenstrual age
  - Retinopathy of prematurity
  - ↑ incidence of sudden death
  - Neurologic impairment in 10-70% (depending on GA)

Treatment
- Prenatal prevention by treatment of mother
  - Efforts to delay delivery, allowing fetus to mature
  - Maternal steroid administration: Steroids will cross placenta & ↑ surfactant production
- Surfactant administration to neonate
  - Injected into trachea via endotracheal tube or catheter
  - May be given prophylactically or after symptoms develop
  - Improves oxygenation & ventilator settings; ↓ rates of barotrauma, intracranial hemorrhage, BPD, & death
  - ↑ risk of PDA & pulmonary hemorrhage
- Mechanical ventilation + positive end-expiratory pressure
- High-frequency oscillatory ventilation

SELECTED REFERENCES

1. Sardesai S et al: Evolution of surfactant therapy for respiratory distress syndrome: past, present, and future. Pediatr Res. 81(1-2):240-248, 2017
2. Liu J: Lung ultrasonography for the diagnosis of neonatal lung disease. J Matern Fetal Neonatal Med. 27(8):856-61, 2014

Neonatal Pneumonia

TERMINOLOGY

- Pneumonia in first 28 days of life
- Early onset: Typically presents within 48 hours
- Late onset: Presents in 2nd-4th weeks of life

IMAGING

- Radiographs
  - Low lung volumes & granular opacities similar to surfactant deficiency (but pleural effusion in up to 67%)
  - Confluent > patchy alveolar or reticular opacities; may be perihilar
  - Complications: Pneumothorax, pneumomediastinum, pneumatocele, pulmonary interstitial emphysema
- Ultrasound may be used in some centers

PATHOLOGY

- Bacterial pathogens most common in early & late onset

- Most common early-onset causes: Group B *Streptococcus* (GBS) (developed countries), *Escherichia coli* (developing countries)
- Transmission
  - Early onset: Transplacental, aspiration of infected amniotic fluid, maternal systemic infection
  - Late onset: Contaminated/colonized equipment or individuals

CLINICAL ISSUES

- Typical presentations: Respiratory distress, sepsis, abnormal WBC with > 20% bands, ↑ CRP, ↑ ESR
- Prevention: Universal screening at 35-37 weeks gestation for maternal GBS colonization
  - Intrapartum antibiotic prophylaxis with penicillin
- Treatment of neonate
  - Early onset: Empiric ampicillin + gentamicin
  - Late onset: Empiric vancomycin + aminoglycoside
  - Consider adding acyclovir until HSV status known

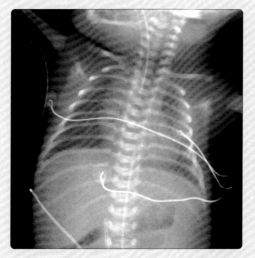
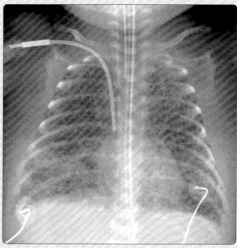

(Left) AP radiograph of the chest in a neonate with group B streptococcal pneumonia shows diffuse, bilateral hazy opacities with low lung volumes. This appearance is very similar to patients with surfactant deficiency disease. (Right) AP radiograph of the chest in a patient with neonatal pneumonia shows increased lung volumes with diffuse nodular pulmonary opacities. Anasarca is also noted.

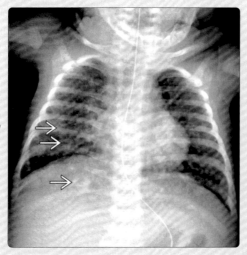
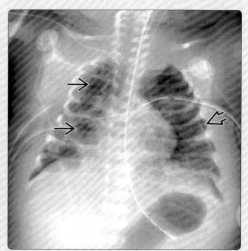

(Left) AP radiograph in a neonate with tuberculosis shows multiple cavitating nodules in the right lung ➡. (Right) AP radiograph in a patient with neonatal pneumonia shows a left pneumothorax ➡ & multiple bilateral pneumatoceles ➡, complications that can be seen with neonatal pneumonia.

Meconium Aspiration Syndrome

KEY FACTS

TERMINOLOGY

- Meconium aspiration syndrome (MAS): Respiratory distress after aspiration of meconium-stained amniotic fluid
  - Causes ↓ lung compliance & hypoxia ± pulmonary hypertension & air leak syndrome

IMAGING

- Coarse, thick, rope-like linear & nodular perihilar opacities
- Patchy, hazy opacities of atelectasis & pneumonitis
- Generalized hyperinflation
- ± pleural effusion
- ± air leak: Pneumomediastinum, pneumothorax, pulmonary interstitial emphysema

TOP DIFFERENTIAL DIAGNOSES

- Congenital heart disease, neonatal pneumonia, transient tachypnea of newborn, surfactant deficiency disease, pulmonary hypoplasia

PATHOLOGY

- Aspirated meconium causes injury by several mechanisms
  - Mechanical obstruction of small airways → air-trapping, air-leak complications
  - Chemical pneumonitis of airways & parenchyma
  - Surfactant inactivation → diffuse atelectasis
  - Pulmonary vasoconstriction → persistent pulmonary hypertension

CLINICAL ISSUES

- Disease of term & postterm neonates
- Meconium staining of amniotic fluid occurs in infants with in utero or intrapartum hypoxia or stress
  - 4-12% with meconium staining develop MAS
- Meconium-stained & distressed infant suctioned immediately ± intubation
- ECMO for severe pulmonary hypertension
- Mortality 7-12%; chronic lung disease 2.5%

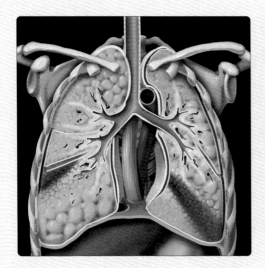

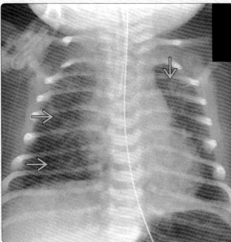

(Left) Graphic demonstrates asymmetric areas of hyperinflation & atelectasis as well as rope-like perihilar densities of aspirated meconium & inflamed airways. (Right) AP chest radiograph in a 41-week gestation newborn with meconium staining of amniotic fluid & respiratory distress shows coarse, reticular, rope-like perihilar opacities ➡, typical of meconium aspiration. There are patchy asymmetric regions of increased hazy lung opacity bilaterally.

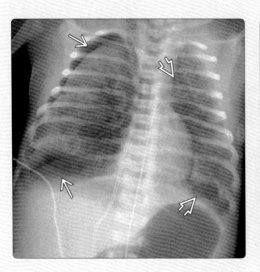

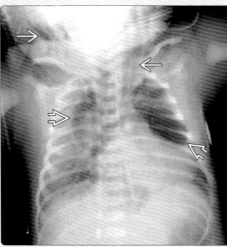

(Left) AP radiograph of the chest in a full-term infant with meconium aspiration demonstrates right ➡ greater than left ➡ pneumothoraces with bilateral lung hyperinflation & diffuse opacification. Pneumothorax is a common complication in these patients. (Right) AP radiograph of a full-term patient with witnessed meconium aspiration shows a large pneumomediastinum ➡. Note the linear lucencies ➡ of subcutaneous emphysema tracking into the neck bilaterally.

Transient Tachypnea of Newborn

TERMINOLOGY

- Caused by delayed evacuation of fetal lung fluid that creates engorgement of pulmonary lymphatics & capillaries
  - Usually occurs after cesarean section due to lack of normal thoracic compression during vaginal delivery
- Synonyms
  - Wet lung disease
  - Retained fetal fluid

IMAGING

- Normal to ↑ lung volumes
- No or minimal cardiomegaly
- Findings similar to pulmonary edema
  - Diffuse, bilateral, & often symmetric ↑ lung markings
  - ± pleural effusion
- Radiographic resolution within 24-48 hours
- Diagnosis of exclusion
  - Not associated with any chronic condition or lung disease
  - Imaging occasionally necessary to exclude other causes

- — Echocardiography for congenital heart disease

CLINICAL ISSUES

- Mild to moderate respiratory distress, usually in term infant
  - Tachypnea occurs early after birth
  - Expiratory grunting, chest retractions, nasal flaring
  - Occasional cyanosis that resolves with minimal oxygen
- Infants usually improve rapidly & are normal on follow-up
  - Occasionally need oxygen for several hours
  - Some fluid restriction may be helpful
  - Typically does not require intubation
  - Respiratory symptoms usually disappear by 3 days
- Diagnosis of exclusion
  - No chorioamnionitis, maternal infection, sepsis
  - No meconium staining of amniotic fluid
  - No premature rupture of membranes

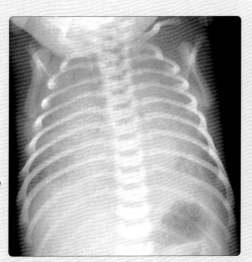
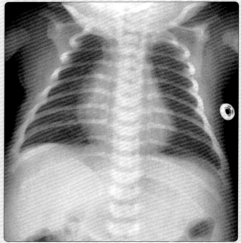

(Left) AP radiograph of the chest in a full-term infant with tachypnea demonstrates diffuse bilateral hazy opacities. The findings & symptoms resolved, & the diagnosis of transient tachypnea of the newborn (TTN) was made. (Right) AP radiograph of the chest in the same patient 48 hours later shows interval clearing of the previously seen diffuse opacification of the lungs. TTN is a diagnosis of exclusion & cannot be confidently diagnosed radiographically unless the findings resolve.

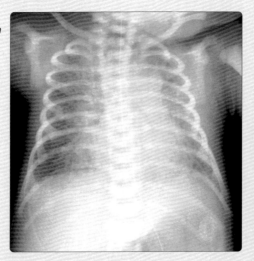
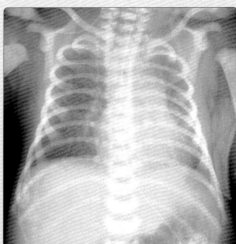

(Left) AP radiograph of the chest in a full-term infant with tachypnea shows diffuse streaky & nodular opacities throughout the lungs. (Right) AP radiograph of the chest in the same patient 48 hours later shows resolution of the previously seen diffuse nodular opacities, consistent with TTN.

Pulmonary Interstitial Emphysema

TERMINOLOGY

- Pulmonary interstitial emphysema (PIE): Air within pulmonary interstitium & lymphatics
- Usually secondary to barotrauma of positive-pressure mechanical ventilation in setting of prematurity, low birth weight, & surfactant deficiency disease (SDD)
  - Not always on mechanical ventilation

IMAGING

- Best clue: New bubbly cystic or linear lucencies within lung of intubated premature infant
- Can be limited to 1 lobe vs. bilateral & symmetric
- Small interstitial lucencies > > large focal/multifocal cysts
- Precursor to pneumothorax or pneumomediastinum
- PIE may rarely endure to form large air-filled cystic mass: "Persistent PIE"
  - CT shows pulmonary vessels as linear (dash) or round (dot) densities within gas collections

TOP DIFFERENTIAL DIAGNOSES

- Surfactant deficiency disease
- Air bronchograms in diffuse lung disease
- Chronic lung disease of prematurity

CLINICAL ISSUES

- 2-3% of neonatal ICU patients
- 20-30% of premature neonates with SDD
- Often asymptomatic, detected on neonatal ICU radiographs
- Usually occurs during first 10 days of life
- Usually transient with adequate therapy
- Primary therapy: ↓ mean airway pressure by switching from conventional positive-pressure to high-frequency ventilation

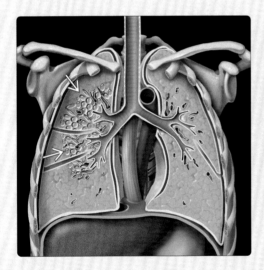

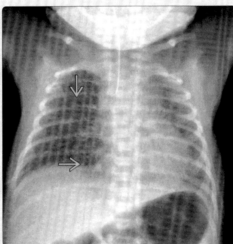

(Left) Coronal graphic depicts round & linear foci of gas ➔ in the right lung parenchyma secondary to air escaping into the pulmonary interstitium. (Right) AP chest radiograph in an intubated, 2-day old former 31-week premature infant with surfactant deficiency disease shows typical diffuse granular pulmonary opacities. There are mild scattered linear & bubbly lucencies of pulmonary interstitial emphysema (PIE) ➔ in the right lung.

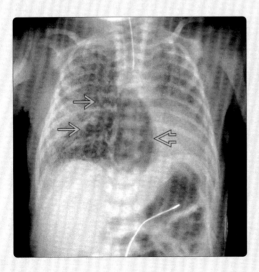

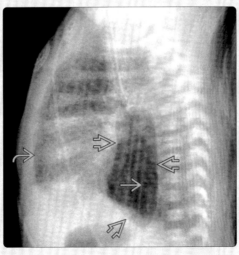

(Left) AP chest radiograph 24 hours later in the same patient shows more extensive bubbly & linear lucencies throughout the right lung ➔, typical of PIE. A large inferomedial gas collection has also developed ➔, shifting the heart leftward. (Right) Cross-table lateral radiograph of the same patient shows localized infraazygous posterior pneumomediastinum ➔. Lucencies from the right lung PIE ➔ are superimposed on the collection. Note that there is no free gas in the nondependent chest ➔ to suggest a pneumothorax.

Neonatal Pneumothorax

IMAGING

- Neonatal chest radiographs typically obtained supine
- Clues to pneumothorax diagnosis on supine study
  - Large, hyperlucent hemithorax
  - Lucency cloaking diaphragm, mediastinum, &/or lung
  - Medial stripe sign: Lucency along mediastinum
  - Deep sulcus sign: Well-defined costophrenic sulcus
  - Gas-filled pleural sac herniated across midline
  - Visualization of anterior junction line if bilateral
- Cross-table lateral view shows air anterior to lung
- Diseased lung may not collapse despite tension (due to decreased lung compliance)
- Ultrasound: Absence of lung sliding & comet-tail artifact

TOP DIFFERENTIAL DIAGNOSES

- Pneumomediastinum, artifact, air-filled mass, recent surgical evacuation of hemithorax

PATHOLOGY

- Overdistention & rupture of alveoli
  - Directly into pleural cavity → pneumothorax
  - Into lung interstitium 1st → interstitial emphysema
- Risk factors: Low birth weight, premature or postmature gestation, male gender, surfactant deficiency disease, meconium aspiration, pulmonary hypoplasia, resuscitation at birth, mechanical ventilation, macrosomia

CLINICAL ISSUES

- Incidence: 1% of term births, 6-7% of preterm births
- Common signs/symptoms: Ipsilateral ↓ breath sounds, respiratory distress, cyanosis, retractions, grunting, nasal flaring, chest asymmetry (↑ on affected side), hypercapnia, hypoxemia; tension pneumothorax → hypotension, shock
- Treatment
  - Expectant/supportive management in asymptomatic patients or those with mild disease
  - Needle aspiration or chest tube drainage if symptomatic

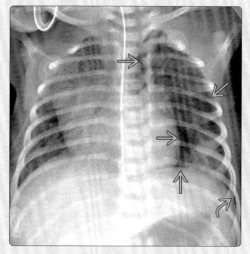
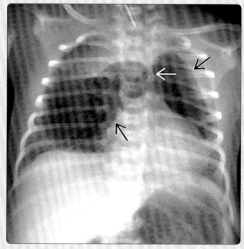

(Left) Supine AP chest radiograph of a 2-day-old neonate born at 34 weeks shows lucency "cloaking" the left hemithorax ⊟ with a well-defined left costophrenic angle ⊿ as compared to the right. This appearance was due to a moderate left pneumothorax that caused mediastinal shift to the right. (Right) Supine AP chest radiograph of a 2-day-old preterm neonate with surfactant deficiency disease shows lucencies ⊟ outlining the anterior junction line ➡, consistent with bilateral pneumothoraces.

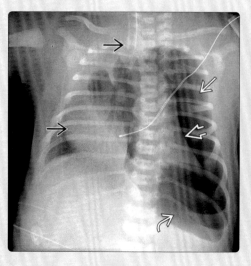
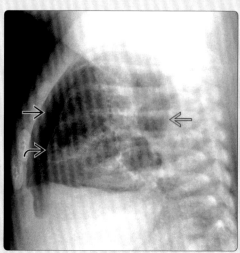

(Left) Supine AP chest radiograph of a 2-day-old term neonate in respiratory distress shows a lucent left hemithorax ➡, collapse of the left lung ➡, depression of the diaphragm ➡, & rightward mediastinal shift ⊡, consistent with a left tension pneumothorax. (Right) Cross-table lateral view of the chest in a 1-day-old full-term girl shows air ➡ anterior to the lung ⊿, consistent with a pneumothorax. Cystic lucencies ⊟ relate to her known congenital pulmonary airway malformation.

Chylothorax

TERMINOLOGY

- Lymphatic fluid in pleural space secondary to congenital or acquired conditions, including obstruction, congenital anomaly, increased vessel pressures, impaired drainage, infection, malignancy, or trauma to thoracic duct

IMAGING

- US, CT, or MR may be done to discover underlying cause of chylothorax & evaluate treatment options
  - Persistent pleural effusion following cardiac surgery
  - Congenital chylothorax from Turner or Noonan syndrome
  - Various associated lymphatic disorders, including conducting channel anomalies, generalized lymphatic anomaly, Gorham-Stout disease, discrete cystic lymphatic malformations, & pulmonary lymphangiectasia
- Lymphangiogram (conventional, nuclear, or MR): Used to investigate suspected central conducting channel anomalies

- Disorders (including atresia, obstruction, disruption, or dysmotility) may show abrupt halt to visualization of normal lymphatic pathways, delayed transit, abnormal accumulations, &/or collaterals

CLINICAL ISSUES

- Symptoms may include tachypnea & dyspnea, generalized edema, chylous ascites, immunosuppression, protein-losing enteropathy (if gut involved)
- Treatment options include: Fat-restricted diet, rapamycin/sirolimus, thoracentesis or drainage procedure, thoracic duct ligation or embolization, microsurgical thoracic duct repair, pleurodesis
  - Thoracic duct injury may resolve spontaneously in 50%
  - Interventions may be indicated with chyle leak > 1 L/day for 5 days or persistent leak for > 2 weeks
  - Treat underlying cause of chylothorax if possible
- Poorer prognosis with syndromes, multiple sites of chylous fluid accumulations, prematurity

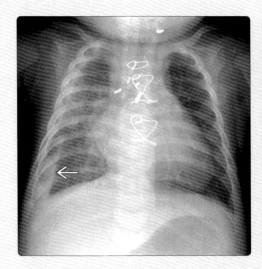

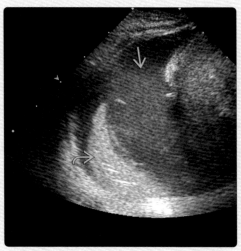

(Left) AP radiograph in a 4-month-old infant status post surgery for congenital heart disease shows a moderate right chylothorax ➡ from a thoracic duct injury. It is not possible to assess the complexity of fluid on radiography. (Right) Transverse US of the right chest in the same 4-month-old patient status post heart surgery & thoracic duct injury shows a large, mildly echogenic pleural effusion ➡. Notice the compressed echogenic right lung ➡ surrounded by the effusion.

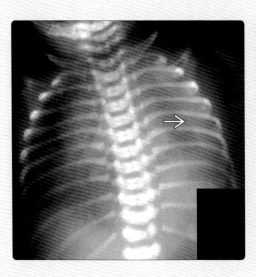

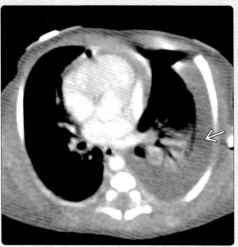

(Left) AP radiograph shows a large congenital left chylous effusion ➡ in a patient with Turner syndrome. (Right) Axial CECT shows a large left pleural effusion ➡ in a patient with Turner syndrome from a congenital chylothorax. Congenital chylothorax is more commonly seen on the left than on the right.

Bronchopulmonary Dysplasia

TERMINOLOGY

- Current definition of bronchopulmonary dysplasia (BPD)
  - Chronic lung disease of premature infants born at < 32-week gestation
  - O_2 dependency for at least 28 days
  - Failure of O_2 challenge at 36-week postmenstrual age
  - Chest radiograph abnormalities no longer required
- Old BPD
  - Larger, later preterm infants with prolonged mechanical ventilation & O_2 therapy
- New BPD
  - More diffuse but overall milder disease of earlier, smaller preterm infants

IMAGING

- Classic old BPD appearance
  - Heterogeneous, hyperinflated lung parenchyma
  - Patchy, small round lucencies separated by coarse, reticular, & band-like opacities

- New BPD
  - Lung appearance may be nearly normal early on with progressive diffuse hazy opacification
  - Severe surfactant deficiency disease patients may follow old imaging patterns
- Similar chronic chest CT findings of old & new BPD
  - Peripheral abnormalities may predominate
  - Cystic/emphysematous change
  - Subpleural cysts & triangular opacities
  - Linear, reticular opacities + parenchymal bands
  - Foci of air-trapping on expiratory images

PATHOLOGY

- Strongest predictors: Prematurity & low birth weight

CLINICAL ISSUES

- Most common chronic pulmonary disease of infancy
- Potentially lifelong complications

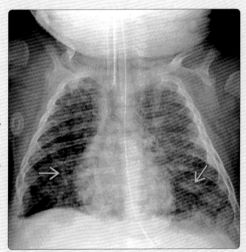
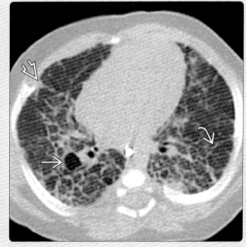

(Left) AP radiograph in a 4-month-old, former 24-week gestation premature infant with bronchopulmonary dysplasia (BPD) shows mild bilateral hyperexpansion with generally coarsened lung markings ➡. There are patchy foci of hazy parenchymal opacity intermixed with foci of hyperlucency due to air-trapping. (Right) Axial NECT in the same patient shows coarse reticular markings with parenchymal bands ➡, triangular subpleural opacities ➡, & scattered cysts ➡.

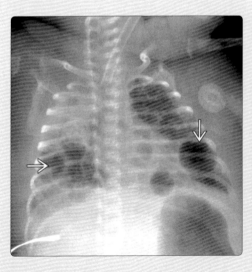
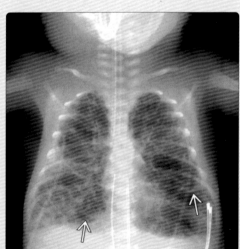

(Left) AP radiograph of the chest in a neonate with chronic lung disease shows development of bilateral pneumatoceles ➡ superimposed on regions of hyperinflation & atelectasis. The background parenchymal markings are coarsened. (Right) AP chest radiograph in a patient with BPD shows marked hyperinflation with coarse interstitial markings ➡ & cystic changes bilaterally.

TERMINOLOGY

Abbreviations

- Bronchopulmonary dysplasia (BPD), chronic lung disease (CLD) of prematurity

Definitions

- Old definition (1979): 28 days of O_2 exposure + characteristic changes on radiographs
- New NIH consensus definition (2001): Chronic disease of premature infants born at < 32-week gestation with O_2 dependency for at least 28 days
  - Assessed at 36-week postmenstrual age (PMA)
  - Chest radiograph abnormalities no longer required
- Physiologic modification (2004): Specific O_2 challenge at 36-week PMA; has lead to more standardized diagnosis
- Classic or old BPD of early descriptions: Larger, later preterm infants with prolonged mechanical ventilation & O_2 therapy leading to inflammation & fibrosis
- New BPD: More diffuse but overall milder disease of earlier, smaller preterm infants in setting of antenatal steroids, postnatal surfactant administration, & reduced ventilator/O_2 intensity yielding less inflammation & fibrosis

IMAGING

Radiographic Findings

- Classic old BPD
  - Characteristic appearance of established BPD
    - Heterogeneous lung parenchyma with patchy focal lucencies separated by coarse, reticular, & band-like opacities of fibrosis, atelectasis
  - More opacities in upper lobes vs. hyperinflation at bases
  - Lateral radiograph may show relatively narrow AP diameter of chest for degree of hyperinflation (differing from bronchiolitis & asthma)
- Current new BPD
  - Lung appearance may be nearly normal early
  - Progressive diffuse hazy opacification that may ultimately lead to cystic foci with air-trapping, parenchymal bands

CT Findings

- NECT/HRCT
  - Overlapping chest CT findings between old & new BPD
    - Findings evolve over time with trend of improvement
  - Subpleural cysts & triangular opacities
  - Linear, reticular opacities
  - Architectural distortion
  - Foci of air-trapping on expiratory images
  - Positive correlation of CT with pulmonary function

Imaging Recommendations

- Best imaging tool
  - Chest radiographs for majority; inspiratory/expiratory chest CT in limited circumstances

PATHOLOGY

General Features

- Etiology
  - Strongest predictors: Prematurity & low birth weight
    - ↑ incidence with earlier gestational ages & ↓ weights

  - Definite risk factors: Fetal growth restriction, mechanical ventilation, higher levels of inspired supplemental O_2, postnatal sepsis

CLINICAL ISSUES

Presentation

- Most common signs/symptoms
  - Sustained O_2 requirement in premature neonate
  - Many new BPD patients have mild respiratory disease initially followed by progressive deterioration

Demographics

- Most common chronic pulmonary disease of infancy
- No significant change in incidence since initial description (due to ↑ survival of very premature infants)
- BPD develops in
  - 25% of infants weighing < 1,500 g at birth, 50% of those weighing < 1,000 g
  - 68% born at 22- to 26-week gestation
  - 10,000-15,000 infants in USA annually

Natural History & Prognosis

- Earlier detection of lung function abnormalities portends worse prognosis, often with lifelong pulmonary problems
- ↑ risk of pulmonary infections in first 2 years of life with ↑ morbidity & mortality, especially with RSV infection
- > 50% hospital readmission rate during infancy
- Pulmonary hypertension in up to 25% of BPD patients
  - Up to 48% 2-year mortality in this group
- Slowly improving pulmonary function with fewer respiratory infections later in childhood
- Abnormal pulmonary function with ↑ airway hyperreactivity & obstruction that may persist into adulthood
  - Clinically similar to asthma: Wheezing, coughing, dyspnea, exercise intolerance
- ↑ risk of emphysema as young adult
- Neurodevelopmental delay, growth failure

Treatment

- Many conflicting results in BPD prevention/therapy trials
- For prevention
  - Prenatal administration of steroids to mother
  - Exogenous surfactant administration
  - Gentle ventilation (pressure limited, volume targeted)
  - Low rather than high inspired O_2 concentrations
  - Closure of patent ductus arteriosus
  - Vitamin A, caffeine, inhaled nitric oxide
- Limited roles for pharmacologic intervention during developing or established BPD: Inhaled vs. systemic steroids, diuretics, bronchodilators, nitric oxide, sildenafil

SELECTED REFERENCES

1. Keszler M et al: Mechanical ventilation and bronchopulmonary dysplasia. Clin Perinatol. 42(4):781-96, 2015
2. Mourani PM et al: Pulmonary hypertension and vascular abnormalities in bronchopulmonary dysplasia. Clin Perinatol. 42(4):839-55, 2015
3. Walkup LL et al: Newer imaging techniques for bronchopulmonary dysplasia. Clin Perinatol. 42(4):871-87, 2015
4. El Mazloum D et al: Chronic lung disease of prematurity: long-term respiratory outcome. Neonatology. 105(4):352-6, 2014
5. Jensen EA et al: Epidemiology of bronchopulmonary dysplasia. Birth Defects Res A Clin Mol Teratol. 100(3):145-57, 2014

TERMINOLOGY

- Viral infection may involve airways &/or lung parenchyma
- Bronchiolitis: Acute inflammation & necrosis of epithelial cells lining small airways with ↑ mucus production
  - Classically < 2 years of age
- Other terms: Viral pneumonia, lower respiratory tract infection, peribronchial pneumonia

IMAGING

- Primary goal of chest radiography: Differentiate viral airway infection from bacterial pneumonia
  - 92% negative predictive value for bacterial pneumonia
- Best imaging clues for viral airway infection
  - ↑ peribronchial markings with radiating linear rope-like or "dirty" perihilar opacities & "doughnuts" of thickened bronchial walls (viewed in cross section)
  - Hyperinflation: Depression of hemidiaphragms with downward sloping on lateral view; ↑ AP chest diameter on lateral view; ± convex bulging of lungs between ribs

- Subsegmental atelectasis, possibly multifocal
- Lack of focal/lobar consolidation or pleural effusion
- Best imaging clues for viral parenchymal involvement
  - Interstitial, nodular, or patchy ground-glass opacities

CLINICAL ISSUES

- Viruses cause majority of chest infections in preschool children; most frequent causative virus differs by age
- Presents with rhinorrhea, cough, tachypnea, wheezing, rales, ↑ respiratory effort (grunting, nasal flaring, intercostal/subcostal retractions)
  - Difficult to differentiate bacterial from viral parenchymal infection based on physical exam or laboratory tests
- Treatment
  - Antibiotics for concomitant bacterial infection
  - No utility for albuterol or steroids
  - Hospitalization if hypoxemia or respiratory distress
  - Antiviral therapy for influenza cases

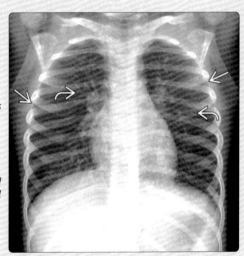

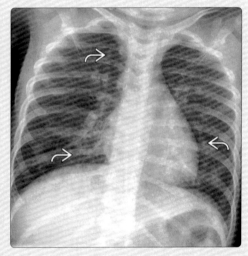

(Left) AP radiograph in a wheezing child shows typical findings of viral airways disease. There are mildly increased perihilar markings with an increased number of "doughnuts" (thickened bronchial walls viewed in cross section) ➔. The lungs show convex bulging between the ribs ➔, typical of hyperinflation. (Right) AP radiograph shows viral airways disease with increased perihilar markings of bronchial wall edema ➔. There is no focal lung consolidation or pleural effusion.

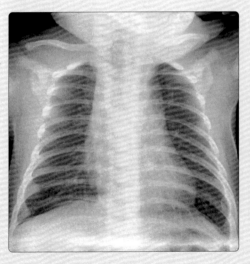

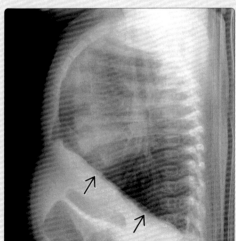

(Left) AP radiograph in a wheezing child shows hyperinflated lungs with increased rope-like perihilar markings, consistent with viral airways disease. There is no focal lung consolidation. (Right) Lateral radiograph in the same patient shows marked hyperinflation with flattening of the hemidiaphragms ➔ (much more evident than on the corresponding frontal view) & widening of the AP diameter of the chest. Also note the increased markings radiating from the hila.

TERMINOLOGY

Definitions

- Bronchiolitis (as defined by AAP): Viral lower respiratory tract infection in infants with "acute inflammation, edema, & necrosis of epithelial cells lining small airways," & ↑ mucus production
- Lower respiratory tract infection may describe findings identical to bronchiolitis in patients ≥ 2 years old but may also refer to any infection of lower airways & parenchyma
- Viral pneumonia may refer to viral infection of lung parenchyma ± airways infection
- Lower airways disease includes viral airways infection as well as asthma

IMAGING

Radiographic Findings

- Primary goal: Differentiate viral airways infection from bacterial pneumonia
- Small airways viral infection
  - Lack of focal dense geographic, round, or fluffy lung consolidation (hallmark of bacterial infection)
  - ↑ peribronchial markings/↑ number of visible bronchi
    - Symmetric, coarse linear markings radiating from hila
    - ↑ thickness of bronchial walls appearing as doughnuts in cross section
    - Central lungs may appear dirty or busy
  - Hyperinflation
    - Hyperlucency with depression of diaphragm > 10 posterior ribs or > 6 anterior ribs
    - Flattening/downward sloping hemidiaphragms (best seen on lateral view)
    - ↑ AP chest diameter on lateral view
    - ± convex bulging of lungs between ribs
    - May not be seen > 2 years old as bronchi larger & less prone to narrowing or obstruction with inflammation
  - Subsegmental atelectasis
    - Wedge-shaped or triangular opacity, often narrow
      - □ Most common in mid or lower lung
      - □ Often multifocal
    - Commonly misinterpreted as bacterial pneumonia
- Parenchymal involvement
  - Interstitial nodular or patchy opacities
  - Lobar consolidation rarely occurs
  - Associated findings of airways infection
- ± mild hilar lymphadenopathy
- Gas-distended bowel from air swallowing

Imaging Recommendations

- Best imaging tool
  - Chest radiographs (frontal & lateral)
    - Performance for bacterial pneumonia
      - □ Positive predictive value: 30%
      - □ Negative predictive value (NPV): 92%
    - Goal: Antibiotic therapy for all children with bacterial pneumonia while minimizing unnecessary antibiotic administration (for isolated viral infection)
      - □ High NPV of chest radiograph helpful

DIFFERENTIAL DIAGNOSIS

Asthma

- Similar ↑ peribronchial markings & hyperinflation

Bacterial Pneumonia

- Focal/lobar lung consolidation > interstitial infiltrate
  - Confluent geographic, round, or fluffy opacities
- Pleural effusions more common with bacterial infection

Bronchial Foreign Body

- Asymmetric hyperinflation characteristic
  - Affected lung volume static throughout respiratory cycle
- Foreign body often radiographically occult

Left-to-Right Cardiovascular Shunts

- In infants, left-to-right shunts may have similar appearance
  - ↑ pulmonary arterial flow may mimic ↑ peribronchial markings; ± hyperinflation
- Shunts have associated cardiomegaly

CLINICAL ISSUES

Presentation

- Signs & symptoms
  - Bronchiolitis: Rhinorrhea, cough, tachypnea, wheezing, rales, ↑ respiratory effort (grunting, nasal flaring, intercostal/subcostal retractions)
  - Community-acquired pneumonia: Cough, fever, anorexia, dyspnea, wheezing (up to 62%)
- Difficult to differentiate bacterial from viral parenchymal infection based on physical exam or laboratory tests

Demographics

- Viruses cause majority of chest infections in preschool children (4 months to 5 years of age)

Natural History & Prognosis

- Resolution of symptoms over time, typically days to weeks

Treatment

- Antibiotics for bacterial infection only (not just viral)
- Bronchiolitis
  - Nebulized hypertonic saline in infants may shorten hospitalization by increasing mucociliary clearance
  - Oxygen supplementation if saturations < 90%
  - Palivizumab (RSV prophylaxis) in select populations
  - Routine use of albuterol & nebulized epinephrine not recommended
  - Corticosteroid use not supported
- Clinical pneumonia with viral pathogen
  - Hospitalization if hypoxemia or respiratory distress
  - Antiviral therapy for influenza cases

SELECTED REFERENCES

1. Rhedin S et al: Respiratory viruses associated with community-acquired pneumonia in children: matched case-control study. Thorax. 70(9):847-53, 2015
2. Ralston SL et al: Clinical practice guideline: the diagnosis, management, and prevention of bronchiolitis. Pediatrics. 134(5):e1474-502, 2014
3. Franquet T: Imaging of pulmonary viral pneumonia. Radiology. Jul;260(1):18-39, 2011
4. Ruuskanen O et al: Viral pneumonia. Lancet; 377(9773):1264-1275, 2011

KEY FACTS

TERMINOLOGY

- Bacterial lung infection with very round, well-defined appearance on chest radiography; simulates mass lesion
- Majority seen in patients < 8 years of age

IMAGING

- Well-circumscribed round opacity ± air bronchograms
- Most common posteriorly in lower lobe superior segments
- No mass effect on or invasion of adjacent tissues
  - No mediastinal or vascular distortion
  - No splaying or erosion of ribs
- Margins of round lung "mass" classically create acute angles with mediastinum or chest wall but can be obtuse

TOP DIFFERENTIAL DIAGNOSES

- Bronchogenic cyst
- Neuroblastoma
- Congenital pulmonary airway malformation
- Bronchopulmonary sequestration

PATHOLOGY

- Collateral pathways of air circulation in lung not well developed until ~ 8 years of age
  - Channels of Lambert, pores of Kohn
- Spread of bacterial infection through lung therefore hindered in young children, predisposing to round appearance
- Typically occurs with *Streptococcus pneumoniae* infection

DIAGNOSTIC CHECKLIST

- Round lung opacity in child < 8 years of age → strongly consider round pneumonia
- With classic symptoms of pneumonia (cough, fever) in this age range, other masses do not need to be excluded
- If any doubt of diagnosis, consider
  - Targeted US or CT through lesion
  - Follow-up radiograph after completion of antibiotic course
    - Resolution of "mass" excludes other etiologies

(Left) *AP radiograph in a young child with cough & fever shows a round, mildly lobulated, well-circumscribed density ⊡ in the medial aspect of the right lower lobe.* (Right) *Lateral radiograph in the same patient confirms that the round "mass" ⊡ is located posteriorly in the right lower lobe. Note that the lesion makes acute angles with the posterior chest wall, consistent with a pulmonary origin. These findings are typical of a round pneumonia.*

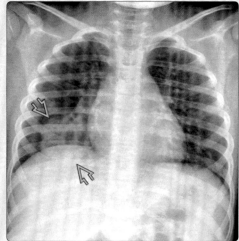
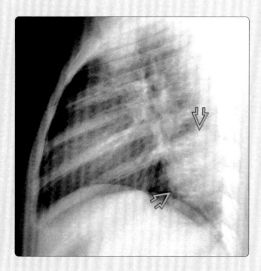

(Left) *Abdominal radiograph of a 7-year-old boy with fever & vomiting shows a round opacity ⊡ projecting over the right hemidiaphragm, suggesting a right lower lobe round pneumonia.* (Right) *Subsequent chest radiograph in the same patient clearly demonstrates a lobulated, well-circumscribed right lower lobe opacity ⊡, consistent with a round pneumonia. Note that the adjacent ribs are normal.*

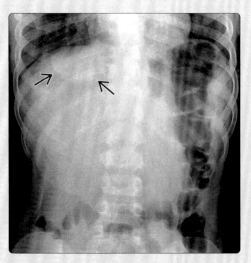
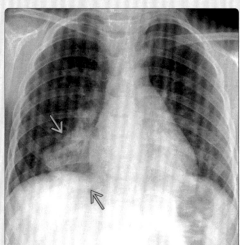

TERMINOLOGY

Definitions

- Bacterial lung infection with very round, well-defined appearance on chest radiography; simulates mass lesion

IMAGING

Radiographic Findings

- Round lung opacity typically marginated by clear lung
  - Paraspinal pneumonia may have acute or obtuse angle borders with posterior mediastinum/spine
- Respects lobar anatomy without crossing fissures
- Does not exert mass effect or invade adjacent tissues
  - No osseous changes (such as splaying or erosion) in adjacent ribs or spine
- Air bronchograms help confirm airspace disease
- Pleural effusion uncommon

Ultrasonographic Findings

- Increasingly used for diagnosis of childhood pneumonia
  - Sensitivity 96%, specificity 93% overall
    - May be lower if round pneumonia completely surrounded by aerated lung
- Abnormality of normally echogenic pleural line: Irregular, coarse, interrupted, or absent
- "Hepatization" of subpleural parenchyma with branching mobile hyperechogenicities (air bronchograms)

CT or MR

- Not advocated for suspected round pneumonia
  - May be obtained if mass lesion of primary concern
- Homogeneous round opacity ± air bronchograms
- No enhancing rim or central cavity
- Normal pulmonary vessels course through consolidated lung without mass effect
- No changes in adjacent bones
- No systemic arterial supply from descending aorta

Imaging Recommendations

- Pediatric Clinical Practice Guidelines for chest radiography in pneumonia
  - Not necessary to confirm suspected community-acquired pneumonia (CAP) in patients well enough to be treated as outpatients; exceptions include hypoxemia, respiratory distress, failed antibiotic therapy
  - Chest radiographs (frontal & lateral) should be obtained in all patients hospitalized for management of CAP
- If child < 8 years old has symptoms of pneumonia + round opacity on radiograph, additional imaging unnecessary
- Follow-up radiograph after antibiotic therapy may be helpful to document resolution of round opacity
  - Particularly helpful for paraspinal round pneumonia that may mimic neuroblastoma

DIFFERENTIAL DIAGNOSIS

Bronchogenic Cyst

- Round, well-defined perihilar mass
- ± mass effect on adjacent structures
- CECT: Water attenuation mass without air bronchograms; ± rim enhancement if infected

Neuroblastoma

- Round or elongated posterior mediastinal/paraspinal mass
  - May only widen paraspinal stripe without focal bulge
- Rib erosion or splaying common
- CT: Ca^{2+} in majority

Bronchopulmonary Sequestration

- Lobulated or triangular mass in lower lobe
- May present as recurrent pneumonias (always in same location)
- CTA: Characteristic systemic feeding artery arises from descending thoracic or abdominal aorta

Lung Abscess

- Round cavity containing air-fluid level
- Surrounded by irregular or poorly defined consolidation

Chest Wall Ewing Sarcoma

- Partially circumscribed mass with definite bony destruction
- Associated pleural effusions frequent
- Typically in children > 8 years of age

PATHOLOGY

General Features

- Exudative opacification of pulmonary airspaces related to bacterial infection
  - *Streptococcus pneumoniae* most common pathogen
- Collateral pathways of air circulation (channels of Lambert & pores of Kohn) not well developed until ~ 8 years of age
  - Hinders spread of bacterial infection, predisposing to round appearance

CLINICAL ISSUES

Presentation

- Most common signs/symptoms
  - Cough & fever
- Other signs/symptoms
  - Abdominal pain, malaise, anorexia

Demographics

- 75% < 8 years old; 90% < 12 years old; mean age: 5 years

Natural History & Prognosis

- With appropriate antibiotic therapy, symptoms & opacity should resolve over days-weeks
  - Resolution on follow-up radiograph confidently excludes other etiologies

SELECTED REFERENCES

1. Jain S et al: Community-acquired pneumonia requiring hospitalization among U.S. children. N Engl J Med. 372(9):835-45, 2015
2. Pereda MA et al: Lung ultrasound for the diagnosis of pneumonia in children: a meta-analysis. Pediatrics. 135(4):714-22, 2015
3. Liu YL et al: Pediatric round pneumonia. Pediatr Neonatol. 55(6):491-4, 2014
4. Restrepo R et al: Imaging of round pneumonia and mimics in children. Pediatr Radiol. 40(12):1931-40, 2010

Parapneumonic Effusion and Empyema

TERMINOLOGY

- Pleural effusions classified as transudative or exudative
- Parapneumonic effusions are exudative secondary to adjacent lung infection & ↑ capillary permeability

IMAGING

- Upright chest radiograph
  - Flattened & elevated hemidiaphragm, lateral shift of diaphragm apex, gastric bubble > 1.5 cm from diaphragm secondary to subpulmonic fluid
  - Blunted posterior costophrenic angle (~ 50 mL)
  - Blunted lateral costophrenic angle (~ 200 mL)
  - Hemidiaphragm inversion (> 2,000 mL)
- Supine chest radiograph may require up to 500 mL
  - Homogeneous vs. gradation of hazy/dense opacification of hemithorax ± pleural cap, mass effect
- CECT: Parietal pleural enhancement & thickening, thickening of extrapleural space, & chest wall edema seen with both transudative & exudative effusions in children

- US: Effusion appears anechoic, echoic, or mixed with floating/swirling/undulating echoes
  - Floating fibrin strands attached to pleural surface, septations, &/or pleural rind/thickening; immobile lung suggests entrapment by pleural rind
  - Loculation: Nonshifting fluid with position change
- Imaging recommendations
  - US if pleural disease suspected on chest radiograph
  - CECT if persistent/progressive illness despite treatment

CLINICAL ISSUES

- Treatment
  - Antibiotics
  - Chest tube drainage if effusion of large volume, loculated, or with worsening/persistent symptoms
  - If empyema: Chest tube + tissue plasminogen activator; video-assisted thoracoscopic surgery if no clinical improvement & pleural disease persists on imaging
- Majority of children make complete clinical recovery

(Left) PA radiograph of a child with a right pneumonia shows opacification of the majority of the right hemithorax with mediastinal shift to the left. (Right) Sagittal US of the right hemithorax in the same patient shows a large pleural effusion ➡ with internal debris & multiple echogenic septa ➡, consistent with a fibrinopurulent parapneumonic effusion.

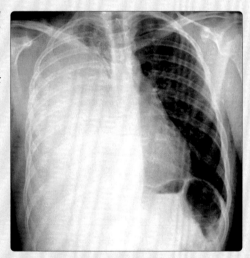
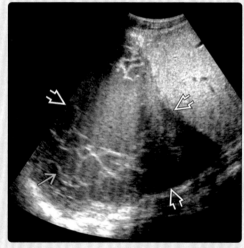

(Left) Axial CECT in the same patient shows the large pleural effusion compressing the right lung ➡. While the rind of enhancement ➡ suggests complexity, the septations demonstrated on the previous US are not visualized on this CT examination. (Right) Longitudinal US of the right lung in a patient with pneumonia shows a right pleural effusion ➡ with multiple areas of echogenic debris & septations. Note the consolidated, echogenic lung ➡. The liver ➡ is shown inferiorly.

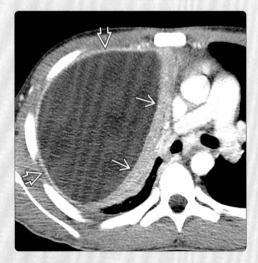
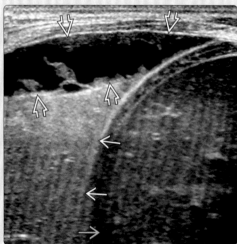

Parapneumonic Effusion and Empyema

TERMINOLOGY

Definitions

- Pleural effusions classified as transudative or exudative
  - Transudative: Due to hydrostatic & oncotic imbalances
  - Exudative: Due to ↑ capillary permeability
- Parapneumonic effusions are exudative
  - Stages of progression: Exudative (simple) → fibrinopurulent (complicated) → organized
  - Empyema is fibrinopurulent parapneumonic effusion

IMAGING

Radiographic Findings

- Pneumonia + adjacent pleural effusion
- Sequence of accumulation on upright image
  - Flattened & elevated hemidiaphragm, lateral shift of diaphragm apex, gastric bubble > 1.5 cm from diaphragm secondary to subpulmonic fluid
  - Blunted posterior costophrenic angle (~ 50 mL)
  - Blunted lateral costophrenic angle (~ 200 mL)
  - Hemidiaphragm inversion (> 2,000 mL)
- Supine images: Sensitivity 70%, may require up to 500 mL
  - Homogeneous vs. gradation of hazy/dense opacification of hemithorax ± pleural cap, mass effect
- Loculation suggested by lenticular shape or nonshifting fluid on decubitus views
- Fissural accumulation may present as thickening or pseudotumor in minor fissure

Ultrasonographic Findings

- Effusion appears anechoic, echoic, or mixed with floating/swirling/undulating echoes
- Fibrin deposition: Floating/flapping strands attached to pleural surface, septations, pleural rind/thickening; lack of lung mobility suggests pleural rind entrapping lung
- Loculation: Nonshifting fluid with position change

CT Findings

- Parietal pleural thickening & enhancement, thickened extrapleural space, & chest wall edema seen with both transudative & exudative effusions in children
- Inferior to US at demonstrating fibrin strands or septations
- Loculation inferred if air in collection separates into bubbles rather than single air-fluid level

Imaging Recommendations

- US if pleural space disease suspected on chest radiograph
  - Must scan dependent & nondependent pleural cavity
- CECT if persistent/progressive illness despite treatment (to evaluate for malpositioned chest tube, lung necrosis or abscess, purulent pericarditis)

DIFFERENTIAL DIAGNOSIS

Malignant Pleural Effusion

- Lymphoma, Ewing sarcoma, pleuropulmonary blastoma
- Look for nodularity/mass &/or rib destruction

Chylothorax

- Birth trauma, lymphangiectasia, lymphatic malformation

Lung Abscess

- Walled-off collection with pneumonia & progressive illness

PATHOLOGY

General Features

- Transudate vs. exudate classification based on fluid analysis
- Light's criteria for exudate (≥ 1 required): Pleural fluid to serum protein ratio > 0.5 or lactate dehydrogenase (LDH) ratio > 0.6; pleural fluid LDH > 2/3 upper limit of normal serum level
- If exudative, then empyema suggested by: pH < 7.2, LDH > 1,000 U, glucose < 40 mg/dL or < 25% blood glucose, positive Gram stain or positive culture, > 10,000 WBC/uL, loculations on imaging
- Common causes include *Streptococcus pneumoniae* & methicillin-resistant *Staphylococcus aureus*
- Test for tuberculosis if lymphocytic exudate
- Stages of parapneumonic effusion progression
  - Precollection: Pleuritis, inflammation
  - Exudative (simple): Free fluid with low white cell count
  - Fibrinopurulent (complicated): Deposition of fibrin & purulent material
  - Organized: Thick pleural peel, which may entrap lung

CLINICAL ISSUES

Presentation

- Fever, cough, chest pain, dyspnea, tachypnea, splinting to affected side, respiratory distress if large volume

Natural History & Prognosis

- Most pediatric patients make complete clinical recovery with almost normal radiograph in 3-6 months
- Pediatric mortality < 3% in 1 study (in contrast to adults, with mortality reported up to 20%)

Treatment

- American Pediatric Surgical Association recommendations
  - Antibiotics
  - Fluid evacuation if effusion of large volume, loculated, or with worsening/persistent symptoms
  - < 14F chest tube recommended; single thoracentesis can be used for older children with free fluid
  - If empyema: 12F chest tube + 3 doses of intrapleural tissue plasminogen activator → video-assisted thoracoscopic surgery if no clinical improvement & pleural disease persists on imaging

SELECTED REFERENCES

1. Long AM et al: 'Less may be best'-Pediatric parapneumonic effusion and empyema management: Lessons from a UK center. J Pediatr Surg. 51(4):588-91, 2015
2. Islam S et al: The diagnosis and management of empyema in children: a comprehensive review from the APSA Outcomes and Clinical Trials Committee. J Pediatr Surg. 47(11):2101-10, 2012
3. Calder A et al: Imaging of parapneumonic pleural effusions and empyema in children. Pediatr Radiol. 39(6):527-37, 2009
4. Kurian J et al: Comparison of ultrasound and CT in the evaluation of pneumonia complicated by parapneumonic effusion in children. AJR Am J Roentgenol. 193(6):1648-54, 2009

Pneumonia With Cavitary Necrosis

TERMINOLOGY

- Complication of bacterial pneumonia where dominant focus of necrosis develops in consolidated lung, resulting in variable number of thin-walled cysts
- Synonyms: Necrotizing pneumonia, pulmonary gangrene
  - Abscess has thick, well-defined wall & is more commonly seen in immunocompromised children

IMAGING

- Not identified radiographically until tissue breakdown leads to communication of cavity with aerated lung/airways
- CECT shows lack of normal lung architecture, ↓ lung enhancement, & thin-walled cysts in midst of consolidation
- No clear role for percutaneous drainage in cases of cavitary necrosis in immunocompetent children

TOP DIFFERENTIAL DIAGNOSES

- Congenital pulmonary airway malformation
- Lung abscess
- Bronchogenic cyst

CLINICAL ISSUES

- Increasingly identified as pediatric pneumonia complication
- *Streptococcus pneumoniae* most common cause followed by MSSA, MRSA, other *Staphylococcus & Streptococcus* species, *Pseudomonas, Fusobacterium*
- Progressive symptoms (fever, respiratory distress, sepsis) in pediatric pneumonia patient despite appropriate medical management suggests complication (such as cavitary necrosis)
  - Patients with cavitary necrosis tend to be intensely ill (ICU)
- Most recover with antibiotics & nonsurgical management; may lead to bronchopleural fistula & development of pneumothorax

(Left) *AP chest radiograph in a child with rapidly progressive symptoms shows complete opacification of the right hemithorax & partial opacification of the medial left lower lobe (LLL). There are bilateral chest tubes in place.* (Right) *Coronal CECT in the same patient shows heterogeneous opacification of the entire right lung with multiple thin-walled, fluid-containing cystic foci ➡, consistent with cavitary necrosis. Also note the LLL opacification. There are no significant pleural effusions.*

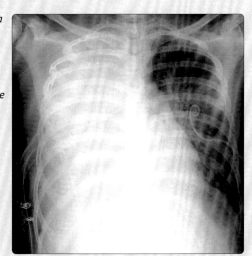
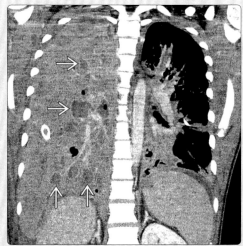

(Left) *Axial CECT shows multiple thin-walled, air-containing cysts ➡ with surrounding consolidation in the LLL. This appearance is very similar to a congenital pulmonary airway malformation. However, follow-up imaging after antibiotics showed the lesions to resolve over time, most consistent with cavitary necrosis.* (Right) *AP radiograph in a young child shows opacification of the right hemithorax with an air-filled cystic focus ➡ in the mid lung, suggesting cavitary necrosis.*

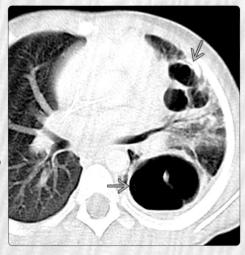
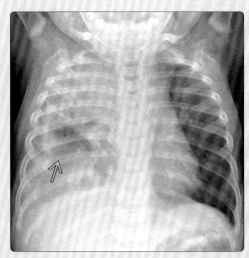

Papillomatosis

TERMINOLOGY

- Recurrent respiratory papillomatosis (RRP): Benign tumors of aerodigestive tract caused by infection with human papillomavirus (HPV)
  - Variable lifelong morbidity; potentially fatal course

IMAGING

- Locations: Junctional sites between respiratory & squamous epithelium
  - Larynx most common site
  - Extralaryngeal spread in ~ 30% of patients
    - Endobronchial spread → pulmonary nodules
      - □ Lung parenchymal involvement in 3%
- Radiographic/CT appearances
  - Airway: Soft tissue nodules protruding into lumen
  - Lung: Multiple solid or cavitated nodules
    - ± postobstructive atelectasis or pneumonia
    - Malignant degeneration of pulmonary disease in 0.5%
      - □ Squamous cell carcinoma

CLINICAL ISSUES

- Most common laryngeal tumor in children
- Perinatal transmission of HPV: Infected mother → child
  - Vast majority caused by HPV-6 & HPV-11
  - ↑ risk: Vaginal delivery, firstborn, mother < 20 years of age; delivery time > 10 hours doubles risk; active condylomata ↑ risk 231x
- Most common symptoms: Hoarseness/voice change
- Mean age at diagnosis: ~ 4 years
- Disease remission can occur spontaneously at any stage; death can occur from large airway obstruction, respiratory failure, or malignant degeneration
- Treatment with resection using powered microdebrider
  - Need for repeated debulking typical
  - Tracheostomy needed in 10-15% due to airway obstruction; delayed as long as possible due to ↑ risk of distal spread
- HPV quadrivalent vaccine protective

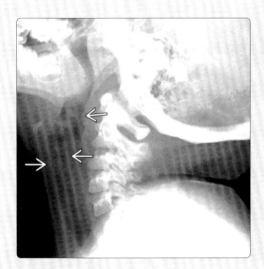

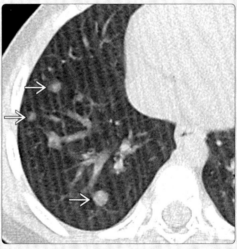

(Left) Lateral radiograph of the airway in a child with recurrent respiratory papillomatosis (RRP) shows multiple nodular filling defects ➡ from papillomas within the pharyngeal, laryngeal, & subglottic airways. RRP most commonly occurs in the larynx. (Right) Axial CT in the same patient shows multiple solid pulmonary nodules ➡ within the right lung. Nearly 30% of patients with RRP have extralaryngeal spread of papillomas. Extension to the lung represents the most serious form of the disease.

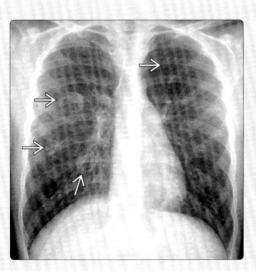

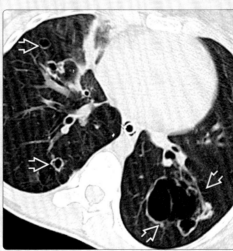

(Left) Chest radiograph in an adolescent with RRP shows multiple cavitary nodules ➡ in the lungs. (Right) Axial NECT shows irregular, thin-walled cavitary lesions ➡ of varying sizes in both lungs. Papillomatosis is generally a benign, self-limited disease. However, severe cases can cause significant morbidity.

TERMINOLOGY

- Lymphoma: Malignant neoplasm arising from constituent cells of immune system or their precursors
- Hodgkin lymphoma (HL), non-Hodgkin lymphoma (NHL)

IMAGING

- Most common thoracic location: Anterior mediastinum
- US can help to distinguish normal thymus from abnormal thymus if nature of prominent anterior mediastinum unclear radiographically
- CECT: Typically used for initial diagnosis
  - Diffuse thymic infiltration: Anterior mediastinal mass with fairly homogeneous enhancement
    - Displaces, encases, & compresses adjacent structures (i.e., vessels & airway)
      - \> 50% area reduction of trachea associated with respiratory failure during induction of anesthesia
  - Other locations in thorax: Hilum, axilla, supraclavicular region, lungs, pleura, pericardium

- PET: Very sensitive & specific (96.5%, 100%) for lymphoma
  - Changes initial stage in 10-23% of patients compared to conventional imaging
  - Can distinguish active disease from residual inactive mass

CLINICAL ISSUES

- Lymphoma 3rd most common pediatric malignancy
  - Accounts for 10-15% of all pediatric malignancies
- 60% of children with lymphoma have respiratory symptoms
- HL may present with painless adenopathy & B symptoms of fever, night sweats, weight loss
- NHL can have life-threatening symptoms due to compression of trachea or superior vena cava &/or large pleural or pericardial effusion
- Treatment
  - HL: Chemotherapy ± radiation; 5-year survival = 91%
  - NHL: Chemotherapy ± bone marrow transplantation or radiation therapy; 5-year survival = 70-76%

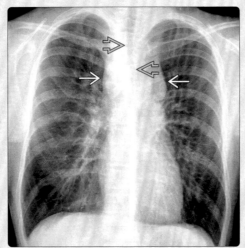
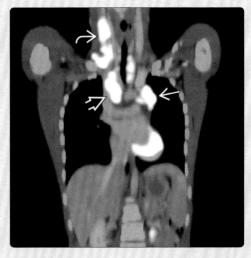

(Left) Frontal chest radiograph in a 14-year-old boy with Hodgkin lymphoma shows a widened mediastinum ➡ with tracheal narrowing & deviation ➡. (Right) Coronal FDG PET/CT in the same patient shows abnormal FDG uptake in the aortopulmonary window ➡, right paratracheal level ➡, & right cervical chain ➡. Approximately 80% of pediatric patients with Hodgkin lymphoma present with painless cervical adenopathy.

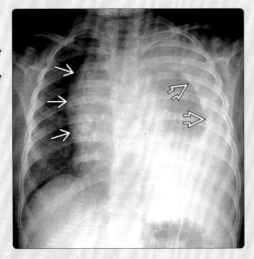
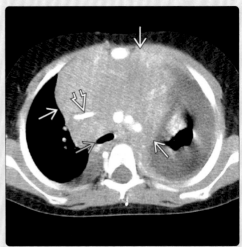

(Left) AP radiograph in a young child with respiratory distress shows a large mediastinal mass ➡ & a large left pleural effusion ➡. (Right) Axial CECT in the same patient shows the large lymphomatous mediastinal mass ➡, left > right pleural effusions, narrowing of the superior vena cava ➡, & compression of the trachea ➡.

Germ Cell Tumors

TERMINOLOGY

- Derived from primordial germ cells that differentiate into embryonic & extraembryonic structures
  - Teratoma: Mature, immature, malignant
  - Seminoma: Germinoma & dysgerminoma
  - Nonseminomatous germ cell tumor (NSGCT): Embryonal cell, yolk sac tumor, choriocarcinoma, & mixed GCT

IMAGING

- Best clue: Heterogeneous anterior mediastinal mass arising within or adjacent to thymus
  - Less common thoracic locations: Posterior mediastinum, heart, pericardium
- Teratoma: Mostly cystic + soft tissue, fat (93%), & calcium (20-40%)
  - CECT sensitive for these components
- Seminoma: Homogeneous, bulky soft tissue mass
  - Often straddles midline & has mass effect
- NSGCT: Heterogeneous with hemorrhage & necrosis

- Irregular margins: Obliterated fat planes & lung invasion
- Pericardial lesions often cause pericardial effusion
- Beware of potential airway collapse from tumor compression during sedation/general anesthesia

CLINICAL ISSUES

- Typical presentations
  - Dyspnea (25-48%), chest pain (23-52%), cough (17-24%), superior vena cava syndrome (6-14%), hoarseness (1-14%), fever (13%), weight loss (11%)
  - Asymptomatic in 50-60% of teratomas, 38% of seminomas, & 10% of NSGCTs
  - α-fetoprotein elevated in 74% of patients with NSGCT; β-HCG elevated in 38%
- 50-300x risk of mediastinal GCT with Klinefelter syndrome
- Treatment
  - Mature teratoma → surgery
  - Seminoma or NSGCT → chemotherapy followed by surgery for residual disease

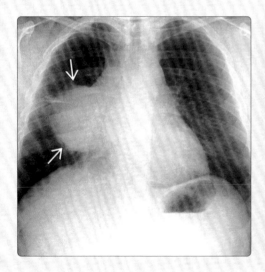

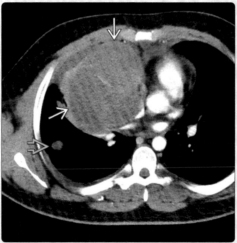

(Left) Frontal chest radiograph in a young adult male patient with a yolk sac tumor shows a large mass ➡ in the right mid chest obscuring the right heart border (& implying an anterior position). (Right) Axial CECT in the same patient shows a round mass ➡ of the anterior mediastinum that is hypodense compared to muscle. There is a solitary pulmonary nodule ➡ in the right lung base. Nonseminomatous germ cell tumors can metastasize to the lymph nodes, lung, & liver.

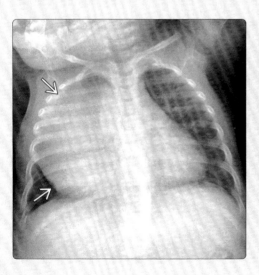

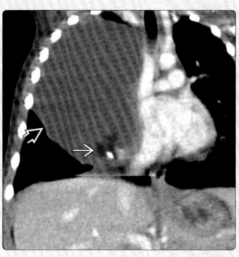

(Left) Chest radiograph in a 1-year-old patient with a mature teratoma shows a large mass ➡ abutting the right heart border & filling much of the right hemithorax. This is larger than typically seen for normal thymus, & the right hemidiaphragm is mildly depressed. (Right) Coronal CECT in the same patient shows a large mass ➡ in the right hemithorax. The mass is mostly fluid density but shows a nodule inferiorly ➡ that contains fat & calcium. The presence of cystic, fatty, & calcific foci is diagnostic of a teratoma.

Child Abuse, Rib Fractures

TERMINOLOGY

- Child abuse: Any act or failure to act by parent/caretaker that causes harm or imminent risk of harm to child

IMAGING

- Posterior rib fractures most common & specific for nonaccidental trauma (NAT)
- Radiography
  - Linear lucency of acute rib fracture often not visible
  - Callus/subperiosteal new bone formation may become visible 7-10 days after injury
    - Ranges from indistinct margins & broadening of rib → sharply marginated nodular/bulbous callus
  - Rib head fracture may appear fragmented with mixed sclerosis & lucency; often no subperiosteal new bone
- Tc-99m MDP bone scan or 18F-NaF PET complementary
  - Focal ↑ radiotracer activity within 24 hours
- CT not advocated for identifying rib fractures but may be used to evaluate intrathoracic or intraabdominal injury

- Indications for initial radiographic skeletal survey
  - < 2 years old with suspicion of NAT
  - < 5 years old with suspicious fracture
  - Suspicion of NAT in any child unable to communicate
- Follow-up skeletal survey, typically after 2 weeks, if
  - Possible fractures present on initial study
  - Normal initial study with persistent suspicion based on clinical or imaging findings

CLINICAL ISSUES

- Presentation: Injury inconsistent with history, multiple injuries in various stages of healing, bruising in nonmobile infant, genitalia injury, cigarette burns, other injuries with high specificity for NAT
- Majority of rib fractures not suspected on clinical exam
  - Overlying bruising in ~ 9%; ± "clicking" or "popping" sound from back or chest on physical exam
- Most common skeletal injury in NAT
  - Only radiographic manifestation of NAT in up to 29%

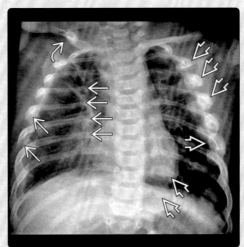
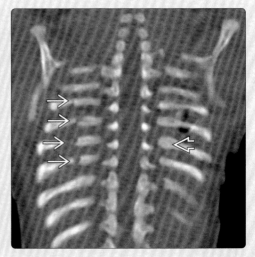

(Left) AP radiograph in an infant with suspected abuse demonstrates multiple left lateral & posterior rib fractures with callus formation ➡ as well as more recent right-sided rib fractures without evidence of healing ➡. Also note the right clavicle fracture ➡ & right pleural effusion. (Right) Coronal CECT (in bone windows) in the same patient obtained shortly after the radiographs shows the acute right posterior rib fractures ➡ & 1 of the healing left posterior rib fractures ➡.

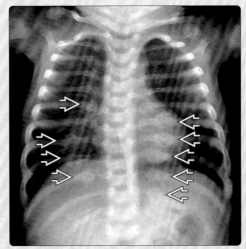
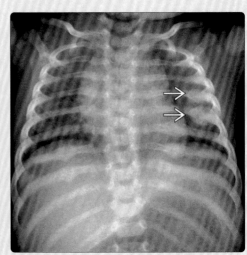

(Left) AP radiograph in this 1 month old shows multiple healing posterior rib fractures with bulbous callus formation ➡. (Right) AP radiograph obtained 2 weeks later in the same patient shows 2 additional healing rib fractures ➡, which, even in retrospect, are difficult to appreciate on the initial study.

TERMINOLOGY

Definitions

- Child abuse: Any act or failure to act by parent/caretaker that causes harm or imminent risk of harm to child
  - Also known as nonaccidental trauma or injury (NAT, NAI)

IMAGING

General Features

- Best diagnostic clue
  - Bulbous callus/subperiosteal new bone formation of multiple adjacent posteromedial ribs in infant
- Location
  - Can occur anywhere along rib
  - Posterior near costovertebral junction most common

Radiographic Findings

- Acute fractures often not visualized radiographically
  - Typically vertical/oblique linear lucency in rib short axis
- Healing fractures may become visible 7-10 days after injury
- Sensitivity 73% in 1 study vs. follow-up radiographs
- Sensitivity only 26% in 1 study vs. postmortem histology

CT Findings

- Greater sensitivity than initial skeletal survey but only performed for suspected thoracoabdominal visceral injuries

MR Findings

- Whole-body MR child abuse evaluations show low sensitivity (57%) for rib fractures vs. radiographs

Nuclear Medicine Findings

- Tc-99m MDP skeletal scintigraphy or 18F-NaF PET complementary to initial survey but not routinely obtained

Imaging Recommendations

- Initial skeletal survey
  - Indications
    - < 2 years old with suspicion of NAT
    - < 5 years old with suspicious fracture
    - Concern for NAT in any child unable to communicate
  - All bones imaged with high detail in at least 1 plane; ribs imaged with AP, lateral, & bilateral oblique views
- Follow-up skeletal survey
  - Typically 2 weeks (not < 10 days) from initial evaluation
  - Indications
    - Concerning fractures on initial study
    - Normal initial study with persistent suspicion based on clinical or imaging findings
  - In 1 study, clarified questionable fractures or identified new fractures (most often of ribs) in 48% of cases

DIFFERENTIAL DIAGNOSIS

Entities Associated With Multiple Fractures

- Osteogenesis imperfecta (OI)
  - Type IV OI most commonly mistaken for abuse
    - Sclera normal in color (not blue)
  - ± osteoporosis, multiple fractures, & wormian bones
- Menkes syndrome
  - Osteoporosis, wormian bones, metaphyseal spurs, brittle hair, tortuous intracranial vessels

- Rickets
  - Widening/lengthening of physes with metaphyseal fraying, cupping, & splaying
- Leukemia
  - Osteoporosis ± lucent metaphyseal bands, permeative destruction, aggressive periosteal new bone formation

Birth Trauma

- Rare but can occur with large babies & difficult deliveries

Trauma From Cardiopulmonary Resuscitation

- Rib fractures very rare in pediatric CPR (< 1%)
- Most such fractures involve anterior ribs

Accidental Trauma

- Age & history must be consistent with injury
- Rib fractures more likely to be anterior & lateral
- Greater likelihood of visceral injury & fewer fractures

PATHOLOGY

General Features

- Assailant holds infant, wrapping hands around chest with finger tips at posterior ribs & thumbs situated anteriorly
- Anteroposterior compression while squeezing & shaking child results in fractures
  - Posterior rib fractures (most common & specific) occur from leveraging posterior ribs on transverse processes

CLINICAL ISSUES

Presentation

- Wide range of clinical presentations for NAT: Injury inconsistent with history, multiple injuries in various stages of healing, bruising in nonmobile infant, genitalia injury, cigarette burns, other injuries with high specificity for NAT (e.g., classic metaphyseal lesion/corner fracture)
- Rib fractures
  - Most common skeletal injury in NAT
    - Present in 10-14% of skeletal surveys performed for suspected abuse
    - Only radiographic finding of NAT in up to 29% of cases
  - Majority not suspected based on clinical exam
    - Associated bruising at fracture site is rare, 9%
    - "Clicking" or "popping" sound from back or chest on physical exam, ± crepitus
  - Associated intrathoracic injury in 12.8% of NAT vs. 55.6% of accidental injuries
  - In children < 3 years of age, 61% associated with abuse vs. 82% if < 1 year of age

Treatment

- Multidisciplinary investigation of maltreatment allegation involves physicians, social worker, legal authorities
- Ensure "at risk" child & siblings placed in safe environment

SELECTED REFERENCES

1. Barber I et al: The yield of high-detail radiographic skeletal surveys in suspected infant abuse. Pediatr Radiol. 45(1):69-80, 2015
2. Kleinman, Paul K. Diagnostic Imaging of Child Abuse. Cambridge University Press, 2015.
3. Darling SE et al: Frequency of intrathoracic injuries in children younger than 3 years with rib fractures. Pediatr Radiol. 44(10):1230-6, 2014

Lung Contusion and Laceration

TERMINOLOGY

- Lung contusion: Hemorrhage + edema in alveoli & interstitium due to traumatic alveolar capillary damage
- Lung laceration: Frank tear of lung parenchyma

IMAGING

- Radiograph: Often sufficient for blunt chest trauma
  - Contusion: Nonsegmental patchy or diffuse opacification
    - May not be radiographically evident < 4-6 hours
  - Laceration: Round lucency ± air-fluid level
    - May be obscured by contusion initially
- CECT: Performed if strong clinical or imaging findings suggest significant thoracic injury
  - ↑ sensitivity for detecting contusion
    - Significance of contusions seen only on CT doubtful → may not be associated with ↑ morbidity
  - Contusion: Confluent, nodular, crescentic, or amorphous consolidative or ground-glass opacities
    - Commonly peripheral with rim of subpleural sparing
  - Laceration: Air-/fluid-filled cavity surrounded by opacity

PATHOLOGY

- Mechanism: Penetrating trauma 10-15%; blunt trauma 85%-90% (consider nonaccidental trauma in young patients)

CLINICAL ISSUES

- Patients with lung injuries typically have ↑ overall injury severity with multisystem trauma → assess for other major organ injuries leading to high morbidity & mortality
  - Associated chest injuries: Heart & great vessels (8%); diaphragm, tracheobronchial tree, esophagus < 5% each
- Presentation: ↓ breath sounds, dull to percussion, tachypnea, chest tenderness, hemoptysis, respiratory failure
- Supportive therapy (pulmonary toilet, pain control, alveolar recruitment maneuvers, etc.) with observation for complications (infection, ARDS, tension pneumothorax, hemopneumothorax, hemoptysis)

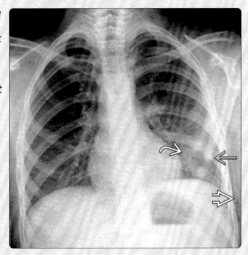

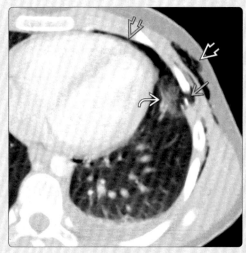

(Left) AP chest radiograph of a 13 year old after a bicycle collision shows an anterior left 5th-rib fracture ➡ with adjacent subcutaneous emphysema ➡ & patchy airspace opacity ➡, consistent with contusion. (Right) Axial CECT in the same patient shows the left 5th-rib fracture ➡, subcutaneous emphysema ➡, a pneumothorax ➡, & adjacent ground-glass lung opacity ➡, consistent with contusion. Associated rib fractures are less frequent in pediatric patients (as compared to adults) due to the pliability of the rib cage.

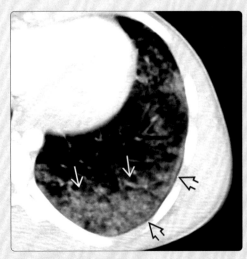

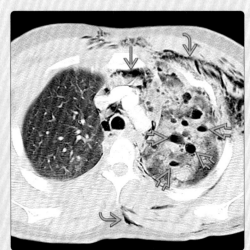

(Left) Axial CECT in a trauma patient shows amorphous density in the left lower lobe ➡. Note the thin crescentic lucency ➡ adjacent to the chest wall. This finding of subpleural sparing is frequently seen in pulmonary contusions. (Right) Axial CECT of a 17 year old after a car accident shows multiple air- & fluid-filled cysts ➡ throughout the left upper lobe, consistent with lung lacerations. Also note the pneumomediastinum ➡ & extensive subcutaneous emphysema ➡.

Pneumomediastinum

IMAGING

- Best tool for pneumomediastinum (PM): Chest radiograph
  - Pleural line lateral to main pulmonary artery & aortic arch
  - Vertical lucencies tracking on either side of superior mediastinum into neck
  - Continuous diaphragm sign: Air between pericardium & diaphragm results in visualization of normally obscured superior surface of central diaphragm
  - Spinnaker sail sign: Thymic elevation by mediastinal air
- CT or esophagram only with radiographic evidence of trauma, risk factors for aerodigestive tract injury (foreign body, surgery, mediastinitis), or respiratory distress

PATHOLOGY

- Spontaneous PM: Extension of air from ruptured alveolus into interstitium & mediastinum, most commonly from asthma or infection
- Secondary PM: Disruption of aerodigestive tract (trauma, foreign body, Boerhaave syndrome), surgery, mediastinitis

CLINICAL ISSUES

- Chest pain, cough, & dyspnea typical, ± crepitus from subcutaneous emphysema
- Secondary PM likely to present with rib fracture, pneumothorax, hemothorax, intracranial injury, respiratory distress, tachycardia
- Isolated spontaneous PM in stable patient: Self-limited → supportive care, emergency department observation
  - With symptom progression: Further evaluate & treat underlying pulmonary cause
- Secondary PM: CT or esophagram if clinical or imaging evidence suggests aerodigestive tract injury
  - Widespread screening of low yield in blunt trauma patients with otherwise normal chest radiograph
- Complications uncommon; can include pseudotamponade, mediastinitis, pneumothorax

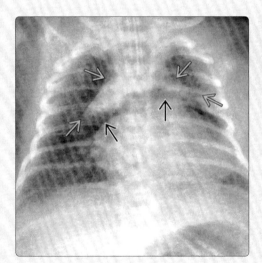

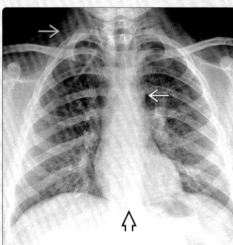

(Left) Supine chest radiograph of a 2 day old demonstrates air ➡ uplifting the thymus ➡, an appearance known as the spinnaker sail sign that is consistent with pneumomediastinum. The diffuse granular lung opacities relate to the patient's known surfactant deficiency. (Right) AP radiograph in this asthmatic child shows a continuous diaphragm sign ➡ due to pneumomediastinum. There is also pneumomediastinum adjacent to the aortic knob ➡. Subcutaneous emphysema is seen in the right neck ➡.

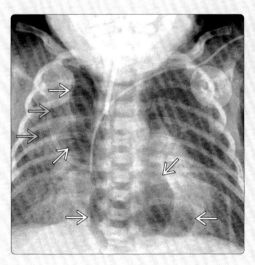

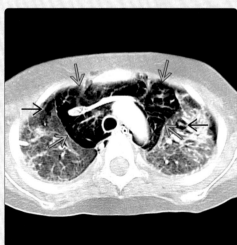

(Left) AP chest radiograph in this intubated neonate demonstrates a large amount of abnormal lucency ➡ throughout the mediastinum, consistent with pneumomediastinum. The thymic tissue ➡ is displaced to the right. (Right) Axial CECT (in lung windows) in a child with pulmonary interstitial emphysema ➡ shows extensive pneumomediastinum ➡.

TERMINOLOGY

- Not single disease; rather, umbrella term for numerous phenotypes in which normally harmless environmental allergens cause airway hyperresponsiveness due to pathologic immune-mediated host response
- Chronic airway hyperresponsiveness → contraction of bronchial wall smooth muscle & cascade of inflammation → acute, reversible airway narrowing & airflow obstruction

IMAGING

- Usually normal; may have symmetric hyperexpansion with flattened hemidiaphragms & ↑ retrosternal clear space
- Often unnecessary; helps exclude complications & mimics
- Consider chest radiographs if response to therapy poor

TOP DIFFERENTIAL DIAGNOSES

- Viral bronchiolitis
- Foreign body aspiration
- Cystic fibrosis

CLINICAL ISSUES

- Typical presentations
  - Chronic &/or recurrent cough, wheezing, shortness of breath, chest tightness, exercise limitation, use of accessory muscles to breathe at rest
  - ↓ peak expiratory flow rates & forced expiratory volume in 1-second (FEV₁) values
- Treatment
  - Avoidance of known precipitating environments
  - Inhaled β-agonists for bronchospasm
  - Inhaled & oral corticosteroids to ↓ inflammation
  - Inhaled mast cell stabilizers prevent release of mediators that cause airway inflammation & bronchospasm
- Prognosis
  - Intermittent wheezing before age 6 is usually benign & typically resolves within few years
  - Severity of asthma symptoms between ages of 7-10 years predicts persistence into adulthood

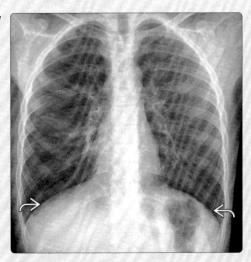
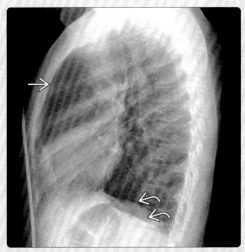

(Left) *AP chest radiograph in a 9-year-old boy with severe asthma who presented with respiratory distress & decreased breath sounds shows generalized lung hyperexpansion & flattening of the hemidiaphragms ➡ typical of air-trapping.* (Right) *Lateral radiograph from the same patient shows an enlarged retrosternal clear space ➡ & flattening of the hemidiaphragms ➡.*

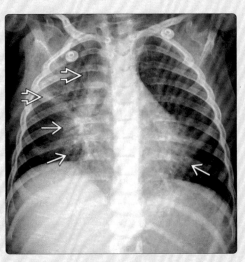
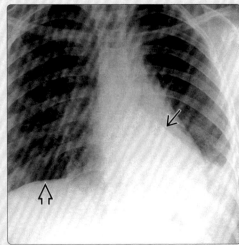

(Left) *Frontal radiograph in a young child with an acute asthma exacerbation shows an irregular cardiac contour ➡ & streaky right upper lobe opacities ➡ due to multifocal subsegmental atelectasis & peribronchial thickening.* (Right) *Frontal chest radiograph in an older child with asthma shows a triangular homogeneous opacity due to left lower lobe collapse ➡. There is loss of visualization of the left hemidiaphragm (as compared to the sharply defined right hemidiaphragm ➡).*

Asthma

TERMINOLOGY

Synonyms
- "Reactive airways disease" may be falling out of favor

Definitions
- Umbrella term for numerous phenotypes in which normally harmless environmental allergens cause airway hyperresponsiveness due to pathologic immune-mediated host response
- Airway hyperresponsiveness → contraction of bronchial wall smooth muscle & cascade of inflammation → acute, reversible airway narrowing & airflow obstruction

IMAGING

Radiographic Findings
- Not part of most acute childhood asthma algorithms; reserved for those with fever, suspected foreign body (FB) aspiration, failure to improve with treatment, or focal findings on physical exam
- Most common finding: Normal chest radiograph
- Next most common: Subtle & nonspecific signs of hyperinflation, usually symmetric
  - Flattening of hemidiaphragms
  - ↑ AP diameter of chest & retrosternal space
  - ± bulging intercostal spaces
- Less common findings
  - Peribronchial thickening/cuffing
  - Atelectasis
- Complications: More frequent in younger children (as smaller bronchi are more easily narrowed or occluded) & those with concurrent viral bronchiolitis
  - Barotrauma (pneumomediastinum, subcutaneous emphysema, & rarely pneumothorax)
  - Secondary allergic bronchopulmonary aspergillosis
  - Pneumonia

CT Findings
- HRCT
  - Generally not indicated, particularly in acute asthma

Imaging Recommendations
- Imaging generally not recommended except in
  - Febrile children (suspected complicating pneumonia)
  - Suspected FB aspiration
  - Those who fail to improve with treatment
  - Suspected barotrauma or lung collapse

DIFFERENTIAL DIAGNOSIS

Viral Bronchiolitis
- Often acts as precipitating trigger for asthma & may be impossible to differentiate radiographically or clinically

Foreign Body Inhalation or Ingestion
- Vast majority of aspirated FBs not radiopaque
- Stable air-trapping or collapse on serial radiographs, usually unilateral
- Static lung volumes on bilateral decubitus or inspiratory/expiratory imaging
- Persistent symptoms that do not respond to bronchodilator therapy

Cystic Fibrosis
- Early bronchial wall thickening that progresses to bronchiectasis
- Mucous plugging of dilated bronchi
- Focal disease most common in upper lobes

Ciliary Dyskinesias
- Situs inversus or dextrocardia (50%), paranasal sinusitis, & bronchiectasis
- Recurrent pneumonias

Pulmonary Sling
- Symptoms often present from birth
- No response to bronchodilator therapy
- Abnormal impression of left pulmonary artery coursing between trachea & esophagus

CLINICAL ISSUES

Presentation
- Most common signs/symptoms
  - Chronic &/or recurrent cough, wheezing, shortness of breath, chest tightness
- Other signs/symptoms
  - Exercise limitation
  - Use of accessory muscles to breathe at rest
  - ↓ peak expiratory flow rates & forced expiratory volume in 1-second (FEV₁) values
  - Improved symptoms with bronchodilator therapy

Demographics
- Most common chronic disease of childhood
  - Prevalence of 1-30% worldwide
  - Prevalence peak between 6-11 years
  - In USA, more common in African American & Hispanic children

Natural History & Prognosis
- Prognosis usually excellent with appropriate treatment
- Wheezing before age 6 often benign, usually resolves within few years
- Severity of asthma symptoms between ages of 7-10 years predictive of persistence into adulthood

Treatment
- Avoidance of known precipitating environments
- Inhaled β-agonists for bronchospasm
- Inhaled & oral corticosteroids to ↓ inflammatory response
- Inhaled mast cell stabilizers prevent release of mediators that cause airway inflammation & bronchospasm

SELECTED REFERENCES

1. Douglas LC et al: RAD: Reactive airways disease or really asthma disease? Pediatrics. 139(1), 2017
2. Narayanan S et al: Relevance of chest radiography in pediatric inpatients with asthma. J Asthma. 51(7):751-5, 2014
3. Szefler SJ et al: Asthma across the ages: knowledge gaps in childhood asthma. J Allergy Clin Immunol. 133(1):3-13; quiz 14, 2014
4. Ober C et al: The genetics of asthma and allergic disease: a 21st century perspective. Immunol Rev. 242(1):10-30, 2011
5. Bisgaard H et al: Long-term studies of the natural history of asthma in childhood. J Allergy Clin Immunol. 126(2):187-97; quiz 198-9, 2010
6. Bush A et al: Management of severe asthma in children. Lancet. 376(9743):814-25, 2010

Bronchial Foreign Body

KEY FACTS

TERMINOLOGY

- Complete or partial bronchial occlusion by aspirated foreign body (FB)

IMAGING

- Vast majority of aspirated FBs are **not** radiopaque
- Look for unilateral static lung volume on chest radiographs
  - In uncooperative patients (most common), obtain frontal view + bilateral decubitus images: Look for lack of passive deflation of dependent lung, suggesting air-trapping
  - In cooperative patients, frontal radiographs can be obtained at maximum inspiration & expiration: Look for static appearance on affected side
- Volume of affected lung segments can be normal, ↑, or ↓
- Consider CT with multiplanar reconstructions & 3D virtual bronchoscopy in cases with persistent clinical suspicion & negative chest radiographs

TOP DIFFERENTIAL DIAGNOSES

- Refractory asthma, viral lower respiratory tract infection, pulmonary sling

CLINICAL ISSUES

- Age: Most common at 1-3 years; peak at 18 months
- Aspiration often unwitnessed or not remembered until later: High degree of suspicion important
  - Delay in diagnosis associated with ↑ complication rate: Bronchopulmonary fistula, bronchial rupture, damage to distal lung, granuloma formation
- Presentation may be acute or delayed
  - Same day (25%): Wheezing, cough, ± fever
  - Days 2-7 (45%) or delayed by > 1 week (30%): Indolent cough, medically refractory wheezing, dyspnea
  - Complete obstruction: Atelectasis & collapse
  - Partial obstruction leads to "ball-valve" effect: Air-trapping & hyperinflation
- Treatment: Bronchoscopic removal of FB

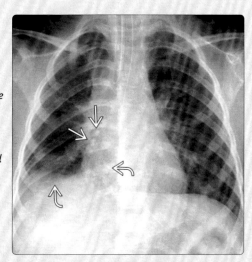

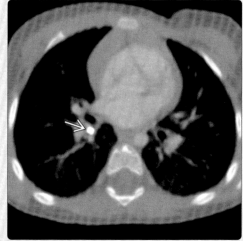

(Left) *Portable chest radiograph of a 3-year-old patient who aspirated glass fragments during a car crash shows 3 small radiopaque foreign bodies in the right lower lobe bronchus ➡. There is resulting airspace opacity ➡ as well as volume loss causing elevation of the right hemidiaphragm & slight mediastinal shift.* (Right) *Axial CECT in the same child shows a square-shaped radiopaque glass foreign body ➡ in a segmental bronchus of the right lower lobe.*

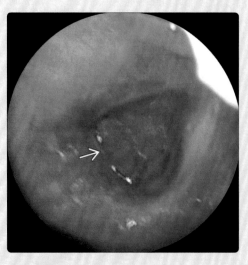

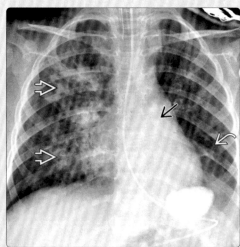

(Left) *Bronchoscopic image from the same patient shows complete occlusion of the segmental bronchus by glass fragments ➡.* (Right) *Frontal radiograph of a toddler found unconscious in a debris pile after a flood shows a small, well-defined opacity in the left main bronchus ➡. The left lower lobe is relatively hyperlucent due to air-trapping ➡, & there are widespread patchy opacities due to aspiration ➡. The bronchial obstruction was due to a small aspirated stone. (Gastric contrast was related to the tube placement.)*

TERMINOLOGY

Abbreviations

- Foreign body (FB), foreign body aspiration (FBA)

Definitions

- Complete or partial bronchial occlusion by aspirated FB

IMAGING

General Features

- Location: Most FBs lodge in main bronchi
  - Bronchial (76%), laryngeal (6%), tracheal (4%)
  - Right bronchi (58%) > left bronchi (42%)
    - Due to straighter course & larger caliber of right vs. left main bronchi

Radiographic Findings

- Best direct evidence: Radiopaque FB
  - However, most FBs are **not** radiopaque
- Best indirect evidence: Static unilateral lung volume on inspiration/expiration or bilateral decubitus imaging
- Volume of affected lung segments can be normal, ↑, or ↓ (i.e., larger lung not always abnormal)
  - Hyperinflation & oligemia from air-trapping
    - ± depressed hemidiaphragm, widening of intercostal spaces, contralateral mediastinal shift
  - Atelectasis from total bronchial obstruction, pneumonia from superinfection
    - ± elevation of hemidiaphragm, narrowing of intercostal spaces, ipsilateral mediastinal shift
- Pneumothorax & pneumomediastinum from tracheobronchial laceration or alveolar rupture
- Reported incidence of chest radiograph findings in FBA
  - Normal: 14-35%
  - Hyperinflation: 21-43%
  - Opacification/atelectasis: 18-29%
  - Mediastinal shift: 10-37%
  - Radiopaque FB: 3-23%
- Bilateral decubitus radiographs: Most appropriate maneuver for infants & toddlers
  - Normal, nonobstructed lung will become smaller & more opaque when dependent
  - Abnormal, obstructed lung will remain inflated & relatively lucent when dependent
- Inspiratory/expiratory radiographs: Requires cooperation
  - Volume of nonobstructed lung ↓ with expiration

CT Findings

- May be obtained for
  - Persistent lung collapse or pneumonia
  - Work-up of suspected extrinsic airway compression
- Some advocate CT with multiplanar reconstructions & 3D virtual bronchoscopy in cases with persistent clinical suspicion & negative chest radiograph
  - May see FB as filling defect in bronchus ± focal hyperinflation or atelectasis

Imaging Recommendations

- Best imaging tool: Chest radiographs
- Protocol advice: Normal inspiratory chest radiograph alone does not exclude aspirated FB

DIFFERENTIAL DIAGNOSIS

Viral Lower Respiratory Tract Infection

- Much more common than FB
- ↑ peribronchial markings + symmetric hyperinflation

Refractory Asthma

- Much more common than FB
- ↑ peribronchial markings + symmetric hyperinflation

Pulmonary Sling

- Chronic; often presents at birth
- Often associated with other congenital heart disease & complete tracheal rings

Extrinsic Tracheal Compression by Mass

- Bronchogenic cysts, lymphadenopathy, & other masses may compress bronchi & present with asymmetric aeration

PATHOLOGY

Gross Pathologic & Surgical Features

- Most FBs organic or plastic & therefore radiolucent
- FB lodged in tracheobronchial tree
  - Dried foods absorb water & may swell
  - Peanuts & tree nuts elicit most airway irritation
  - Leukocyte infiltration & edema in bronchial wall
  - Chronic FB leads to granuloma formation
- May have "ball valve" effect leading to
  - Air-trapping & hyperinflation
  - Complete obstruction leading to atelectasis & collapse

CLINICAL ISSUES

Presentation

- Most common signs/symptoms
  - FBA may present acutely or in delayed fashion; event often unwitnessed or not remembered until later
    - Same day (25%): Wheezing, cough, ± fever
    - Days 2-7 (45%): Indolent cough, medically refractory wheezing, dyspnea
    - Delayed by > 1 week (30%): Same as above
  - High degree of suspicion important

Demographics

- Age: Most common at 1-3 years; peak: 18 months

Natural History & Prognosis

- Delay in diagnosis → ↑ risk of major complications
  - Complications: 4% if > 4 days, 91% if > 30 days
    - Bronchopulmonary fistula, bronchial rupture, damage to distal lung
- Death rare, ~ 100 per year in USA

Treatment

- Endobronchial removal of FB

SELECTED REFERENCES

1. Adramerina A et al: How parents' lack of awareness could be associated with foreign body aspiration in children. Pediatr Emerg Care. 32(2):98-100, 2016
2. Salih AM et al: Airway foreign bodies: a critical review for a common pediatric emergency. World J Emerg Med. 7(1):5-12, 2016
3. Darras KE et al: Imaging acute airway obstruction in infants and children. Radiographics. 35(7):2064-79, 2015

Cystic Fibrosis, Pulmonary

TERMINOLOGY

- Autosomal recessive multisystem disorder caused by dysfunctional chloride ion transport across epithelial surfaces → thickening of secretions (e.g., mucus, digestive fluids, sweat)
- In lungs, abnormal mucus & degraded WBCs → chronic airway impaction → recurrent inflammation & infections → chronic airway damage (in progressively worsening cycle)

IMAGING

- Most common in upper lobes, superior lower lobes
  - Peribronchial thickening (early finding)
  - Mosaic attenuation due to air-trapping, best seen on expiratory CT
  - Bronchiectasis with signet ring sign (bronchus larger than adjacent artery)
  - Mucus plugging within dilated bronchi (finger-in-glove appearance)
  - Tree-in-bud centrilobular nodular opacities on CT

PATHOLOGY

- Most common lethal genetic disorder in Caucasians
  - ~ 1 in 2,500 affected
- Mutation in both copies of CF transmembrane conductance regulator (*CFTR*) gene at chromosome 7q31.2 → defective chloride transport → abnormal water regulation
- > 1,000 genetic defects can result in CF; ΔF508 mutation of *CFTR* most common (~ 90%)

CLINICAL ISSUES

- 70% present < 1 year of age: GI symptoms more common
- 90% by 12 years of age: Respiratory more typical
  - Often have asthma-type symptoms
- Median survival: 41.1 years

DIAGNOSTIC CHECKLIST

- Annual chest radiograph or low-dose surveillance CT
  - CT best assesses progressive disease & predicts future exacerbations vs. pulmonary function tests, radiographs

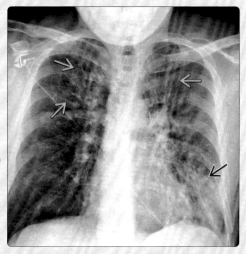
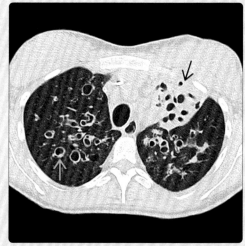

(Left) Frontal radiograph in a patient with cystic fibrosis (CF) shows prominent bronchiectasis ⇨ in the upper lobes + left lower lobe consolidation with nodularity ⇨. (Right) Axial NECT in a CF patient shows bilateral upper lobe bronchiectasis with consolidation ⇨ of the anterior segment of the left upper lobe. Note the signet ring sign (or pearl ring sign) ⇨ in the right upper lobe with the dilated bronchus forming the ring & the adjacent artery forming the attached jewel.

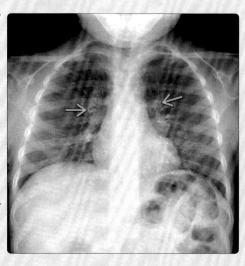
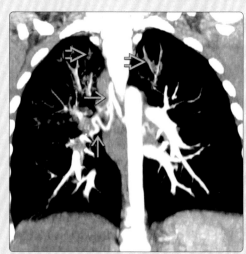

(Left) Frontal radiograph in a 7 year old with CF shows mild peribronchial thickening in the perihilar regions ⇨, an early finding of CF that is indistinguishable from common viral bronchiolitis. (Right) Coronal CTA in a 12-year-old CF patient with hemoptysis shows an enlarged right bronchial artery ⇨. Evaluation of the more distal branches & adjacent parenchyma (for alveolar hemorrhage & extravasation) may help localize the source of bleeding. There is also upper lobe bronchiectasis & mucus plugging bilaterally ⇨.

TERMINOLOGY

Definitions

- Cystic fibrosis (CF): Autosomal recessive multisystem disorder caused by dysfunctional chloride ion transport across epithelial surfaces → thickening of secretions (e.g., mucus, digestive fluids, sweat)

IMAGING

General Features

- Best diagnostic clue
  - Upper lobe predominant bronchiectasis & bronchial wall thickening with respiratory (± gastrointestinal) symptoms
- Location
  - In lungs, more common in upper lobes & superior segments of lower lobes
  - Also affects sinuses, pancreas, hepatobiliary system, GI tract, & sex organs

Radiographic Findings

- Radiographs insensitive to early changes of CF
- Late changes on radiographs include bronchiectasis, bronchial wall thickening, mucoid impaction, hyperinflation, lobar collapse, & pulmonary arterial enlargement due to pulmonary artery hypertension

CT Findings

- HRCT
  - Peribronchial thickening (early finding)
  - Bronchiectasis with signet ring sign
    - Ectatic bronchus > adjacent pulmonary artery
  - Mosaic attenuation due to air-trapping, best seen on expiratory scan
  - Tree-in-bud centrilobular nodular opacities
    - Bronchiolar impaction of mucus &/or infectious/inflammatory debris
  - Finger-in-glove appearance of mucus plugging within dilated bronchi
- CTA
  - ± bronchial artery hypertrophy &/or aberrant/collateral arterial supply in setting of hemoptysis

Imaging Recommendations

- Best imaging tool
  - High-resolution CT with full inspiration & expiration

PATHOLOGY

General Features

- Mutation in both copies of CF transmembrane conductance regulator gene (CFTR) at chromosome 7q31.2
  - > 1,000 genetic defects can result in CF; ΔF508 mutation most common (~ 90%)
- CFTR protein malfunction → lack of chloride ion secretion → ↑ sodium retention & fluid resorption → ↑ viscosity of luminal secretions → obstruction of ducts of solid organs & hollow viscera
- In lungs, abnormal mucus & WBC degradation products (including DNA) → stasis in airways → recurrent infection & inflammation → chronic airway damage with worsening susceptibility to infection & inflammation

CLINICAL ISSUES

Presentation

- Most common signs/symptoms
  - 1st symptoms may be delayed passage of meconium with bowel obstruction in newborn with meconium Ileus
  - In childhood, patients often look similar to asthma patients, presenting with chronic cough & wheezing
- Other signs/symptoms
  - Chronic constipation, recurrent pancreatitis, hepatobiliary disease
- Clinical profile
  - Most now detected on neonatal screening
  - After symptom development, testing by sweat chloride (> 60 mEq/mL = + for CF)

Demographics

- Age
  - 70% present < 1 year: GI symptoms more common
  - 90% by 12 years: Respiratory more typical
- Epidemiology
  - Most common lethal gene defect in Caucasians (1 in 2,500 affected)
    - Much less common with African or Asian ancestry

Natural History & Prognosis

- Infancy: Often only mild or absent pulmonary symptoms
- Early childhood: Present similar to asthma patients with cough, wheezing, & bronchitis
- Late childhood & adolescence: Recurrent pneumonias, bronchitis, & bronchiectasis with mucus plugging
- End-stage lung disease occurs at variable ages but often in late adolescence to early adulthood
- Exact timing of progression in CF unpredictable
- Median survival: 41.1 years

Treatment

- Goal: ↓ lung damage from mucus plugging & infection
- Various internal & external airway clearance techniques
- Prophylactic antibiotics to ↓ chance of infection
- ± long-term IV (Port-a-Cath) for recurrent lung infections
- New medicines targeted at specific CFTR mutations
- ± lobectomy for patients with single lobe complications
- End-stage lung disease may require lung transplantation

DIAGNOSTIC CHECKLIST

Consider

- Annual chest radiograph or low-dose CT surveillance of bronchiectasis complications
- Pulmonary MR showing promise for future utility

Image Interpretation Pearls

- CT more accurate in assessing progressive lung disease than pulmonary function tests or radiographs
- CT improves with treatment of acute exacerbations

SELECTED REFERENCES

1. Murphy KP et al: Imaging of cystic fibrosis and pediatric bronchiectasis. AJR Am J Roentgenol. 206(3):448-54, 2016
2. Sanders DB et al: Chest computed tomography predicts the frequency of pulmonary exacerbations in children with cystic fibrosis. Ann Am Thorac Soc. 12(1):64-9, 2015

Sickle Cell Disease, Acute Chest Syndrome

TERMINOLOGY

- New pulmonary opacity on chest radiograph + ≥ 1 additional symptom (such as fever, cough, sputum production, tachypnea, dyspnea, or hypoxia) in setting of sickle cell disease (SCD)

IMAGING

- Upper & middle lobe opacities more common in children
- Lower lobe disease more common in adults
- Initial chest radiograph may be normal (46%)
  - Opacity may not appear until 2-3 days after symptoms develop
- Opacities on CT may be more extensive than on radiograph

PATHOLOGY

- Potential causes: Infection (30%), pulmonary fat embolism (9%), pulmonary infarction (18%), & rib infarction

CLINICAL ISSUES

- Acute chest syndrome (ACS) most common in patients aged 2-4 years; incidence ↓ with age
  - Fever, cough, & tachypnea most common symptoms in patients < 10 years of age
  - Pain (chest, extremity, abdominal) more common in adolescents & adults
  - Risk factors: Asthma, smoking, abdominal surgery, trauma
- ACS 2nd most common cause of hospitalization in patients with SCD after pain crisis
- ACS most common cause of premature death in patients with SCD
  - Mortality 4-9x higher in adults than in children
- Treatment
  - Supportive: Oxygen, antibiotics, pain control, IV fluids, incentive spirometry, & blood transfusions
  - Prevention: Pneumococcal vaccine, *Haemophilus influenzae* vaccine, & hydroxyurea

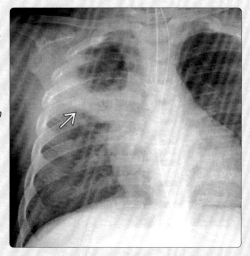
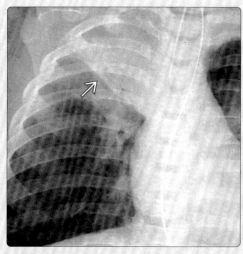

(Left) *AP radiograph of the chest shows an opacity in the right upper lobe* ➡ *in a 1 year old with sickle cell disease presenting with fever & dyspnea.* (Right) *AP radiograph of the chest in the same patient 12 hours later shows worsening opacification & volume loss of the right upper lobe* ➡. *Acute chest syndrome is defined as a new pulmonary opacity in a symptomatic patient with sickle cell disease. In children, it occurs more commonly in the upper & middle lobes.*

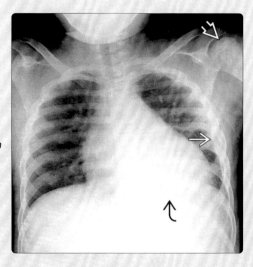
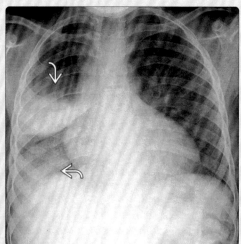

(Left) *AP radiograph shows common thoracic findings in sickle cell disease: Cardiomegaly, a left lower lobe opacity* ➡, *& a pleural effusion* ➡. *Note the avascular necrosis in the left humeral head* ➡. (Right) *AP radiograph shows multifocal right lung opacities* ➡ *in this sickle cell disease patient with respiratory distress & fever, consistent with acute chest syndrome. Note the cardiomegaly.*

TERMINOLOGY

Definitions

- New pulmonary opacity on chest radiograph + ≥ 1 additional symptom (such as fever, cough, sputum production, tachypnea, dyspnea, or hypoxia) in setting of sickle cell disease (SCD)

IMAGING

Radiographic Findings

- Acute chest syndrome (ACS)
  - Initial chest radiograph may be normal (46%)
    - Radiograph lags behind physiological changes
    - Opacity may not appear until 2-3 days after symptoms
  - Opacity mimics pneumonia ± volume loss
  - Pleural effusions present in > 50% of patients
- Other findings of SCD
  - Cardiomegaly due to chronic anemia
  - Avascular necrosis of humeral heads
  - H-shaped or biconcave vertebrae
  - Enlarged ribs due to marrow expansion
  - Small spleen (autosplenectomy) identified by lateralization of stomach bubble
  - Cholecystectomy clips in right upper quadrant

CT Findings

- CTA
  - Pulmonary embolism 3rd most common cause of ACS
    - Accounts for 16-17% of ACS episodes
    - Occurs in segmental/subsegmental pulmonary arteries
    - No associated lower extremity deep vein thrombosis

Nuclear Medicine Findings

- Bone scan
  - Foci of abnormal radiotracer uptake in ribs
    - ↓ or ↑ uptake: Acute or subacute bone infarcts
  - May have other bone infarcts vs. osteomyelitis

PATHOLOGY

General Features

- Etiology
  - Infection in 38-54% of ACS
    - Most common pathogens: *Chlamydia pneumoniae*, *Mycoplasma pneumoniae*, RSV
    - Pulmonary opacity persists longer than cases where infection not documented
  - Pulmonary fat embolism in 9-16% of ACS
    - Etiology: Vasoocclusive crisis → edema & infarction of marrow compartment → marrow necrosis → fat cells enter venous bloodstream → embolize in branches of pulmonary artery
    - Frequently have bone pain
    - Lab findings: Thrombocytopenia, anemia; ↑ LDH, lipase, phospholipase A2, & uric acid; ↓ serum calcium
  - Pulmonary infarction in 16-17% of ACS
    - Occurs in segmental & subsegmental pulmonary arteries
    - No associated lower extremity deep vein thrombosis suggests in situ thrombosis
  - Rib infarction with hypoventilation from pain &/or analgesics
    - High correlation between rib infarction & pulmonary opacity
    - Pain may lead to splinting & atelectasis
    - Incentive spirometry helps prevent pulmonary complications of ACS
    - Analgesics may ↓ splinting but may cause hypoventilation

CLINICAL ISSUES

Presentation

- Most common signs/symptoms
  - Fever, cough, & tachypnea most common in patients < 10 years of age
  - Pain (chest, extremity, abdominal) more common in adolescents & adults

Demographics

- Age
  - Most common in patients aged 2-4 years
  - Lower incidence in patients < 2 years due to higher fetal hemoglobin concentrations
  - Incidence gradually declines with age
    - Excess mortality in group with ACS
    - Fewer viral illnesses due to acquired immunity
- Ethnicity
  - In USA, almost exclusively seen in African Americans
- Epidemiology
  - Overall incidence of 12.8 episodes per 100 patient-years
  - ACS most common cause of premature death in patients with SCD
  - ACS 2nd most common cause of hospitalization in patients with SCD after pain crisis
    - ~ 50% admitted with diagnosis other than ACS
    - Diagnosed with ACS 2-3 days after admission

Natural History & Prognosis

- More severe in patients > 20 years
  - Mortality 4-9x higher in adults than in children
- Features associated with poor prognosis
  - Physical exam: Altered mental status, tachycardia > 125 beats/minute, tachypnea > 30 breaths/minute, temperature > 40°C, hypotension
  - Lab findings: Arterial pH < 7.35, O_2 saturation < 88%, hemoglobin concentration ↓ by ≥ 2 g/dL, platelet count < 200,000, multiorgan failure
- Risk factors: Asthma, smoking, abdominal surgery, trauma

Treatment

- Supportive: Oxygen, antibiotics, pain control, IV fluids, incentive spirometry, & blood transfusions
- Prevention: Pneumococcal & *Haemophilus influenzae* vaccinations, hydroxyurea, transfusion therapy

SELECTED REFERENCES

1. Knight-Madden J et al: Acute pulmonary complications of sickle cell disease. Paediatr Respir Rev. 15(1):13-6, 2014
2. Abbas HA et al: A review of acute chest syndrome in pediatric sickle cell disease. Pediatr Ann. 42(3):115-20, 2013
3. Desai PC et al: The acute chest syndrome of sickle cell disease. Expert Opin Pharmacother. 14(8):991-9, 2013

Pectus Excavatum

TERMINOLOGY

- Pectus excavatum: Depression of sternum posteriorly → sunken appearance of midline anterior inferior chest wall
- Nuss procedure: Minimally invasive pectus repair
  - Transverse curved metal bar surgically inserted deep to sternum & ribs

IMAGING

- Radiographs: Right heart border blurring with vertical anterior ribs; degree of depression best seen on lateral view
- Pre-Nuss procedure evaluation with CT/MR
  - Haller index
    - Ratio of transverse (left-right) diameter divided by sagittal (anterior-posterior) diameter of chest
    - Haller index > 3.25 considered enough deformity for surgical candidacy (by most insurance agencies)
  - MR: Single cardiac MR can replace echocardiogram & CT
    - ± ↓ right ventricular ejection fraction & hemodynamically insignificant pericardial effusion

- Post Nuss procedure
  - Assess for complications → bar displacement/rotation, pneumothorax, pleural effusion, sternal infection

CLINICAL ISSUES

- Concerns about physical appearance common
- Exercise intolerance (82%), chest pain (68%), poor endurance (67%), shortness of breath (42%)
- Palpable bony asymmetry associated with mild pectus deformity may be mistaken for soft tissue mass
- Less common symptoms include cardiac (pulmonic murmur, mitral valve prolapse, syncope, Wolff-Parkinson-White syndrome), restrictive lung disease, central airway compression
- Treated conservatively unless symptomatic
- Surgical treatment with Nuss procedure provides excellent results in > 85% of patients

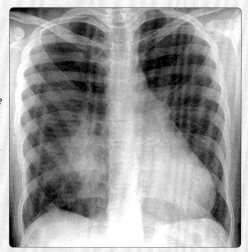

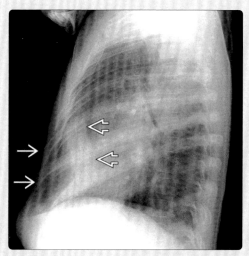

(Left) *AP radiograph shows a silhouette sign with an apparent opacity obscuring the right heart border (mimicking middle lobe disease). Note the vertically oriented anterior ribs.* (Right) *Lateral radiograph in the same patient shows posterior positioning of the sternum ➡ as compared to the anterior ribs ➡, consistent with pectus excavatum. There is no middle lobe pathology.*

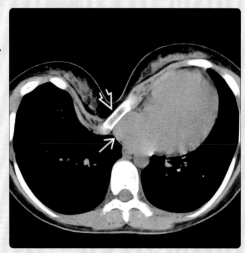

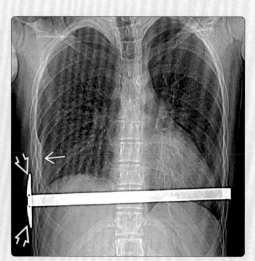

(Left) *Axial NECT of the chest shows marked pectus excavatum with posterior displacement & rotation of the sternum ➡ as compared with the anterior chest wall. Note the position of the right atrium ➡ immediately behind the sternum.* (Right) *Scout CT image after a Nuss procedure shows the transverse metal bar with a T-shaped stabilization device ➡ at one end. Note the small right pleural effusion ➡. No pneumothorax is seen.*

Askin Tumor/Ewing Sarcoma of Chest Wall

KEY FACTS

TERMINOLOGY

- Askin tumor: Extraskeletal Ewing sarcoma of chest
  - Part of Ewing sarcoma family of tumors

IMAGING

- Unilateral thoracic opacification
  - Large, lobular mass may occupy much of hemithorax, often with pleural effusion
- Rib destruction common (> 50%)
- Mass effect on mediastinal structures: Displacement rather than encasement or invasion of vessels, airway
- Mediastinal lymphadenopathy: 25% at presentation
- Pulmonary metastasis: 38% at presentation
- CT & MR can be complimentary
  - CT better detects small pulmonary metastases
  - MR better evaluates involvement of chest wall
- PET/CT: Useful in staging
  - ↑ metabolic activity in primary tumor & metastases

TOP DIFFERENTIAL DIAGNOSES

- Round pneumonia
- Other malignancies: Lymphoma, neuroblastoma, neural tumors, germ cell tumor, rhabdomyosarcoma

PATHOLOGY

- Classically arises in chest wall soft tissues; less commonly from bone or periphery of lung
- Small round blue cells identical to other Ewing sarcomas
  - Positive immunohistochemical stain for *MIC2* gene product (CD99): 90%
  - Classic chromosomal translocation of t[11;22][q24;q12]: 85-95%

CLINICAL ISSUES

- Large pleural-based mass ± pain, fever, anorexia, weight loss, shortness of breath
- Median age: 14.5 years (range: 4 months to 20 years)
- Poor prognosis: Recurrence > 50%; 6-year survival of 14%

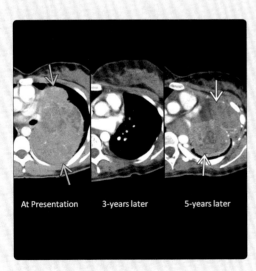
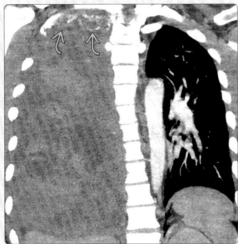

(Left) PA radiograph shows a 15-year-old girl with a chest wall Ewing sarcoma. There is complete opacification of the right hemithorax with mass effect on the mediastinum ➡. Note the lucency, expansion, permeation, & erosion of the right 2nd rib ➡. (Right) Coronal CECT in the same patient shows a heterogeneous mass occupying the right hemithorax. There is expansion & destruction of the right 2nd rib ➡.

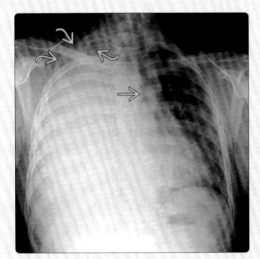
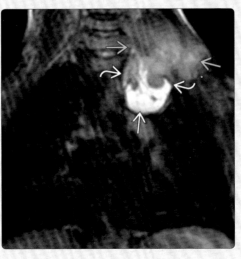

At Presentation   3-years later   5-years later

(Left) Initial axial CECT of a girl with an Askin tumor at presentation (L) shows a large heterogeneous mass in the left upper hemithorax ➡. After chemotherapy, resection, & radiation, no tumor was detectable on the 3-year follow-up CT (M). Tumor recurrence is present at 5 years ➡ (R). (Right) Coronal T2 FS MR shows a 3-year-old patient with an Askin tumor. A heterogeneous mass in the left upper hemithorax ➡ appears partly cystic ➡ & extends into the soft tissues of the left lower neck ➡.

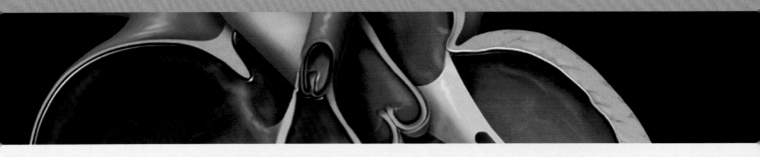

SECTION 3
Cardiac

Imaging Modalities

Radiography

The days in which congenital heart disease (CHD) was characterized by chest radiography & defined by angiography are gone. Both still play some role in the diagnosis & management of CHD. However, with echocardiography & cardiac MR & CT, we now have robust imaging modalities that can provide detailed anatomic & functional evaluation in patients with complex cardiovascular issues.

The chest radiograph still retains value in separating patient presentations into cardiac vs. pulmonary etiologies. Patients with signs & symptoms suspected to be of cardiovascular origin (such as chest pain, syncope, shortness of breath, or cyanosis) should undergo chest radiography as an initial imaging study, typically in conjunction with electrocardiography & possibly laboratory markers of cardiac pathology.

Several fundamental assessments of the cardiovascular system must be made on the initial chest radiograph, including the size & orientation of the heart, the complement of pulmonary vascularity, & the position of the trachea & aortic arch.

Cardiac size is best evaluated on an upright view of the chest with full inspiration, though this is often not possible in the uncooperative or unstable patient. With ideal parameters, the cardiothoracic ratio (or widest transverse dimension of the heart relative to the widest transverse dimension of the chest on a frontal view) should be less than 50% for most of childhood. During infancy, accounting for the likelihood of a supine image obtained in expiration, the cardiothoracic ratio can be up to 70%. It should be noted that thymic size, which can be relatively large in the infant, may affect the assessment of the heart size. Additionally, the "cardiac size" actually reflects the contents of the pericardial sac, such that a pericardial effusion can cause enlargement of the heart shadow without true cardiomegaly. As these structures may be inseparable radiographically, the term "cardiomediastinal" or "cardiothymic silhouette" may be used to reflect the central chest anatomy.

An assessment of the orientation of the heart is also required. The cardiac apex should be left-sided, though it can be deviated by thoracic pathologies pushing or pulling it to one side (such as a congenital diaphragmatic hernia shifting the mediastinum into the contralateral hemithorax & rotating the heart). Additionally, the stomach bubble (which is typically visible on a chest radiograph) should be on the same side as the cardiac apex; opposite positions indicate a disorder of situs (heterotaxy) that has a high association with CHD.

Alterations in cardiac morphology can be difficult to discern due to variations in thymic size & shape. Additionally, recognition of radiographic patterns of chamber & vessel enlargement (or even absence) requires experience &, at best, lacks sensitivity & specificity in many instances.

Increased vascular flow may be detected radiographically, though increased arterial flow (from a cardiac shunt) may not be distinguishable from increased pulmonary venous congestion (as seen with heart failure). In some circumstances, both patterns may be present.

Abnormalities of aortic arch position can often be detected with careful radiographic assessment. The aortic knob should mildly indent the left aspect of the mid to distal trachea & shift the airway slightly to the right. Alterations may indicate a right-sided or double aortic arch that can cause airway problems &/or be associated with underlying CHD.

Other Modalities

The next imaging step in patients with suspected heart disease is usually echocardiography, though this is typically performed in consultation with the cardiologist. (Very limited cardiac ultrasound, such as to detect pericardial fluid in the emergent setting, may be used by other practitioners in some circumstances.)

The routine congenital heart patient with a simple lesion (such as an atrial or ventricular septal defect) would likely never undergo cardiac CT or MR as echocardiography provides excellent delineation of the intracardiac anatomy, great artery relationships, & function of the heart. Cardiac CT & MR are generally reserved for problem solving in difficult echocardiography cases. CT & MR are frequently done to evaluate the pulmonary veins, pulmonary arteries, systemic veins, & aorta as the extracardiac anatomy can be difficult to completely evaluate by echocardiography. Heterotaxy patients also often have abnormalities involving the extracardiac anatomy & airways & may routinely undergo cardiac CT or MR.

Basic functional evaluation of the heart can be performed by both CT & MR cardiac exams, including calculating the volumes & ejection fractions of both ventricles, left ventricular muscle mass, & regurgitant fractions across valves.

3D images of the heart can be segmented & exported to 3D printers to create physical models of the heart. These models can be used in educating parents, patients, & other health professionals. Additionally, patient-specific models can be used in presurgical planning to test devices on the patient's anatomy before performing the actual procedure. This method has proven effective in decreasing procedure times.

With regards to choosing cardiac CT or MR, several factors should be considered. With higher temporal resolution, cardiac MR is superior to cardiac CT for functional imaging of the heart & evaluation of intracardiac anatomy. With higher spatial resolution, cardiac CT is superior to MR for extracardiac anatomy as well as airway & coronary artery evaluation. However, there is significant overlap between the 2 modalities. As with other regions of the body, cardiac MR requires longer sedation times than CT, & cardiac CT exposes the patient to ionizing radiation.

Selected References

1. Cantinotti M et al: Three-dimensional printed models in congenital heart disease. Int J Cardiovasc Imaging. 33(1):137-144, 2017
2. Rajiah P et al: Update on the role of cardiac magnetic resonance imaging in congenital heart disease. Curr Treat Options Cardiovasc Med. 19(1):2, 2017
3. Dacher JN et al: CT and MR imaging in congenital cardiac malformations: Where do we come from and where are we going? Diagn Interv Imaging. 97(5):505-12, 2016
4. Lapierre C et al: Segmental approach to imaging of congenital heart disease. Radiographics. 30(2):397-411, 2010

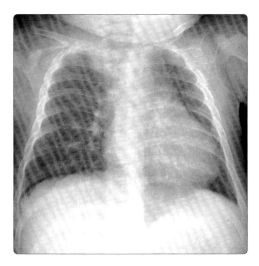

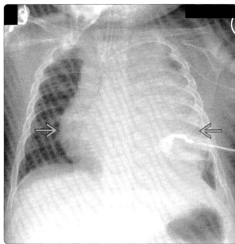

(Left) *Frontal radiograph in a 9 month old with fever & bacteremia shows a normal size, orientation, & morphology to the cardiac silhouette for a supine infant. The pulmonary vascularity is within normal limits.* (Right) *Frontal radiograph in the same patient 5 days later shows marked interval enlargement of the cardiac silhouette ⇨ due to a large pericardial effusion (which was confirmed with echocardiography & subsequently drained).*

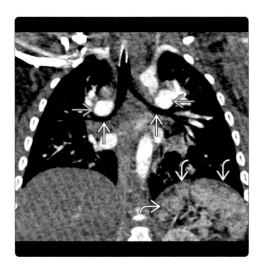

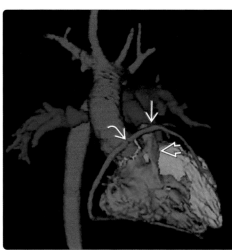

(Left) *Coronal cardiac CTA image shows bilateral left-sided bronchial morphologies ⇨ & pulmonary artery positions ⇨ with multiple spleens ⇨ in this patient with the polysplenia form of heterotaxy.* (Right) *Anterior 3D color-coded cardiac CTA in a patient with tetralogy of Fallot (TOF) shows the left coronary artery ⇨ arising from the right coronary sinus ⇨ & passing anterior to the right ventricular outflow tract (RVOT). Notice the infundibular narrowing ⇨ of the RVOT. These features are common in TOF.*

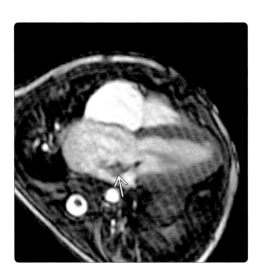

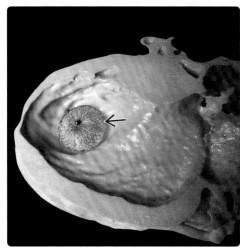

(Left) *Single image from a 4-chamber view SSFP cine cardiac MR shows dephasing artifact ⇨ directed back into the left atrium from the mitral valve in this patient with mitral regurgitation.* (Right) *Resin 3D-printed model looking from within the left ventricle at the interventricular septum shows placement of a closure device ⇨ within an intramuscular ventricular septal defect. This 3D printing was performed for procedural planning.*

Atrial Septal Defect

TERMINOLOGY

- ASD: Defect(s) in cardiac atrial septum; may be isolated anomaly or associated with other congenital heart lesions
- L → R shunt: Blood from left heart bypasses systemic circulation to enter right heart
  - Most ASD sequelae related to long-term L → R shunting
- Types of ASD
  - L → R shunts: Ostium secundum (70-90%), ostium primum, sinus venosus, unroofed coronary sinus defects
  - Patent foramen ovale only allows R → L shunting, usually transient given normal atrial pressures
    - Increased stroke risk; unclear migraine association

IMAGING

- L → R shunting leads to chronic volume overload of right heart, eventual enlargement of RA, RV, & PA
  - Secondary findings & symptoms uncommon in children
- Diagnosis primarily made by echocardiography
- Cardiac MR can depict function, flow, & anatomy

CLINICAL ISSUES

- ASD: 10% of congenital heart disease (CHD) in children, yet 30% of CHD in adults
- Secundum ASD: Majority of patients asymptomatic; detected due to murmur or other medical work-up
  - Spontaneous closure occurs in many children
  - Rarely presents in childhood with failure to thrive, respiratory infection, tachypnea
  - Subtle symptoms more likely in 2nd decade, though large defects frequently do not present until adulthood
    - Fatigue, exercise intolerance, syncope, shortness of breath, palpitations
    - ASD leading to severe pulmonary hypertension: Median age of detection is 51 years
  - Repair indicated if shunt ratio > 1.5:1 or defect > 10 mm
    - Percutaneous closure with occlusion device
- Primum/atrioventricular septal defect more severe; requires early surgical repair
- Sinus venosus ASDs require surgery for complex anatomy

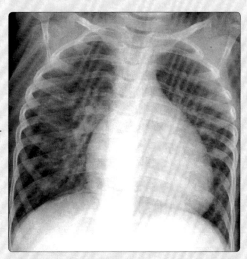
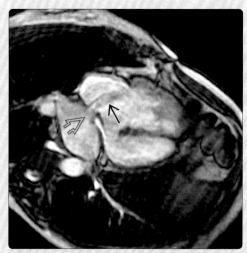

(Left) Single frontal chest radiograph in a 4-year-old child demonstrates cardiomegaly & increased pulmonary vascularity. The patient had a large, untreated atrial septal defect (ASD). (Right) Four-chamber view from an SSFP (bright blood) cardiac MR shows a secundum-type defect of the atrial septum ➡. Note the L → R flow across the ASD causing dephasing artifact ➡ in the right atrium (RA).

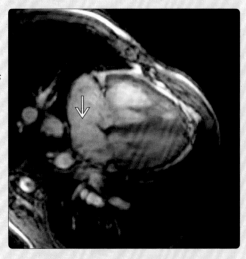
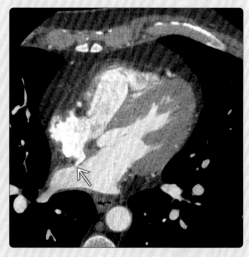

(Left) Four-chamber view from an SSFP (bright blood) cardiac MR shows a sinus venosus ASD with the defect in the superolateral aspect of the atrial septum ➡. This defect is nearly always associated with right upper lobe partial anomalous pulmonary venous return. (Right) Axial image from a coronary CTA shows a patent foramen ovale ➡ with a typical oblique defect & flap in the atrial septum. This is seen in 25% of the population. Note that the size of the RA is normal as L → R shunting does not occur.

Ventricular Septal Defect

TERMINOLOGY

- Cardiac anomaly with communication(s) between left & right ventricles through septum
  - Perimembranous septal defect (80%)
  - Posterior or inlet defect associated with atrioventricular septal defect (8-10%)
  - Muscular or trabecular septal defect (5-10%)
  - Outlet septal defect or supracristal ventricular septal defect (VSD) (5%)
- Complex cardiac anomalies with VSD: TOF, truncus, DORV

IMAGING

- Cardiomegaly with ↑ size of main pulmonary artery, ↑ pulmonary artery flow, left atrial enlargement, & usually small aorta
- Hyperinflation in large shunts from abnormal lung compliance & bronchial compression by dilated pulmonary arteries
- Echo, CT, & MR delineate anatomy

- Multiple muscular VSDs: "Swiss cheese" septum
- Shunt volume estimated by velocity encoded cine MR imaging

TOP DIFFERENTIAL DIAGNOSES

- Atrioventricular canal defects
- Patent ductus arteriosus
- Double outlet right ventricle

CLINICAL ISSUES

- Small VSD: Children asymptomatic but have heart murmur
  - May close spontaneously
- Moderate or large shunts often asymptomatic early until pulmonary vascular resistance drops
  - Children develop tachypnea, tachycardia, diaphoresis, & failure to thrive
  - Treated medically with subsequent surgical approach
    - Muscular lesions require more difficult surgical approach; VSD catheter closure devices often used

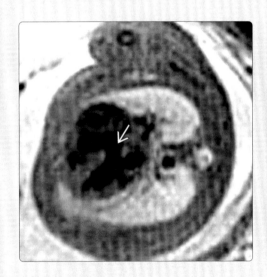
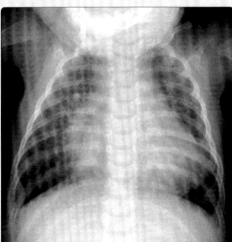

(Left) Axial SSFSE T2 fetal MR shows a perimembranous-type ventricular septal defect (VSD) ➡ in this fetus with tetralogy of Fallot. (Right) AP radiograph of a 2 month old shows cardiomegaly & increased pulmonary vascularity. This patient had multiple muscular-type VSDs.

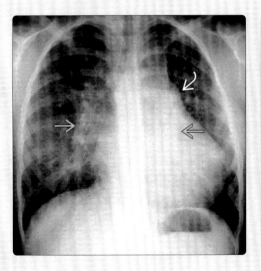
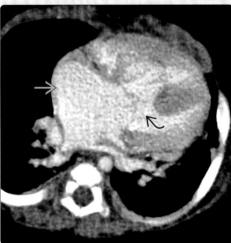

(Left) AP radiograph shows an elevated (or upturned) apex of the heart. The branch pulmonary arteries (PAs) are enlarged ➡. There is a convex main PA segment ➡ with pruning of peripheral vessels in this patient who had an unrepaired large VSD & pulmonary hypertension. (Right) Axial CTA shows marked right atrial enlargement ➡ in a young patient with a VSD ➡.

Atrioventricular Septal Defect

TERMINOLOGY

- Atrioventricular septal defect: Complete atrioventricular canal (AVC) defect, endocardial cushion defect
- Broad spectrum of defects characterized by involvement of atrial septum, ventricular septum, & 1 or both atrioventricular valves
- Ostium primum defect: Partial AVC defect or partial atrioventricular septal defect

IMAGING

- Large right atrium, right ventricle, & pulmonary artery with ↑ pulmonary artery flow
- Large defect in anterior inferior portion of atrial septum (ostium primum defect)
- Large defect in ventricular septum (posterior type most common)
- Anterior & superior aortic position with elongation + dysplastic common 5-leaflet AV valve narrowing subvalvular LVOT → "gooseneck" deformity on angiography

- When AV valve opens toward 1 ventricle → unbalanced canal defect (right ventricular or left ventricular dominance can occur with single ventricle physiology)
- Pulmonary hypertension patients have abnormal lung compliance: Lungs often hyperinflated
- Mitral insufficiency may occur both pre- & postoperatively

CLINICAL ISSUES

- Presentation
  - Large shunts → tachypnea, tachycardia, & failure to thrive
  - Small shunts may be asymptomatic & well tolerated through 1st decade
  - Mitral insufficiency adds complexity & earlier symptoms
- Associations: Trisomy 21, heterotaxy, tetralogy of Fallot
- Treatment: Medical management until surgery (depending on lesion & severity)
  - Partial AVC closed by pericardial patch
  - Single ventricle physiology may necessitate staged procedure (e.g., Glenn → Fontan for unbalanced AVC)

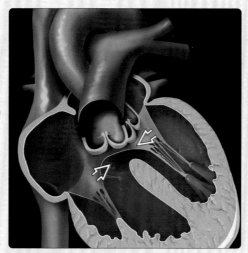

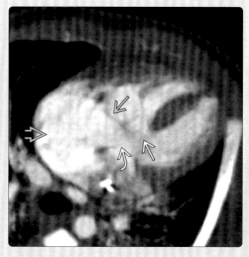

(Left) Graphic shows a defect ➡ in the atrioventricular (AV) septum connecting the right atrium & right ventricle to the left atrium & left ventricle. (Right) Axial image from a cardiac CTA in a newborn with Down syndrome shows a large ventricular septal defect (VSD) ➡, septum primum atrial septal defect (ASD) ➡, & a common AV valve ➡, consistent with an atrioventricular septal defect (AVSD). Notice the large right atrium ➡.

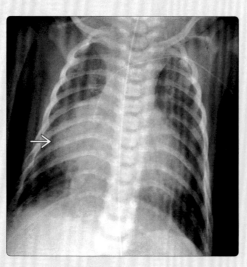

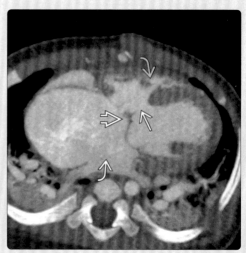

(Left) Frontal chest radiograph in a 2 month old with Down syndrome shows cardiomegaly, increased pulmonary vascularity, & venous congestion. Notice the massive enlargement of the right atrium ➡. (Right) Axial image from a cardiac CTA shows an AVSD. There is a common dysplastic AV valve ➡ with an inlet-type VSD ➡ & a septum primum ASD ➡. Notice the enlargement of the right atrium & the small right ventricle ➡ in this unbalanced AV canal defect.

Patent Ductus Arteriosus

KEY FACTS

TERMINOLOGY

- Persistent postnatal patency of normal prenatal connection from pulmonary artery (PA) to proximal descending aorta
- Hemodynamics: L → R shunt between aorta & PA
- PDA frequently essential in complex congenital heart disease: L → R or R → L flow, depending on other anomalies
- PDA in persistent fetal circulation syndrome: R → L flow

IMAGING

- Best radiographic clue: Cardiomegaly & heart failure once pulmonary vascular resistance drops in premature infant recovering from surfactant deficiency disease
- Echocardiography primary modality for imaging
- Well demonstrated by CTA & MRA: Usually linear, directed anterior to posterior, of variable size
  - PDA may be tortuous vessel connecting aorta &/or innominate artery with PA
  - CTA modality of choice for showing airway compression from tortuous PDA or vascular ring

- When closed: Forms ligamentum arteriosum, ± Ca^{2+}

PATHOLOGY

- With normal drop of pulmonary vascular resistance after birth, L → R shunting to PA through PDA
  - Volume overload of left-sided cardiac chambers
  - Associated diastolic flow reversal in aorta can lead to renal & intestinal hypoperfusion → renal dysfunction, necrotizing enterocolitis
  - Pressure overload of right ventricle eventually causes reversal of shunt (R → L) → cyanosis (Eisenmenger physiology)

CLINICAL ISSUES

- To close ductus in premature infants: Indomethacin
- To keep ductus open in cyanotic heart disease: Prostaglandin E1
- Term infants, older children: Surgical clipping or ligation vs. endovascular closure with duct occluder devices &/or coils

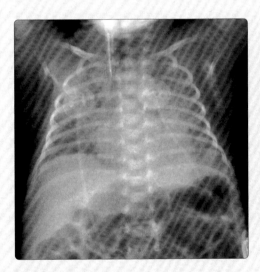
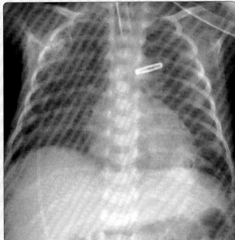

(Left) AP chest radiograph in a 7-day-old premature infant shows diffuse bilateral hazy opacification of the lungs. An echocardiogram showed a patent ductus arteriosus (PDA) with L → R flow. (Right) AP chest radiograph in the same patient shows a surgical clip due to interval ligation of the PDA. There is increased aeration of the lungs & decreased pulmonary edema.

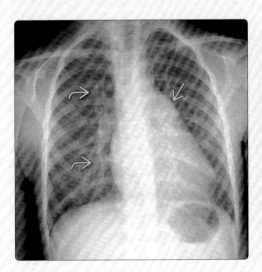
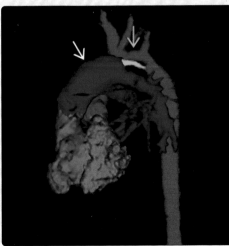

(Left) Frontal view of the chest in an 8-year-old patient with a persistent PDA shows increased (shunt) vascularity ⬈ with prominence of the main pulmonary artery ⬈. A chronic PDA can cause Eisenmenger syndrome. (Right) Oblique lateral view of a 3D color-coded cardiac CTA shows a PDA (green) with a mildly hypoplastic aortic arch ⬈. Note the enlarged size of the main pulmonary artery ⬈ caused by increased L → R shunting.

Cardiac

TERMINOLOGY

- Most common cyanotic congenital heart lesion
- Tetralogy: 4 heart defects from embryological anterocephalad deviation of conoventricular septum
  - Infundibular or subpulmonary narrowing
  - Anterior malalignment ventricular septal defect (VSD)
  - Aorta overriding VSD
  - Secondary right ventricular hypertrophy (RVH)
- Spectrum of tetralogy of Fallot disease
  - "Blue Tet": More subpulmonary obstruction → VSD shunts R → L → cyanotic appearance
  - "Pink Tet": Less subpulmonary obstruction → VSD shunts L → R (normal) → acyanotic appearance
  - Tetralogy with pulmonary atresia & major aortopulmonary collaterals (MAPCAs): Severe cyanosis if MAPCAs restrictive
  - Tetralogy with absent pulmonary valve: "To-fro" flow in pulmonary artery (PA) leading to massively dilated branch PAs, tracheobronchial compression

IMAGING

- Radiography: Normal heart size, concave PA segment, ↓ pulmonary vascularity (oligemia)
  - RVH → upturned cardiac apex → boot-shaped heart
  - Right-sided aortic arch in 25%
- Echocardiography: Initial diagnosis, often prenatal
  - Coronary artery anomalies important for surgical planning: Left anterior descending artery may arise from right coronary & cross right ventricular outflow tract (RVOT) (4%)
- Cardiac MR: ↑ use for postoperative assessment; critical for timing of pulmonary valve replacement (PVR)

CLINICAL ISSUES

- Typical repair within 1st year to life: VSD closure, relieve RVOT obstruction with patch
- Pulmonary regurgitation → RV dilation over time → ↓ exercise tolerance, RV dysfunction, ventricular arrhythmias
- PVR increasingly utilized to prevent RV dilation

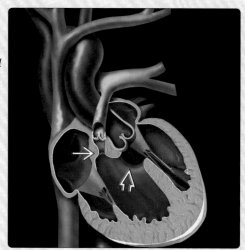

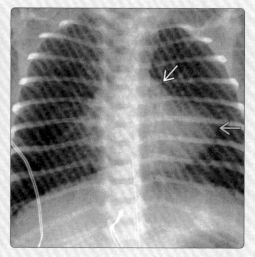

(Left) *Coronal graphic shows common features of tetralogy of Fallot (TOF), including subvalvular (infundibular) pulmonary stenosis* ➡, *a small pulmonic valve, an aorta overriding a high ventricular septal defect (VSD)* ➡, *right ventricular hypertrophy, & a right-sided aortic arch.* (Right) *AP radiograph in a patient with TOF shows classic features, including a concave pulmonary artery segment* ➡ *& an upturned cardiac apex* ➡, *creating the "coeur en sabot" (boot-shaped heart) appearance. Note the pulmonary oligemia.*

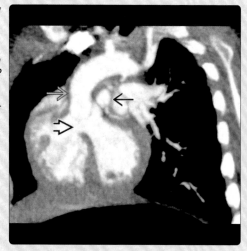

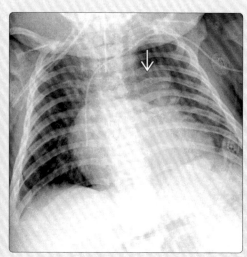

(Left) *Coronal oblique CTA in a patient with TOF shows a hypoplastic main pulmonary artery* ➡ *& a high (membranous) VSD* ➡ *with an overriding aorta* ➡. (Right) *AP radiograph in an infant with TOF & pulmonic valve absence shows marked enlargement of the pulmonary arteries, most pronounced on the left* ➡. *This patient was difficult to manage because of severe airway narrowing.*

Pulmonary Atresia

TERMINOLOGY

- 2 distinct entities, differentiated by presence or absence of ventricular septal defect (VSD)
  - Pulmonary atresia (PAt), intact VS: Normal-sized pulmonary arteries (PAs) supplied by patent ductus arteriosus (PDA), patent foramen ovale (PFO)
  - PAt, VSD, multiple aortopulmonary collateral arteries (MAPCAs): Hypoplastic/absent PAs; MAPCAs supply 1 or both lungs
    - At extreme end of spectrum of RVOT-obstructive (Fallot-type) heart lesions, with complex & highly variable PA anatomy

IMAGING

- Extreme boot-shaped appearance of heart
- Right-sided aortic arch common
- PAt, intact VS: Severe cardiomegaly from massive right atrial dilation
- Initial diagnosis with echocardiography

- Cardiac CTA delineates PAs, MAPCAs, & coronary artery fistulas & sinusoids
- CT or MR postoperatively for shunt/conduit patency
- Cardiac catheterization for hemodynamic assessment, selective injection studies, & catheter-based interventions

CLINICAL ISSUES

- Progressive cyanosis after birth at closure of PDA
  - Prostaglandin E1 to maintain PDA
- Congestive heart failure with large, unobstructed, high-flow MAPCAs
- Progressive cyanosis due to development of pulmonary vascular disease → irreversible pulmonary hypertension
  - Life expectancy when untreated < 10 years
- Treatment
  - PAt, intact VS: Type of repair dependent on RV size & RV-dependency on coronary circulation
  - PAt, VSD, MAPCAs: Unifocalization of MAPCAs & true PAs (if existent, to allow for PA growth)

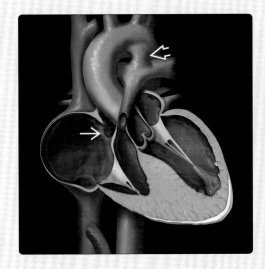

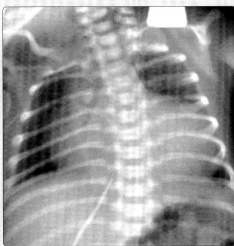

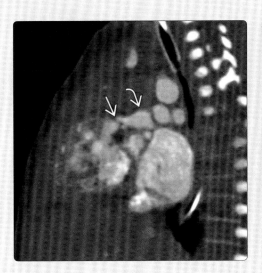

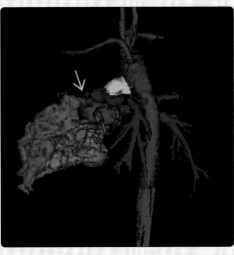

(Left) Graphic shows pulmonary atresia with an intact ventricular septum. Note the patent foramen ovale ➡, dilation of the right atrium, & right ventricular hypertrophy. The pulmonary arteries are perfused by flow from the aorta through a patent ductus arteriosus (PDA) ➡. (Right) Frontal view of the chest in a neonate with pulmonic atresia shows cardiomegaly with decreased pulmonary vascularity. The differential diagnosis for this appearance includes pulmonic atresia, Ebstein anomaly, & tricuspid atresia.

(Left) Sagittal MIP from a cardiac CTA shows an atretic thickened pulmonary valve ➡. A PDA ➡ feeds the main pulmonary artery. This patient is considered ductal dependent as survival is not possible without the PDA. (Right) Left lateral oblique view of a color-coded 3D CTA shows complete pulmonic atresia with a gap ➡ seen between the right ventricle (purple) & the pulmonary artery (blue). Notice the large PDA (green) that provides flow to the lungs.

KEY FACTS

TERMINOLOGY

- Downward/apical displacement of septal & posterior leaflets of tricuspid valve with tricuspid regurgitation
- Cyanotic congenital heart disease with cardiomegaly & ↓ pulmonary vascularity

IMAGING

- Classic radiographic appearance: Massive right-sided cardiomegaly (box-shaped heart)
- All cross-sectional modalities can show right atrial enlargement, apical displacement of tricuspid septal leaflet, & "atrialized" portion of right ventricle

PATHOLOGY

- Patent foramen ovale (PFO), secundum atrial septal defect in 90%
- Massive tricuspid regurgitation → volume overload to right side of heart → R → L shunt through PFO → cyanosis

- Left ventricular diastolic dysfunction may result from massive right-sided cardiac enlargement
- Arrhythmias due to conduction abnormalities

CLINICAL ISSUES

- 1st presentation can range from prenatal or neonatal periods through old age (average: 14 years)
  - Wide spectrum of findings: Cyanotic neonate, chronic right heart failure, arrhythmias, thrombosis with paradoxical embolus, asymptomatic
  - Prenatal: Hydrops fetalis or pulmonary hypoplasia
- Prognosis dependent on hemodynamic significance of tricuspid regurgitation & presence of cyanosis, arrhythmias
  - Cyanosis improves in 1st weeks of life: ↓ in pulmonary vascular resistance→ ↓ in R → L shunt
- Supportive treatment in cyanotic neonate: Oxygen, nitric oxide ventilation to lower pulmonary vascular resistance
- Definitive repair procedure: Tricuspid valve replacement &/or reconstruction (valvuloplasty)

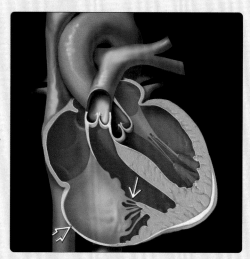
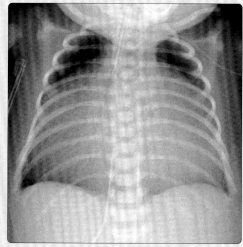

(Left) Graphic depicts downward displacement of the tricuspid valve posterior leaflet ➡, which has become incorporated into the right ventricular (RV) wall ➡, leading to "atrialization" of the inflow portion of the RV. (Right) Single frontal view of the chest shows massive cardiomegaly (the box-shaped heart) with decreased pulmonary vascularity, typical of patients with Ebstein anomaly.

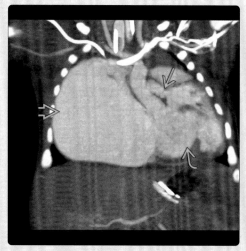
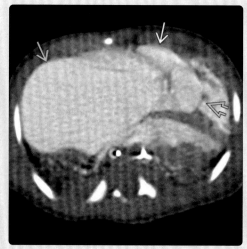

(Left) Coronal MIP image from a cardiac CTA shows massive dilation of the right atrium ➡ with enlargement of the RV ➡ in a patient with Ebstein anomaly. Note the narrowed pulmonary outflow tract ➡. (Right) Axial cardiac CTA shows a massively dilated right atrium ➡ with the septal leaflet ➡ of the tricuspid valve deviated toward the apex of the heart. Notice the atrialized (smooth) right ventricular wall ➡.

D-Transposition of Great Arteries

TERMINOLOGY

- Ventriculoarterial discordance with atrioventricular concordance: Aorta arises from right ventricle & pulmonary artery (PA) arises from left ventricle
- Complete separation of pulmonary & systemic circulations; lethal without flow admixture via patent foramen ovale, ventricular septal defect (VSD), &/or patent ductus arteriosus (PDA)

IMAGING

- Preoperative
  - Great vessels lie parallel & almost in same sagittal plane, with aortic valve in anterior position & slightly to right (D-loop) of pulmonary valve; coronary anomalies common
  - Classic radiographic appearance: Narrow mediastinum with cardiomegaly ("egg on string/egg on its side" heart) + ↑ pulmonary vascularity
- Postoperative (after arterial switch/Jatene procedure)
  - Classic alterations of great vessel anatomy

- – PA now anterior with posterior aorta in same sagittal plane; right & left PAs drape over ascending aorta
  - Transposed coronary arteries
  - Traction on both branch PAs may lead to stenosis

CLINICAL ISSUES

- Presents with severe cyanosis not improving with oxygen but little respiratory distress
  - If large VSD: Congestive heart failure as neonate
  - If large VSD + (sub-) pulmonic stenosis: Mild symptoms, may survive for years without treatment
- Potential treatments: Prostaglandin E1 to maintain PDA preoperatively; emergency balloon atrial septostomy (Rashkind); early surgery (preferred): Arterial switch with transposition of coronaries (Jatene); late surgery: Rerouting of venous flow in atria with pericardial baffle (Mustard) or reorientation of atrial septum (Senning)
- Simple transposition has good prognosis with early switch; prognosis determined by potential coronary anomalies

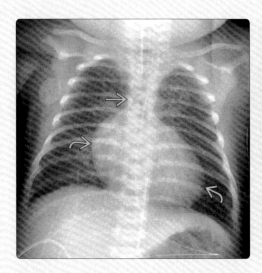
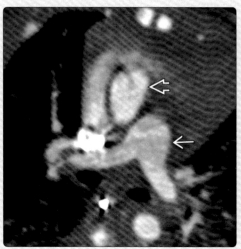

(Left) Frontal radiograph of the chest shows cardiomegaly & increased pulmonary vascularity in a patient with D-transposition of the great arteries (D-TGA). The superior mediastinum is narrow ➡, & the heart is globular in shape ➡. This combination is referred to as the egg-on-a-string appearance. (Right) Axial cardiac CTA shows the pulmonary artery (PA) ➡ posterior & slightly to the left of the ascending aorta ➡. This is the classic relationship of the great vessels seen with D-TGA.

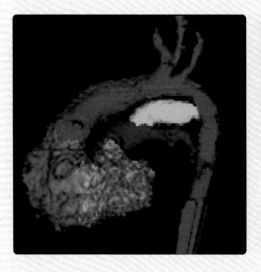
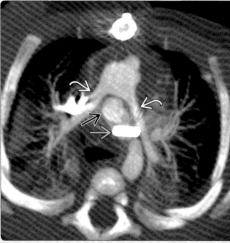

(Left) Lateral color-coded 3D CTA reformation in a D-TGA patient shows that the aorta (red) arises from the right ventricle (purple) & the PA (blue) arises from the left ventricle (pink). A large patent ductus arteriosus (PDA) (green) connects the aortic arch to the PA (blue). (Right) Axial MIP of a cardiac CTA status post arterial switch procedure shows typical postoperative anatomy with the PAs ➡ draped over the ascending aorta ➡. Most D-TGA patients have a persistent large PDA that needs to be ligated ➡.

L-Transposition of Great Arteries

TERMINOLOGY

- "Congenitally corrected transposition" (misnomer)
- Inversion of ventricles & great arteries: Atrioventricular (AV) discordance & ventriculoarterial discordance
  - Right atrium connects via mitral valve to right-sided morphologic left ventricle (LV), which connects to pulmonary circulation
  - Left atrium connects via tricuspid valve to left-sided morphologic right ventricle (RV), which connects to systemic circulation
- Category: Dependent on associated anomalies
  - Ventricular septal defect (VSD) (60-80%): Acyanotic, ↑ pulmonary vascularity
  - LV outflow tract (subpulmonary) obstruction (30-50%): Cyanotic
  - Only 1% have no associated anomalies: True congenitally corrected transposition

IMAGING

- Classic radiograph: Straight upper left heart border
- CT & MR demonstrate complex anatomy

PATHOLOGY

- VSD: Up to 80%; LV outflow tract (subpulmonary) obstruction: 30-50%; left-sided tricuspid valve dysplasia, Ebstein anomaly, regurgitation: 30%

CLINICAL ISSUES

- Congestive heart failure (VSD, systemic AV valve dysfunction); cyanosis (subpulmonary stenosis); rarely completely asymptomatic
- Guarded prognosis due to progressive systemic AV valve & RV dysfunction after corrective surgery: 50% mortality after 15 years
- Patients with true congenitally corrected transposition may have normal life expectancy

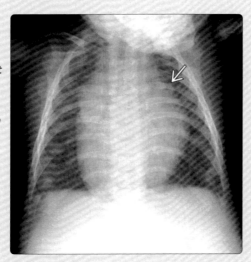
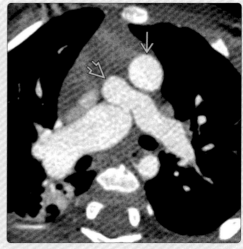

(Left) Frontal radiograph of the chest shows a straightened left upper heart border ➡ in a patient with levo-transposition of the great arteries (L-TGA). (Right) Axial image from a cardiac CT angiogram shows the typical position of the great vessels in L-TGA. The aorta (Ao) ➡ is anterior & to the left of the pulmonary artery (PA) ➡ (whereas the PA lies anterior & to the left of the Ao normally).

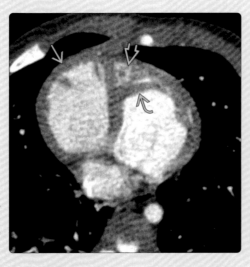
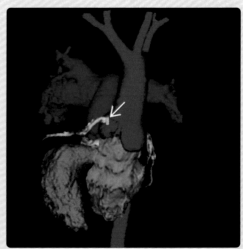

(Left) Axial cardiac CT angiogram in a patient with L-TGA shows a smooth-walled morphologic left ventricle (LV) ➡ on the right. The morphologic right ventricle (RV) ➡ is on the left, showing a characteristic moderator band ➡. (Right) Frontal 3D color-coded cardiac CT angiogram shows the morphologic LV (pink) on the right giving rise to the PAs (blue) & the morphologic RV (purple) on the left giving rise to the Ao (red). Right coronary artery ➡ arises from the right coronary sinus & branches into the LAD & circumflex.

Tricuspid Atresia

TERMINOLOGY

- Congenital absence or agenesis of tricuspid valve & inlet portion of right ventricle

IMAGING

- Type I: Normally related great arteries (70-80%)
- Type II: D-transposition of great arteries (12-25%)
- Type III: L-transposition of great arteries/malposition (3-6%)
- Small ventricular septal defect (VSD) → heart usually normal in size, right ventricle hypoplastic, pulmonary flow diminished
- Large VSD → heart usually large with ↑ flow or transposition of great arteries
- MR: Excellent for postoperative left ventricular functional assessment & anatomy of caval-pulmonary artery anastomosis
- CTA: Useful to assess for pulmonary artery embolus & collateral vessels in children who have increasing cyanosis

  ○ Knowledge of previous surgical procedure is critical to correctly prescribing protocol & interpreting imaging, particularly in Glenn anastomosis & Fontan procedures (as unopacified blood can mimic thrombus)

TOP DIFFERENTIAL DIAGNOSES

- Ebstein anomaly
- Tetralogy of Fallot

CLINICAL ISSUES

- 50% of neonates present with cyanosis in first 24 hours
- 30% present with signs of congestive heart failure
- Left axis deviation on newborn electrocardiography suggestive with cyanotic presentation
- Staged surgical approach, similar to single ventricle
  ○ Modified Blalock-Taussig shunt with systemic artery to pulmonary flow → bidirectional Glenn anastomosis with superior vena cava to pulmonary artery → modified Fontan procedure with inferior vena cava conduit to pulmonary artery

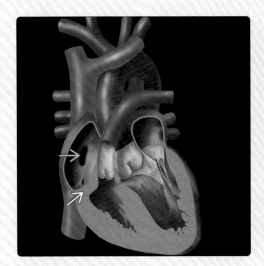

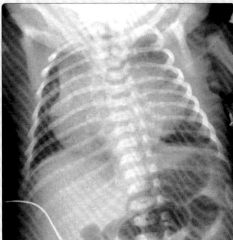

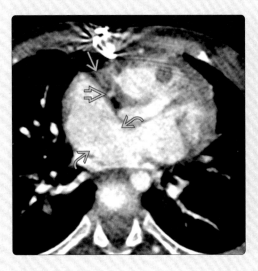

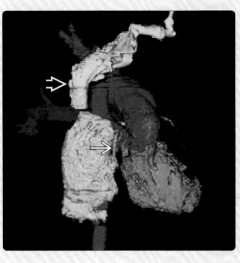

(Left) Coronal graphic shows tricuspid atresia where there is no forward flow into the right ventricle due to obstruction at the level of the right atrioventricular (AV) groove ➡. There is an atrial septal defect (ASD) ➡, a ventricular septal defect, & a hypoplastic right ventricle. (Right) Single frontal radiograph of the chest shows cardiomegaly with decreased pulmonary vascularity in an infant with tricuspid atresia.

(Left) Cardiac CTA shows fat & soft tissue ➡ in the right AV groove where the tricuspid valve is normally located. Note the right coronary artery ➡ deep within the groove. A large ASD (between the ➡) is also seen. (Right) 3D cardiac CTA image shows a Glenn shunt with the SVC ➡ directly connected to pulmonary arteries (dark blue). Note the appearance of tricuspid atresia with wide separation of the right atrium (light blue) & hypoplastic right ventricle (purple). The right coronary artery ➡ lies in the AV groove at the atretic tricuspid valve.

TERMINOLOGY

- Common arterial vessel (trunk) arising from heart; gives rise to aorta, pulmonary arteries (PAs), & coronaries
- Congenital heart lesion most commonly associated with right aortic arch (30-40%)

IMAGING

- Classic radiograph: Cardiomegaly, ↑ pulmonary vascularity, narrow mediastinum, right aortic arch
- Echo: High (outlet) ventricular septal defect (VSD) immediately below truncal valve

PATHOLOGY

- Collett & Edwards classification
  - Type I: Separation of common trunk into ascending aorta & main PA
  - Type II: Common take-off of branch PAs from trunk
  - Type III: Both branch PAs originate separately from posterolateral aspect of ascending aorta

- Type IV: "Pseudotruncus": PA supply from major aortopulmonary collateral arteries (MAPCAs) arising from descending aorta; (controversial entity, misnomer for pulmonary atresia with VSD & MAPCAs)
- Strong association with chromosomal deletion at 22q11 (CATCH-22 syndrome with cardiac anomalies, abnormal facies, thymic hypoplasia, cleft palate, & hypocalcemia)

CLINICAL ISSUES

- Intractable congestive heart failure → pulmonary hypertension → shunt reversal → increasing cyanosis
  - Untreated: 65% 6-month & 75% 1-year mortality
- Early complete repair (at 2-6 weeks of life) favored by most surgeons: Placement of conduit between right ventricle & PA with closure of VSD
  - Postoperative course determined by function of PA conduit & need for conduit replacement
  - Truncal valve dysfunction (regurgitation) common → need for valvuloplasty, prosthesis

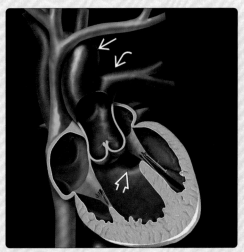
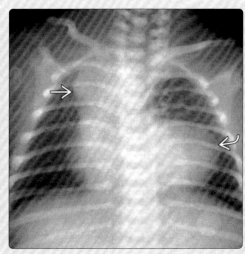

(Left) Coronal graphic shows a type I truncus with a high ventricular septal defect ➡ & a common truncal valve giving rise to the aorta ➡ & the main pulmonary artery (PA) ➡. Cyanosis is due to flow admixture within the ventricles & truncus. (Right) AP radiograph shows cardiomegaly with a right aortic arch ➡ & increased pulmonary vascularity in an infant with truncus arteriosus. The apex of the heart is upturned ➡. This appearance is often mistaken for tetralogy of Fallot.

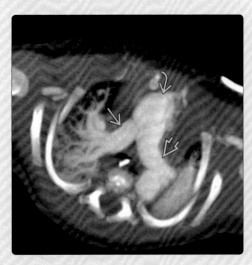
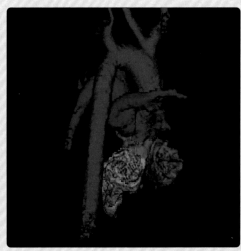

(Left) Axial CTA MIP of an infant with truncus arteriosus shows both right ➡ & left ➡ PAs coming off of a central common trunk ➡ that includes the aorta. (Right) Posterior lateral oblique image from a 3D color-coded cardiac CTA reconstruction shows the PAs (blue) arising from the posterior aspect of the ascending aorta (red), consistent with truncus arteriosus.

Total Anomalous Pulmonary Venous Return

KEY FACTS

TERMINOLOGY

- Total anomalous pulmonary venous return (TAPVR) or "drainage": Failure of connection between pulmonary veins (PVs) & left atrium
  - All PV return goes to right heart (extracardiac L → R shunt)
- Supracardiac TAPVR (type I, 40-50%): "Vertical" common PV joins left innominate vein
- Cardiac TAPVR (type II, 20-30%): Common PV joins coronary sinus or right atrium
- Infracardiac TAPVR (type III, 10-30%): Common PV joins portal vein, ductus venosus, or inferior vena cava

IMAGING

- Cardiomegaly (types I, II); small heart (type III)
- Shunt vascularity (types I, II); pulmonary edema (type III)
- Type I: "Snowman" heart
- Type II: Indistinguishable from atrial septal defect (ASD)
- Type III: Small heart, reticular pattern in lungs (edema)

PATHOLOGY

- All types have patent foramen ovale (PFO) to allow for obligatory R → L flow → varying degrees of cyanosis
- Type III: Common PV obstructed by diaphragmatic hiatus → PV congestion & edema
- Left-sided cardiac chambers may be underdeveloped, especially in type III
- Associations: Single ventricle, atrioventricular septal defect, truncus arteriosus, tetralogy of Fallot, anomalous systemic venous connection, heterotaxy syndromes

CLINICAL ISSUES

- Types I, II: Congestive heart failure
- Type III: Severe cyanosis at birth
- Prostaglandin E1 improves systemic perfusion followed by early surgical anastomosis of PV confluence to left atrium
- Complications include anastomotic PV stenosis → irreversible pulmonary hypertension

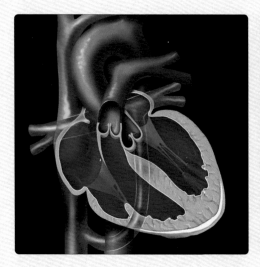

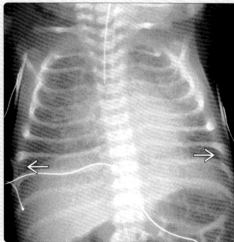

(Left) Graphic shows an infradiaphragmatic total anomalous pulmonary venous return (TAPVR) (type III) to the inferior vena cava, constituting an obligatory extracardiac L → R shunt. Mixed blood flows to the left atrium through a patent foramen ovale. (Right) Frontal radiograph in a newborn shows diffuse pulmonary edema with small bilateral pleural effusions ➡. Notice that the heart size is normal in this patient with type III TAPVR.

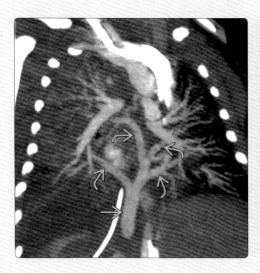

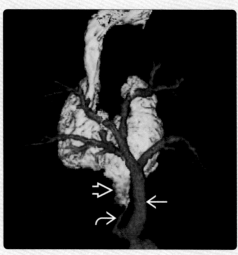

(Left) Coronal MIP CTA of an infant with an obstructed type III TAPVR shows that the pulmonary veins ➡ connect to a large vertical vein ➡ that then drains below the diaphragm. (Right) Posterior view of a color-coded 3D CTA shows the pulmonary veins (purple) emptying into a large inferior vertical vein ➡ in a patient with obstructed infracardiac TAPVR. Only a small venous connection ➡ was seen to the inferior vena cava ➡. Notice the symmetric atria (light blue) in this patient with heterotaxy.

TERMINOLOGY

- Hypoplasia/atresia of ascending aorta, aortic valve, left ventricle (LV), & mitral valve
- Secondary findings: Patent ductus arteriosus, juxtaductal aortic coarctation

IMAGING

- Chest radiograph shows cardiomegaly, large right atrium, pulmonary venous congestion with interstitial fluid
- Postnatal echocardiogram sufficient for treatment planning
  - Diminutive ascending aorta < 5 mm
  - Small, thick-walled LV
  - Dilation of right cardiac chambers & pulmonary artery
  - Unrestricted atrial level shunt critical for immediate postnatal care; may require emergent balloon atrial septostomy; saturations dependent on degree of atrial level shunting
  - Abnormal ventricular wall motion
- CTA & MR used between surgical stages

CLINICAL ISSUES

- Most severe congenital heart lesion: Death within days/weeks when untreated; prognosis improves substantially with intervention
  - Presents in neonatal period with congestive heart failure, cardiogenic shock, cyanosis, poor systemic perfusion, metabolic acidosis
- Treatment
  - Medical: Prostaglandins initiated at birth/time of diagnosis to keep patent ductus arteriosus open (provides R → L flow to descending aorta)
  - Palliative repair: Norwood 3-stage approach
  - In some centers: Cardiac transplantation
- Prognosis determined by complications, residua, & sequelae of staged Norwood repair & Fontan operation (right ventricular dysfunction, venous hypertension)

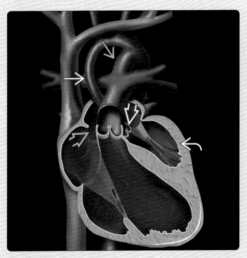

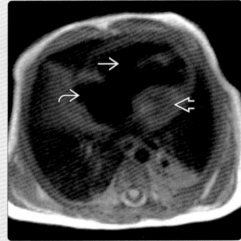

(Left) *Anterior graphic of hypoplastic left heart syndrome (HLHS) shows hypoplasia of the left atrium, mitral valve, left ventricle* ➤, *aortic valve* ➤, *& ascending aorta* ➤. *Systemic blood flow depends on the patency of the ductus arteriosus* ➾ *in the setting of an atrial septal defect* ➾. (Right) *Axial T1 MR at the level of the ventricles in an HLHS patient shows a large right ventricle* ➤ *& diminutive left ventricle* ➤. *Note the large right atrium* ➤.

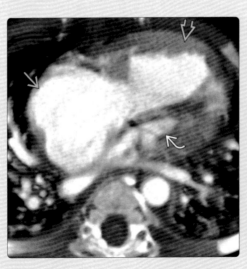

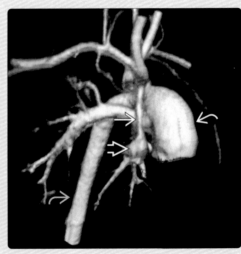

(Left) *Axial CTA MIP in a newborn with HLHS shows hypoplasia of the left ventricle* ➤ *with dilation of the right atrium* ➾ *& right ventricle* ➾. (Right) *Anterior oblique 3D reformation of a CTA in the same patient shows the very small ascending aorta* ➤ *& coronary sinuses* ➤. *The pulmonary artery is enlarged* ➤ *& supplies the descending aorta* ➾ *by a patent ductus arteriosus. Blood flow to the coronary sinuses occurs retrograde via the hypoplastic aorta.*

Left Coronary Artery Anomalous Origin

KEY FACTS

TERMINOLOGY

- Anomalous origin of left coronary artery from pulmonary artery: Most common congenital coronary artery anomaly presenting in children

IMAGING

- Chest radiograph demonstrates cardiomegaly
- Echocardiogram (~ 90% diagnostic accuracy) demonstrates
  - Abnormal left coronary artery (LCA) ostium arising from pulmonary trunk
  - Retrograde flow in LCA toward pulmonary artery
  - Right coronary artery dilation & abundant intercoronary septal collaterals
  - Depressed left ventricle (LV) systolic function & dilated LV chamber
  - Significant mitral regurgitation from ischemic papillary muscle dysfunction & mitral annular dilation
- CTA/MRA to identify coronary origins when echo limited (~ 100% diagnostic accuracy)

CLINICAL ISSUES

- Rare congenital anomaly; up to 90% mortality if not identified & surgically corrected
  - Causes cardiac ischemia & infarction, poor LV systolic function, & significant mitral regurgitation
- Up to 90% present in infancy with nonspecific symptoms of irritability, failure to thrive, wheezing (from mitral regurgitation), diaphoresis, ↓ oxygenation & perfusion (severe cyanosis or grayish appearance)
  - ECG shows anterior lateral wall infarct pattern
- Older children often asymptomatic until sudden event with syncope, dysrhythmia, & occasional sudden cardiac death
- Coronary artery anomalies can be isolated or associated with other defects → must identify for surgical planning
- Surgical therapy: Up to 90% mortality if left unrepaired; prognosis related to degree of preoperative LV systolic dysfunction
  - Surgical options include coronary reimplantation to aorta, bypass grafting, Takeuchi baffle

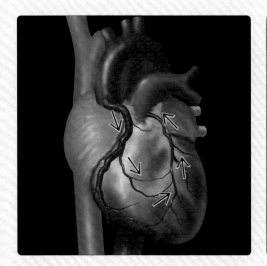

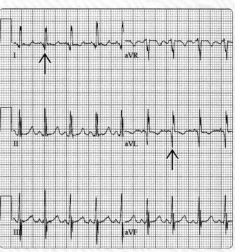

(Left) Graphic shows an anomalous origin of the left coronary artery (LCA) from the main pulmonary artery (PA). Collateral flow develops from the normal right coronary artery to the LCA, allowing retrograde flow through the LCA to the low-resistance PA (with flow direction denoted ⇨). This flow bypasses the high-resistance myocardial bed of the left ventricle (LV). (Right) ECG of a neonate shows pathologic deep Q-waves in leads I & aVL ⇨, consistent with a diagnosis of ALCAPA & myocardial ischemia.

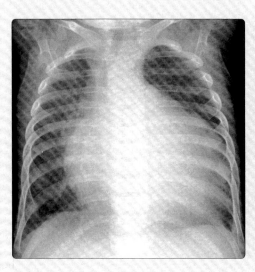

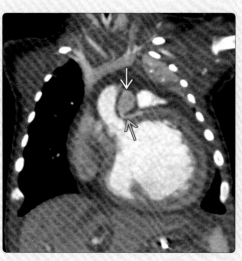

(Left) AP radiograph from an 8 month old with wheezing, grunting, & weight loss (& a normal radiograph 4 months prior) shows a markedly enlarged cardiac silhouette. Echocardiography showed the LCA arising from the PA. (Right) Coronal projection of a CT angiogram demonstrates an anomalous LCA ⇨ originating from the underside of the PA trunk ⇨, consistent with ALCAPA. The LV is markedly dilated.

Double Outlet Right Ventricle

TERMINOLOGY

- Double outlet right ventricle (DORV): Form of abnormal ventriculoarterial connection in which both great arteries arise completely or predominately from morphologic right ventricle
  - 16 variants based on relationship of great arteries & position/location of ventricular septal defect (VSD)
- May be part of complex congenital heart disease coexisting with ventricular anomalies, valve stenosis or atresia, abnormal atrioventricular valve, aortic valve anomalies, coarctation, coronary anomalies, & anomalies of systemic or pulmonary venous return

IMAGING

- Radiographic pulmonary flow dependent on site of VSD & degree of outflow or pulmonary valve stenosis
- Beyond echocardiography, 3D CTA/MR imaging can help define complex intracardiac relationships for presurgical planning

- Side-by-side relationship of aorta & pulmonary artery with aorta on right in 50-64%

CLINICAL ISSUES

- May be diagnosed in utero; usually has clinical symptoms at birth or in 1st month
  - DORV with pulmonic stenosis: Cyanosis, failure to thrive, tachypnea
  - DORV with subaortic VSD without pulmonic stenosis: Symptoms of large L → R shunt & early evidence of pulmonary hypertension
- Surgery depends on anatomy
  - Closure of VSD & placement of conduit from right ventricle to pulmonary artery
  - Norwood/Fontan procedure if there is hypoplasia of ventricle
- Mortality rate after operation higher for complex lesions; 15-year survival rate for noncomplex lesions: 85-90%

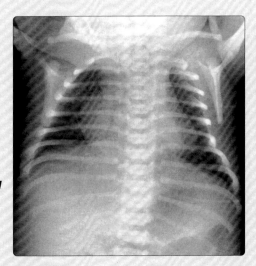

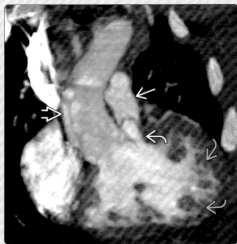

(Left) AP chest radiograph in an infant with double outlet right ventricle (DORV) shows decreased pulmonary vascularity & mild cardiomegaly. Pulmonic stenosis in this patient makes the radiographic appearance similar to that of a patient with tetralogy of Fallot. (Right) Coronal MIP image from a cardiac CTA in a newborn with DORV shows both the pulmonary artery ➡ & aorta ⮕ arising from the trabeculated right ventricle ➲. Notice the subpulmonic stenosis ➤ of the right ventricular outflow tract.

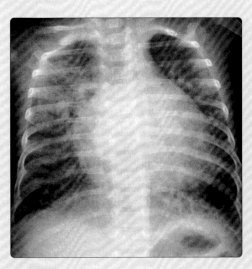

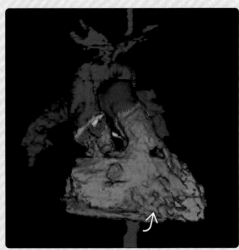

(Left) AP chest radiograph in an infant shows cardiomegaly with a significant increase in pulmonary artery flow plus signs of venous edema. This patient had DORV with no pulmonic stenosis, which explains the increased blood flow to the lungs. (Right) Frontal view of a 3D cardiac CTA in a patient with DORV shows both the aorta (red) & pulmonary artery (blue) arising from the trabeculated ➡ right ventricle (purple).

Aortic Coarctation

TERMINOLOGY

- Narrowing of aortic lumen with obstruction to blood flow

IMAGING

- Locations: Preductal, typically hypoplastic (infantile); juxtaductal or postductal, typically focal (adult); abdominal, middle aortic syndrome (rare)
  - May have diffuse hypoplasia of aortic isthmus + focal coarctation (important for surgical planning)
- Can be simple (isolated coarctation in adult) or complex (additional cardiac anomalies, presenting in infancy)
- Classic radiographic findings
  - Poststenotic dilatation of proximal descending aorta (figure 3 sign)
  - Rib notching (age > 5 years)
  - Left ventricular hypertrophy: Rounded cardiac apex
- Echocardiography for primary diagnosis in infancy

PATHOLOGY

- Most common additional cardiac anomalies: Ventricular septal defect (33%), PDA (66%), bicuspid aortic valve (50%)
- Turner syndrome: 20-36% have coarctation

CLINICAL ISSUES

- Presentations include
  - Infancy: Congestive heart failure (due to aortic arch interruption, associated anomalies)
  - Older child, adult: Hypertension, diminished femoral pulses, differential BP between upper & lower extremities (arm-leg gradient)
- Treatment: Resection + end-to-end anastomosis, interposition graft, patch + aortoplasty, balloon angioplasty
  - Complications: Recoarctation (< 3%; ↑ if operation in infancy), postoperative aneurysms (24% after patch aortoplasty)
- ↓ long-term survival (late hypertension, coronary artery disease)

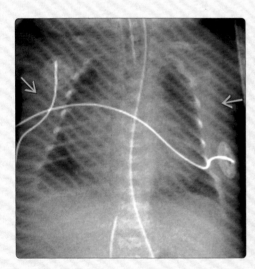

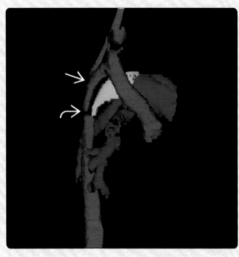

(Left) Frontal chest radiograph in a 2-week-old infant with congestive heart failure & severe coarctation of the aorta shows cardiomegaly & anasarca ➡. (Right) Lateral oblique view of a 3D color-coded cardiac CTA shows a preductal hypoplastic-type coarctation ➡ of the aorta with a periductal focal coarctation ➡. Notice that the patent ductus arteriosus (green) is beginning to close with severe narrowing near the aortic connection. (The pulmonary arteries are shaded blue for reference.)

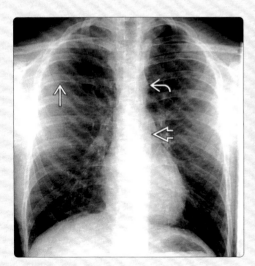

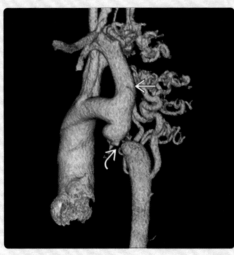

(Left) Frontal chest radiograph in a teenage patient with coarctation of the aorta shows prominence of the aortic knob ➡ & descending aorta ➡ straddling the level of the narrowing, creating a figure 3 sign. Note the sclerosis & undulation of the undersurface of the ribs ➡ from collateral vessels causing rib notching. (Right) Lateral oblique 3D image from a cardiac CTA shows a focal coarctation ➡ of the aorta with the formation of multiple large arterial collaterals. Note the massive enlargement of the left subclavian artery ➡.

TERMINOLOGY

- Spectrum of aortic valve abnormalities that ranges from asymptomatic bicuspid aortic valve to thickened & obstructed aortic valve stenosis to severe neonatal aortic atresia & hypoplastic left heart syndrome: 3-5% of all congenital heart defects
- Aortic stenosis (AS) may be valvar, supravalvar, or subvalvar
  - Valvar stenosis most common at 80%

IMAGING

- Varies by location, etiology, & severity of stenosis
- Chest radiographs range from cardiomegaly & edema in severely affected infants to normal in adolescents
- Poststenotic dilation of ascending aorta in valvar stenosis
  - Due to flow jet through stenotic valve
- Supravalvar shows hourglass shape of ascending aorta
- Subaortic stenosis may have hypertrophic cardiomyopathy
- Cardiac enlargement may not be seen in childhood
- MR & echo allow quantitative assessments

- Cardiac catheterization for interventional treatment with balloon valvotomy; leads to aortic regurgitation

PATHOLOGY

- Grading of AS: Jet velocity, gradient across valve, valve area
  - Mild has gradient < 20 mmHg
  - Moderate has gradient from 20-40 mmHg
  - Severe has gradient > 40 mmHg
- Associations include Williams syndrome, hypoplastic left heart syndrome, bicuspid aortic valve, hypertrophic cardiomyopathy, endocarditis

CLINICAL ISSUES

- 10-20% of AS presents in 1st year of life
- Neonatal: Signs of poor or low cardiac output with tachypnea & feeding problems
- Childhood: Usually asymptomatic but may have systolic murmur or suprasternal thrill
  - 1% of sudden deaths may be due to undetected AS; usually occurs during exercise

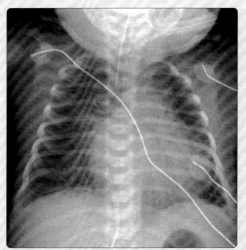
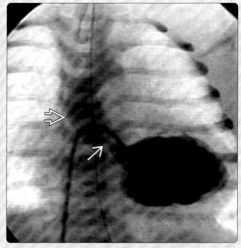

(Left) Frontal chest radiograph shows a 2-week-old infant in heart failure with perihilar pulmonary edema & cardiomegaly. This patient had critical aortic stenosis. (Right) Single frontal image from a left ventricular angiogram shows a jet across the aortic valve ➡ from severe aortic stenosis in a 2-week-old infant. Notice the dilation of the ascending aorta ➡.

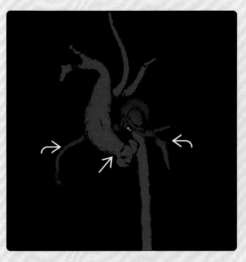
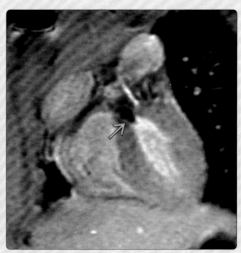

(Left) Frontal image from a 3D color-coded cardiac CTA shows supravalvular aortic stenosis ➡ in a patient with Williams syndrome. Notice the hypoplastic pulmonary arteries ➡, which are often seen in this syndrome. (Right) Oblique coronal bright blood GRE cine cardiac MR along the left ventricular outflow tract in a patient with a subvalvular membrane shows dephasing signal void artifact ➡ from stenosis below the aortic valve.

Pulmonary Artery Stenosis

KEY FACTS

TERMINOLOGY

- Stenosis at level of infundibulum, pulmonary valve, supravalvar main pulmonary artery (PA), or branches of PA
- Pulmonary valvar stenosis most common (> 90%)

IMAGING

- Valvar stenosis: Normal heart size with dilated main pulmonary artery segment in ~ 80%
  - Thickened valve leaflets, doming of valve, systolic high-velocity flow jet in pulmonary outflow tract
- Supravalvar PA stenosis (PS) in Williams syndrome
- Alagille syndrome has valvar PS & peripheral PA stenosis
- Infundibular narrowing in tetralogy of Fallot & complex malformations
- Right ventricular hypertrophy occurs secondary to ↑ work

PATHOLOGY

- Associations include Williams, Noonan, & Alagille syndromes

CLINICAL ISSUES

- PS often diagnosed between 2-6 years of age during routine physical exam
- Mild stenosis: Usually asymptomatic with systolic ejection murmur
- Moderate stenosis: Exertional dyspnea, easy fatigability
- Severe stenosis: Infants may present with severe cyanosis
- Treatment: Medical management for mild valvar gradients < 25 mm Hg; balloon valvuloplasty for moderate to severe gradients > 50 mm Hg
  - Not as effective in dysplastic valves, which may require surgery
- Newborns with critical PS: Immediate valvotomy with prostaglandin to maintain ductus arteriosus flow
  - May need surgical valvotomy or palliative Blalock-Taussig shunt

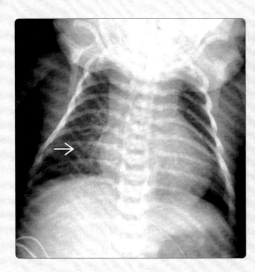

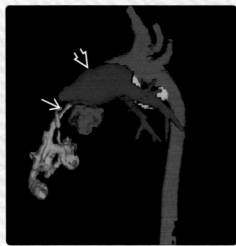

(Left) Frontal radiograph shows mild cardiomegaly & perihilar pulmonary edema in a patient with severe pulmonic stenosis. Notice how the interstitial edema makes the pulmonary vessels indistinct ➡. (Right) Lateral image from a 3D color-coded cardiac CTA shows severe pulmonic stenosis ➡ with poststenotic dilation of the main pulmonary artery ➡. Notice the large patent ductus arteriosus (PDA) (green) extending from the aorta (red) to the pulmonary artery (blue).

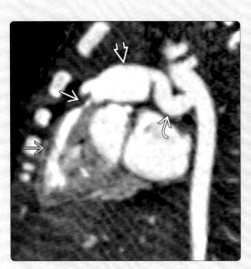

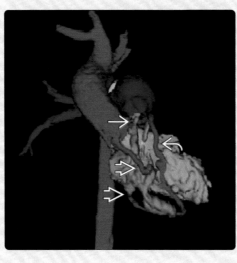

(Left) Sagittal MIP from a cardiac CTA shows severe pulmonic stenosis ➡ with poststenotic dilation of the main pulmonary artery ➡ & right ventricular (RV) hypertrophy ➡. Notice the tortuous PDA ➡ extending from the descending aorta to the main pulmonary artery. (Right) Frontal view from a 3D color-coded cardiac CTA shows severe pulmonic stenosis ➡ with a hypoplastic RV (purple). Notice that the coronary arteries ➡ communicate with the RV ➡, consistent with coronary artery fistulas.

KEY FACTS

IMAGING

- Chest radiograph: Many cases normal
  - Cardiomegaly &/or pericardial effusion in setting of cardiac dysfunction
  - Pulmonary edema in more severe cases
- Echocardiography: Identifies cardiac dysfunction &/or pericardial effusion
- Cardiac catheterization & endomyocardial biopsy: Historical gold standard (but invasive & can miss patchy inflammation)
- Cardiac MR: Increasingly utilized for diagnostic capabilities
  - Cardiac volumes & functional assessment: ↓ ejection fraction with wall motion abnormality, ± pericardial effusion
  - Myocardial tissue characterization (edema, hyperemia, & fibrosis): ↑ T2 signal, early & late gadolinium enhancement, native T1 values > 990 ms
  - ≥ 2 positive criteria in acute phase: 80% sensitivity, 90% specificity

TOP DIFFERENTIAL DIAGNOSES

- Ischemic heart disease, inheritable cardiomyopathy, Kawasaki disease, septic shock, & sarcoidosis

PATHOLOGY

- Infectious etiology (typically viral): Most common in otherwise healthy individuals
- Toxins/drug reactions: Antibiotics, antiepileptics, carbon monoxide, illegal drugs (cocaine)
- Autoimmune: Lupus, sarcoidosis, Takayasu arteritis
- Ischemic: Acute coronary syndrome/myocardial infarction

CLINICAL ISSUES

- Nonspecific symptoms: Fever, fatigue, malaise, dyspnea, muscle aches, poor feeding, unexplained sinus tachycardia
  - May imitate acute myocardial infarction
- Most cases: Mild symptoms, need only supportive care
- Rarely, fulminant with cardiovascular collapse & shock
  - May account for 10% of sudden death in young

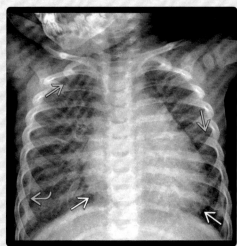
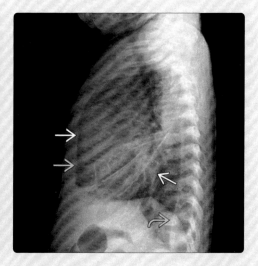

(Left) PA chest radiograph in a previously healthy 18 month old with respiratory distress shows enlargement of the cardiac silhouette ➡ with engorgement of the central pulmonary vascularity & peripheral interstitium ⇨, typical of pulmonary edema. Small pleural effusions ▱ are also present. (Right) Lateral radiograph in the same patient shows cardiomegaly ➡, interstitial edema ⇨, & pleural effusions ▱, suggesting cardiac dysfunction in this patient found to have parvovirus myocarditis.

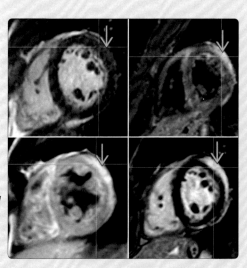
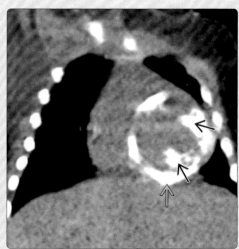

(Left) Short axis MR tissue characterization in a patient with myocarditis shows a region of interest with increased signal in the anterolateral segment ⇨ on SSFP (upper left), T2 (upper right), early gadolinium (lower left), & late gadolinium (lower right) enhancement images. (Right) Coronal NECT demonstrates significant dystrophic calcification of the left ventricular myocardial wall ⇨ & papillary muscles ⇨ in a neonate with prior enterovirus myocarditis.

Hypertrophic Cardiomyopathy

TERMINOLOGY

- Familial cardiomyopathy characterized by thickened but nondilated left ventricle (LV) & no identifiable systemic or cardiac cause

IMAGING

- Echocardiography primary diagnostic/screening tool
- Cardiac MR increasingly utilized for ventricular dimensions, left ventricular outflow tract (LVOT) obstruction, & fibrosis [shown by late gadolinium enhancement (LGE)]
  - Asymmetric septal hypertrophy, typically basal septum
  - Dynamic LVOT obstruction
    - Severe thickening of septum during systole causing midcavitary obstruction
    - Systolic anterior motion of mitral valve
  - Systolic & diastolic dysfunction variable
  - Patchy or focal LGE of basal & midventricle septal segments

- Risk factor for ventricular arrhythmia & sudden cardiac death

CLINICAL ISSUES

- Most common genetic cardiomyopathy (1 in 500)
  - Primary: Typically autosomal dominant inheritance
  - Secondary: Associated with syndromic, neuromuscular, & metabolic disorders
  - Idiopathic: ~ 50% of affected children < 1 year old
- Typically asymptomatic but symptoms may include dyspnea, chest pain, or syncope, especially with exertion
  - Ventricular arrhythmias common
  - Systolic heart murmur increases in intensity with Valsalva, positional change (standing/squatting), or exercise; prominence of LV apical impulse
- Variable clinical course with 1% annual mortality
  - Leading cause of sudden cardiac death in youth
- Treatment: Medical: β-blockers, antiarrhythmics; invasive: Pacemaker, septal ablation, myomectomy

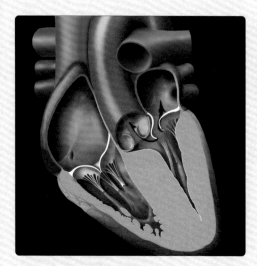

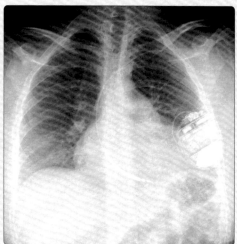

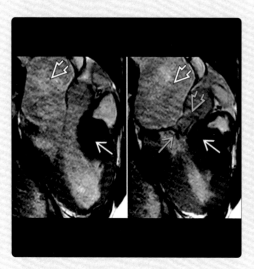

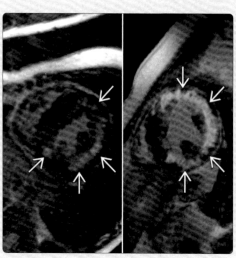

(Left) "Five-chamber" graphic demonstrates concentric hypertrophic obstructive cardiomyopathy (HOCM). Septal hypertrophy & systolic anterior motion (SAM) of the mitral valve leaflet combine to cause left ventricular outflow tract (LVOT) obstruction & mitral regurgitation. (Right) AP chest radiograph in an 18-year-old girl with HOCM shows cardiomegaly & a ventricular pacing device (which was placed due to a high number of risk factors for a sudden cardiac event).

(Left) Three-chamber SSFP MRs during diastole (left) & systole (right) demonstrate LVOT obstruction ⇥ from severe septal hypertrophy ➡ & SAM of the mitral valve apparatus ⇥. Also note the left atrial enlargement ➡. (Right) Short axis late gadolinium enhanced MRs of the same patient show progression of fibrosis on a follow-up study. The delayed enhancement ➡ is severe (though patchy) on the 1st image (left), becoming more extensive on the follow-up exam (right).

KEY FACTS

TERMINOLOGY

- Disturbance of normal left-right asymmetry in position of thoracic & abdominal organs; typically described in terms of right atrial isomerism vs. left atrial isomerism

IMAGING

- Best diagnostic clue: Abnormal symmetry in chest & abdomen
- Classic radiographic appearance: Transverse midline liver, discrepancy between position of cardiac apex & stomach, bilateral left- or right-sidedness in chest, cardiomegaly or other findings of congenital heart disease
- Echo: Initial characterization of intracardiac anomalies & abnormal systemic &/or pulmonary venous connections
- Multiplanar MR for segmental analysis of intracardiac connections & defects
- CTA: Rapid examination of chest & abdomen for abnormalities of situs, systemic & pulmonary venous connections, tracheobronchial anatomy

- Upper GI study: Malrotation frequently associated
- Best imaging tools: Echocardiography, followed by MR

PATHOLOGY

- Any arrangement other than situs solitus or inversus is termed situs ambiguous
- Heterotaxy syndrome represents spectrum with overlap between classic asplenia & polysplenia manifestations & other anomalies

CLINICAL ISSUES

- Asplenia
  - Neonate with severe cyanosis, susceptibility for infections, severe congenital heart disease
- Polysplenia
  - Less severe cardiac disease (i.e., systemic venous malformations, atrial septal defect); often presents later
- 1st year mortality: 85% asplenia, 65% polysplenia

(Left) PA chest radiograph demonstrates a left-sided cardiac apex ➡️, a left-sided aortic arch ➡️, & a right-sided stomach bubble ➡️ in this patient with situs ambiguous. (Right) Axial CECT through the upper abdomen in a child with heterotaxy shows a right-sided stomach ➡️ & multiple spleens ➡️. An enlarged azygous vein is noted ➡️ but no intrahepatic inferior vena cava (IVC) is visualized, consistent with azygous continuation of the IVC.

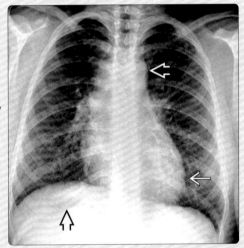

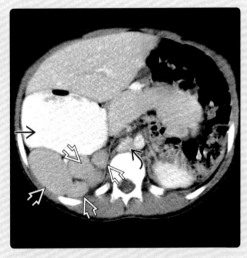

(Left) Axial CECT through the upper abdomen in a child with heterotaxy demonstrates a midline liver ➡️, a left-sided stomach ➡️, multiple spleens ➡️, & an enlarged azygous vein ➡️ without an intrahepatic IVC, consistent with azygous continuation of the IVC. (Right) Coronal CTA shows symmetric bilateral eparterial bronchi ➡️ above the visualized pulmonary arteries ➡️, consistent with right isomerism. The bronchi both have a configuration typical of right main bronchi.

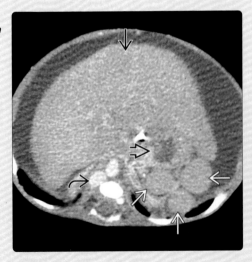

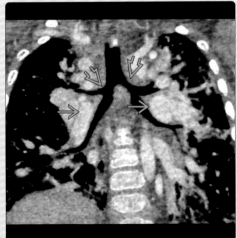

TERMINOLOGY

Synonyms

- Situs ambiguous, right/left isomerism

Definitions

- Disturbance of normal left-right asymmetry in position of thoracic & abdominal organs

IMAGING

Radiographic Findings

- Classic appearance: Transverse midline liver, discrepancy between position of cardiac apex & stomach, bilateral left- or right-sidedness in chest, cardiomegaly or other findings of congenital heart disease (CHD)
- Asplenia syndrome or right atrial isomerism
  - Bilateral minor fissures
  - Symmetrical short main bronchi with right-sided morphology (narrow carinal angle, early take-off of upper lobe bronchus)
  - Bilateral eparterial bronchi: Main bronchus is superior to branch pulmonary artery (eparterial bronchus)
  - Cardiomegaly, pulmonary edema
- Polysplenia syndrome or left atrial isomerism
  - No minor fissure on either side
  - Symmetrical long main bronchi with left-sided morphology (wide carinal angle)
  - Bilateral hyparterial bronchi: Main bronchus is inferior to branch pulmonary artery (hyparterial bronchus)
  - Absent inferior vena cava (IVC) shadow on lateral film, prominent azygous shadow on AP
- Both syndromes
  - Cardiac malposition (40%: Mesocardia, dextrocardia)
  - Transverse liver
  - Right stomach bubble with levocardia, left stomach bubble with dextrocardia, or midline stomach

Other Modality Findings

- Upper GI study: Malrotation frequently associated

Imaging Recommendations

- Best imaging tool
  - Echocardiography, followed by MR
  - CTA for anatomic study in postoperative patients

DIFFERENTIAL DIAGNOSIS

Situs Inversus Totalis

- Mirror image of normal
- Low association with CHD (3-5%)
- May be associated with immotile cilia syndrome (Kartagener): Sinusitis, bronchiectasis, infertility

True Dextrocardia + Abdominal Situs Solitus or Levocardia + Abdominal Situs Inversus

- Both have high association with CHD (95-100%)

Dextroversion of Heart

- Heart in right chest with apex & stomach on left
  - Right lung hypoplasia (scimitar syndrome)
  - Left-sided mass lesions (diaphragmatic hernia, congenital pulmonary airway malformation)

PATHOLOGY

General Features

- Spectrum with overlap between asplenia & polysplenia
  - Pathophysiology determined by associated CHD
- No specific genetic defect in majority (usually sporadic)

Staging, Grading, & Classification

- 2 major subtypes
  - Asplenia syndrome = right atrial isomerism or double/bilateral right-sidedness
    - Absence of spleen
    - IVC & aorta on same side
    - Bilateral superior vena cavae (~ 36%)
    - Bilateral trilobed lungs with eparterial bronchi
    - Right isomerism of atrial appendages
    - Associated with severe cyanotic CHD (atrioventricular septal defect, common atrioventricular valve, double-outlet right ventricle, transposition of great arteries, pulmonary stenosis/atresia)
    - Abnormalities of pulmonary venous connections
      - Total anomalous pulmonary venous return, > 80%; often obstructed, below diaphragm
  - Polysplenia syndrome = left atrial isomerism or double/bilateral left-sidedness
    - Multiple spleens, anisosplenia, multilobed spleen (functional asplenia)
    - Bilateral bilobed lungs with hyparterial bronchi
    - Bilateral superior vena cavae (~ 41%)
    - Left isomerism of atrial appendages
    - Associated with less severe CHD (common atrium, ventricular septal defect)
    - Abnormalities of systemic venous connections: Interrupted IVC with azygous continuation (> 70%), hepatic veins drain separately into common atrium

CLINICAL ISSUES

Presentation

- Most common signs/symptoms
  - Asplenia: Male neonate with severe cyanosis, susceptibility for infections
  - Polysplenia: More variable, often presents later
- Other signs/symptoms
  - Malrotation, volvulus, extrahepatic biliary atresia

Natural History & Prognosis

- 1st year mortality: 85% asplenia, 65% polysplenia

Treatment

- Prostaglandins (if CHD lesion has inadequate pulmonary blood flow or aortic arch interruption/obstruction)
- Various surgical procedures depending on nature of underlying cardiac disease
- Antibiotic prophylaxis (for functional asplenia)

SELECTED REFERENCES

1. Teele SA et al: Heterotaxy syndrome: proceedings from the 10th international PCICS meeting. World J Pediatr Congenit Heart Surg. 6(4):616-29, 2015
2. Kothari SS: Non-cardiac issues in patients with heterotaxy syndrome. Ann Pediatr Cardiol. 7(3):187-92, 2014

Kawasaki Disease

TERMINOLOGY

- Inflammatory disease of small- & medium-sized blood vessels of unknown etiology, mainly in young children
  - Widespread but characteristic manifestations
  - Coronary artery aneurysms most feared complication

IMAGING

- Chest radiography usually normal
- Echocardiography has sufficient sensitivity & specificity in detecting proximal coronary artery aneurysms
  - Remains 1st-line modality
- CTA can demonstrate aneurysms, stenoses, & Ca^{2+} of coronary or other arteries
- Cardiac MR protocol includes function, coronary artery imaging, 1st-pass perfusion, & late gadolinium enhancement for myocardial viability
- MRA with large field of view can show aneurysms of peripheral arteries

TOP DIFFERENTIAL DIAGNOSES

- Exanthematous infections, allergies or hypersensitivity reactions, vasculitides

PATHOLOGY

- Etiology unclear, but clinical & epidemiologic features suggest abnormal immune response to toxin or infection

CLINICAL ISSUES

- Acute febrile phase (days 1-11): Fever for ≥ 5 days, bilateral nonpurulent conjunctivitis, rash, extremity erythema/edema, oral mucosa becomes red & cracked, cervical lymphadenopathy (usually unilateral), gallbladder hydrops; myocarditis (36%) & pericarditis (16%)
- Subacute phase (days 11-21): Thrombocytosis, desquamation of digits, aneurysms develop; fever resolved
- Chronic phase (> 60 days): Cardiac complications
- Favorable outcome with early recognition & treatment with intravenous gamma globulin + aspirin

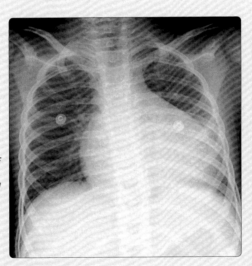
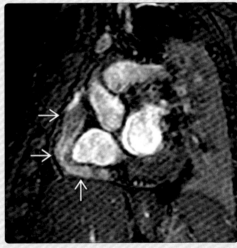

(Left) AP radiograph of a 5-year-old boy with persistent fever shows an enlarged cardiac silhouette due to cardiomegaly. A chest radiograph obtained 6 days earlier (not shown) demonstrated a normal cardiac silhouette. (Right) Sagittal bright blood SSFP MR of the same patient shows a large fusiform aneurysm ➡ of the right coronary artery. This patient had already developed a myocardial infarction.

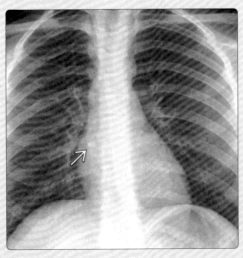
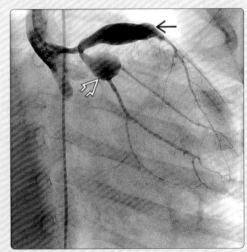

(Left) PA radiograph of an older child shows a curvilinear Ca^{2+} ➡ projecting inferior to the right hilum. The patient's history revealed that the child had been diagnosed with Kawasaki disease at the age of 4 years, confirming that this abnormality is due to a calcified aneurysm. (Right) Oblique angiography of the left main coronary artery in a patient with Kawasaki disease shows fusiform aneurysmal dilation of the proximal left anterior descending coronary artery ➡ & a bulbous aneurysmal dilation of the left circumflex coronary artery ➡.

TERMINOLOGY

Synonyms

- Mucocutaneous lymph node syndrome; acute febrile mucocutaneous syndrome

Definitions

- Inflammatory disease of small & medium blood vessels of unknown etiology, occurring in characteristic phases

IMAGING

Radiographic Findings

- Chest radiography usually normal initially
- Occasionally, may have large cardiac silhouette due to pericardial effusion or cardiomegaly
- ± Ca^{2+} of coronary or other arteries

Echocardiographic Findings

- Sufficient sensitivity (80-85%) & specificity for proximal coronary artery ectasia & aneurysms → 1st-line modality
  - Evaluates ventricular function, valvar function, & pericardial effusion

CT Findings

- CTA can demonstrate aneurysms, stenoses, & Ca^{2+} of coronary or other arteries

MR Findings

- T2WI: Can show edema secondary to myocarditis acutely
- GRE MR stress imaging: Quantifies perfusion
- MRA: Accurately images coronary artery aneurysms, occlusions, & stenoses; can be used to depict & follow other aneurysms of thorax & abdomen or peripheral involvement
- Steady-state free precession cine MR: Shows regional wall motion abnormalities; can measure cardiac function with end diastolic volumes & ejection fraction
- Late gadolinium enhancement: Can show infarcted myocardium

Ultrasonographic Findings

- Lymphadenopathy usually nonsuppurative, unilateral, & in anterior triangle of neck
- Gallbladder may be hydropic
- ± nephromegaly
- Aneurysms may be identified outside of chest

Imaging Recommendations

- Best imaging tool
  - Echocardiography for initial & sequential studies
  - Cardiac MR in older children for assessing function, myocardial ischemia, myocardial viability, & aneurysms

DIFFERENTIAL DIAGNOSIS

Exanthematous Infections: Viral or Bacterial

- Toxic shock syndrome, rheumatic fever, mononucleosis

Allergic or Hypersensitivity Reactions

- Stevens-Johnson syndrome, erythema multiforme

Vasculitides

- Systemic lupus erythematosus, polyarteritis nodosa, Takayasu arteritis

CLINICAL ISSUES

Presentation

- Most common signs/symptoms
  - Acute febrile phase (days 1-11)
    - Temperature elevated ≥ 5 days
    - Bilateral nonpurulent conjunctivitis
    - Rash
    - Hands & feet develop erythema & edema
    - Tongue & oral mucosa become red & cracked
    - Cervical lymphadenopathy, usually unilateral
    - Myocarditis (36%) & pericarditis (16%)
  - Subacute phase (days 11-21): Fever has resolved
    - Persistent irritability, anorexia, conjunctivitis
    - Thrombocytosis develops
    - Desquamation of fingers & toes
    - ± aneurysms (greatest risk for sudden death)
  - Convalescent phase (days 21-60): Symptoms resolved
  - Chronic phase (> 60 days): Cardiac complications
- Other signs/symptoms
  - Dilation of gallbladder (hydrops) early in disease (15%)
  - Hepatic enlargement & jaundice can occur
  - Diarrhea, vomiting, abdominal pain

Demographics

- Peak incidence: 6 months to 2 years
- Another peak occurs after 5 years of age
- Japan: Incidence 50/100,000 children < 4 years of age (10x that of USA)

Natural History & Prognosis

- Self-limited disease in majority of cases
- Favorable outcome with early recognition & treatment
- With development of coronary artery aneurysms
  - Thrombosis, arrhythmia, infarct, or delayed rupture
  - Persistent wall abnormalities after aneurysm regression
  - Chronic coronary insufficiency, premature atherosclerosis in < 4%
  - Death in > 1% due to arrhythmias

Treatment

- High-dose aspirin used as antiinflammatory agent early in disease until fever has decreased
- Intravenous gamma globulin given in acute phase to reduce coronary artery abnormalities
- Low-dose aspirin used in children for 6-8 weeks & for prolonged period in children with confirmed aneurysms
- Transcatheter coronary intervention if thrombosis occurs: Thrombolysis with tissue plasminogen activator
- Long-term treatment directed by degree of coronary involvement: Coronary bypass surgery or cardiac transplantation may be necessary

SELECTED REFERENCES

1. Newburger JW et al: Kawasaki disease. J Am Coll Cardiol. 67(14):1738-49, 2016
2. Mavrogeni S et al: How to image Kawasaki disease: a validation of different imaging techniques. Int J Cardiol. 124(1):27-31, 2008

Rheumatic Heart Disease

TERMINOLOGY

- Acute rheumatic fever: Multisystem disease affecting heart, joints, skin, & brain 1-5 weeks following infection with group A β-hemolytic *Streptococcus*
  - Due to autoimmune response
  - 40% of acute rheumatic fever patients develop cardiac involvement (rheumatic heart disease)

IMAGING

- Acute rheumatic fever: Large heart, left atrial enlargement, pulmonary edema (due to left ventricular dysfunction with mitral insufficiency)
  - "Rheumatic pneumonia" rarely seen
  - Pericardial effusion
- Chronic RHD: Ca^{2+} of valves, especially mitral or aortic
- Echocardiogram during acute disease quantitates degree of mitral insufficiency & left ventricular function
- Echocardiogram in chronic disease shows progression of valve stenosis with thickened leaflets, which calcify

CLINICAL ISSUES

- Acute disease occurs in young children 3-15 years who present with streptococcal infection (usually pharyngitis)
  - RHD develops after 0.3% of such infections in USA
- Initial treatment: Therapy aimed at preventing acute rheumatic fever by treating group A streptococcal pharyngitis & eradicating reservoir for transmission
  - Disease has dramatically ↓ in USA where sore throat from *Streptococcus pyogenes* is treated
  - Disease now most common in overcrowded, poor areas of world where *S. pyogenes* can spread in dry, hot climate
- Jones criteria for rheumatic fever: Diagnosis with 2 major or 1 major + 2 minor criteria with evidence of streptococcal infection
  - Major: Carditis, polyarthritis, chorea, subcutaneous nodules, & erythema marginatum
  - Minor: Fever, arthralgia, elevated acute phase reactants, ↑ sedimentation rate

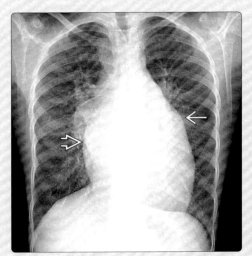
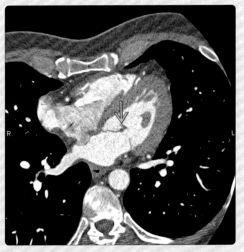

(Left) *PA radiograph in an adult with rheumatic heart disease (RHD) shows cardiomegaly with dilation of the left atrial appendage ➡, creating a broad bump on the lateral margin of the heart below the level of the pulmonary artery. The left atrium splays the carina & creates a double shadow over the right heart border ➡.* (Right) *Axial CECT in a young adult shows irregular thickening of the mitral valve ➡ due to RHD.*

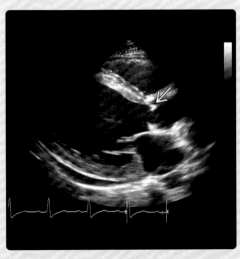
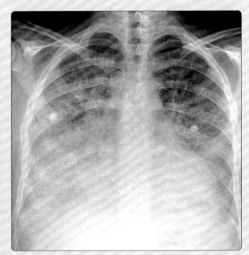

(Left) *Left ventricular outflow tract (3 chamber) view echocardiogram of a 17 year old with prior acute rheumatic fever shows the aortic valve ➡ to be thickened & destroyed with moderate to severe regurgitation (on Doppler, not shown). Vegetations were visualized, confirming endocarditis complicating RHD.* (Right) *AP radiograph in the same patient shows pulmonary edema due to progressive aortic insufficiency from acute bacterial endocarditis complicating rheumatic aortic valve disease.*

Marfan Syndrome

TERMINOLOGY

- Inherited autosomal dominant connective tissue disorder due to *FBN1* mutation → abnormal fibrillin-1

IMAGING

- Cardiovascular: Aortic root dilation (75%), ascending aortic dissection, mitral valve prolapse (50-70%), main pulmonary artery dilation, mitral annulus Ca²⁺, abdominal aorta dilation
- Skeletal: Pectus excavatum, pectus carinatum, long arms & legs, arachnodactyly, joint hypermobility, scoliosis, thoracic lordosis, pes planus, protrusio acetabuli
- Pulmonary: Spontaneous pneumothorax, apical blebs
- Dural: Ectasia (enlarged nerve sleeves & posterior vertebral body scalloping)
- Best imaging tools
  o CTA in acute setting to exclude dissection &/or rupture
  o Echocardiography or cardiac MR for routine follow-up of aortic root dilation & valvular disease

PATHOLOGY

- 2010 revised Ghent nosology for diagnosis
  o Based on family history, aortic root size/dissection, ectopia lentis, *FBN1* mutation, systemic score

CLINICAL ISSUES

- Presentation: Heart murmurs, chest pain, visual disturbances, tall with extended arm span, long fingers & toes, pectus excavatum
  o 90% of deaths from cardiovascular complications
    – Progressive aortic dilation → highest risk of dissection
      □ Chest pain radiating down back in Marfan syndrome patient → suspect aortic dissection
- Treatment
  o Medical: β-blocker or angiotensin II receptor blocker for prophylaxis of progressive aortic root dilation
  o Surgery: Prophylactic aortic root surgery when diameter at sinuses of Valsalva exceeds 5 cm

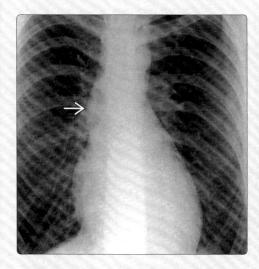

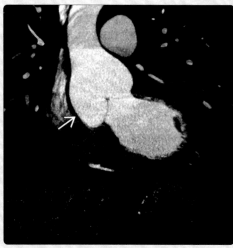

(Left) *Single frontal view of the chest in a patient with Marfan syndrome shows a dilated ascending aorta ➡ along the right side of the mediastinum.* (Right) *Coronal MR angiogram of the chest in a patient with Marfan syndrome shows aortic dilation at the sinuses of Valsalva ➡. This is commonly seen in patients with Marfan syndrome & causes soft tissue prominence along the right side of the mediastinum on the chest radiograph.*

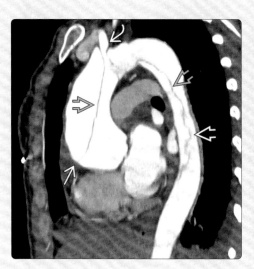

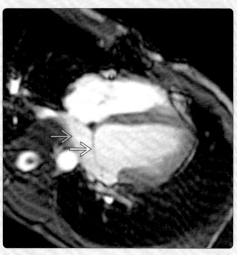

(Left) *Sagittal oblique chest CTA in a patient with Marfan syndrome demonstrates an extensive dissection ➡ of the aorta, which extends from the ascending aorta ➡ to the descending aorta ➡. Note the involvement of the brachiocephalic artery ➡.* (Right) *Four-chamber view from a cine bright blood SSFP cardiac MR demonstrates mitral valve prolapse with ballooning of the septal leaflet of the mitral valve ➡ into the left atrium ➡.*

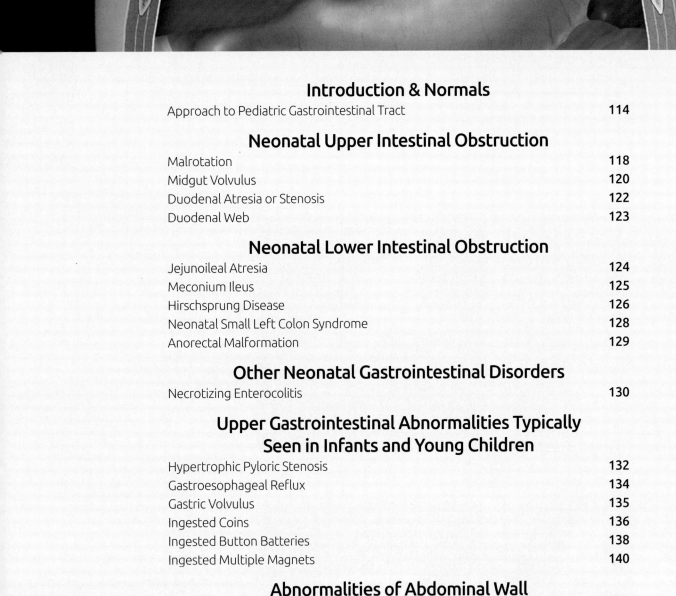

SECTION 4
Gastrointestinal

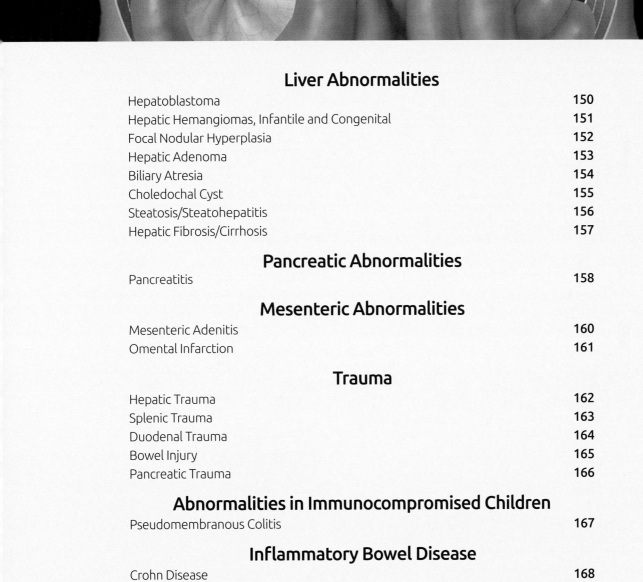

Liver Abnormalities

Pancreatic Abnormalities

Mesenteric Abnormalities

Trauma

Abnormalities in Immunocompromised Children

Inflammatory Bowel Disease

Miscellaneous

Imaging Modalities

Radiography

Generalized abdominal pain, vomiting, & constipation are the most common indications for plain radiographs in the pediatric patient. A patient with a palpable mass may also benefit from plain radiographs if a stool ball is a consideration. Abdominal pain that is able to be localized more clearly (either by suggestive history, physical exam, or laboratory tests) often leads directly to a cross-sectional imaging exam, particularly ultrasound or CT.

A mnemonic for recalling key points in assessing abdominal radiographs is "stones, bones, mass, gas." While attention is typically given primarily to the detection of free air or an abnormal bowel gas pattern, this mnemonic helps us remember other findings of the pediatric abdomen that may be radiographically detectable (with "stones" being due to abnormal calcifications of any kind and "mass" generally as a distortion of the normal bowel gas distribution). "Gas" also helps remind us to look at the lung bases on abdominal radiographs (as pneumonia can present with abdominal pain).

One question that frequently arises is the need for 1 vs. 2 views of the abdomen. A single supine view is generally sufficient if the primary concern is for constipation, or if the bowel gas is being followed serially in an inpatient after an initial 2-view exam. However, an additional view that dependently shifts bowel contents (such as an upright, left-side down decubitus, or cross-table lateral view) is particularly helpful in further discerning bowel gas patterns & detecting free intraperitoneal air.

Assessment of the bowel gas pattern is core to the interpretation of the abdominal plan radiograph. Beyond the neonatal period, mild to moderate amounts of gas & stool are scattered throughout the colon to the level of the rectum. Mild amounts of gas will be also scattered throughout the small bowel.

When there are focally lesser or greater amounts of bowel gas than expected in 1 region, the phrases "nonspecific" or "paucity of bowel gas" may be applied. These should not be interpreted by the clinician as normal (& should not be used as such by the radiologist), but these terms generally represent mild to moderate deviations from normal without other concerning imaging features (such as frankly dilated gas-filled bowel loops, small bowel air-fluid levels, or bowel wall thickening) that would allow further characterization radiographically.

A commonly seen (& occasionally initially frightening) bowel gas pattern in young children with air swallowing (typically in the setting of a respiratory infection or asthma) is generalized gaseous distention of bowel. However, this gaseous distention/mild dilation should not be localized to just 1 segment (such as the stomach, which would imply gastric outlet or duodenal obstruction).

One of the most common bowel gas patterns in the pediatric patient is that of gastroenteritis. Typically, there are scattered or multiple gas-distended bowel loops with mild dilation. Numerous air-fluid levels may be present on an upright or decubitus view, and colonic air-fluid levels are particularly suggestive of gastroenteritis. Ileus can overlap this appearance, though clinical findings (such as lack of bowel sounds) would be typical (unlike gastroenteritis or obstruction). A distal small bowel obstruction might also overlap the appearance of gastroenteritis, but colonic distention & air-fluid levels would not be typical. Focally or diffusely dilated bowel loops are particularly concerning for obstruction or (rarely) ischemic ileus, though it should be noted that both of these concerning entities may have a relatively innocuous plain film appearance.

Radiographs are rarely of value when the pain is secondary to blunt abdominal trauma, though iatrogenic trauma (such as an endoscopic biopsy that leads to pain) may benefit from upright or decubitus radiography as an initial exam to look for free intraperitoneal air.

Ultrasound

In most children, ultrasound provides excellent visualization of the abdominal viscera, including solid & hollow organs. However, an appropriate "nothing by mouth" (NPO) preparation may be required to limit the bowel gas that can obscure adjacent organs. The exact NPO time required prior to the study is determined by individual departments & varies according to the type of scan requested.

The hepatobiliary system is well characterized by sonography, including hepatic lesions, biliary dilation, & gallbladder pathology. The detection of collections (localized or free) is also served well by ultrasound. The evaluation of certain gut pathologies in the child has largely changed from fluoroscopy to ultrasound in the last 20 years, including evaluations for hypertrophic pyloric stenosis & ileocolic intussusceptions. Many institutions also now use ultrasound as the primary modality for evaluating appendicitis (with CECT or MR serving as a backup modality for unclear cases). Some centers are also using ultrasound for a variety of other bowel pathologies, including inflammatory bowel disease, midgut volvulus, & necrotizing enterocolitis, though these uses are highly institution specific.

Sonography remains an excellent choice in the initial evaluation of a pediatric patient with a suspected abdominal mass, be it a cyst or neoplasm. Further cross-sectional imaging, such as with CECT or MR, will ultimately be required for most confirmed masses to determine the extent of the lesion & relationship to critical nearby structures (such as vessels).

Fluoroscopy

A variety of fluoroscopic studies with contrast are used to examine the pediatric GI tract.

The video swallow study (a.k.a. the modified barium swallow) is typically employed in patients with anomalies of the airway, upper GI tract, &/or nervous system that impair swallowing &/or predispose to aspiration. These studies are typically performed in conjunction with speech pathologists who may be evaluating the patient in other ways as well.

Common indications for an esophagram include dysphagia, acute food impaction, & complications of prior or ongoing esophageal disease (such as repaired esophageal atresia & tracheoesophageal fistula with postoperative stricture). The esophagram is rarely useful in the setting of spontaneous pneumomediastinum (which typically results from alveolar rupture rather than esophageal perforation). However, patients with pneumomediastinum after penetrating injury, blunt trauma with other thoracic injuries, or severe vomiting may require a contrast evaluation of the esophagus.

The upper GI series is most commonly used to evaluate vomiting patterns outside of the young infant with suspected pyloric stenosis (where ultrasound is preferred). The upper GI has traditionally served as the 1st-line tool for suspected malrotation, but this is not a perfect test. There are numerous variations in the appearance of the proximal GI tract on fluoroscopic imaging, & there has been increasing recognition that cross-sectional studies demonstrating the relationship of the duodenum to the superior mesenteric artery may be more sensitive & specific for malrotation, though even these studies are limited compared to the surgical gold standard. The upper GI series generally remains widely accepted as the modality of choice for the acute onset of bilious emesis where midgut volvulus is suspected, though ultrasound can be a helpful adjunct for unclear cases.

Small bowel follow-through (SBFT) exams can be helpful in evaluating gut dysmotility or suspected partial obstructions. SBFT exams are now less commonly used for the evaluation of acute small bowel pathology (such as inflammatory bowel disease).

One of the most commonly listed indications for a contrasted enema in pediatric patients is to "rule out Hirschsprung disease." While the contrasted enema can show features suggestive of Hirschsprung disease, Hirschsprung disease can have a variety of appearances, including normal. Therefore, the value of the enema is actually to exclude other pathologies. That is to say, if Hirschsprung disease is being considered as a cause for a distal obstruction or chronic constipation, the enema will not rule out Hirschsprung disease; this can only be done by rectal biopsy.

Computed Tomography

Due to its availability & speed, CECT is an extremely valuable tool in the setting of blunt abdominal trauma in which concerning mechanisms (such as motor vehicle accidents or falls) &/or symptoms require a rapid assessment for visceral injury. It excels at the evaluation of solid organ trauma, though bowel injury is more problematic & often relies on secondary clues (such as focal thickening or mesenteric fluid). Oral contrast is rarely useful in this setting & only delays the scan.

CECT can be helpful in evaluating other acute abdominal pathologies, including bowel obstruction, ischemia, inflammatory bowel disease, & appendicitis. The use of oral contrast in these settings can be helpful but is not without controversy. If the region of interest (such as the point of bowel obstruction) is distal to numerous dilated bowel loops, it will often not yet be opacified with oral contrast in a typical 1- to-2 hour window, potentially delaying the scan for many hours. Additionally, oral contrast may impede critical assessments of bowel wall enhancement (such as with ischemia or inflammatory bowel disease). In such settings, it is best to discuss the use of oral contrast with the radiologist &/or surgeon

Acute & chronic pancreatitis generally employs some type of cross-sectional imaging to look for necrosis & complications, though MR may provide additional tools in this arena. The evaluation of a newly detected abdominal mass by CECT vs. MR remains debated, though MR offers some advantages, particularly for the child who will require numerous follow-up studies (thereby eliminating the radiation associated with multiple CT scans).

As a general rule, NECT has no virtually no role in the evaluation of GI pathologies.

Magnetic Resonance

MR use has gained momentum in the setting of acute bowel inflammation, particularly inflammatory bowel disease & appendicitis. It has also made significant gains in imaging the hepatobiliary system, though not typically in the acute setting. Useful techniques in this arena include determinations of fat fraction (the most quantitative noninvasive way to measure liver fat) & iron content (typically in patients with chronic transfusions), MRCP to look at the biliary system, & hepatobiliary phase contrast agents (where enhancement patterns can give greater sensitivity & specificity to liver lesions than other modalities).

Nuclear Medicine

Nuclear imaging of the pediatric GI tract has few indications. The function of the hepatobiliary system (particularly with HIDA scan) can be used to evaluate gallbladder pathologies (such as acute & chronic cholecystitis) or absence of a normal hepatobiliary system (such as biliary atresia). In the patient with lower GI tract bleeding, the Meckel scan can be quite useful, having a high sensitivity & specificity for Meckel diverticula that contain ectopic gastric mucosa (which are most common overall & typically account for those causing bleeding). However, Meckel diverticula causing problems in other ways (such as inflammation or obstruction) may not be visible on these scans. Gastric emptying can also be assessed by nuclear medicine in patients with suspected dysmotility.

Selected References

1. ACR Appropriateness Criteria: Vomiting in Infants up to 3 Months of Age. https://acsearch.acr.org/docs/69445/Narrative/. Published 1995. Reviewed 2014. Accessed March 27, 2017
2. Carroll AG et al: Comparative effectiveness of imaging modalities for the diagnosis of intestinal obstruction in neonates and infants: a critically appraised topic. Acad Radiol. 23(5):559-68, 2016
3. Dillman JR et al: Equivocal pediatric appendicitis: unenhanced MR imaging protocol for nonsedated children-a clinical effectiveness study. Radiology. 279(1):216-25, 2016
4. Pugmire BS et al: Magnetic resonance imaging of primary pediatric liver tumors. Pediatr Radiol. 46(6):764-77, 2016
5. Sanchez TR et al: Sonography of abdominal pain in children: appendicitis and its common mimics. J Ultrasound Med. 35(3):627-35, 2016
6. Hernanz-Schulman M: Pyloric stenosis: role of imaging. Pediatr Radiol. 39 Suppl 2:S134-9, 2009
7. Chang PT et al: Diagnostic errors of right lower quadrant pain in children: beyond appendicitis. Abdom Imaging. 40(7):2071-90, 2015
8. Tackett JJ et al: Malrotation: Current strategies navigating the radiologic diagnosis of a surgical emergency. World J Radiol. 6(9):730-6, 2014
9. Bongers ME et al: The value of the abdominal radiograph in children with functional gastrointestinal disorders. Eur J Radiol. 59(1):8-13, 2006
10. Strouse PJ: Sonographic evaluation of the child with lower abdominal or pelvic pain. Radiol Clin North Am. 44(6):911-23, 2006

(Left) Supine radiograph in a 16 year old with abdominal pain shows what is essentially a normal bowel gas pattern with moderate amounts of stool & gas throughout the colon ⮕ to the level of the rectum ➡. There is nonspecific prominence of a few small bowel loops centrally ⮕. (Right) Upright radiograph in the same patient shows normal gas & stool in the colon ⮕. There is no dilation, thickening, or air-fluid level of the small bowel ⮕ to suggest pathology. There is a normal air-fluid level in the stomach ⮕.

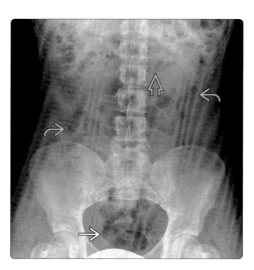

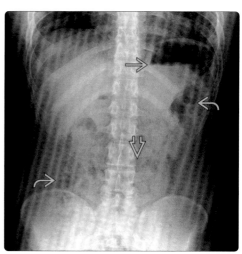

(Left) Upright radiograph in a 17 year old with abdominal pain shows free intraperitoneal air under the right hemidiaphragm ⮕ & over the liver. The free air under the left hemidiaphragm ⮕ is more difficult to see due to the adjacent stomach bubble ⮕. Contrast remains within the colon ⮕ from a previous upper GI series. (Right) Cross-table lateral radiograph in the same patient confirms free intraperitoneal air ⮕ overlying the liver, strongly suggesting a bowel perforation.

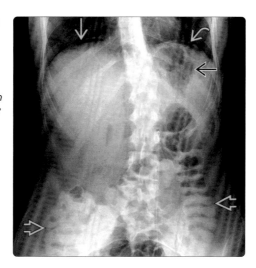

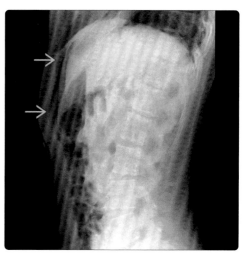

(Left) Supine radiograph in a 6 year old with constipation shows a large stool burden throughout the colon ⮕, most pronounced at the rectum ⮕. (Right) Upright radiograph in a 4 year old with fever & upper abdominal pain shows generalized gaseous distention of small & large bowel with numerous predominantly colonic air-fluid levels ⮕, a pattern than can be seen with gastroenteritis or ileus. Also note the retrocardiac left lower lobe pneumonia ⮕ & pleural effusion ⮕.

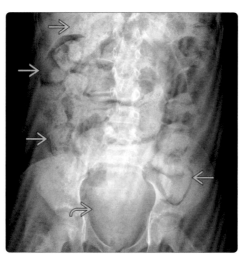

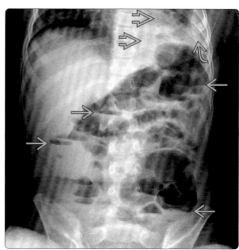

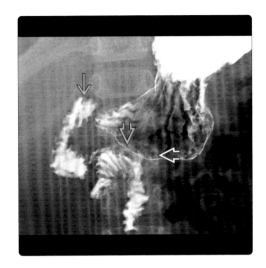

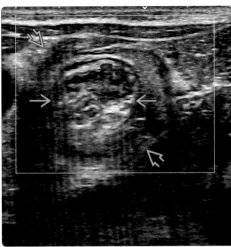

(Left) *Supine upper GI series in a 3 year old with malrotation shows the duodenojejunal junction ⇨ below the level of the duodenal bulb ⇥ & right of the left vertebral pedicle ⇉. This anomaly predisposes children to midgut volvulus.* (Right) *Transverse US of the right lower quadrant in a 16 month old with intermittent abdominal pain, bilious emesis, & bloody stools shows the target sign of an ileocolic intussusception. The concentric circles of the target sign are made up from the inner intussusceptum ⇨ & the outer intussuscipiens ⇨.*

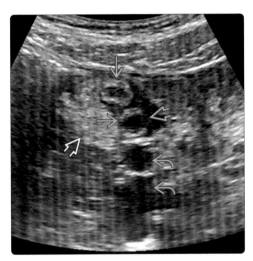

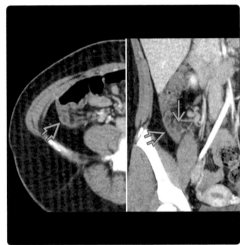

(Left) *Transverse right lower quadrant US in an adolescent with appendicitis shows interruption ⇨ of the wall of the coiled & dilated appendix ⇥ (viewed in cross sections). The appendix overlies the iliac vessels ⇥. Note the induration/inflammation of the periappendiceal fat ⇉.* (Right) *Abdominal CECT images in an 11 year old with right lower quadrant pain, vomiting, & leukocytosis show a dilated retrocecal appendix ⇥ with enhancement & adjacent fat stranding ⇥, consistent with acute appendicitis.*

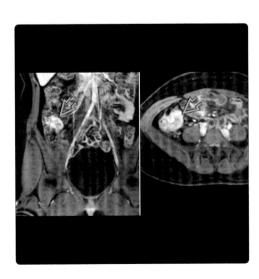

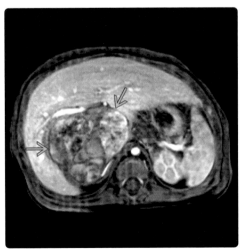

(Left) *T1 C+ FS MR enterography images in a 15 year old with newly diagnosed Crohn disease show mucosal hyperenhancement & wall thickening of the terminal ileum ⇥, consistent with active inflammation.* (Right) *Axial T1 C+ FS MR in a 16 month old with hepatoblastoma shows a heterogeneously enhancing mass ⇥ arising from the right lobe of the liver.*

KEY FACTS

TERMINOLOGY

- Malrotation: Any abnormal rotation of small or large bowel, which rotate separately during development
- Malfixation: Abnormal position or length of bowel fixation by mesentery, typically associated with malrotation
  - Short mesenteric fixation predisposes to midgut volvulus [twisting of midgut about superior mesenteric artery (SMA) → vascular occlusion & potential bowel ischemia]

IMAGING

- Fluoroscopic GI findings
  - 3rd duodenum (D3) never crosses midline, often extends anteriorly on lateral view of upper GI
  - Duodenojejunal junction lies right of left pedicle & below duodenal bulb on true frontal view of upper GI
  - Variable degrees of colonic malrotation with abnormal cecal position on enema or small bowel follow-through
- US/CT/MR

- Duodenal nonrotation: D3 segment fails to pass between SMA & aorta when crossing to left of midline
- Reversal of normal SMA/superior mesenteric vein position (not reliable)
- Best imaging tool
  - Fluoroscopic upper GI vs. ultrasound debated

PATHOLOGY

- Typically isolated but common in congenital diaphragmatic hernia, gastroschisis, omphalocele, & heterotaxy

CLINICAL ISSUES

- Majority present in infancy with nonbilious or bilious emesis, recurrent abdominal pain, or poor weight gain; may be asymptomatic
- Treated with Ladd procedure: Untwist volvulus if present, divide Ladd bands if present, reposition small & large intestine into right & left abdomen, respectively

(Left) Anterior graphic shows abnormal positions of the small & large bowel. The duodenojejunal junction (DJJ) lies low & midline ➡, very close to the malpositioned cecum ⇨. This results in a short mesenteric fixation that predisposes to midgut volvulus. (Right) Lateral upper GI image in a 3-year-old child with a history of nonbilious vomiting shows an anterior, intraperitoneal course of the D3 segment with a low position of the DJJ ➡ below the duodenal bulb ⇨, indicating abnormal rotation.

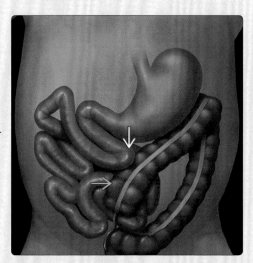
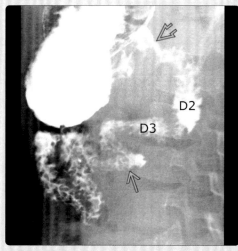

(Left) Supine front view of the same patient shows a low DJJ ➡ (below the duodenal bulb ⇨) that fails to cross the midline, consistent with malrotation. Note that there is no twisting or dilation of the duodenum to suggest midgut volvulus or obstructing Ladd bands. (Right) Supine SBFT was continued in the same patient to determine the cecal position & estimate the length of the mesenteric pedicle. The cecum (C) is high & just left of the midline, suggesting a very short mesenteric pedicle that is at high risk of future midgut volvulus.

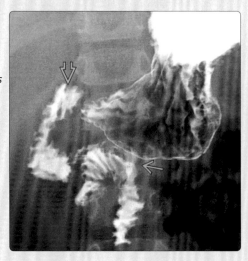
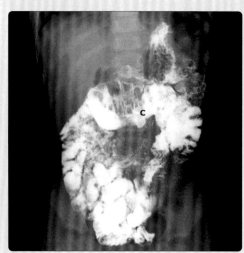

TERMINOLOGY

Definitions

- Malrotation: Varying degrees of abnormal positioning of small &/or large bowel due to abnormal rotation during development
  - Small & large bowel rotate separately in utero
  - Abnormalities of rotation may affect either or both
- Malfixation: Abnormal position or length of bowel fixation by mesentery, typically associated with malrotation
  - Predisposes to midgut volvulus (MV)

IMAGING

General Features

- Best diagnostic clue
  - Upper GI: Nonretroperitoneal position of duodenum + abnormal duodenojejunal junction (DJJ) position at or to right of midline
  - US/CT/MR: Failure of 3rd duodenum (D3) to pass between aorta & superior mesenteric artery (SMA)
  - Enema or cross-sectional imaging: Abnormal configuration of colon

Fluoroscopic Findings

- Upper GI
  - D3 never crosses midline; often extends anteriorly on lateral view
  - DJJ to right of left pedicle on true frontal view
  - Jejunum often in right abdomen
  - ± bowel obstruction due to Ladd bands or MV
- Contrast enema
  - Variable degrees of colonic malrotation
    - High &/or midline cecum of partial rotation
    - Left-sided colon of nonrotation
    - Anything in between

Imaging Recommendations

- Best imaging tool
  - Fluoroscopic upper GI to visualize DJJ

PATHOLOGY

General Features

- Etiology
  - Failure of normal embryonic 270° counterclockwise rotation of midgut & colon, resulting in malposition of bowel to varying degrees
    - Ranges from complete nonrotation to nearly normal
    - Length of mesenteric fixation from DJJ to cecum determines risk for MV
  - Ladd (peritoneal fibrous) bands attempt to fix abnormal duodenal &/or colonic positions
    - Can occur anywhere, frequently across D2 or D3
    - Potentially lead to extrinsic obstruction
- Associated abnormalities
  - Congenital diaphragmatic hernia, gastroschisis, & omphalocele will virtually always have malrotation
    - Rarely volvulize due to adhesions
  - Malrotation commonly associated with duodenal atresia spectrum, small bowel atresia & stenosis, & heterotaxy syndromes (asplenia & polysplenia), among others

Gross Pathologic & Surgical Features

- Ligament of Treitz: Muscle that can be stretched
  - Normal position of DJJ can be displaced by
    - Adjacent dilated bowel loops
    - Adjacent masses, cysts, organomegaly
    - Enteric tube distorting duodenum

CLINICAL ISSUES

Presentation

- Most common signs/symptoms
  - Children: Nonbilious or bilious emesis, recurrent abdominal pain, poor weight gain; may be asymptomatic
  - Adults: Nonspecific → chronic vomiting, intermittent colicky abdominal pain, diarrhea

Demographics

- Majority present in 1st month of life
  - Vast majority present by 1st few years of life
- 1/200 live births have asymptomatic rotational anomaly
  - 1/6,000 live births have symptomatic malrotation

Natural History & Prognosis

- Complications of malrotation
  - MV: Twisting of midgut about SMA → vascular occlusion & potential bowel ischemia
  - Bowel obstruction due to Ladd bands
  - Internal hernia: Rare, usually due to duodenal malrotation with normal colonic rotation
    - Sac-like mass of malfixed bowel herniates posterior to right colic vein into right upper quadrant

Treatment

- Ladd procedure
  - Untwist volvulus if present
  - Divide Ladd bands if present
  - Reposition small & large intestine into right & left abdomen, respectively
    - Adhesions expected to secure bowel in place
  - ± appendectomy

SELECTED REFERENCES

1. Abbas PI et al: Evaluating a management strategy for malrotation in heterotaxy patients. J Pediatr Surg. 51(5):859-62, 2016
2. Carroll AG et al: Comparative effectiveness of imaging modalities for the diagnosis of intestinal obstruction in neonates and infants: a critically appraised topic. Acad Radiol. 23(5):559-68, 2016
3. Drewett M et al: The burden of excluding malrotation in term neonates with bile stained vomiting. Pediatr Surg Int. 32(5):483-6, 2016
4. Koch C et al: Redefining the projectional and clinical anatomy of the duodenojejunal flexure in children. Clin Anat. 29(2):175-82, 2016
5. Raitio A et al: Malrotation: age-related differences in reoperation rate. Eur J Pediatr Surg. 26(1):34-7, 2016
6. Graziano K et al: Asymptomatic malrotation: diagnosis and surgical management: an American Pediatric Surgical Association outcomes and evidence based practice committee systematic review. J Pediatr Surg. 50(10):1783-90, 2015
7. Landisch R et al: Observation versus prophylactic Ladd procedure for asymptomatic intestinal rotational abnormalities in heterotaxy syndrome: A systematic review. J Pediatr Surg. 50(11):1971-4, 2015
8. Lodwick DL et al: Current surgical management of intestinal rotational abnormalities. Curr Opin Pediatr. 27(3):383-8, 2015
9. Zhou LY et al: Usefulness of sonography in evaluating children suspected of malrotation: comparison with an upper gastrointestinal contrast Study. J Ultrasound Med. 34(10):1825-32, 2015

KEY FACTS

TERMINOLOGY

- Ligament of Treitz: Suspends duodenojejunal junction (DJJ), defines normal duodenal rotation
- Malrotation: Abnormal rotation & fixation of small bowel (SB) mesentery that can lead to complications
  - Bowel obstruction by Ladd bands
  - Midgut volvulus (MV) due to short mesenteric base, prone to twisting
- MV: Twisting of SB about superior mesenteric artery → bowel obstruction, ischemia/necrosis

IMAGING

- Radiographs: Most common appearance is normal
  - Distended stomach & proximal duodenum with ↓ distal bowel gas very suggestive
  - May rarely show diffuse distal bowel distention/ileus from ischemia/necrosis
- Upper GI: Dilated duodenum to D2-D3 segment with corkscrew/spiral sign just beyond duodenal "beak"

- US or CT: Whirlpool sign

TOP DIFFERENTIAL DIAGNOSES

- Malrotation with obstructing Ladd band
- Spectrum of congenital duodenal obstructions

PATHOLOGY

- If bowel malrotated, DJJ-cecal distance (mesenteric base) is short, predisposing to twisting (volvulus)

CLINICAL ISSUES

- Classic presentation: Infant with bilious vomiting
  - > 90% present within first 3 months of life
  - Requires emergent upper GI (best imaging tool)
- Delayed diagnosis can lead to diffuse bowel necrosis
- Treatment: Surgical emergency (Ladd procedure)
  - Reduce volvulus, resect nonviable bowel, transect Ladd bands (if present), place SB in right & colon in left abdomen

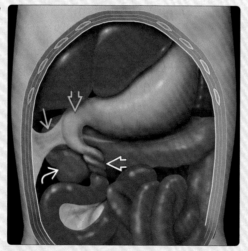

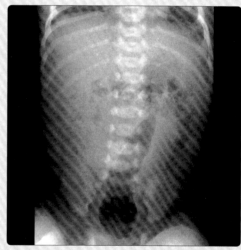

(Left) *Anterior graphic shows a midgut volvulus (MV) with dilation of the proximal duodenum* ⇨ *that tapers into a coil of twisted, narrowed loops* ⇱. *The cecum* ⇱ *is malpositioned within the right upper quadrant medially & fixed by a Ladd band* ⇨. *Note the purple discoloration & dilation of the remaining small bowel due to an ischemic ileus.* (Right) *AP radiograph shows a nonobstructive bowel gas pattern in a patient with bilious emesis who was ultimately found to have MV on a subsequent upper GI series.*

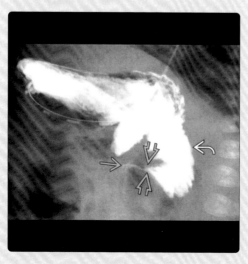

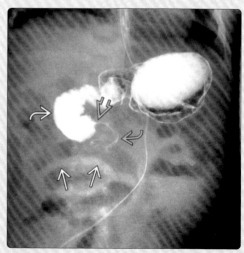

(Left) *Lateral upper GI in a 3-day-old boy with bilious vomiting shows a dilated duodenum* ⇱ *up to D3, which ends in a beak-like configuration* ⇨ *with a wisp of contrast* ⇨ *extending distally, highly suggestive of MV.* (Right) *Frontal upper GI image in the same patient (a few seconds later) shows proximal duodenal dilation* ⇱ *with partial obstruction at D3* ⇨. *The corkscrew/spiral sign* ⇨ *is diagnostic of MV. Thickened loops* ⇱ *in this context suggest bowel ischemia.*

TERMINOLOGY

Definitions

- Ligament of Treitz: Suspends duodenojejunal junction (DJJ), defines normal duodenal rotation
- Malrotation: Abnormal rotation & fixation of small bowel (SB) mesentery that can lead to complications
  - Bowel obstruction by Ladd (peritoneal) bands
  - Midgut volvulus (MV) due to short mesenteric base prone to twisting
- MV: Abnormal twisting of SB about superior mesenteric artery (SMA) that can lead to bowel obstruction & ischemia/necrosis

IMAGING

Radiographic Findings

- Distended stomach & proximal duodenum with ↓ distal bowel gas very suggestive
  - Different from marked longstanding bulbous dilation without distal gas, as seen in duodenal atresia
- May rarely show diffuse distal bowel distention/ileus from ischemia/necrosis
  - Such children often extremely ill
- Most common early finding: Normal

Fluoroscopic Findings

- Upper GI
  - Dilated duodenum to D2-D3
    - Degree of proximal duodenal dilation depends on chronicity
  - Often beaked appearance at level of twist, ± complete obstruction
  - Usually spiral/corkscrew appearance distal to beak
  - May see malrotation without MV
    - In patients with bilious emesis, this may reflect intermittent volvulus

Ultrasonographic Findings

- Proximal duodenum usually dilated
- Whirlpool sign of swirling vessels (SMV) & SB mesentery around SMA on grayscale & color Doppler

CT Findings

- CECT
  - Whirlpool sign of swirling vessels (SMV) & SB mesentery around SMA
  - Potentially ↓ or no enhancement of SB due to obstruction of SMA (causing ischemia/necrosis)
  - May have SB distention due to ischemic ileus

Imaging Recommendations

- Best imaging tool
  - Infant with bilious vomiting → emergent upper GI

DIFFERENTIAL DIAGNOSIS

Malrotation With Obstructing Ladd Bands

- May be completely obstructive with beaking, mimicking MV

Spectrum of Congenital Duodenal Obstruction

- Duodenal atresia, duodenal stenosis, annular pancreas, duodenal web

- Atresia has double bubble sign: Marked proximal duodenal dilation with **no** distal gas
- Stenosis or web usually has transition to normal distal duodenum & normal DJJ

PATHOLOGY

General Features

- Etiology
  - With normal rotation, DJJ positioned in left upper quadrant & cecum positioned in right lower quadrant
    - Results in long fixed mesenteric base between ligament of Treitz & cecum that keeps mesentery from twisting
  - If bowel malrotated, DJJ-cecal distance (mesenteric base) is short, predisposing to twisting (volvulus)

CLINICAL ISSUES

Presentation

- Most common signs/symptoms
  - Bilious emesis in 1st month of life
    - Green/yellow vomit typically from obstruction of duodenum distal to ampulla of Vater
- Other signs/symptoms
  - Acute abdominal pain
  - Patients may be asymptomatic or have atypical or chronic symptoms

Demographics

- > 90% present within first 3 months of life
- 39% present within first 10 days of life
- Can occur at any age

Natural History & Prognosis

- Delay in diagnosis can lead to diffuse bowel necrosis

Treatment

- Surgical emergency
  - Ladd procedure: Reduce volvulus, resect nonviable bowel, transect Ladd bands (if present), place SB in right & colon in left abdomen

SELECTED REFERENCES

1. Carroll AG et al: Comparative effectiveness of imaging modalities for the diagnosis of intestinal obstruction in neonates and infants: a critically appraised topic. Acad Radiol. 23(5):559-68, 2016
2. Drewett M et al: The burden of excluding malrotation in term neonates with bile stained vomiting. Pediatr Surg Int. 32(5):483-6, 2016
3. Dumitriu DI et al: Ultrasound of the duodenum in children. Pediatr Radiol. 46(9):1324-31, 2016
4. Horsch S et al: Volvulus in term and preterm infants - clinical presentation and outcome. Acta Paediatr. 105(6):623-7, 2016
5. Shrimal PK et al: Midgut volvulus with whirlpool sign. Clin Gastroenterol Hepatol. 14(2):e13, 2016
6. Mitsunaga T et al: Risk factors for intestinal obstruction after Ladd procedure. Pediatr Rep. 7(2):5795, 2015
7. Marine MB et al: Imaging of malrotation in the neonate. Semin Ultrasound CT MR. 35(6):555-70, 2014
8. Nehra D et al: Intestinal malrotation: varied clinical presentation from infancy through adulthood. Surgery. 149(3):386-93, 2011

Duodenal Atresia or Stenosis

TERMINOLOGY

- Most common upper intestinal obstruction in neonate
- Atresia: Congenital occlusion of intestinal lumen
- Stenosis: Fixed narrowing of intestinal lumen

IMAGING

- Newborn radiographic double bubble sign essentially diagnostic
  - Markedly dilated duodenum implies chronic in utero obstruction (with duodenal atresia as most common cause), especially with no distal gas
  - May not be seen on initial radiographs if stomach or duodenum decompressed by tube or vomiting
- If duodenum mildly to moderately dilated with some distal gas → emergent upper GI to exclude midgut volvulus

TOP DIFFERENTIAL DIAGNOSES

- Midgut volvulus, duodenal web, jejunal atresia, annular pancreas

PATHOLOGY

- Associated anomalies in > 50% of patients
  - Malrotation, annular pancreas, choledochal cyst or other biliary anomalies, esophageal atresia/tracheoesophageal fistula, imperforate anus, cardiac defects, renal anomalies, VACTERL association
  - 30-46% have Down syndrome (trisomy 21)

CLINICAL ISSUES

- Diagnosis often made prenatally by ultrasound
- After birth, bilious > nonbilious (80:20) vomiting
  - Determined by site of atresia relative to ampulla of Vater
- Untreated: Dehydration, electrolyte abnormalities, death
- With surgical treatment, survival rate > 90%
  - Duodenoduodenostomy most common operation
  - Complications: Megaduodenum, motility issues, adhesions

(Left) Coronal graphic shows the types of duodenal atresia: Internal membrane (I), fibrous cord (II), & complete discontinuity (III). (Right) AP radiograph shows dilation of the stomach ⊿ & duodenum ⊳ with no distal bowel gas, the so-called double bubble sign of duodenal atresia. No upper GI series is required prior to surgery.

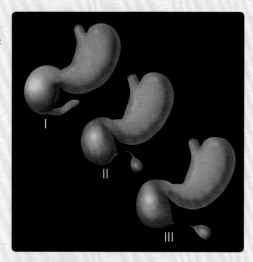
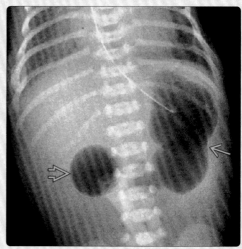

(Left) Coronal SSFP MR of a 33-week gestation fetus shows moderate dilation of the stomach ⊿ & marked dilation of the proximal duodenum ⊳. (Right) AP postnatal radiograph of the same patient shows marked dilation of the duodenum ⊿, which has a rounded configuration when viewed en face. The stomach is moderately dilated ⊿. There is no distal bowel gas ⊿. This is the classic double bubble appearance of duodenal atresia.

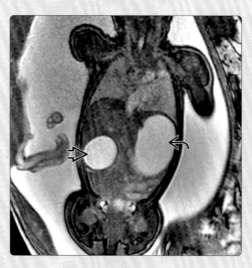
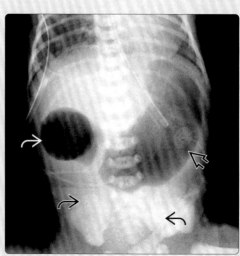

KEY FACTS

TERMINOLOGY

- Incomplete diaphragm of duodenal lumen causing partial or intermittent complete duodenal obstruction (spectrum of duodenal atresia)

IMAGING

- Web found in 2nd to 4th portion of duodenum
  - Usually adjacent to ampulla of Vater
- Aperture size determines degree of obstruction, age of presentation, imaging appearance
- Early presentation: Dilated stomach & proximal duodenum up to D2/D3; distal gas typically present
- Late presentation: Thin, ballooned "windsock" membrane in distal duodenum; variable duodenal caliber (depends on orifice size)
- Web may not be visualized on any imaging study
- Best modality: Upper GI with barium

TOP DIFFERENTIAL DIAGNOSES

- Duodenal atresia or stenosis, midgut volvulus, gastrointestinal duplication cysts, annular pancreas, superior mesenteric artery syndrome

PATHOLOGY

- Failed recanalization: Spectrum of duodenal atresia
- Associated anomalies: Down syndrome (30%), malrotation (28%), annular pancreas (33%), other intestinal atresias, biliary anomalies, pyloric stenosis, preduodenal portal vein; cardiac anomalies

CLINICAL ISSUES

- Early presenters (late in 1st week of life & early infancy): Feeding intolerance, vomiting (bilious > nonbilious)
- Late presenters (childhood to adulthood): Nausea, abdominal pain, progressive vomiting, acute pancreatitis
- Prognosis excellent with treatment
  - Surgical vs. endoscopic excision

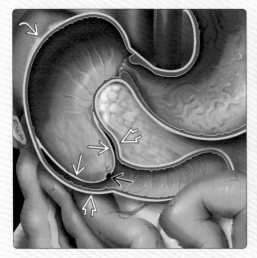

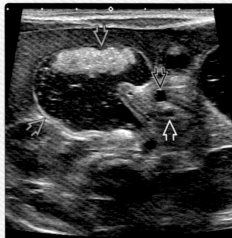

(Left) Graphic shows a web ➡ with a windsock shape in the duodenal lumen ➡ with a pinhole opening ➡ distally. The proximal duodenum ➡ is moderately dilated from this longstanding partial obstruction. (Right) Transverse US performed for pyloric stenosis in a 3-week-old boy with recurrent emesis showed a normal pylorus. However, there is marked dilation of the duodenum ➡ to D2-D3 with no findings of midgut volvulus (i.e., there is absence of the swirl sign & a normal superior mesenteric artery ➡/vein ➡ relationship).

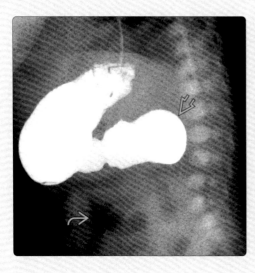

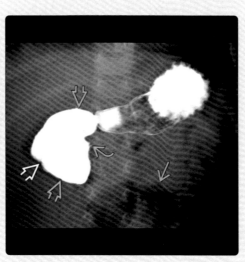

(Left) Lateral upper GI in the same patient immediately after the US shows no barium passing from the dilated proximal duodenum ➡, but bowel gas ➡ is seen distally. The patient was brought straight to the operating room where a tight duodenal web was found. (Right) Supine upper GI shows a dilated duodenum ➡ with distal gas ➡ & a tiny orifice ➡, as well as the dimple sign ➡ at the attachment of the proximal aspect of the web (which puckers when the web is stretched distally).

Jejunoileal Atresia

TERMINOLOGY

- Congenital occlusion of jejunal or ileal lumen; ranges from membrane to long-segment intestinal & mesenteric gaps

IMAGING

- Site of obstruction (atresia) determines radiographic & fluoroscopic patterns
- Proximal jejunal atresia
  - Dilated stomach + duodenum + 1-2 loops of jejunum; microcolon less likely on contrast enema
- Midjejunal to distal ileal atresia
  - Numerous dilated loops; enema shows microcolon
- Protocol advice in newborns
  - Abdominal radiograph 1st
  - Water-soluble contrast enema for suspected distal bowel obstructions
  - Upper GI series for acute proximal obstructions; if chronic, no preoperative study may be necessary

TOP DIFFERENTIAL DIAGNOSES

- Meconium ileus, neonatal small left colon, Hirschsprung disease, anorectal malformation, inguinal hernia

PATHOLOGY

- Associated anomalies in 10-52%: Gastroschisis (up to 20%), meconium ileus/cystic fibrosis, malrotation, volvulus

CLINICAL ISSUES

- Presentations in newborn
  - Atresia presents in utero to first 1-2 days of life
    - Distal ileal atresia: Failure to pass meconium + abdominal distention, bilious emesis
    - Jejunal or proximal ileal atresia: Bilious emesis
  - Stenosis or web: Early vs. delayed presentation with intermittent emesis, failure to thrive
- Treated by resection of atretic segment + anastomosis
- Complications: Short gut (14%), dysmotility, adhesions

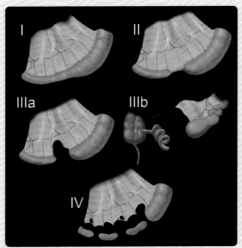

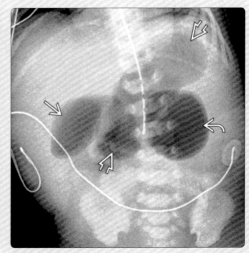

(Left) Coronal graphic shows the classification of jejunoileal atresias: Membrane (I), fibrous cord without mesenteric defect (II), complete separation with mesenteric defect (IIIa), long segment with "apple peel" morphology (IIIb), & multiple atresias (IV). (Right) AP radiograph shows the classic triple bubble sign of jejunal atresia due to a dilated stomach ➡, duodenum ➡, & proximal jejunum ➡ with no distal bowel gas.

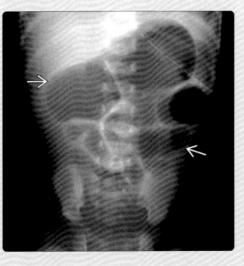

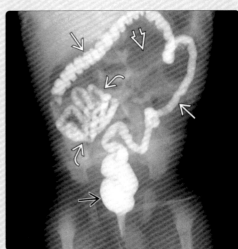

(Left) AP radiograph in a newborn with bilious emesis shows numerous dilated bowel loops ➡, suggestive of a mid to distal small bowel obstruction. (Right) Supine contrast enema in the same patient shows a typical microcolon ➡ with a preserved rectal caliber ➡. Numerous tiny loops of distal ileum are opacified ➡ without filling defects. Contrast does not pass proximally to the dilated, gas-distended small bowel loops ➡. These findings strongly suggest a mid ileal atresia (confirmed at surgery).

Meconium Ileus

KEY FACTS

TERMINOLOGY

- Neonatal obstruction of distal ileum due to abnormally thick, tenacious meconium, usually in setting of cystic fibrosis (CF)
- Poorly named disease (not actually ileus)

IMAGING

- Multiple dilated bowel loops on abdominal radiograph
- If complicated in perinatal period by superimposed segmental volvulus, atresia, necrosis, &/or perforation, radiographs can show
  - Soft tissue mass or gasless abdomen
  - Ca^{2+} of meconium peritonitis
- Microcolon + meconium-filled terminal ileum on water-soluble contrast enema (WSCE)

TOP DIFFERENTIAL DIAGNOSES

- Ileal atresia, Hirschsprung disease, small left colon/meconium plug syndrome, anorectal malformation

PATHOLOGY

- Complicated meconium ileus (MI): 50%
- Up to 90% of all MI patients have CF; MI is presenting illness in 10-20% of CF patients
  - CF incidence: 1 in 2,500 Caucasian live births (much less common in other races)
  - Mutation of *CFTR* gene (chromosome 7)

CLINICAL ISSUES

- Presents in newborn with failure to pass meconium, abdominal distention, bilious emesis
- Treatment
  - Serial hyperosmotic WSCE for uncomplicated MI
    - Requires adequate IV resuscitation due to fluid shifts
  - Surgery typically required in complicated MI or uncomplicated MI refractory to hyperosmotic WSCE

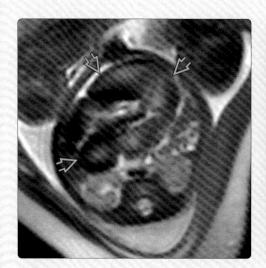
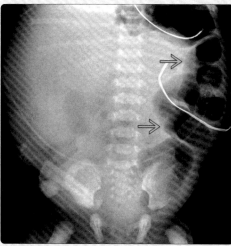

(Left) Axial SSFSE T2 fetal MR at 33-week gestation shows dilated small bowel (SB) ⇨ filled with intermediate to low signal intensity meconium. A tiny-caliber colon was best seen on sagittal images (not shown), consistent with a distal SB obstruction. The mother was noted to be a carrier of the cystic fibrosis (CF) gene. (Right) Supine abdominal radiograph of the same patient several hours after birth shows a large soft tissue mass displacing dilated bowel ⇨ towards the left, worrisome for a complicated meconium ileus (MI).

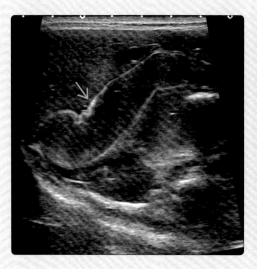
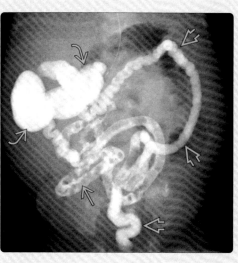

(Left) US immediately following the radiograph in the same patient shows dilated, debris-filled bowel with echogenic walls, consistent with bowel obstruction ⇨. Ascites was scattered in the abdomen. However, no pseudocyst or other sign of perforation was seen. (Right) WSCE in the same patient on the same day shows a microcolon ⇨ without significant meconium. Reflux into the terminal ileum (TI) shows obstructing meconium pellets ⇨ before reaching dilated SB ⇨. The findings confirm MI.

KEY FACTS

TERMINOLOGY

- Congenital disorder of enteric nervous system: Absence of ganglion cells in intestinal myenteric & submucosal plexus
  - Lack of peristalsis → functional bowel obstruction
- Aganglionic segment extends retrograde from anus for variable length with gradual transition to normal innervation

IMAGING

- Newborn radiograph: Numerous loops of dilated bowel
- Radiograph outside neonatal period: Large stool burden with variable colonic dilation
- Contrast enema especially useful in evaluating neonate with distal bowel obstruction; findings suggestive of Hirschsprung disease (HD) include
  - Rectosigmoid ratio < 1
  - Transition zone from small distal colon to dilated proximal colon

TOP DIFFERENTIAL DIAGNOSES

- Neonatal small left colon (meconium plug syndrome)
- Ileal atresia
- Meconium ileus
- Anorectal malformation
- Milk allergy colitis

CLINICAL ISSUES

- Neonate: Failure to pass meconium, abdominal distention, bilious emesis, enterocolitis
- Older child: Constipation since birth, enterocolitis
- Diagnosis by rectal biopsy
- Treatment: Resect affected colon & pullthrough of normal bowel to anus

DIAGNOSTIC CHECKLIST

- **Contrast enema cannot rule out HD** (but can suggest HD or other diagnoses)
- Frank colitis in term newborn: HD until proven otherwise

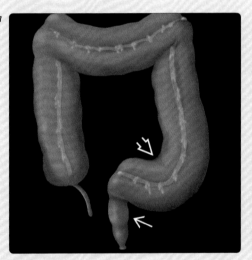

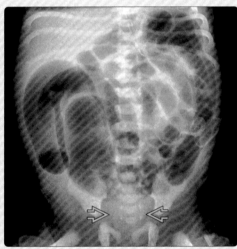

(Left) Anterior graphic shows a narrow caliber distal colon ➡ with a transition ⮕ to a dilated proximal colon at the sigmoid-descending colonic junction, characteristic of short-segment Hirschsprung disease (HD). (Right) AP radiograph of a 2-day-old boy with failure to pass meconium shows multiple dilated loops of bowel, suggesting a distal bowel obstruction. No air is seen in the rectum ➡. One cannot differentiate small bowel from colonic loops on this exam. A contrast enema is required to elucidate the etiology of obstruction.

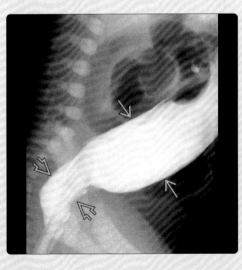

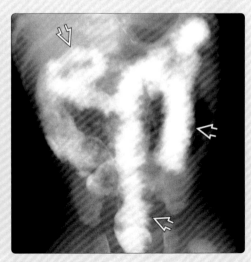

(Left) Lateral view of a water-soluble contrast enema (WSCE) in the same patient shows a small caliber rectum ➡ relative to the dilated sigmoid ➡, suggesting short-segment HD. This was confirmed by rectal biopsy. (Right) Frontal view of a WSCE in a newborn with bilious emesis shows severe mucosal irregularity ⮕ throughout the colon, suggesting colitis in HD. Biopsies showed total intestinal aganglionosis.

TERMINOLOGY

Definitions

- Hirschsprung disease (HD): Congenital anomaly of enteric nervous system
  - Absence of ganglion cells in myenteric & submucosal plexus of intestine
    - Lack of peristalsis → functional bowel obstruction
  - Aganglionic segment extends retrograde from anus for variable length with gradual transition to innervated colon; level of transition may be
    - Rectosigmoid: Short-segment HD (70-80%)
    - Proximal to rectosigmoid: Long-segment HD (15-25%)
    - Entire colon: Total colonic HD (4-13%)
    - Colon & small bowel (SB): Total intestinal HD (very rare)
    - Just above anorectal verge: Ultrashort-segment HD (very rare)

IMAGING

General Features

- Best diagnostic clue
  - Rectosigmoid ratio < 1 on contrast enema
    - Requires well-distended lateral view from rectum to splenic flexure
- Morphology
  - Small caliber of aganglionic distal colon
  - Dilation of innervated proximal colon above transition

Radiographic Findings

- In newborn
  - Numerous dilated bowel loops suggesting distal obstruction
  - ± irregular, thickened bowel wall with enterocolitis
    - Rarely pneumatosis
- Outside neonatal period
  - Large stool burden with varying degrees of dilation
  - Rarely, free air from perforation in 1st year of life
    - Perforation usually at proximal colon or appendix

Fluoroscopic Findings

- Contrast enema
  - Short- or long-segment HD
    - Rectosigmoid ratio classically < 1 (but not always)
    - Transition zone: Level at which small distal colon becomes dilated proximal colon
    - ± sawtooth pattern of distal mucosa (spasm)
    - ± irregular mucosa/thickened wall of enterocolitis
    - Delayed (> 24-48 hours) evacuation of contrast
    - Near normal enema in ultrashort-segment HD
  - Total colonic HD
    - May appear normal vs. microcolon vs. shortened length with round flexures (question mark- or comma-shaped)

Imaging Recommendations

- Best imaging tool
  - Water-soluble contrast enema (WSCE)

PATHOLOGY

General Features

- Associated abnormalities
  - 5-32% of HD overall
    - Down syndrome (7-15%)
    - Neurocristopathy syndromes
    - Congenital central hypoventilation ("Ondine curse")

Microscopic Features

- Diagnosis by rectal biopsy
  - Suction biopsy: Bedside, less reliable
  - Full-thickness biopsy: In operating room, definitive
- Absent ganglia in myenteric & submucosal plexus
- Hypertrophic nerve fibers (acetylcholinesterase positive)
- Disease generally contiguous without skip areas
- Radiologic-pathologic correlation of transition zone site
  - Short-segment HD: 75% correlation
  - Long-segment HD: 25% correlation

CLINICAL ISSUES

Presentation

- Most common signs/symptoms
  - Failure to pass meconium by 24-48 hours (60-90%)
  - Abdominal distention (63-91%)
  - Bilious vomiting (19-37%)
  - Enterocolitis (5-44%)

Demographics

- 90% diagnosed in newborn period
- 10% diagnosed later, rarely adolescent or adult
- M > F = 4:1 (long-segment & total colonic HD → 1:1)

Natural History & Prognosis

- Untreated HD may lead to constipation, enterocolitis, toxic megacolon, sepsis, death
- Treated: Up to 40% with chronic soiling, constipation
  - Must assess for failure of pull-through procedure

Treatment

- Resection of aganglionic colon
- Pull-through of normal bowel to anus

DIAGNOSTIC CHECKLIST

Consider

- Contrast enema cannot rule out HD
  - With clinical suspicion, must biopsy
- WSCE most useful in assessing distal obstruction in neonates
  - Only up to 80% sensitive for HD in newborns

SELECTED REFERENCES

1. Aworanti OM et al: Does functional outcome improve with time postsurgery for Hirschsprung disease? Eur J Pediatr Surg. 26(2):192-9, 2016
2. Frongia G et al: Contrast enema for Hirschsprung disease investigation: diagnostic accuracy and validity for subsequent diagnostic and surgical planning. Eur J Pediatr Surg. 26(2):207-14, 2016
3. Gosain A: Established and emerging concepts in Hirschsprung's-associated enterocolitis. Pediatr Surg Int. 32(4):313-20, 2016
4. Putnam LR et al: The utility of the contrast enema in neonates with suspected Hirschsprung disease. J Pediatr Surg. 50(6):963-6, 2015
5. Langer JC: Hirschsprung disease. Curr Opin Pediatr. 25(3):368-74, 2013

Gastrointestinal

TERMINOLOGY

- Transient functional colonic obstruction of newborn
  - Retained colonic plugs of normal meconium are secondary to functional obstruction in this scenario (not an underlying cause of mechanical obstruction)
- Synonyms: Functional immaturity of colon, meconium plug syndrome

IMAGING

- Numerous dilated loops of bowel on newborn radiograph
  - Difficult to radiographically distinguish small vs. large bowel in neonate
- Water-soluble contrast enema (WSCE)
  - Small-caliber left colon (sigmoid + descending segments) up to splenic flexure with abrupt or gradual transition to normal/mildly dilated transverse colon
    - Normal rectosigmoid ratio
  - Scattered meconium filling defects in colon
    - May be proximal or distal to level of caliber change

TOP DIFFERENTIAL DIAGNOSES

- Hirschsprung disease
- Ileal atresia
- Meconium ileus
- Anorectal malformation

PATHOLOGY

- ↑ incidence in infants of diabetic mothers or mothers who received magnesium sulfate

CLINICAL ISSUES

- Presents with abdominal distention, delayed passage of meconium, bilious emesis
  - Most frequently encountered diagnosis in neonates with failure to pass meconium
- Temporary phenomenon: Usually resolves within several days (hastened by enemas or rectal stimulation)
- Rectal biopsy to exclude Hirschsprung disease if symptoms persist; some advocate biopsy for all

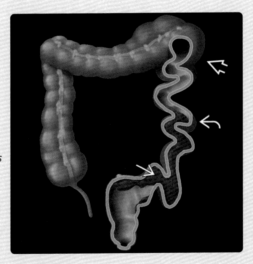

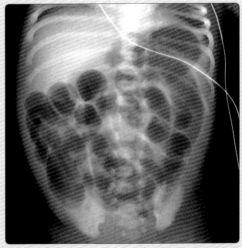

(Left) Frontal graphic shows a neonatal small left colon ➡ extending up to the splenic flexure ➡. A plug of meconium ➡ is shown in the small sigmoid colon, but this normal meconium does not cause the obstruction (unlike meconium ileus). (Right) AP radiograph of the abdomen in a term neonate with abdominal distention & emesis shows diffuse dilation of bowel but no rectal gas, suggesting a distal intestinal obstruction. The patient's mother had received magnesium late in pregnancy.

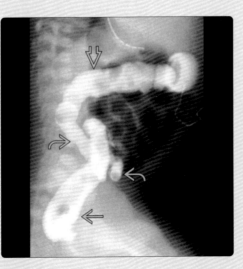

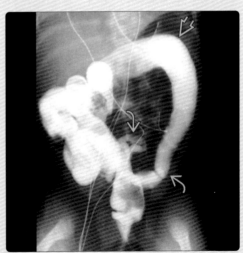

(Left) Lateral water-soluble contrast enema (WSCE) in the same patient shows a normal-caliber rectum ➡ with small sigmoid & descending colonic segments ➡. There is a gradual transition to a normal-caliber distal transverse colon ➡. (Right) Supine frontal image from the same WSCE shows the gradual transition from small sigmoid & descending colonic segments ➡ to a normal splenic flexure ➡. Meconium was passed with stimulation, & biopsy was negative for Hirschsprung disease, typical of small left colon syndrome.

Anorectal Malformation

KEY FACTS

IMAGING

- Neonatal clinical exam + AP abdominal radiograph
  - Many dilated bowel loops, ± rectal gas, ± bowel Ca²⁺
- Evaluate additional anomalies (VACTERL or syndromes)
  - Renal & spine US
  - Pelvic US for females with cloaca
    - Urgent drainage of hydrocolpos required to prevent rupture & alleviate bladder/ureteral obstruction
- Delayed distal colostogram for classification of anorectal malformation (ARM) & preoperative planning
- ± pelvic MR prior to, during, &/or after operative repair

TOP DIFFERENTIAL DIAGNOSES

- Neonatal distal bowel obstruction (with normal anus): Hirschsprung disease, meconium ileus, jejunoileal atresia

PATHOLOGY

- Imperforate anus types
  - Rectoperineal fistula (male or female)

- Rectovestibular fistula: 25% of female ARMs
- Rectourethral fistula: 50% of male ARMs
- Rectobladder neck fistula: 10% of male ARMs
- No fistula: 5% of ARMs (male or female)
- Cloacal malformation: Only females
- Rectal atresia or stenosis: 1% of ARMs

CLINICAL ISSUES

- Typical presentation: Absent/misplaced rectal opening & abdominal distention in newborn
- Most ARMs require
  - Diverting colostomy within days of birth
  - Posterior sagittal anorectoplasty for definitive repair months later
  - Goals: Maximize continence of feces & urine, preserve sexual function
- Prognosis dependent on type of malformation, degree of sacral insufficiency, spine anomalies, surgical technique

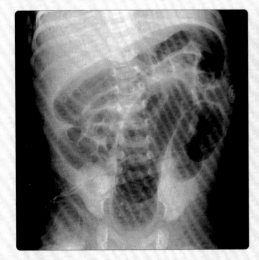
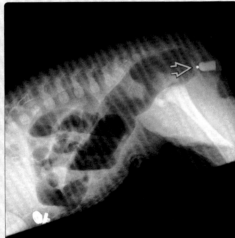

(Left) AP radiograph in a newborn (24 hours old) boy with imperforate anus & no clinical signs of a fistula (i.e., no meconium per urethra or perineum) shows multiple dilated bowel loops to the pelvis with a dilated rectum. (Right) Prone cross-table lateral view with a BB on the anus in the same patient shows the rectal pouch ⇨ adjacent to the anus, a type of low anorectal malformation (ARM) that is unlikely to have a rectourinary fistula & can be repaired as a neonate without colostomy.

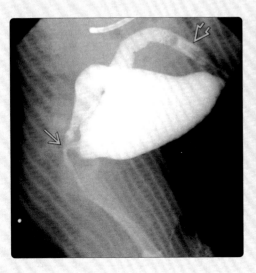
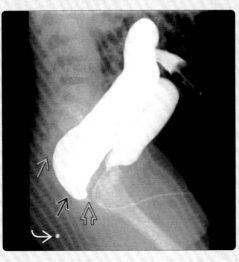

(Left) Colostogram in a 3-month-old boy with an ARM shows injection of the distal colonic segment ⇨. A rectoprostatic urethral fistula ⇨ is located anterior to the spine, which will require laparoscopy as well as a posterior sagittal anorectoplasty (PSARP). (Right) Colostogram in a 3-month-old boy with an ARM shows a rectobulbar urethral fistula ⇨ with a rectal pouch ⇨ well below the tip of spine ⇨. The distal colonic segment is adequate in length to bring the pouch to the anal region ⇨ by a PSARP.

TERMINOLOGY

- Necrotizing enterocolitis (NEC): Life-threatening condition of neonatal GI tract characterized by inflammation, ischemia, & translocation of bacteria into bowel wall

IMAGING

- Diagnosis based on clinical & imaging findings
- Mainstay of imaging for suspected NEC: Radiography
  - Findings range from nonspecific (paucity of bowel gas) to suggestive (thickened, dilated bowel loops) to diagnostic [pneumatosis, portal venous gas (PVG), & free peritoneal gas]
  - Duke Abdominal Assessment Scale for radiographs
    - Standard lexicon for reporting NEC findings
    - Strong intraobserver & interobserver agreement
    - ↑ scores correlate with need for surgery
- Ultrasound excellent adjunct
  - Radiographically occult necrosis requiring surgery suggested by absent vascularity + ↓ peristalsis
- Additional findings include focal fluid collections, echogenic ascites, ↑ bowel wall echogenicity, intramural gas, bowel wall thickening or thinning, PVG, & free air
- Contrast enema not used acutely; useful to localize strictures after treatment of acute episode

CLINICAL ISSUES

- Most common in very low birth weight (< 1,500 g) premature infants 2-3 weeks after delivery
  - 10% in term infants (usually with underlying diseases)
- Typical history: Feeding intolerance with emesis, ↑ gastric residuals, bloody stools
  - Other frequent clinical findings include abdominal distention &/or discoloration, apnea & bradycardia, lethargy, temperature instability
- Treatment: IV nutrition + antibiotics ± surgery
- Overall mortality 10-50%
  - Death secondary to sepsis from bowel perforation
- Delayed bowel strictures in 10-20% of survivors

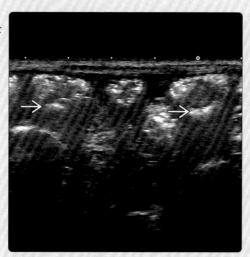

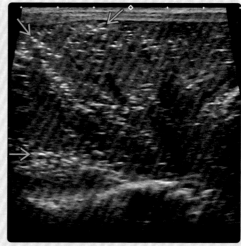

(Left) *Longitudinal US of the abdominal left lower quadrant (LLQ) in a former 34-week premature infant shows numerous bowel loops with circumferential nodular echogenicity to their walls. Many of the echogenic foci* ➡ *demonstrate "dirty" shadowing posteriorly, typical of pneumatosis.* (Right) *Transverse US of the liver in the same patient shows numerous branching linear & nodular echogenic foci* ➡ *in the parenchyma, particularly peripherally, typical of portal venous gas (PVG).*

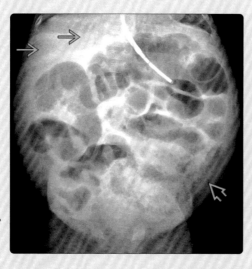

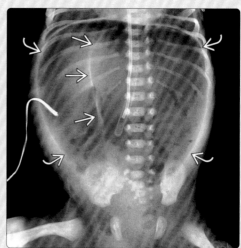

(Left) *Subsequent supine AP radiograph (same patient) shows bubbly lucencies of pneumatosis in the LLQ* ➡. *Branching foci of PVG* ➡ *are seen in the liver. This patient was managed conservatively for medical necrotizing enterocolitis (NEC).* (Right) *Abdominal radiograph in a premature infant with NEC shows a large amount of pneumoperitoneum causing abnormal lucency throughout abdomen* ➡. *The falciform ligament* ➡ *is outlined by air; this appearance resembles the laces of an American-type football (the football sign).*

TERMINOLOGY

Definitions

- Necrotizing enterocolitis (NEC): Poorly understood condition of neonatal GI tract with inflammation, ischemia, & translocation of bacteria into bowel wall
- Very low birth weight (VLBW) infant: < 1,500 g
- Extremely low birth weight (ELBW) infant: < 1,000 g

IMAGING

Radiographic Findings

- Nonspecific findings
  - Paucity of bowel gas
  - Loss of normal mosaic bowel gas pattern
- Suggestive findings
  - Asymmetric bowel dilation
  - Fixed, "unfolded" bowel loops on serial radiographs
  - Separation of bowel loops
    - Due to bowel wall thickening vs. intervening collapsed or fluid-filled bowel vs. free fluid
- Definitive findings
  - Pneumatosis (50-75% of patients)
    - Bubbly or curvilinear lucencies of bowel wall
    - Can mimic formed stool
  - Portal venous gas (PVG)
    - Branching lucencies over liver
  - Free intraperitoneal air
    - Overall ↑ upper abdominal lucency
    - Football sign: Lucent, distended abdomen with gas outlining vertical falciform ligament on supine view
    - Cupola sign: Gas under midline diaphragm if supine
    - Rigler sign: Gas outlining both sides of bowel wall
    - Crescentic lucency overlying right hepatic margin on left lateral decubitus view or anterior hepatic margin on cross-table lateral view
    - Triangles of lucency anteriorly on cross-table lateral view or peripherally on supine AP view

Ultrasonographic Findings

- Grayscale ultrasound
  - Focal fluid collections, echogenic ascites, aperistaltic bowel with thickening or thinning, & ↑ echogenicity of bowel wall all suggest NEC
  - Pneumatosis: Nodular echogenicities around entire circumference of bowel wall ± "dirty" shadowing posteriorly
  - PVG: Branching linear & punctate echogenicities in liver periphery; may see echogenic foci coursing through portal veins in real time
  - Free intraperitoneal air: Linear echogenicities with "dirty" shadowing immediately deep to peritoneal surface
- Color Doppler
  - ↓ vascularity indicates necrosis/perforation
  - ↑ vascularity may be seen in earlier stages

Fluoroscopic Findings

- Acute: Enema contraindicated in acute NEC
- Chronic: Strictures create obstruction in "older" NICU babies; causative NEC episode not always clinically apparent
  - Single or multiple strictures found 4-8 weeks after NEC

Imaging Recommendations

- Best imaging tool
  - Serial radiography: Fixed, dilated loops predict necrosis
  - Sonography up to 100% sensitive, 95% specific for necrosis (primarily by absent vascularity + ↓ peristalsis)

PATHOLOGY

General Features

- Associated abnormalities: Lung disease of prematurity, congenital heart disease, intracranial hemorrhage, periventricular leukomalacia

CLINICAL ISSUES

Presentation

- Most common signs/symptoms
  - Signs of feeding intolerance (emesis, ↑ gastric residuals, bloody stools)
  - Abdomen may become distended, discolored, erythematous, &/or shiny
  - Apnea & bradycardia, lethargy, temperature instability
- Other signs/symptoms
  - 1/3 have fulminant course with bowel perforation
  - 1/3 develop septic shock

Demographics

- Premature VLBW or ELBW newborns have highest incidence (90% of cases)
  - Affects 3-13% < 1,500 g; rate in ELBW 3x VLBW
  - Onset of NEC peaks at 29-31 weeks postmenstrual age, especially 2-3 weeks after delivery
- Term newborns make up 10% of cases
  - Earlier age onset of NEC (1-3 days after delivery)
  - Often have 1 or more risk factors

Natural History & Prognosis

- Overall mortality 10-50%
  - Death secondary to sepsis from bowel perforation
- Morbidity in survivors includes: Delayed bowel strictures (10-20%), short gut syndrome, neurodevelopmental delays

Treatment

- Prevention: Probiotics ↓ NEC incidence & mortality in VLBW infants
- When NEC suspected: IV nutrition + antibiotics
- Indications for surgery: Clinical ± radiologic findings
  - Free air considered absolute indication
  - Clinical deterioration, bowel necrosis

SELECTED REFERENCES

1. He Y et al: Ultrasonography and radiography findings predicted the need for surgery in patients with necrotising enterocolitis without pneumoperitoneum. Acta Paediatr. 105(4):e151-5, 2016
2. Lau CS et al: Probiotic administration can prevent necrotizing enterocolitis in preterm infants: A meta-analysis. J Pediatr Surg. 50(8):1405-12, 2015
3. Yikilmaz A et al: Prospective evaluation of the impact of sonography on the management and surgical intervention of neonates with necrotizing enterocolitis. Pediatr Surg Int. 30(12):1231-40, 2014
4. Muchantef K et al: Sonographic and radiographic imaging features of the neonate with necrotizing enterocolitis: correlating findings with outcomes. Pediatr Radiol. 43(11):1444-52, 2013
5. Sharma R et al: A clinical perspective of necrotizing enterocolitis: past, present, and future. Clin Perinatol. 40(1):27-51, 2013

Hypertrophic Pyloric Stenosis

TERMINOLOGY

- Hypertrophic pyloric stenosis (HPS): Idiopathic pyloric muscle thickening in young infants → progressive gastric outlet obstruction

IMAGING

- Near complete gastric outlet obstruction due to abnormally elongated & thickened pyloric muscle
  - Pylorus fails to relax/open → minimal gastric emptying → gastric overdistention → emesis
- Ultrasound shows hypertrophied circumferential hypoechoic muscle & elongated pyloric canal filled with echogenic mucosa
  - Commonly accepted sonographic criteria for HPS
    - Pyloric channel length > 15-16 mm
    - Single wall thickness of pyloric muscle > 3 mm
    - Failure of thickened pylorus to change during exam
      □ May still see trickle of passage of gastric contents

- Upper GI shows minimal barium traversing narrowed & elongated pyloric channel, mass effect on gastric antrum & duodenum by hypertrophied muscle, hyperperistaltic gastric contractions, & gastroesophageal reflux/emesis

CLINICAL ISSUES

- Typically seen in infants 2-12 weeks old; peaks at 5 weeks
  - Progressive nonbilious projectile vomiting: Feedings previously tolerated (i.e., HPS not congenital)
  - Weight loss, hypokalemic-hypochloremic metabolic alkalosis, dehydration
  - Palpable "olive" on physical exam: 97% specific in experienced hands; less common now due to earlier imaging diagnosis
- HPS in 1/5 infants imaged for vomiting
  - Gastroesophageal reflux > > HPS
- Surgical treatment: Pyloromyotomy; excellent prognosis

DIAGNOSTIC CHECKLIST

- Pylorospasm mimics HPS (but typically transient)

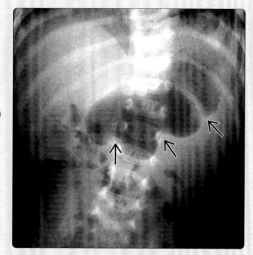

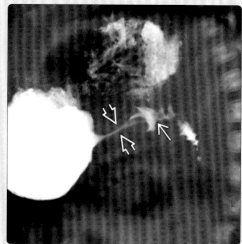

(Left) AP radiograph in a vomiting patient with hypertrophic pyloric stenosis (HPS) shows hyperperistalsis of a gas-filled stomach as muscular contractions ⤐ try to push gastric contents through the narrowed, hypertrophied pylorus. (Right) Lateral upper GI image shows a thin "string" of barium extending through the narrowed, elongated pyloric channel ⮕, opacifying the duodenal bulb ⮕. The thickened pyloric muscle creates rounded indentations on the gastric antrum & base of the duodenal bulb.

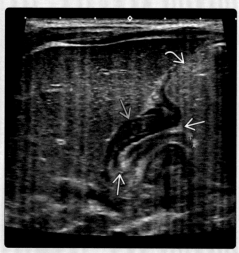

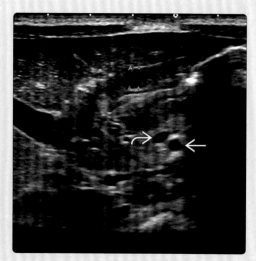

(Left) Transverse oblique ultrasound in a 3-week-old boy with HPS shows elongation of the pyloric channel ⮕ at 22.5 mm in length. The hypoechoic muscle is thickened ⮕, & there is a large amount of retained formula in the stomach ⤐. (Right) Transverse oblique ultrasound in a different baby with HPS shows thickening of the pyloric muscle at 4.5 mm between the cursors. Note the normal relationship of the superior mesenteric artery ⮕ & superior mesenteric vein ⮕ (which suggests normal rotation of the midgut).

TERMINOLOGY

Definitions

- Idiopathic pyloric muscle thickening → progressive gastric outlet obstruction

IMAGING

Radiographic Findings

- Overdistended stomach with ↓ distal bowel gas
- Stomach may be collapsed if infant has recently vomited
- Benign gastric pneumatosis & portal venous gas rarely reported in association with hypertrophic pyloric stenosis (HPS)

Ultrasonographic Findings

- Threshold for abnormal measurements of pyloric muscle thickness & channel length vary by study
  - In general, ↑ threshold measurements ↑ specificity but ↓ sensitivity
- Commonly accepted threshold values for HPS
  - Single wall of pyloric muscle > 3-mm thick
  - Pyloric channel > 15- to 16-mm long
- Hypertrophied & redundant echogenic mucosal lining
- Gastric hyperperistalsis & persistently obliterated pyloric lumen on dynamic exam

Fluoroscopic Findings

- Overdistended "caterpillar stomach": Undulations of wall due to exaggerated gastric motility (hyperperistalsis)
- Tram-track or string sign of contrast within narrowed pyloric channel
- Shoulders of thickened pyloric muscle create impressions on distal antrum
- "Beak" where contrast encounters narrowed pyloric canal
- Contrast in duodenal bulb (covering hypertrophied muscle impressions at base of duodenal bulb) + contrast in narrowed & elongated pyloric channel: Mushroom sign

Imaging Recommendations

- Best imaging tool
  - Ultrasound when HPS suspected
    - Excellent sensitivity & specificity; no ionizing radiation
  - Upper GI with atypical history (including bilious emesis)

DIFFERENTIAL DIAGNOSIS

Pylorospasm

- Typically seen in irritable infants; resolves with time
- Rarely as thick or elongated as true HPS

Gastroesophageal Reflux

- Cause of vomiting in > 2/3 infants referred to radiology
- Presumed diagnosis when pyloric ultrasound normal

Malrotation With Midgut Volvulus

- Surgical emergency due to risk of midgut ischemia
- Emesis classically bilious (greenish) from bile
- Mildly dilated proximal duodenum with abrupt beaking near junction of 2nd-3rd duodenum
- Distal contrast passage shows "corkscrew" or swirling contrast in typically narrowed bowel

Gastric Bezoar

- Caused by accumulation of undigested matter in stomach
- Contrast in interstices of large filling defect on upper GI

Other Causes of Gastric Outlet Obstruction

- Duodenal stenosis or antral web
- Antral polyps, antritis, annular pancreas

PATHOLOGY

General Features

- Idiopathic hypertrophy of circular muscles in pylorus
  - May be prostaglandin or erythromycin induced, neural mediated, familial
  - Slightly ↑ incidence in preterm infants vs. full term
    - Presents at later chronological age in preemies
  - Higher incidence in mothers < 20 years old, nulliparous, smokers, & formula-fed babies

CLINICAL ISSUES

Presentation

- Most common signs/symptoms
  - Progressive vomiting in previously healthy infant
  - Palpable "olive" on physical exam: 97% specific in experienced hands
    - Less common finding due to earlier imaging diagnosis
- Other signs/symptoms
  - Weight loss, alkalosis, & dehydration

Demographics

- Age: 2-12 weeks or later if premature; peaks at 5 weeks
- Gender: M:F = 5:1
- Incidence: 2.5-3 per 1,000 infants

Natural History & Prognosis

- Gradual progression; spontaneous remission can occur over weeks
- Excellent prognosis following surgery or conservative medical management

Treatment

- Surgical: Pyloromyotomy
  - Splits thickened muscle longitudinally (without breaching mucosa), opening channel
  - Laparoscopic pyloromyotomy & open procedures have equal success rates
- Nonsurgical alternative: Medications & frequent small feeds
  - Requires several weeks before resuming normal feeding without medications
  - Medications used include Botox, IV atropine
- Complications
  - Failed surgery due to inadequate pyloromyotomy
  - Gastroduodenal myotomy or enterotomy

SELECTED REFERENCES

1. Bakal U et al: Recent changes in the features of hypertrophic pyloric stenosis. Pediatr Int. 58(5): 369-71, 2016
2. Raske ME et al: ACR appropriateness criteria vomiting in infants up to 3 months of age. J Am Coll Radiol. 12(9):915-22, 2015
3. Aboagye J et al: Age at presentation of common pediatric surgical conditions: Reexamining dogma. J Pediatr Surg. 49(6):995-9, 2014
4. Hernanz-Schulman M: Infantile hypertrophic pyloric stenosis. Radiology. 227(2):319-31, 2003

Gastroesophageal Reflux

TERMINOLOGY

- Gastroesophageal reflux (GER): Retrograde flow of gastric contents into esophagus
- GER disease (GERD): GER causes clinical symptoms or tissue damage

IMAGING

- Retrograde passage of gastric contents into esophagus
  - Can see on US, fluoroscopic upper GI, radionuclide scintigraphy
- Reflux esophagitis (GERD)
  - Best seen fluoroscopically
  - Esophageal dysmotility often earliest sign
  - Distal esophageal mucosal irregularity/thickening/stricture
  - Barrett esophagus (rare in children)
- Upper GI to exclude anatomic/functional abnormalities, not to identify GER
  - Esophageal dysmotility
    - Hiatal hernia
    - Gastric outlet/duodenal obstruction
    - Malrotation
- Radionuclide scintigraphy: Most sensitive imaging test to detect GER

CLINICAL ISSUES

- Infants: Recurrent vomiting/regurgitation, excessive irritability, feeding difficulty, poor weight gain/failure to thrive, sleep disturbances, brief resolved unexplained event
- Children: Poorly localized abdominal or chest pain, heartburn, recurrent vomiting/regurgitation, dysphagia, respiratory symptoms (e.g., wheezing, cough)
- Most infantile GER resolves by age 1-2 years: 50% at 4 months ↓ to 5-10% at 12 months; ~ 4% have persistent GER, 1% require surgery (fundoplication)

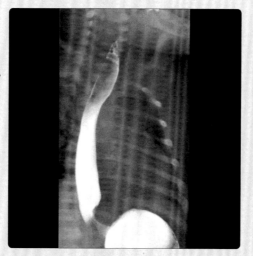

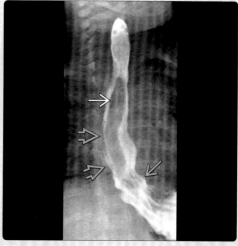

(Left) *Upper GI of a 3 day old with severe regurgitation shows almost no peristalsis of an otherwise normal, completely distended esophagus. Hypomotility is the earliest finding in reflux esophagitis & gastroesophageal reflux disease.* (Right) *Upper GI in a 7 month old with worsening gastroesophageal reflux shows a mild hiatal hernia with gastric folds ➡ above the diaphragm & thickened folds in the distal esophagus ➡, consistent with reflux esophagitis & dysmotility. Note air ➡ in the esophagus.*

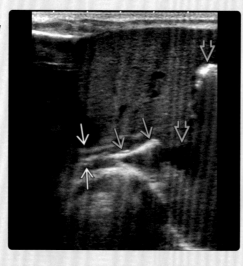

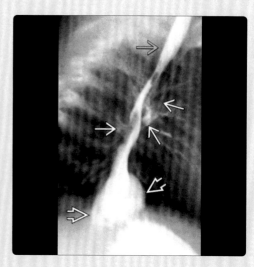

(Left) *Longitudinal US of the gastroesophageal junction in a 20 day old with recurrent nonbilious vomiting shows a column of echogenic air ➡ that, in real-time scanning, was moving from the fluid-filled stomach ➡ in a retrograde direction into the esophagus ➡.* (Right) *Lateral upper GI image in a patient with a hiatal hernia ➡ demonstrates significant reflux of contrast ➡ with aspiration ➡, requiring placement of an enteric suction tube into the esophagus to prevent further aspiration.*

Gastric Volvulus

KEY FACTS

TERMINOLOGY

- Twisting of all or part of stomach on its axes at least 180°
  - Organoaxial volvulus (OAV): Rotation along long axis
  - Mesenteroaxial volvulus (MAV): Rotation along short axis

IMAGING

- Radiographic findings: Round gas-distended viscus under &/or above left hemidiaphragm that decompresses with nasogastric (NG) tube
  - Dependent image may show 2 air-fluid levels
- Upper GI vs. CECT to confirm diagnosis
  - OAV: Horizontal stomach with pylorus directed inferiorly; greater curvature superior to lesser curvature
  - MAV: Vertical stomach with pylorus superior to fundus; pylorus close to or overlaps gastroesophageal junction

PATHOLOGY

- Primary volvulus: Absent, failed, or lax ligamentous fixation

- Secondary volvulus: Disorder of gastric anatomy/function (e.g., ulcer, prior surgery) or adjacent organ (e.g., diaphragm eventration, wandering spleen, intestinal malrotation)

CLINICAL ISSUES

- 58% present within 1st year of life
- Symptoms: Retching, nonbilious emesis, pain, & distention
  - Acute: Respiratory distress & cyanosis
  - Chronic: Failure to thrive & colic
  - Complete Borchardt triad uncommon (unproductive retching, epigastric distention, inability to pass NG tube)
- Natural history: Obstruction, ischemia, perforation
- Treatment
  - Resuscitation required in 23-60% of acute presentations
  - Gastric decompression with NG tube
  - Open or laparoscopic reduction + gastropexy &/or gastrostomy tube
  - Repair of associated defects in secondary volvulus

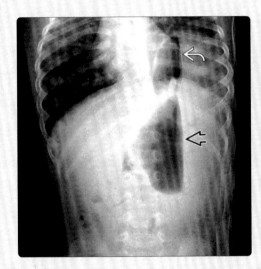

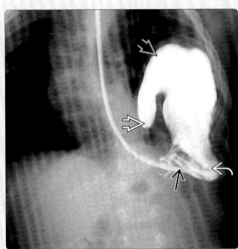

(Left) Left side down decubitus radiograph of a 6-month-old patient with vomiting shows 2 large air-fluid levels in the left lower hemithorax ➜ & left upper quadrant of the abdomen ➔. (Right) Frontal upper GI image in the same patient shows the stomach lying largely in the left hemithorax. The stomach is inverted with the antrum ➔ & gastric outlet ➔ lying above the fundus ➔. Note the twisting of rugal folds ➔ in the cardia. Acute mesenteroaxial volvulus was found at surgery with a chronic diaphragmatic hernia.

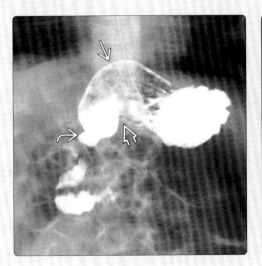

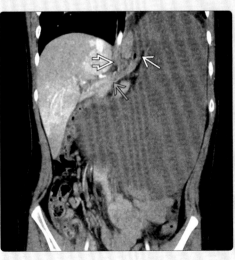

(Left) Frontal upper GI image in a 4 month old with ↓ oral intake shows that the greater curvature ➔ of the stomach lies superior to the lesser curvature ➔. The pylorus is directed inferiorly ➔. The findings are consistent with an organoaxial volvulus. (Right) Coronal CECT in an 11 year old with vomiting shows a narrow pylorus ➔ above the level of the gastroesophageal junction ➔. The proximal duodenum is stretched ➔. The abdominal contents extend abnormally into the lower left hemithorax. A mesenteroaxial volvulus was found at surgery.

Ingested Coins

IMAGING

- Disc-shaped metallic density without circumferential beveled edge/step-off
- Most common sites of impaction
  - Upper esophagus at thoracic inlet
  - Midesophagus at aortic arch impression
  - Lower esophageal sphincter at gastroesophageal junction
- Other sites of impaction include pylorus, duodenum, ileocecal valve
- Imaging recommendations
  - Screening frontal radiographs of neck through pelvis ± lateral view of upper airway
  - Targeted lateral radiograph if foreign body identified

TOP DIFFERENTIAL DIAGNOSES

- Button battery ingestion
- Magnet ingestion
- Various other foreign bodies

CLINICAL ISSUES

- Majority of ingestions by children < 5 years old
- Most common symptoms
  - Asymptomatic: Witnessed ingestion or incidental finding
  - Symptomatic: Drooling, chest/neck pain, vomiting, dysphagia, cough, respiratory distress, stridor
- 25-30% of esophageal coins pass spontaneously: More likely if further distal in esophagus on early imaging
- Treatment of esophageal coins: Urgent endoscopic removal if symptomatic; endoscopic removal within 24 hours if asymptomatic (with repeat radiograph prior to endoscopy to verify position)
- Treatment of coins in stomach: Monitor stools for passage; repeat radiograph in 2 weeks → endoscopic removal if not passed in 2-4 weeks
- Treatment of small bowel coins: Observation; endoscopic/surgical removal if symptomatic
- Complications uncommon: Esophageal stricture, perforation, aortoesophageal or tracheoesophageal fistulas

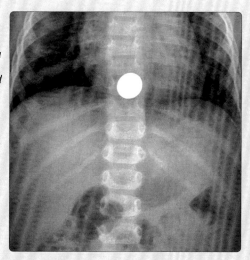

(Left) Frontal radiograph of the lower chest in a 2 year old with emesis shows a 19.5-mm metallic disc, consistent with a coin, projecting over the distal esophagus. The disc was found to be a dime at endoscopy. Radiographs cannot accurately identify coin types based on size. (Right) AP radiograph shows a coin lodged in the cervical esophagus. Note that the coin is wider than the trachea, indicative of an esophageal location. The erosions ➡ are due to gastroesophageal reflux reaching a zinc-based coin.

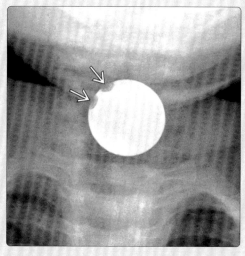

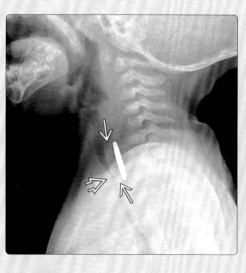

(Left) Lateral radiograph demonstrates a metallic coin in the proximal esophagus at the thoracic inlet. There is soft tissue swelling ➡ between the coin and the trachea with associated tracheal narrowing ⇒. These findings suggest a more chronic foreign body that may be difficult to remove. (Right) Lateral airway radiograph in a 2 year old after a witnessed ingestion shows 2 directly apposed coins ➡ projecting over the upper esophagus at the thoracic inlet. This appearance can mimic the edge step-off of a button battery.

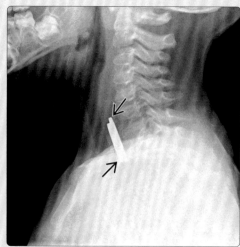

IMAGING

General Features

- Location
  - Most common sites of impaction
    - Upper esophagus at thoracic inlet
    - Midesophagus at aortic arch impression
    - Lower esophageal sphincter (LES) at gastroesophageal junction
  - Other sites of impaction include pylorus, duodenum, ileocecal valve
- Size
  - United States coins
    - Penny (1 cent): 19 mm
    - Nickel (5 cents): 21 mm
    - Dime (10 cents): 18 mm
    - Quarter (25 cents): 25 mm
  - Radiographic measurements may not allow accurate coin identification due to magnification & small differences in coin diameters

Radiographic Findings

- Disc-shaped metallic foreign body without circumferential beveled edge/step-off/halo
- Typically seen en face (oriented in coronal plane) on frontal radiograph
- Rarely oriented in sagittal plane on frontal radiograph
- May exert mass effect on trachea secondary to size of coin or associated soft tissue swelling

Imaging Recommendations

- Ingested foreign body screening radiographs: Frontal views to include neck through pelvis ± lateral view of upper airway
- Targeted lateral radiograph if foreign body identified
  - Helps confirm location
  - Helps determine type of foreign body

DIFFERENTIAL DIAGNOSIS

Button Battery Ingestion

- Disc-shaped metallic foreign body
  - Lateral view: Circumferential beveled edge/step-off
  - Frontal view: Circumferential halo or double ring sign
- Esophageal impaction requires emergent removal

Magnet Ingestion

- Metallic densities of variable shapes & sizes
- Multiple magnets or magnets with other metallic foreign bodies may attract through different bowel loops → fistulization, perforation, obstruction

Other Metallic Foreign Bodies

- Buttons, jewelry, toy parts

Aspirated Coin in Trachea

- Classic teaching that sagittally oriented coin on frontal radiograph likely in trachea: Incorrect
  - Coin impacted in esophagus much more likely regardless of orientation (coronal or sagittal)
  - Coin may lie in coronal or sagittal plane in trachea or esophagus

CLINICAL ISSUES

Presentation

- Most common signs/symptoms
  - Asymptomatic: Witnessed ingestion or incidental finding
  - Symptomatic: Drooling, chest/neck pain, vomiting, dysphagia, cough, respiratory distress, stridor

Demographics

- Majority of patients < 5 years old
- Penny ingestions most common: 44%

Natural History & Prognosis

- 25-30% of esophageal coins pass spontaneously
  - Likelihood of spontaneous passage correlates with location in esophagus: Proximal 14%, middle 43%, distal 67%
- Complications uncommon
  - Esophageal stricture, perforation, aortoesophageal or tracheoesophageal fistulas
  - Post-1982 copper-plated zinc penny: 97.5% zinc
    - Gastric acid may erode coin margins
    - Gastric acid reacts with zinc to form zinc-chloride
    - Ingestion of large number may cause zinc toxicity

Treatment

- North American Society for Pediatric Gastroenterology, Hepatology, & Nutrition guidelines
  - Esophageal coin
    - Symptomatic: Urgent endoscopic removal
    - Asymptomatic: Endoscopic removal within 24 hours; repeat radiograph prior to endoscopy to look for interval progression
  - Gastric coin
    - Monitor stools for passage; repeat radiograph in 2 weeks
    - Endoscopic removal if not passed within 2-4 weeks
    - Repeat radiograph prior to endoscopy
  - Small bowel coin
    - Clinical observation
    - Enteroscopy/surgical removal if symptomatic
- Use of glucagon (to relax LES) controversial: May cause vomiting & aspiration
- Fluoroscopic-guided retraction with Foley catheter may result in acute airway obstruction if coin moves into airway
- Pushing coin into stomach by dilator (bougienage) does not allow esophagus to be evaluated

SELECTED REFERENCES

1. Kramer RE et al: Management of ingested foreign bodies in children: a clinical report of the NASPGHAN Endoscopy Committee. J Pediatr Gastroenterol Nutr. 60(4):562-74, 2015
2. Pugmire BS et al: Review of ingested and aspirated foreign bodies in children and their clinical significance for radiologists. Radiographics. 35(5):1528-38, 2015
3. Wright CC et al: Updates in pediatric gastrointestinal foreign bodies. Pediatr Clin North Am. 60(5):1221-39, 2013
4. Schlesinger AE et al: Sagittal orientation of ingested coins in the esophagus in children. AJR Am J Roentgenol. 196(3):670-2, 2011
5. Chen X et al: Pediatric coin ingestion and aspiration. Int J Pediatr Otorhinolaryngol. 70(2):325-9, 2006
6. Waltzman ML et al: A randomized clinical trial of the management of esophageal coins in children. Pediatrics. 116(3):614-9, 2005
7. O'Hara SM et al: Gastric retention of zinc-based pennies: radiographic appearance and hazards. Radiology. 213(1):113-7, 1999

Ingested Button Batteries

TERMINOLOGY

- Ingestion of disc-shaped battery, typically by young child
  - Increasingly of more injurious lithium cell type
- Esophagus particularly susceptible to injury by lodged battery with potentially catastrophic consequences

IMAGING

- Frontal radiograph: Margin shows double halo/ring en face
- Lateral radiograph: Rim of step-off/beveled edge
  - Negative pole (narrower side): Site of anticipated most severe injury
- North American Society for Pediatric Gastroenterology, Hepatology, & Nutrition imaging guidelines
  - Radiographic coverage from nasopharynx to anus
    - Lateral view at least at site of confirmed foreign body
  - After emergent removal of esophageal battery
    - CTA/MR if esophageal injury present to evaluate proximity/involvement of vascular structures
      - CTA safest & most efficient vessel assessment
    - Esophagram to exclude leak prior to advancing diet
  - Battery distal to esophagus: Management varies based on battery size & patient age

CLINICAL ISSUES

- Caustic injury due to hydroxide radical production in tissues adjacent to negative pole
- Unwitnessed ingestion more likely to present in delayed fashion with nonspecific symptoms: Vomiting, difficulty feeding, cough, chest or abdominal pain, drooling, stridor
- ↑ risk of major complications: Unwitnessed ingestion, size ≥ 20 mm (majority lithium; radiographs overestimate size), age < 5 years old, multiple batteries ingested
  - Unwitnessed ingestion accounts for 92% of associated fatalities & 56% of major outcome cases
  - Complications include tracheoesophageal fistula, esophageal perforation, esophageal stricture, vocal cord paralysis, aortoenteric fistula (high fatality rate)
- Injury evolves weeks after battery removal

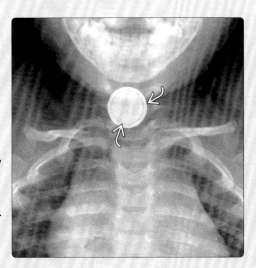

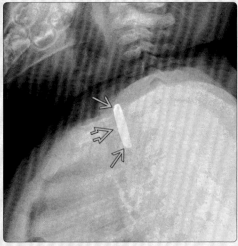

(Left) *Frontal radiograph of a 1 year old with acute cough, gagging, & emesis (but no witnessed ingestion) shows a 23-mm diameter disc-shaped foreign body with a double ring/halo ➦ appearance in the proximal esophagus, consistent with a button battery.* **(Right)** *Lateral radiograph of a 10 month old with a witnessed foreign body ingestion & subsequent drooling & emesis shows the circumferential edge step-off ➥ typical of a button battery. The negative pole is the narrower anterior side ➥.*

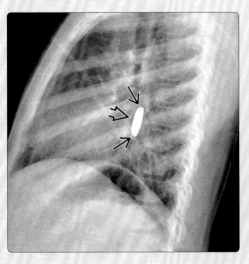

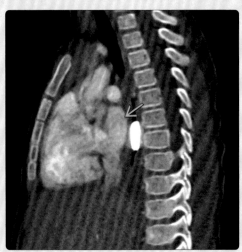

(Left) *Lateral radiograph from a 7 year old after the known ingestion of a button battery (> 20 mm in diameter) > 12 hours prior to presentation shows that the button battery is impacted in the mid to distal esophagus. Beveled edges are seen ➥ with the negative pole ➦ directed anteriorly toward the left atrium.* **(Right)** *Sagittal CECT from the same patient shows the esophageal battery posterior to the left atrium ➥. There is soft tissue thickening (inflammation) without evidence of fistula.*

TERMINOLOGY

Definitions

- Ingestion of disc-shaped battery, typically by young child
- Esophagus particularly susceptible to injury by lodged battery with potentially catastrophic consequences

IMAGING

General Features

- Most common sites of impaction in esophagus
  - Upper esophagus at thoracic inlet
  - Mid esophagus at aortic arch
  - Lower esophageal sphincter at GE junction

Radiographic Findings

- Metallic density disc of variable size
  - Size ≥ 20 mm: ↑ risk for worse outcome (but radiograph overestimates size)
- Frontal view: Margin shows double halo/ring en face
- Lateral view: Rim of step-off/beveled edge in tangent
  - Step-off may not be visible on new thinner batteries
  - Negative pole: Narrower side on lateral view; site most likely for most severe injury
  - Soft tissue edema surrounding battery may cause anterior tracheal displacement or narrowing
- Complications may show mediastinal widening (from edema or fluid collections) &/or gas
- Metallic fragments may remain after battery removal

CT

- CTA to look for aortic/vascular injury
  - Wall irregularity/outpouching or wall edema
  - Active extravasation
  - Mediastinal edema/fluid collections
- No established findings (at this time) predictive of subsequent vascular catastrophes

Esophagram

- Irregularity/edema of mucosa with luminal narrowing
- Leak of contrast into mediastinum or trachea
- Long-term stricturing

Imaging Recommendations

- Initial "foreign body screening" frontal radiographs to include neck through pelvis
- Lateral radiographs of
  - Upper airway to include nasopharynx
  - Any site where foreign body is identified
    - Distinguish battery from coin & identify negative pole
- Follow-up imaging as per North American Society for Pediatric Gastroenterology, Hepatology, & Nutrition (NASPGHAN) guidelines
  - CTA safest & most efficient tool to assess vessels

DIFFERENTIAL DIAGNOSIS

Coin Ingestion

- Flat metallic disc (no beveled edge or double ring sign)

Magnet Ingestion

- > 1 magnet or 1 magnet + other metallic foreign body may cause bowel injury by attraction through bowel walls

PATHOLOGY

General Features

- Lithium cell → caustic injury after impaction in esophagus
  - Mucosa contacts both poles, completes circuit
  - Electrolytic current generates hydroxide radicals in tissue adjacent to negative pole → ↑ pH
  - Injury evolves weeks after removal
- Non-lithium types injure mainly via alkaline leakage

CLINICAL ISSUES

Presentation

- Ingestion may be witnessed (often without symptoms) or unwitnessed with symptoms: Vomiting, difficulty feeding, cough, chest or abdominal pain, drooling, stridor

Natural History & Prognosis

- Unwitnessed ingestion accounts for 92% of associated fatalities & 56% of major outcome cases
- ↑ risk of major complications: Size ≥ 20 mm (majority lithium), age < 5 years old, multiple batteries ingested
- Major complications
  - Tracheoesophageal fistula in 48%
  - Esophageal perforation in 23%
  - Esophageal stricture in 38%
  - Vocal cord paralysis in 10%
  - Aortoenteric fistula in 46% of fatal cases (1977-2015)
    - Can occur weeks after battery removal

Treatment

- NASPGHAN guidelines based on battery location & size, clinical stability, & patient age
  - Esophageal & stable: Immediate endoscopic removal
  - Esophageal & unstable/active bleeding: Immediate endoscopic removal in OR with surgeon present
    - CTA or MR to evaluate involvement/proximity of aorta
    - Negative CTA, MR → esophagram to exclude leak
    - Injury close to aorta (≤ 3 mm) → serial CTA or MR every 5-7 days until injury recedes
  - Distal to esophagus, ≥ 20 mm, < 5 years old
    - Assess for esophageal injury + endoscopic removal within 24-48 hours
    - If esophageal injury → CTA, MR
  - Distal to esophagus, < 20 mm, &/or ≥ 5 years old
    - May consider outpatient observation with repeat radiograph (48 hours ≥ 20 mm or 10-14 days < 20 mm)
    - Endoscopic removal if GI symptoms develop or battery not passed at time of repeat radiograph

SELECTED REFERENCES

1. Leinwand K et al: Button battery ingestion in children: A paradigm for management of severe pediatric foreign body ingestions. Gastrointest Endosc Clin N Am. 26(1):99-118, 2016
2. Kramer RE et al: Management of ingested foreign bodies in children: a clinical report of the NASPGHAN Endoscopy Committee. J Pediatr Gastroenterol Nutr. 60(4):562-74, 2015
3. Pugmire BS et al: Review of ingested and aspirated foreign bodies in children and their clinical significance for radiologists. Radiographics. 35(5):1528-38, 2015
4. Jatana KR et al: Pediatric button battery injuries: 2013 task force update. Int J Pediatr Otorhinolaryngol. 77(9):1392-9, 2013
5. Litovitz T et al: Emerging battery-ingestion hazard: clinical implications. Pediatrics. 125(6):1168-77, 2010

Ingested Multiple Magnets

TERMINOLOGY

- Ingestion of multiple magnets or single magnet + additional metallic foreign bodies
  - Potential for significant bowel complications
- Rare-earth magnets 5-10x stronger than traditional magnets

IMAGING

- Metallic density foreign bodies; shapes variable
- Magnets attract through bowel walls
  - Multiple "stacked" magnets may simulate single rectangular or cylindrical foreign body
- Entrapment of interposed bowel wall suggested with
  - Gap between otherwise closely apposed magnets or magnet & adjacent metallic foreign body
  - Failure of magnet to move on sequential radiographs
- Abnormal bowel gas patterns from complications
  - Ulceration, perforation, fistulae, obstruction, volvulus
- Foreign body ingestion radiographic series includes

- Frontal views of neck through anus, ± lateral view of upper airway
- Targeted lateral views if foreign body identified

CLINICAL ISSUES

- Symptoms: None, abdominal pain/vomiting, choking
- Management depends on number of magnets, location in GI tract, & symptoms
  - Single magnet: Remove vs. follow radiographic passage
  - Multiple magnets or magnet + metal in esophagus/stomach: Endoscopic or surgical removal
  - Multiple magnets or magnet + metal beyond stomach
    - With symptoms &/or abnormal bowel gas pattern: Operative exploration with magnet removal
    - Without symptoms or abnormal bowel gas pattern: Consider careful, frequent clinical & radiographic evaluation until passage vs. removal

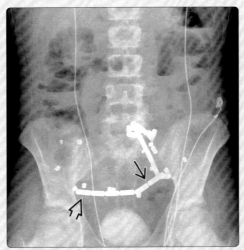
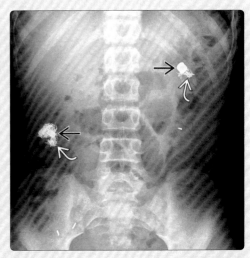

(Left) *Frontal upright abdominal radiograph of a 12-year-old autistic boy with abdominal pain & bilious emesis shows multiple rod-shaped metallic foreign bodies ➡, most of which appear linked. Small gaps ➡ between the magnets may represent entrapped intervening bowel. Numerous small bowel perforations & fistulae were noted at surgery.* (Right) *Frontal radiograph shows 2 clusters of magnets ➡ that attracted additional ingested metallic foreign bodies ➡. Associated bowel perforations were present at surgery.*

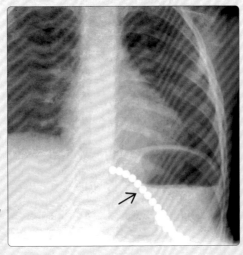
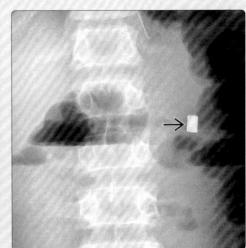

(Left) *Frontal upright chest radiograph in an asymptomatic 2 year old suspected to have swallowed magnets shows a chain of magnets ➡ projecting over the stomach. The magnets were removed endoscopically.* (Right) *Frontal upright abdominal radiograph from an asymptomatic 13 year old who swallowed 6 magnets shows a stack of metallic foreign bodies ➡ in the left abdomen. Jejunal & colonic perforations due to the magnets attracting across bowel walls were found at surgery.*

TERMINOLOGY

Synonyms

- Postgastric magnetopathy

Definitions

- Ingestion of multiple magnets or single magnet + additional metallic foreign bodies
  - Potential for significant bowel complications due to attraction through bowel loops
- Newer rare-earth magnets composed of iron, boron, & neodymium: 5-10x stronger than traditional magnets

IMAGING

Radiographic Findings

- Metallic density foreign bodies; shapes variable
  - Rods, discs, spheres/ball bearings, others
- May have larger nonradiopaque component
- Multiple attracted "stacked" magnets may simulate single rectangular or cylindrical foreign body
  - Magnification helps delineate individual components
- Entrapment of interposed bowel wall suggested with
  - Gap between otherwise closely apposed magnets or magnet & adjacent metallic foreign body
  - Failure of magnet to move on sequential radiographs
- Abnormal bowel gas patterns from complications
  - Ulceration, perforation, fistulae, obstruction, volvulus

Imaging Recommendations

- NASPGHAN guidelines recommend imaging if
  - Known magnet ingestion
  - Unexplained GI symptoms with rare-earth magnets in environment
- Screening foreign body ingestion radiographs
  - Frontal views from neck through anus, ± lateral view of upper airway
  - Targeted lateral view if foreign body identified
    - Assists in localization & characterization (such as attached metal or magnets not seen on 1 view)

DIFFERENTIAL DIAGNOSIS

Coin Ingestion

- Most common ingested radiopaque foreign body
- Metallic disc without beveled edge

Button Battery Ingestion

- Metallic disc with beveled edge on lateral view, double ring on frontal view
- Esophageal location requires emergent removal

PATHOLOGY

General Features

- Magnets attract to each other through bowel walls
  - Powerful rare-earth magnets attract through up to 6 bowel walls
    - Rare-earth magnets banned from toys in 2009
    - Now commonly sold as adult desk toys, faux piercings
- Produce pressure ulcers, ischemic injury, fistulae, necrosis, perforations, &/or obstruction
  - Mucosal ulcerations may occur in < 8 hours

CLINICAL ISSUES

Presentation

- 54.7% < 5 years old
- Suspicion of magnet ingestion critical: Only 1% of cases between 2000-2012 had witnessed ingestion [US Consumer Product Safety Commission (CPSC) data]
- Common symptoms (single center study, 56 cases): None: 57.1%; abdominal pain/vomiting: 32.1%; choking: 10.7%

Natural History & Prognosis

- CPSC data: 72 cases in United States (2000-2012)
  - No adverse effect: 33%; > 1 perforation & necrosis: 34%; 1 perforation: 6%; ulcer: 5%; fistula: 3%; volvulus: 2%
  - Surgery: 70%; endoscopic removal: 8%; passed naturally: 21%; death: 1%

Treatment

- NASPGHAN published guideline algorithm
  - Single magnet
    - Esophagus/stomach: Remove if risk of more ingestions or consider outpatient serial radiographs until passage ensured
    - Beyond stomach: Removal if possible or outpatient serial radiographs until passage
  - > 1 magnet or 1 magnet + metal in esophagus/stomach
    - If < 12 hours: Pediatric GI consult for endoscopic removal
    - If > 12 hours: Consult surgery prior to endoscopic removal; surgical removal if endoscopy unsuccessful
  - > 1 magnet or 1 magnet + metal beyond stomach
    - Consult pediatric gastroenterologist & surgery
    - Symptomatic: Surgical removal
    - Asymptomatic & no obstruction/perforation on imaging
      - Entero/colonoscopic removal vs. serial radiographs
      - Radiographs every 4-6 hours in emergency department
      - Progression on radiographs: Confirm passage (may educate parents & continue as outpatient)
      - No progression on radiographs: Admit → continue serial radiographs every 8-12 hours if asymptomatic vs. surgical/endoscopic removal
  - Parent education: No other metal or magnets near child

SELECTED REFERENCES

1. Kramer RE et al: Management of ingested foreign bodies in children: a clinical report of the NASPGHAN Endoscopy Committee. J Pediatr Gastroenterol Nutr. 60(4):562-74, 2015
2. Pugmire BS et al: Review of ingested and aspirated foreign bodies in children and their clinical significance for radiologists. Radiographics. 35(5):1528-38, 2015
3. Brown JC et al: Pediatric magnet ingestions: the dark side of the force. Am J Surg. 207(5):754-9; discussion 759, 2014
4. Abbas MI et al: Magnet ingestions in children presenting to US emergency departments, 2002-2011. J Pediatr Gastroenterol Nutr. 57(1):18-22, 2013
5. De Roo AC et al: Rare-earth magnet ingestion-related injuries among children, 2000-2012. Clin Pediatr (Phila). 52(11):1006-13, 2013
6. Otjen JP et al: Imaging pediatric magnet ingestion with surgical-pathological correlation. Pediatr Radiol. 43(7):851-9, 2013
7. Hussain SZ et al: Management of ingested magnets in children. J Pediatr Gastroenterol Nutr. 55(3):239-42, 2012
8. Oestreich AE: The usefulness of magnification in postgastric magnetopathy. Pediatr Radiol. 37(12):1268-9, 2007

KEY FACTS

TERMINOLOGY

- Hernia: Protrusion of contents from normally encasing body cavity through normal or abnormal opening
- Inguinal hernia: Protrusion of abdominal contents through defect in inguinal region
  - Indirect inguinal hernia: Contents protrude into open deep inguinal ring, extend through patent processus vaginalis, & exit superficial inguinal ring
    - 15% of inguinal hernias bilateral
    - In females, ovary may herniate through canal of Nuck
- Umbilical hernia: Contents extend into open umbilical ring
- Femoral hernia: Contents extend through femoral ring
- Amyand hernia: Inguinal hernia contains appendix ± inflammation
- Internal hernia: Extends through defect in abdominal cavity
- Traumatic: Extends through posttraumatic abdominal wall defect
- Incarcerated hernia: Contents cannot be reduced without special maneuvers, sedation, anesthesia, or surgery

- Strangulated hernia: Contents ischemic due to compression by hernia channel

IMAGING

- US excellent modality to investigate palpable abnormality
  - Can characterize hernia contents & evaluate blood flow to contents & adjacent tissues
    - Bowel: Peristalsis, swirling contents, gut signature
  - Standing &/or Valsalva maneuver help reproduce reduced hernia to confirm diagnosis
- Obstructive hernia: Dilated bowel loop enters abdominal wall defect, decompressed bowel loop exits hernia defect
- Signs of strangulation: Bowel wall thickening &/or ↓ enhancement/flow, engorged vasa recta, mesenteric stranding/fluid on CECT or US

CLINICAL ISSUES

- Surgery for most hernias due to risk of incarceration

(Left) AP radiograph in a neonate with abdominal distention shows a loop of gas-filled bowel extending into the left hemiscrotum ⇨ through the left inguinal canal ⇨. The dilation of proximal bowel loops in the abdomen suggests an associated obstruction. (Right) Frontal image from a small bowel follow-through in a neonate shows a loop of small bowel ⇨ extending into the right inguinal canal. The bowel upstream is not dilated. Inguinal hernias are more common in premature infants due to a patent processus vaginalis.

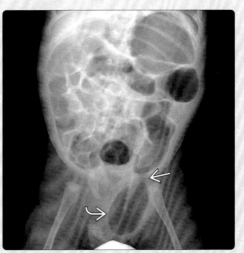 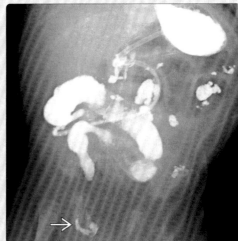

(Left) Coronal CECT in a 1-year-old boy shows the cecum ⇨ & appendix ⇨ herniating into the right hemiscrotum. The appendix contains a fecalith but was not inflamed. When an inguinal hernia contains the appendix, it is termed an Amyand hernia. (Right) Longitudinal power Doppler US in a 1-month-old boy shows bowel ⇨ herniating through the inguinal canal. There is ischemia of the ipsilateral testis ⇨ from spermatic cord compression, a phenomenon limited to neonates.

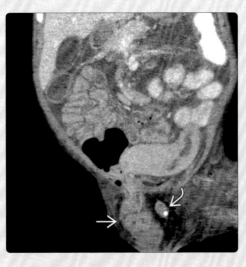 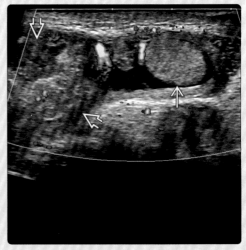

TERMINOLOGY

Definitions

- Hernia: Protrusion of contents from normally encasing body cavity through normal or abnormal opening
  - Inguinal: Protrusion of abdominal contents through defect in inguinal region
    - Indirect inguinal: Protrusion of abdominal contents into open deep inguinal ring → patent processus vaginalis (PPV) → superficial inguinal ring
      □ Canal of Nuck: Term for PPV in females; extends into labia majoris
    - Direct inguinal: Abdominal contents pass through wall of inguinal canal (due to weak abdominal musculature), exiting superficial inguinal ring
  - Umbilical: Protrusion of abdominal contents through open umbilical ring
  - Femoral: Protrusion of abdominal contents through femoral ring
  - Incisional: Protrusion of abdominal contents through defect caused by surgical incision
  - Ventral: Protrusion of abdominal contents through defect along anterior abdominal wall
  - Amyand: Inguinal hernia containing appendix
  - Internal: Hernia through fossa or foramen within abdominal cavity; defect congenital or acquired
  - Traumatic: Hernia into traumatic abdominal wall defect
- Incarcerated: Hernia in which contents cannot be reduced without special maneuvers, sedation, anesthesia, or surgery
- Strangulated: Hernia in which contents become ischemic due to vascular compression by hernia channel

Associations

- Indirect inguinal: Prematurity
- Umbilical: Prematurity, Down syndrome, Beckwith-Wiedemann syndrome
- Acquired internal: Abdominal surgery requiring Roux-en-Y reconstruction
- Recent repair of large congenital hernia (omphalocele, gastroschisis, diaphragmatic hernia)
  - ↑ intraabdominal pressure status post reduction of abdominal contents + defect repair can lead to recurrent or new hernias

IMAGING

Radiographic Findings

- Inguinal: Soft tissue or air-filled mass extending beyond pelvis inferiorly
  - 60% on right; 15% bilateral
- Umbilical: Round soft tissue or air-filled mass at umbilicus
- ± signs of obstruction with dilated air-filled loops of bowel & multiple air-fluid levels

CT Findings

- Protrusion of abdominal contents through defect in abdominal wall
- Obstructive hernia: Dilated loop of bowel entering abdominal wall defect & decompressed loop of bowel exiting hernia defect
- Signs of impending strangulation: Free fluid within hernia, bowel wall thickening, or luminal dilation

- Signs of strangulation: Bowel wall thickening, ↓ enhancement of bowel wall, engorged vasa recta, & mesenteric stranding

Ultrasonographic Findings

- Inguinal: Abdominal contents entering scrotum or labia
  - Confirm bowel presence with peristalsis, visualization of swirling bowel contents, gut signature in bowel wall
  - Use color Doppler to confirm blood flow to bowel
  - In females, may see herniated ovary
  - In male neonates, may see ↓ to absent color Doppler flow to ipsilateral testis

Imaging Recommendations

- Best imaging tool
  - Diagnosis often based on clinical exam
  - US to diagnose etiology of unknown abdominal bulges
    - Standing or Valsalva can help reproduce hernia
    - Can characterize hernia contents
    - Can evaluate blood supply to hernia contents & adjacent tissues compressed by hernia
  - CT may be useful for obstruction or pain

CLINICAL ISSUES

Presentation

- Most common signs/symptoms
  - Hernia: Painless, easily reducible bulge
  - Incarcerated: Hernia not easily reduced
  - Obstructed: Vomiting, abdominal distension
  - Strangulated: Pain, peritonitis, shock

Demographics

- Inguinal hernias in 0.8-4.4% of children
  - Occurs at any age; ↑ incidence in premature infants
    - 13% of infants born < 32 weeks & 30% of infants weighing < 1,000 g will have inguinal hernia
    - 40% of PPV close during 1st months of life
  - Incarceration 2nd most common cause of bowel obstruction after postsurgical adhesions
    - 10-30% become incarcerated in premature infants
    - Up to 15% become incarcerated in older children
- Umbilical: Most common in infants & toddlers
  - 75% of infants < 1,500 g have umbilical hernia
  - Most umbilical hernias spontaneously close by age 5
  - Low risk of incarceration
- Traumatic: Mean age = 9.5 years

Treatment

- Surgery for most hernias due to risk of incarceration
- Complications of inguinal hernia repair: Recurrence, infection, testicular atrophy, injury to vas deferens, infertility

SELECTED REFERENCES

1. Cigsar EB et al: Amyand's hernia: 11 years of experience. J Pediatr Surg. 51(8):1327-9, 2016
2. Kelly KB et al: Pediatric abdominal wall defects. Surg Clin North Am. 93(5):1255-67, 2013
3. Orth RC et al: Acute testicular ischemia caused by incarcerated inguinal hernia. Pediatr Radiol. 42(2):196-200, 2012
4. Brandt ML: Pediatric hernias. Surg Clin North Am. 88(1):27-43, vii-viii, 2008

TERMINOLOGY

- Acute obstruction of appendiceal lumen → distention → ↑ intraluminal pressure → venous obstruction → ischemia → superimposed infection of appendiceal wall → eventual perforation

IMAGING

- US 1st-line modality in child with RLQ pain
  - Noncompressible, dilated, tubular blind-ending structure (appendix) in RLQ with induration of surrounding fat
    - ± echogenic, shadowing appendicolith
  - US diameter of appendix ≥ 6 mm (during compression) suggestive of acute appendicitis
- CT diameter of appendix > 6 mm found in 40% of normal patients; look for other inflammatory features
  - Appendiceal wall thickening & hyperenhancement
  - Periappendiceal inflammation with fat stranding & poorly defined fluid
  - RLQ focal ileus

- MR findings similar to CECT
- Features of perforation
  - Discontinuity of appendiceal wall
  - Appendicolith surrounded by inflammatory change but no well-defined appendix
  - Adjacent bowel wall thickening, moderate free fluid, & localized complex collections
- Staged approach gaining traction: US/MR > US/CT

CLINICAL ISSUES

- Classic presentation: RLQ pain, anorexia, nausea, & vomiting
  - Periumbilical pain migrating to RLQ over 12-24 hours
  - Tenderness at McBurney point
  - Fever, guarding, rebound tenderness
- Clinical presentation nonspecific in up to 1/3 of patients
  - Especially young children (more likely to present after perforation)
- Typically benign course if classic history leads to prompt surgery; morbidity & mortality ↑ with perforation

(Left) AP radiograph in a 9 year old with right lower quadrant (RLQ) pain & vomiting shows an ovoid RLQ calcification ⟹, suggesting an appendicolith. A few mildly prominent small bowel loops ⟹ with air-fluid levels are noted in the left upper quadrant, concerning for focal ileus. (Right) Transverse RLQ ultrasound in the same patient shows the round echogenic appendicolith ⟹ with complete posterior acoustic shadowing (typical of calcification). Thickening & increased echogenicity of the surrounding fat ⟹ is noted.

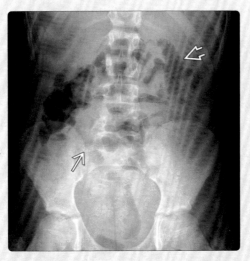
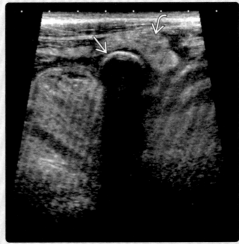

(Left) Transverse ultrasound in this same patient shows a poorly defined, heterogeneous RLQ fluid collection ⟹, concerning for abscess. (Right) Axial CECT in the same patient shows the appendicolith ⟹ & a thick-walled rim-enhancing abscess ⟹ with surrounding inflammation. A similar posterior collection ⟹ was also seen along the rectum. Adjacent bowel loops are displaced with wall thickening ⟹. These findings are typical of perforated appendicitis.

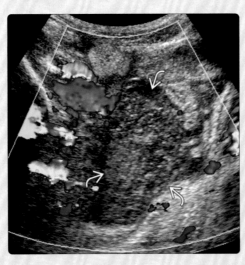
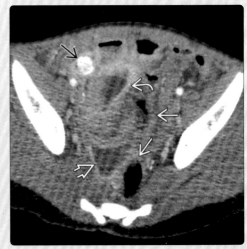

IMAGING

Radiographic Findings

- ± calcified appendicolith, air-fluid levels with paucity of bowel gas in right lower quadrant (RLQ), splinting/scoliosis
- Abnormalities more likely with perforation
  - More diffuse bowel dilation with obstruction or ileus
  - Displacement of bowel loops from RLQ by abscess
  - Thickening of adjacent bowel wall
- Study may be normal

Ultrasonographic Findings

- Grayscale ultrasound
  - Noncompressible blind-ending tubular structure (extending from cecum) ≥ 6 mm in diameter
  - Echogenic appendicolith with posterior shadowing
  - Echogenic thickened periappendiceal fat
    - May be best independent predictor
  - Free fluid in RLQ/pelvis (may be normal finding if small, anechoic, & isolated) vs. localized complex phlegmon or abscess (suggesting perforation)
  - US findings most suggestive of perforation include dilated or thick-walled adjacent bowel, loss of appendiceal wall integrity, fluid in at least 2 locations, complex fluid, & discrete abscess
  - Assessment may be limited by rigid abdomen, overlying bowel gas, or gas in abscess
- Color Doppler
  - ± hyperemia of appendiceal wall

CT Findings

- CECT
  - Dilated appendix (> 6-8 mm)
  - Appendiceal wall thickening & hyperenhancement
  - Periappendiceal inflammation with fat stranding & mild poorly defined fluid
  - Lack of appendiceal filling by enteric contrast despite oral or rectal contrast in cecum
  - Calcified appendicolith
  - RLQ lymphadenopathy
  - RLQ focal ileus
  - With perforation
    - Discontinuity of appendiceal wall
    - Appendicolith surrounded by inflammatory change without well-defined appendix
    - Localized phlegmon or fluid collections in RLQ or dependent pelvis (cul-de-sac) ± rim enhancement to suggest abscess
    - Extraluminal gas
    - Adjacent bowel wall thickening
    - Small bowel obstruction or diffuse ileus
    - Moderate free fluid & peritoneal enhancement with generalized peritonitis
  - Negative predictive value of normal CT with nonvisualized pediatric appendix ~ 99%

MR Findings

- Attractive alternative to CT due to lack of ionizing radiation
- Appendicitis features similar to CT
- Published appendix protocols vary regarding IV contrast administration; sensitivity/specificity > 94% regardless

Imaging Recommendations

- Best imaging tool
  - Staged approach gaining traction with US as 1st modality in patient with RLQ pain
    - US accurate in experienced hands
    - No ionizing radiation exposure
    - Negative predictive value > 90% with visualized normal appendix or nonvisualization of appendix without secondary findings of inflammation
  - Staged US/CT with contrast: Sensitivity ~ 99%, specificity > 90%; negative appendectomy rate of 8.1%
  - Staged US/MR with contrast: Sensitivity ~ 100%, specificity ~ 99%; negative appendectomy rate of 1.4%
  - Considerations include radiation risks, available staffing, scan time, patient size
    - US provides excellent assessment of pathology of female reproductive organs for alternative diagnosis

CLINICAL ISSUES

Presentation

- Most common signs/symptoms
  - RLQ abdominal pain, anorexia, nausea, & vomiting
- Other signs/symptoms
  - Classic symptoms in older children without perforation
    - Periumbilical pain migrating to RLQ over 12-24 hours
    - Tenderness at McBurney point
    - Fever, guarding, rebound tenderness
  - Clinical presentation nonspecific in up to 1/3 of patients
    - Delay of diagnosis, higher perforation rate
    - More common in younger children

Natural History & Prognosis

- Typically benign course if classic history leads to prompt surgery; morbidity & mortality ↑ with perforation
  - Up to 40% perforated at presentation
- Delayed abscesses present weeks to years later with retained infected appendicoliths
  - Appendicolith can migrate/erode to extraperitoneal sites

Treatment

- Appendectomy by laparoscopy for early appendicitis
  - Limited data to support IV antibiotics without surgery in some cases of nonperforated appendicitis
- Perforated appendicitis with abscesses managed with IV antibiotics, percutaneous drainage, delayed appendectomy
  - Must remove appendicolith to prevent future abscess
- Open laparotomy for peritoneal washout if frank peritonitis

SELECTED REFERENCES

1. Duke E et al: A systematic review and meta-analysis of diagnostic performance of MRI for evaluation of acute appendicitis. AJR Am J Roentgenol. 206(3):508-17, 2016
2. Moore MM et al: Magnetic resonance imaging in pediatric appendicitis: a systematic review. Pediatr Radiol. 46(6):928-39, 2016
3. Betancourt SL et al: The 'wandering appendicolith' Pediatr Radiol. 45(7):1091-4, 2015
4. Kulaylat AN et al: An implemented MRI program to eliminate radiation from the evaluation of pediatric appendicitis. J Pediatr Surg. 50(8):1359-63, 2015
5. Tulin-Silver S et al: The challenging ultrasound diagnosis of perforated appendicitis in children: constellations of sonographic findings improve specificity. Pediatr Radiol. 45(6):820-30, 2015
6. Aspelund G et al: Ultrasonography/MRI versus CT for diagnosing appendicitis. Pediatrics. 133(4):586-93, 2014

TERMINOLOGY

- Invagination of distal small bowel (intussusceptum) into colon (intussuscipiens) in telescope-like manner

IMAGING

- US: Best diagnostic modality if clinically suspected
  - Round mass with target sign in right abdomen
  - Mean diameter of 2.6 cm (vs. 1.5 cm for purely small bowel intussusceptions)
  - Sweeping transducer proximal & distal shows relationship to small & large intestine
  - May see entrapped lymph nodes, appendix, other pathologic lead points (such as duplication cyst)
  - Entrapped fluid: ↑ failure rate of enema reduction
  - ↓ vascularity associated with ↑ likelihood of bowel necrosis & ↑ failure rate of reduction
- Radiography: Often abnormal, not always perceived
  - Paucity of right abdominal colonic gas ± round mass
    - ± fat density (from entrapped mesentery) in mass

- Crescent sign: Curvilinear mass-gas interface
- Lateralization of ileum to expected cecal location
- ± small bowel obstruction
- Air enema reduction: Rush of air into small bowel → success

CLINICAL ISSUES

- Most common from ages 3 months to 3 years
  - ~ 90% idiopathic; ~ 5-10% from lead points (Meckel diverticulum > duplication cyst > polyp > lymphoma)
- Presentation: Lethargy & irritability, colic, crampy abdominal pain, intermittent fussiness, palpable right-sided abdominal mass, "currant jelly" stools, vomiting (may be bilious)
- Treatment: Urgent as bowel can infarct if not reduced
  - Reduction: Air enema under fluoroscopy vs. hydrostatic with US guidance
  - Surgery if enema fails or contraindicated
  - Recurs after reduction in ~ 5-15%

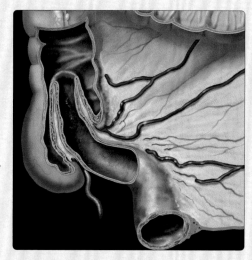
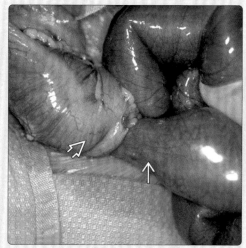

(Left) Coronal graphic shows an ileocolic (IC) intussusception with the terminal ileum invaginating into the cecum & ascending colon. Note the vascular congestion of the intussusceptum. (Right) Photograph from an intraoperative IC intussusception reduction (after a failed air enema reduction attempt) shows the distal ileum ⟹ invaginating into the cecum ⟹.

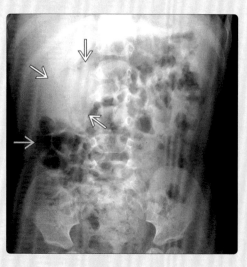
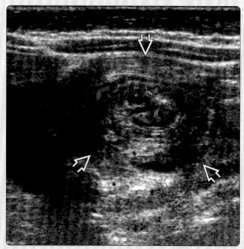

(Left) AP radiograph shows a typical case of IC intussusception with a right upper quadrant soft tissue mass ⟹ overlying the hepatic flexure. Note the lateralization of ileum ⟹ into the right lower quadrant. (Right) Transverse power Doppler US of the right lower quadrant in this 1 year old with abdominal pain shows the classic target sign of intussusception ⟹. The target is composed of the various bowel wall layers of the intussuscipiens & intussusceptum as well as intervening fat.

TERMINOLOGY

Definitions

- Invagination of distal small bowel (intussusceptum) into colon (intussuscipiens) in telescope-like manner

IMAGING

General Features

- Location
  - Always involves proximal colon, extends distally to variable degrees

Radiographic Findings

- Paucity of colonic gas in right abdomen ± round mass
  - May see layers of lucent fat density (from intussuscepted mesentery) in mass
  - Crescent sign: Curvilinear gas outlining round soft tissue mass (intussusceptum) within right or transverse colon
- ± small bowel obstruction

Ultrasonographic Findings

- Target sign: Cross section of intussusception shows round mass with layers of hyper- & hypoechogenicity (due to bowel walls & mesenteric fat)
  - May see entrapped lymph nodes, appendix, other pathologic lead points (such as intestinal duplication cyst)

Fluoroscopic Findings

- Air-contrast enema
  - Apex of intussusceptum appears as round soft tissue mass against distal colonic air column

Imaging Recommendations

- Best imaging tool
  - US for diagnosis (high sensitivity & specificity)
  - Air enema for treatment

DIFFERENTIAL DIAGNOSIS

Appendicitis

- Inflammatory collection can mimic soft tissue mass

Ovarian Torsion

- US may show avascular mass with peripheral cysts
- Only 1 normal ovary visualized

Gastroenteritis

- Air-fluid levels throughout colon suggest gastroenteritis

Isolated Small Bowel Intussusception

- Mean diameter smaller than ileocolic intussusception
- Variable location (as colon not involved)

PATHOLOGY

General Features

- Etiology
  - ~ 90% idiopathic (likely from reactive lymphoid hyperplasia)
    - May be preceded by viral illness
  - ~ 5-10% caused by pathologic lead points in children
    - Meckel diverticulum > duplication cyst, polyp, etc.
    - More likely outside of typical age range

CLINICAL ISSUES

Presentation

- Most common signs/symptoms
  - Alternating lethargy & irritability
  - Colic or "intermittent fussiness"
  - Palpable right-sided abdominal mass
- Other signs/symptoms
  - Bloody diarrhea (red "currant jelly" stools classic)
  - Crampy abdominal pain
  - Vomiting, may be bilious

Demographics

- Most common cause of pediatric small bowel obstruction
- Seasonal occurrence (classically winter, spring) with viral illnesses
- Classic age: 3 months to 3 years

Natural History & Prognosis

- Medical urgency: Bowel can infarct if not reduced
  - Necrosis → perforation → peritonitis, shock, & death
- Can rarely spontaneously reduce

Treatment

- 1st line: Image-guided pressure reduction
  - Air insufflation with fluoroscopic guidance most common: ~ 80% success rate
  - Liquid contrast under fluoroscopy less frequent
  - US-guided hydrostatic reduction gaining acceptance
- Contraindications: Peritonitis (relative), pneumoperitoneum
- Risk of perforation with air enema: 0.5-1.0%
- Preparation guidelines: Adequate hydration, IV access, physical examination, surgery consultation
- With air insufflation, intussusception encountered as round mass that moves retrograde toward cecum
- Intussusceptum most likely to get "stuck" at ileocecal valve
- Success confirmed visually by rush of gas into small bowel + resolution of soft tissue mass
- If mass progresses on initial attempts but does not reduce beyond ileocecal valve, rest for ~ 60 minutes may ↓ edema & ↑ chance of success
  - Repeat attempts acceptable if patient stable & head of intussusceptum progresses more toward cecum with each attempt
- Surgery reserved for cases of enema reduction failure or when enema contraindicated
- Intussusception recurs after successful reduction: 5-15%
  - Most recurrences occur within 48-72 hours
  - Recurrences typically treated by enema up to 3x prior to considering surgical exploration for pathologic lead point

SELECTED REFERENCES

1. Doniger SJ et al: Point-of-care ultrasonography for the rapid diagnosis of intussusception: a case series. Pediatr Emerg Care. 32(5):340-2, 2016
2. Flaum V et al: Twenty years' experience for reduction of ileocolic intussusceptions by saline enema under sonography control. J Pediatr Surg. 51(1):179-82, 2016
3. Tareen F et al: Abdominal radiography is not necessary in children with intussusception. Pediatr Surg Int. 32(1):89-92, 2016
4. Sadigh G et al: Meta-analysis of air versus liquid enema for intussusception reduction in children. AJR Am J Roentgenol. 205(5):W542-9, 2015
5. Applegate KE: Intussusception in children: evidence-based diagnosis and treatment. Pediatr Radiol. 39 Suppl 2:S140-3, 2009

Gastrointestinal

TERMINOLOGY

- Most common omphalomesenteric duct remnant

IMAGING

- Classic imaging appearance (in patient with GI bleeding): Focal persistent accumulation of radiotracer in right lower quadrant on nuclear pertechnetate scan (Meckel scan)
  - Coincident with & isointense to gastric uptake as ~ 65% of symptomatic Meckel diverticula contain ectopic gastric mucosa
- Other modalities (US, CT, MR)
  - Blind-ending tubular structure may be inconspicuous
  - May present as cyst, even with gut signature (due to US appearance of bowel wall)
  - With inflammation, findings similar to appendicitis
    - Thick-walled tubular structure, hyperemic bowel loops
    - Rare perforation
  - Intraluminal mass as lead point in intussusception
  - May only see bowel obstruction without clear cause

TOP DIFFERENTIAL DIAGNOSES

- GI bleeding with positive pertechnetate scan
  - Strong accumulation in GI duplication cyst
  - Hyperemia of Crohn disease, appendicitis, or vascular lesion may cause mild accumulation
- Small bowel obstruction
  - Appendicitis, adhesions, intussusception, inguinal hernia, malrotation (mnemonic of AAIIMM)
- Right lower quadrant inflammation
  - Appendicitis, Crohn disease, omental infarct, mesenteric adenitis, ovarian torsion

CLINICAL ISSUES

- Rule of 2s: 2% of general population; found within 2 feet of ileocecal valve; most have symptoms < 2 years of age
- Presents with bleeding (occult or frank), inflammation, intussusception, bowel obstruction, volvulus (including torsion of diverticulum), or perforation
- Treated with surgical resection

(Left) Axial graphic shows an inflamed Meckel diverticulum ➡ growing off of the antimesenteric border of the intestine with the obliterated remnant of the omphalomesenteric duct ➡ extending from its tip. (Right) Axial CECT in a 10-year-old boy with vague, intermittent abdominal pain shows a rim-enhancing cystic lesion ➡ just deep to the umbilicus. This cyst did not appear to communicate with bowel. A Meckel diverticulum distended with secretions was found at surgery.

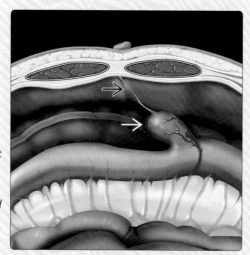
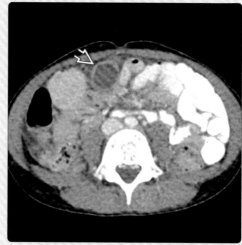

(Left) AP radiograph in a young child shows dilated small bowel loops with differential air-fluid levels & a paucity of colonic gas consistent with a small bowel obstruction. An obstructing omphalomesenteric duct remnant was found at surgery. (Right) Anterior images from a Tc-99m pertechnetate scan in a child with lower GI bleeding show progressive, intense, focal radioisotope accumulation in the lower abdominal Meckel diverticulum ➡.

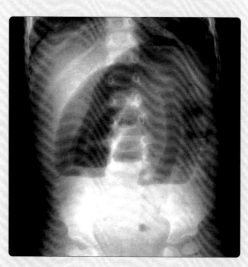
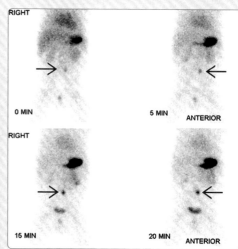

Meckel Diverticulum

TERMINOLOGY

Definitions

- Most common remnant of omphalomesenteric duct

IMAGING

General Features

- Location
  - Right lower quadrant (RLQ) or midline/periumbilical location
  - Most within 2 feet of ileocecal valve

Radiographic Findings

- Abdominal films may be normal or show
  - RLQ mass
  - Displacement of bowel loops
  - Small bowel obstruction
  - Enterolith or ingested foreign body (rare)

Ultrasonographic Findings

- Thick-walled tubular structure or hyperemic bowel in RLQ
- Heterogeneous mass in RLQ, may mimic appendicitis
  - Look for normal appendix
- May present as cyst, even with trilaminar gut signature of wall (due to hypoechoic muscularis between echogenic mucosa & serosa)
  - Walls often heterogeneous & thick with inflammation
- Intraluminal mass as lead point in intussusception (inverted Meckel)

CT Findings

- CECT
  - Incidentally, may be collapsed & blind-ending or appear cystic with trapped secretions
  - If inflamed, similar to appendicitis: Thick-walled blind-ending structure near cecum with surrounding inflammation
    - If perforated, may see abscess & free air
    - Normal appendix clue to diagnosis
  - May cause small bowel obstruction with no clear explanation on imaging
  - If intussuscepted, may be occult
  - If bleeding, CTA may show ↑ flow locally

Nuclear Medicine Findings

- Tc-99m pertechnetate scan
  - Most specific test for Meckel diverticulum: ~ 90% accuracy
  - Pertechnetate accumulates in ectopic gastric mucosa of most Meckel diverticula
    - ~ 65% of symptomatic Meckel diverticula have ectopic gastric mucosa
    - ~ 1/2 of negative scans repeated for high clinical suspicion are positive on 2nd study
  - Diverticulum typically does not communicate with bowel lumen, so radiotracer does not appear to move downstream in bowel unless there is active bleeding

Imaging Recommendations

- Best imaging tool
  - Tc-99m pertechnetate scan for GI bleeding
  - US or CECT for other presentations

PATHOLOGY

General Features

- Omphalomesenteric duct remnant (OMDR) found in 2-3% of autopsy series
  - Connection between yolk sac & primitive digestive tract in early fetal life
  - Meckel diverticulum most common end of spectrum of OMDRs, which also include umbilicoileal fistula, umbilical sinus or cyst, or fibrous cord connecting ileum to umbilicus
- Small percentage of Meckel diverticula become symptomatic, typically due to presence of ectopic gastric mucosa
  - Rarely, diverticulum contains rests of pancreatic tissue

CLINICAL ISSUES

Presentation

- Most common signs/symptoms
  - GI bleeding: Bleeding occult or frank
- Other signs/symptoms
  - Abdominal pain with small bowel obstruction, intussusception, volvulus (including torsion of diverticulum), bowel perforation

Demographics

- Age
  - Most become symptomatic before 2 years of age
    - Older patients more likely to present with intussusception or small bowel obstruction rather than GI bleeding

Treatment

- Surgical resection; incidental appendectomy usually also performed
- Meckel diverticula generally removed when found incidentally on imaging or in operating room

DIAGNOSTIC CHECKLIST

Image Interpretation Pearls

- Tc-99m pertechnetate scan: Positive in Meckel diverticula containing gastric mucosa
- Consider OMDR in small bowel obstruction otherwise unexplained on imaging & history

SELECTED REFERENCES

1. Francis A et al: Pediatric Meckel's diverticulum: report of 208 cases and review of the literature. Fetal Pediatr Pathol. 35(3):199-206, 2016
2. Sanchez TR et al: Sonography of abdominal pain in children: appendicitis and its common mimics. J Ultrasound Med. 35(3):627-35, 2016
3. Gezer HÖ et al: Meckel diverticulum in children: evaluation of macroscopic appearance for guidance in subsequent surgery. J Pediatr Surg. 51(7):1177-80, 2015
4. Kawamoto S et al: CT detection of symptomatic and asymptomatic Meckel diverticulum. AJR Am J Roentgenol. 205(2):281-91, 2015
5. Vali R et al: The value of repeat scintigraphy in patients with a high clinical suspicion for Meckel diverticulum after a negative or equivocal first Meckel scan. Pediatr Radiol. 45(10):1506-14, 2015
6. Huang CC et al: Diverse presentations in pediatric Meckel's diverticulum: a review of 100 cases. Pediatr Neonatol. 55(5):369-75, 2014

KEY FACTS

TERMINOLOGY
- Malignant embryonal hepatic tumor

IMAGING
- US to evaluate palpable mass; MR vs. CT for further characterization & determination of extent
- Single round, lobulated mass (80%), usually > 10 cm
  - May be multifocal (20%)
  - **Pret**reatment **ext**ent of disease (PRETEXT) image-based staging system evaluates number of contiguous sectors free of tumor
- Heterogeneous; usually enhances less than normal liver on all phases
- Displacement/compression/effacement of adjacent vessels vs. true vascular invasion
- Chest CT to evaluate for pulmonary metastases
  - Metastases in 20% at diagnosis: Lung >> bone, brain

CLINICAL ISSUES
- Most common primary liver malignancy of childhood
- Presents as painless abdominal mass or hepatomegaly, usually with markedly ↑ AFP levels
- Diagnosed in young children; median age: 19 months
  - Only 5-10% occur in children > 4 years of age
  - Only 4% congenital
- Increased risk in very low birth weight (20x risk), Beckwith-Wiedemann syndrome (2,280x risk), familial adenomatous polyposis (847x risk)
- Treatment: Resection ± neoadjuvant chemotherapy
  - Resection alone can be curative
  - Primary transplant if unresectable after neoadjuvant therapy (& clear of metastases)
  - Posttherapy AFP levels: Tumor marker for surveillance
- Event-free survival/overall survival
  - Standard risk: Up to 83%/95%
  - High risk: Up to 65%/69%

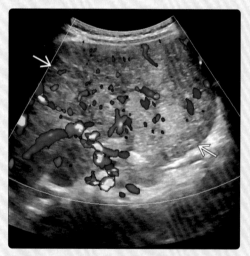 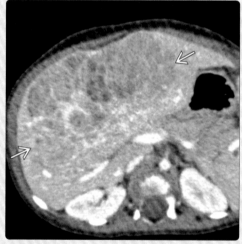

(Left) Transverse color Doppler US of the liver in a 1 year old with hepatoblastoma shows a heterogeneously hyperechoic, moderately vascular mass ➡ in the liver. (Right) Axial CECT in the same patient shows the mass ➡ occupying segments 4b & 5. Assuming that the tumor is confined to these 2 central sectors, this would represent a pretreatment extent of disease (PRETEXT) III tumor (as 3 sectors would need to be resected in order to completely excise the tumor).

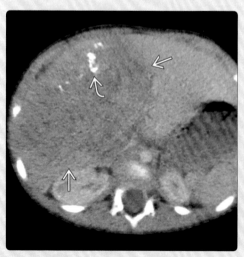 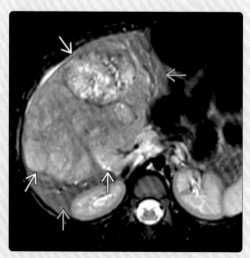

(Left) Axial CECT in a 2 year old shows a hypodense mass ➡ in the liver. The mass has a small area of calcification ➡. Calcification is present in up to 50% of hepatoblastomas. (Right) Axial T2 FS MR in the same patient shows a heterogeneous mass in the inferior liver. The mass ➡ is of intermediate signal intensity overall but is mildly hyperintense compared to the background liver ➡.

Hepatic Hemangiomas, Infantile and Congenital

TERMINOLOGY

- Hemangioma: Benign endothelial neoplasm of neonates/infants in soft tissues or viscera (especially liver)
  - **Not** hemangioendothelioma (more aggressive tumor)
  - **Not** cavernous hemangioma (venous malformation)
- Congenital hemangioma (CH): Found in perinatal period, does not proliferate beyond birth
  - Rapidly involuting (RICH) vs. noninvoluting (NICH) types
- Infantile hemangioma (IH): Develops in 1st few weeks of life with characteristic proliferating & involuting phases

IMAGING

- Pediatric hepatic hemangiomas considered as 3 types
  - Focal (CH): Solitary large heterogeneous mass
  - Multifocal (IHs): Multiple small to moderate homogeneous masses
  - Diffuse (IHs): Liver enlarged & replaced by masses
- US to screen liver, MR for further characterization
  - Hepatic IHs often found in infants with ≥ 5 cutaneous IHs

CLINICAL ISSUES

- Hepatic CH & IHs may be asymptomatic or can present with hepatomegaly &/or heart failure
  - CH may have transient consumptive coagulopathy (**not** Kasabach-Merritt phenomenon)
  - Diffuse IHs may present with hypothyroidism, liver failure, abdominal compartment syndrome
- AFP trends down (not up) in infants with CH or IHs
- Natural history
  - CH: RICH ↓ in size over early months
  - IHs: Will ↑ in infancy but gradually involute over years
    - Mortality: 38% for diffuse IHs, 9% for multifocal IHs
      - ↓ with liver US screening for ≥ 5 cutaneous IHs
- Treatment required if complications develop
  - CH: Embolization, resection
  - IHs: Medical therapies initially (propranolol, steroids; rarely vincristine); embolization, liver transplant in extreme cases

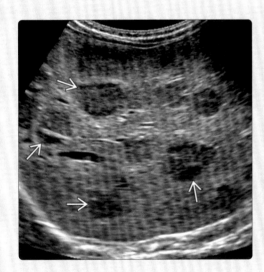

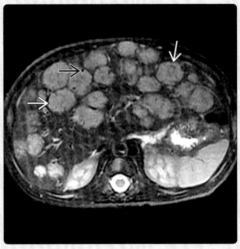

(Left) Longitudinal US in a 7 month old with a history of cutaneous infantile hemangiomas (IHs) shows multiple, round, well-circumscribed hypoechoic masses ⊇ throughout the liver. (Right) Axial T2 FS MR in this patient shows the typical appearance of IHs: Multiple, round, well-circumscribed small- to moderate-sized, hyperintense (but not fluid-bright) lesions ⊇, some of which contain high-flow vessels ⊡.

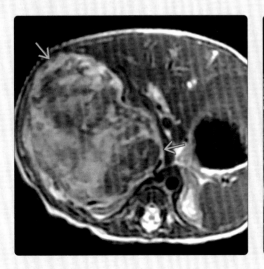

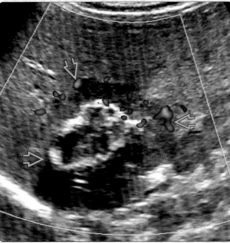

(Left) Axial T2 MR in a 10 day old with abdominal distention shows a large, heterogeneous, solitary mass ⊡ occupying the right lobe of the liver, typical of a congenital hemangioma. (Right) Longitudinal color Doppler US through the same mass 5 months later shows a marked interval decrease in the size of the lesion ⊡ (going from 9 cm to 4 cm) without therapy. This degree of involution in the 1st few months of life is typical of a rapidly involuting congenital hemangioma.

Focal Nodular Hyperplasia

TERMINOLOGY

- Benign epithelial tumor composed of hepatocytes, Kupffer cells, abnormal bile ducts, & vessels

IMAGING

- Well-defined round or ovoid mass with smooth or mildly lobulated margins; central scar in 50-70%
- Ultrasound: Can be ↑, ↓, or ↔ echogenicity relative to liver
  - Doppler shows spoke-wheel pattern with hypervascular central scar & radiating vessels
- CECT: Homogeneous arterial enhancement ± hypoenhancing central scar
- MR with hepatobiliary phase contrast agent (best tool)
  - T1WI: Iso- to slightly hypointense; ± hypointense scar
  - T2WI: Slightly hyperintense; ± hyperintense scar
  - Arterial phase: Hyperenhancing mass ± hypoenhancing central scar
  - Venous phase: Iso- to slight hyperenhancement of mass ± hyperenhancing central scar

- Delayed hepatobiliary phase: Mild hyperenhancement relative to normally enhancing background liver
  - Usually homogeneous (can be heterogeneous)

PATHOLOGY

- Hyperplastic response to preexisting vascular malformation within central scar
- ↑ prevalence after chemotherapy &/or stem cell transplant
  - Often multiple lesions, smaller with no central scar

CLINICAL ISSUES

- 2% of primary hepatic tumors in children
- Often asymptomatic; occasionally causes palpable mass &/or vague abdominal pain
- Normal lab values, including α-fetoprotein
- No known malignant potential
- Managed conservatively in asymptomatic patients, surgically in symptomatic patients

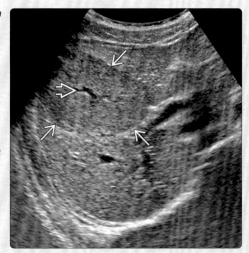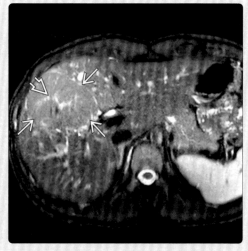

(Left) Transverse ultrasound in a 17-year-old girl with right upper quadrant pain demonstrates a well-defined, slightly hypoechoic hepatic mass ➡ with a central anechoic scar ⮞ typical of focal nodular hyperplasia (FNH). (Right) Axial T2 FS MR in the same patient demonstrates a well-defined right lobe liver mass ➡ that is slightly hyperintense relative to the surrounding parenchyma & shows a hyperintense central scar ⮞. This lesion was ultimately proven to be FNH.

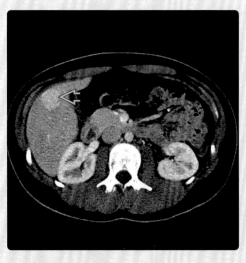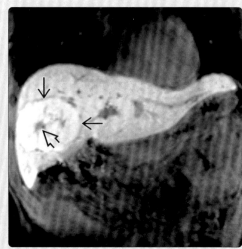

(Left) Axial CECT in a 14-year-old girl shows a homogeneous liver mass ⮞ with mild hyperenhancement. On the subsequent multiphase MR with a hepatocyte-specific contrast agent, the lesion was consistent with FNH. (Right) Twenty-minute delayed coronal T1 C+ FS MR using a hepatocyte-specific contrast agent in a patient with a hepatic lesion demonstrates hyperenhancement of the mass ➡ relative to the surrounding normally enhanced liver parenchyma. There is a nonenhancing central scar ⮞, typical of FNH.

Hepatic Adenoma

KEY FACTS

TERMINOLOGY

- Benign neoplasm arising from hepatocytes
- Subtypes include
  - Inflammatory ~ 35-50%
  - Hepatocyte nuclear factor 1α (*HNF1a*) mutated ~ 35-40%
  - β-catenin activated ~ 10-19%
    - ↑ malignant potential
  - Undifferentiated ~ 5-10%

IMAGING

- May be uniform vs. heterogeneous on US/CT/MR due to fat, hemorrhage, necrosis, Ca^{2+}
- Subtypes may have different MR features
  - Inflammatory: Peripheral ↑ on T2WI, ↑ arterial enhancement
  - *HNF1a*: ↓ on T1 opposed-phase (due to ↑ lipid), ↑ to ↔ arterial enhancement
  - β-catenin & undifferentiated subtypes: Variable features

- Hepatobiliary phase MR contrast agents may help differentiate from focal nodular hyperplasia
  - Adenomas rarely retain contrast on hepatobiliary phase
- CT: Arterial phase → heterogeneous hyperenhancement
  - ↑ attenuation subcapsular or peritoneal fluid if tumor rupture/hemorrhage occurs

TOP DIFFERENTIAL DIAGNOSES

- Focal nodular hyperplasia
- Hepatocellular carcinoma

CLINICAL ISSUES

- Adenomas more likely with oral contraceptive use, steroid use, glycogen storage disease
  - May regress if oral contraceptives discontinued
- May hemorrhage/rupture; rare malignant potential (~ 5%)
  - ↑ risk of hemorrhage with ↑ size of mass
- Surgical excision if large or symptomatic

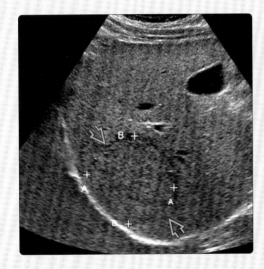
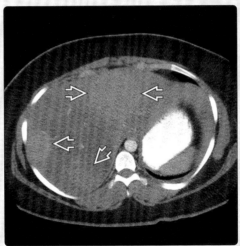

(Left) *Longitudinal oblique ultrasound in a teenager with Fanconi anemia who is on androgen therapy shows an isoechoic but relatively well-defined round mass* ⇨ *in the right lobe of the liver. Biopsy confirmed a hepatic adenoma.* (Right) *Axial arterial phase CECT in a 16-year-old girl with vague abdominal pain shows 3 liver masses with mild early enhancement* ⇒*, later found to be hepatic adenomas at biopsy.*

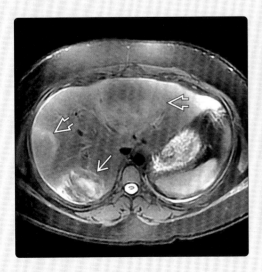
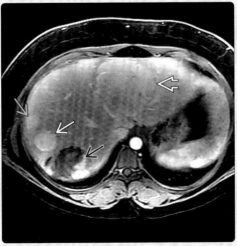

(Left) *Axial T2 FS MR in the same 16-year-old girl shows 2 of the adenomas to be mildly hyperintense* ⇒*. The 3rd mass is heterogeneous with hypointense foci* ⇒ *due to prior hemorrhage.* (Right) *Arterial phase T1 C+ FS MR in the same 16-year-old girl shows mild enhancement in the largest adenoma* ⇒*, homogeneous enhancement in a smaller adenoma* ⇒*, & heterogeneous enhancement with low signal in a 3rd adenoma* ⇒*. Additional smaller enhancing adenomas are also present* ⇨*.*

Biliary Atresia

TERMINOLOGY

- Biliary atresia (BA): Absent or severely deficient extrahepatic biliary tree

IMAGING

- US classically used to exclude other causes of neonatal jaundice; however, characteristic findings can be very suggestive of BA
  - Absent or abnormal small irregular gallbladder in vast majority (gallbladder ghost sign)
  - Echogenic fibrous tissue (triangular cord sign) anterior to portal vein at site of obliterated extrahepatic biliary duct
  - No biliary ductal dilation
  - Liver echotexture typically normal (early)
  - ↑ liver stiffness (by elastography) may be more specific for BA
- Nuclear medicine hepatobiliary (HIDA) scan: No radiotracer excretion into intestines; gallbladder visible in up to 25%
- Intraoperative cholangiogram: No biliary-enteric channel

TOP DIFFERENTIAL DIAGNOSES

- Neonatal hepatitis, bile-plug syndrome, Alagille syndrome, choledochal malformation

PATHOLOGY

- Hypoplastic, atretic, or fibrosed extrahepatic ducts that worsen in perinatal period
- Associations: Preduodenal portal vein, interrupted IVC, congenital heart disease, situs anomalies, polysplenia (or asplenia) in BA splenic malformation syndrome (10-15%)

CLINICAL ISSUES

- Neonatal jaundice with conjugated (direct) hyperbilirubinemia, evident in immediate perinatal period
- Hepatocytes function well initially with gradual deterioration → fibrosis → portal hypertension
- Kasai portoenterostomy temporarily effective in 90% if performed < 2 months of age; ↓ to < 50% if > 3 months
- Liver transplant ultimately required in most by adulthood

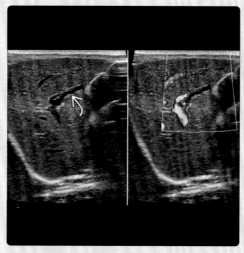
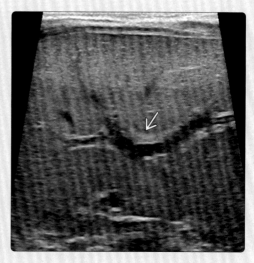

(Left) Split-screen grayscale & color Doppler US show a very small & irregularly shaped gallbladder ⊅ along the inferior margin of the liver in a newborn with jaundice, despite adequate fasting. This crenulated appearance is sometimes called the ghost gallbladder. (Right) Transverse US shows echogenic tissue ➡ at the expected location of the common hepatic duct anterior to the portal vein, the triangular cord sign. This sign & the ghost gallbladder strongly suggest biliary atresia (BA).

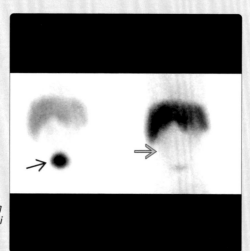
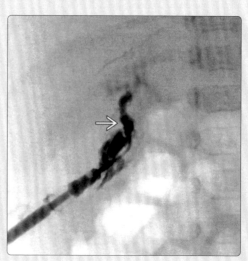

(Left) Hepatobiliary scintigraphy in a jaundiced infant shows no intestinal excretion of mebrofenin. The hepatic radiotracer is slowly excreted by the kidneys into the urinary bladder ➡. A 24-hour delayed image also shows no intestinal radiotracer ➡, typical of BA. (Right) Intraoperative cholangiogram through a hypoplastic gallbladder shows a short segment of common hepatic duct ➡ but no intestinal drainage, confirming BA. A portoenterostomy (Kasai procedure) followed.

Choledochal Cyst

KEY FACTS

TERMINOLOGY

- Spectrum of malformations involving extrahepatic & intrahepatic bile ducts

IMAGING

- US in child with jaundice & elevated liver enzymes
  - Round or tubular cystic right upper quadrant mass separate from gallbladder
    - CBD dilation > 10 mm very suggestive in child
- MRCP for detailed preoperative assessment of ductal anatomy & pancreaticobiliary maljunction

PATHOLOGY

- Etiology may be due to pancreaticobiliary maljunction with pancreatic duct joining CBD proximal to sphincter of Oddi → biliary reflux of pancreatic enzymes
- Classification modified by Todani in 1977
  - Type I cyst: Segmental or diffuse fusiform dilation of CBD; most common variety (75-95% of cases)

- Type II cyst: Diverticulum of duct
- Type III cyst: Choledochocele protruding into duodenum
- Type IV: Discontinuous extrahepatic bile duct cysts, isolated (type IVb) or Caroli type (type IVa)
- Type V: Intrahepatic cystic dilations (Caroli disease)

CLINICAL ISSUES

- Presentation: 2/3 diagnosed before 10 years of age
  - Infants: Jaundice, acholic stools, hepatomegaly, & palpable abdominal mass
  - Adults: Upper abdominal pain, jaundice, cholangitis, & pancreatitis
- Complications: Bile duct perforation, biliary stone formation, bacterial cholangitis with subsequent hepatic abscess & sepsis, biliary strictures, low-grade biliary obstruction → cirrhosis & portal hypertension, development of bile duct carcinomas
- General treatment: Cyst resection & biliary diversion/portoenterostomy

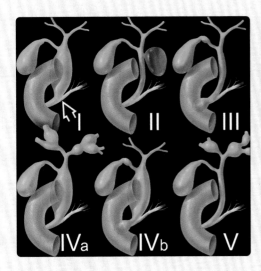
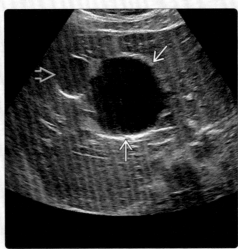

(Left) Graphic shows various types of choledochal malformations. Note the anomalous pancreaticobiliary junction ⇨ with the pancreatic duct inserting into the common bile duct proximal to the sphincter of Oddi. (Right) Transverse US of the liver in a 9 year old shows a large, simple-appearing cyst ⇨ adjacent to the gallbladder ⇨.

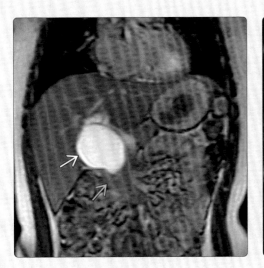
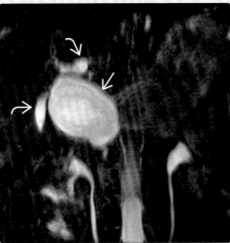

(Left) Coronal SSFP MR of the same child shows the elliptical cyst ⇨ in the porta hepatis extending into the pancreatic head ⇨, typical of a choledochal cyst. (Right) Coronal MIP image from an MRCP in the same patient shows a severely enlarged common hepatic/bile duct ⇨ & focally dilated central intrahepatic bile ducts ⇨ in this case of a type IVa choledochal cyst.

KEY FACTS

TERMINOLOGY

- Simple steatosis: Fat infiltration of > 5% of hepatocytes
- Nonalcoholic fatty liver disease (NAFLD): Steatosis with metabolic syndrome &/or abnormal liver function enzymes
- Nonalcoholic steatohepatitis (NASH): Abnormal hepatic fat content with inflammatory activity or fibrosis

IMAGING

- Ultrasound shows diffusely ↑ hepatic echogenicity
  - Liver much more echogenic than right kidney
  - Poor through transmission of sound waves
    - ↓ visualization of echogenic portal triads & right hemidiaphragm
- NECT: ↓ liver attenuation relative to spleen
  - Normal liver slightly > spleen
- CECT: Difficult to assess steatosis due to variable enhancement of liver & spleen depending on phase
- MR: Only imaging test that can quantify hepatic fat
  - Steatosis defined as fat fraction > 5%

TOP DIFFERENTIAL DIAGNOSES

- Cirrhosis
- Cystic fibrosis

CLINICAL ISSUES

- Most common cause of chronic liver disease in children
  - NAFLD present in 38-40% of obese patients
  - Most commonly presents between 11-13 years of age
    - Obesity, abdominal pain, fatigue, hepatomegaly
- Risk factors
  - Modifiable: Obesity, sedentary lifestyle, high intake of sugar-sweetened beverages, sleep apnea
  - Nonmodifiable: Male, Hispanic origin, family history, parental obesity, low birth weight
- Thought to represent progression from simple steatosis → NAFLD → NASH → cirrhosis
- Treatment: Weight loss with dietary modification & exercise

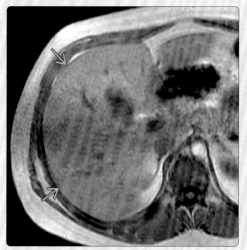
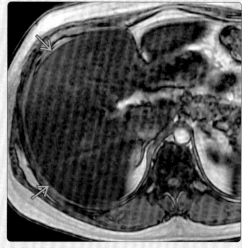

(Left) Axial T1 MR in-phase image of the liver in an adolescent with nonalcoholic steatohepatitis shows a normal contour & signal intensity of the liver ➡. (Right) Axial T1 MR opposed-phase image in the same patient shows considerable loss of signal (i.e., dropout) of the liver ➡, typical of steatosis. In this case, the fat fraction was measured at 30%. There are multiple methods to detect & quantify hepatic fat content via MR, including MR spectroscopy & chemical shift imaging.

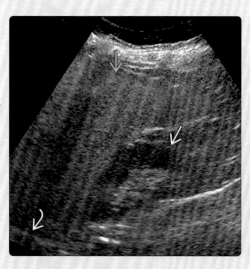
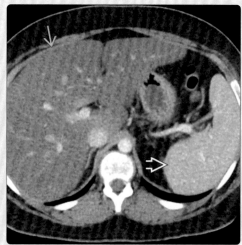

(Left) Ultrasound in the same patient shows diffusely increased echogenicity of the liver ➡ as compared to the right kidney ➡. In addition, there is poor through transmission of the sound beam with nonvisualization of the normally echogenic portal triads & poor visualization of the right hemidiaphragm ➡. (Right) Axial CECT in the same patient shows the liver ➡ to have diffusely lower attenuation than the spleen ➡, consistent with hepatic steatosis.

KEY FACTS

TERMINOLOGY

- Cirrhosis: Liver disease characterized by bridging fibrosis
  - Variety of underlying disorders may lead to cirrhosis

IMAGING

- Nodular contour of liver, easiest to see along free margin
- US: Liver has coarsened echotexture
- MR: Lace-like ↓ T1 signal of fibrosis
  - MR can detect underlying deposition (fat, iron, etc.)
  - Hepatocyte-specific contrast agents allow characterization of nodules
- MR or US elastography can determine liver stiffness as marker of fibrosis
- Progressive fibrosis leads to ↓ hepatic size
- Signs of portal hypertension: Ascites, splenomegaly, varices

TOP DIFFERENTIAL DIAGNOSES

- Biliary atresia, Alagille syndrome, progressive familial intrahepatic cholestasis, viral hepatitis, α-1 antitrypsin deficiency, cystic fibrosis, Wilson disease, nonalcoholic fatty liver disease, autoimmune hepatitis, primary sclerosing cholangitis, post-Fontan physiology

CLINICAL ISSUES

- Symptoms generally include anorexia, fatigue, weakness, nausea, & vomiting
- Patients with end-stage liver disease may have jaundice, pruritus, gastrointestinal bleeding, ascites, & hepatic encephalopathy
- Early stages of fibrosis can be reversed by treating underlying condition
- Treatment for end-stage liver disease: Liver transplant
- Cirrhotic patients typically screened every 6 months for hepatocellular carcinoma

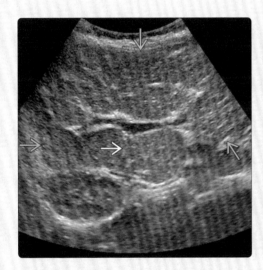
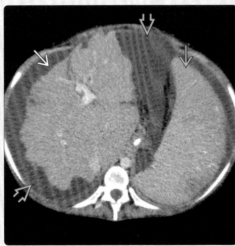

(Left) Transverse ultrasound shows a markedly abnormal appearance of the liver ➡ with a macronodular contour & coarsened echotexture. Note the fine echogenic regions of fibrosis ➡. (Right) Axial CECT shows a small, cirrhotic liver ➡ with a macronodular contour. There are signs of portal hypertension, including ascites ➡ & splenomegaly ➡.

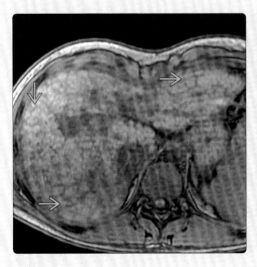
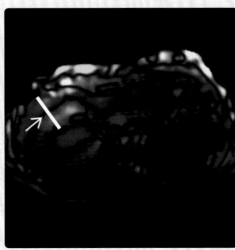

(Left) Axial T1 opposed-phase MR in an adolescent with autoimmune hepatitis shows an abnormal lace-like pattern of fibrosis throughout the liver ➡. (Right) Axial MR elastogram of the liver shows abnormal increased thickness ➡ of the sound waves traversing the liver. The liver stiffness was measured at 4.92 kPa in this patient (with advanced fibrosis > 2.71 kPa).

KEY FACTS

TERMINOLOGY

- Acute pancreatitis (AP): Acute inflammation of pancreas with variable involvement of local tissues/remote organs
  - 2 of 3 features required for diagnosis: Abdominal pain consistent with disease, 3x rise in serum amylase or lipase, or imaging findings consistent with AP
  - 2 types of AP: Interstitial edematous vs. necrotizing
  - Fluid collections
    - Pancreatic pseudocyst: Fluid collection associated with interstitial edematous pancreatitis after first 4 weeks
    - Walled-off necrosis: Collection containing fluid & necrotic material after first 4 weeks
- Chronic pancreatitis (CP): Relapsing or continuing inflammation with destruction of parenchyma & ducts

IMAGING

- Interstitial edematous pancreatitis: Gland enlargement with edema & homogeneous (± mildly decreased) enhancement
  - Acute peripancreatic fluid collection: Nonencapsulated collections of variable size & shape
  - Pancreatic pseudocyst: Encapsulated cystic lesion with no internal solid component, > 4 weeks from onset
- Necrotizing pancreatitis: Heterogeneous enhancement (moderately to severely decreased)
  - Acute necrotic collection: Nonencapsulated collection with heterogeneous contents
  - Walled-off necrosis: Well-circumscribed cavity containing necrotic tissue, > 4 weeks from onset
- CP: Atrophic pancreas with dilated duct & pancreatic Ca^{2+}
- Best imaging modalities
  - CECT vs. MR + MRCP acutely
  - US for following known pancreatitis or fluid collection

CLINICAL ISSUES

- Epigastric abdominal pain, ↑ amylase & lipase > 3x normal
- Treated with fluid resuscitation, pain management, early enteral nutrition, ± collection drainage

(Left) Transverse US of the pancreas in an adolescent with abdominal pain & acute interstitial pancreatitis shows a poorly defined hypoechoic pancreas ➡. The head of the pancreas ➡ is enlarged to a greater degree than the remainder of the gland, & the border is not distinct. (Right) Coronal CECT in the same patient shows enlargement of the head of the pancreas ➡ with surrounding peripancreatic edema ➡. Interstitial edematous pancreatitis is characterized by homogeneous enhancement of the gland.

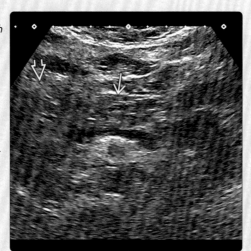
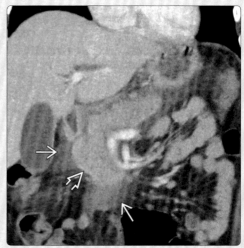

(Left) Transverse US of the right upper quadrant in an adolescent boy with a 2-week history of pancreatitis shows cholelithiasis ➡ within the gallbladder lumen. There is a large fluid collection ➡ medial & posterior to the gallbladder consistent with an acute peripancreatic collection. (Right) Axial 2D SSFP FS MR in the same patient shows the pancreatic duct ➡ extending to the large peripancreatic fluid collection ➡. If the collection lasts > 4 weeks after the onset of symptoms, it would be considered a pseudocyst.

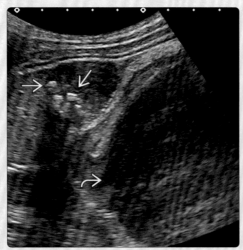
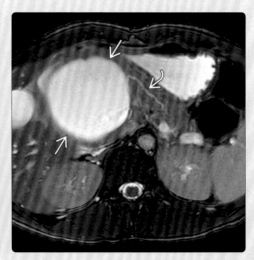

TERMINOLOGY

Definitions

- Acute pancreatitis (AP): Acute inflammation of pancreas with variable involvement of local/regional tissues
  - 2 of 3 features required for diagnosis
    - Abdominal pain consistent with disease
    - Rise in serum amylase or lipase ≥ 3x normal
    - Imaging findings consistent with AP
  - 2 types of AP
    - Interstitial edematous pancreatitis
    - Necrotizing pancreatitis
- Acute recurrent pancreatitis: ≥ 2 distinct episodes of AP with complete resolution of pain for ≥ 1 month or normalization of enzyme levels
- Chronic pancreatitis (CP): Relapsing/continuing pancreatic inflammation leading to irreversible destruction of parenchyma & ducts with ↓ exocrine function
- Fluid collections
  - Acute peripancreatic fluid collection: Fluid collection associated with interstitial edematous pancreatitis during first 4 weeks
  - Pancreatic pseudocyst: Fluid collection associated with interstitial edematous pancreatitis after first 4 weeks
  - Acute necrotic collection: Collection containing fluid & necrotic material during first 4 weeks
  - Walled-off necrosis: Collection containing fluid & necrotic material after first 4 weeks

IMAGING

CT Findings

- Interstitial edematous pancreatitis
  - Focal or diffuse pancreatic enlargement
  - Homogeneous enhancement, often mildly decreased, of edematous pancreatic parenchyma
  - ± surrounding fat inflammation
  - Acute peripancreatic fluid collection: Homogeneous fluid collection without defined capsule
  - Pancreatic pseudocyst: Fluid density cyst with well-defined capsule > 4 weeks from onset
- Necrotizing pancreatitis
  - Area of moderately to severely decreased enhancement within pancreas or peripancreatic mesentery
  - Walled-off necrosis: Fluid density collection in area of prior necrosis > 4 weeks from onset
- CP: Atrophic pancreas ± Ca^{2+}, dilation of pancreatic duct

MR Findings

- T1, T2 FS, T1 C+ FS: Generally follow CECT findings
- MRCP
  - AP: Look for congenital anomalies (pancreas divisum, pancreatobiliary maljunction)
  - CP: Look for sequelae of pancreatitis (dilation or strictures of pancreatic duct)

Ultrasonographic Findings

- AP: Enlarged, hypoechoic pancreas
  - Look for gallstones, biliary dilation
- CP: Atrophic pancreas with echogenic areas of Ca^{2+} & dilated pancreatic duct

Imaging Recommendations

- Best imaging tool
  - CECT or MR with MRCP acutely
  - US for following known pancreatitis or fluid collection

PATHOLOGY

General Features

- Etiology
  - AP: Caused by acinar cell injury & premature activation of trypsinogen to trypsin in pancreas; etiologies include
    - Anatomic: Pancreas divisum, pancreatobiliary maljunction, choledochal cyst, annular pancreas
    - Biliary obstruction: Gallstones
    - Systemic illness: Sepsis, shock, hemolytic uremic syndrome, systemic lupus erythematosus
    - Drugs: L-asparaginase, valproic acid, azathioprine, mercaptopurine, mesalamine
    - Trauma: Motor vehicle accident, handlebar injury, nonaccidental trauma
    - Idiopathic
    - Metabolic disorders: Cystic fibrosis, hyperlipidemia, hyperparathyroidism
    - Genetic/hereditary
    - Autoimmune
  - CP: Pancreatic injury followed by sustained immune activation where fibrosis dominates
    - Cystic fibrosis: Most common cause of CP
    - Hereditary pancreatitis: Autosomal dominant disorder associated with recurrent bouts of pancreatitis
    - Anatomic causes: Pancreas divisum, annular pancreas, choledochal cyst

CLINICAL ISSUES

Presentation

- Most common signs/symptoms
  - Epigastric abdominal pain
  - Elevated amylase & lipase to level > 3x normal
- Other signs/symptoms
  - Vomiting, anorexia, & nausea
  - Patient appears ill, irritable, & quiet
  - Tachycardia, fever, hypotension, abdominal signs

Natural History & Prognosis

- Pseudocyst most common complication of AP
- Mortality rate from AP: 2-10%
  - Mortality ↓ in children vs. adults
- ~ 50% of patients with hereditary pancreatitis develop CP
- With CP, pain may be transient & not severe
  - End-stage disease → endocrine & exocrine dysfunction

Treatment

- Current mainstays of therapy: Fluid resuscitation, pain management, early enteral nutrition, ± collection drainage

SELECTED REFERENCES

1. Zhao K et al: Acute pancreatitis: revised Atlanta classification and the role of cross-sectional imaging. AJR Am J Roentgenol. 205(1):W32-41, 2015
2. Meyer A et al: Contrasts and comparisons between childhood and adult onset acute pancreatitis. Pancreatology. 13(4):429-35, 2013
3. Srinath AI et al: Pediatric pancreatitis. Pediatr Rev. 34(2):79-90, 2013

KEY FACTS

TERMINOLOGY

- Self-limited benign inflammation of lymph nodes in bowel mesentery; diagnosis of exclusion

IMAGING

- Best diagnostic clue: Cluster of ≥ 3 enlarged lymph nodes, each ≥ 5 mm in size (short axis)
- Ultrasound
  - Enlarged lymph nodes often retain normal nodal architecture with fatty hilum & radiating vessels
  - Pain with compression over nodes
  - ± fat induration; no abscess or phlegmon
  - Normal appendix (< 6-mm diameter & compressible)
- CECT findings
  - Mildly enlarged lymph nodes, most commonly anterior to right psoas muscle
  - Ileal or colonic wall thickening in < 1/3
    - More common < 5 years of age
  - Normal appendix without surrounding inflammation

TOP DIFFERENTIAL DIAGNOSES

- Appendicitis
- Omental infarction
- Crohn disease
- Burkitt lymphoma

PATHOLOGY

- Majority likely secondary to viral or bacterial infection (*Yersinia enterocolitica* classic)
- Recent URI in up to 25%

CLINICAL ISSUES

- Most commonly occurs < 15 years of age
- Mimics appendicitis: Similar clinical presentation
  - Most frequent alternative diagnosis to appendicitis
  - Diffuse or focal right lower quadrant abdominal pain
  - ± nausea, vomiting, diarrhea, leukocytosis
- Treatment conservative for primary mesenteric adenitis
  - Symptoms typically resolve by 2 weeks

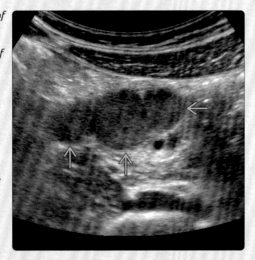

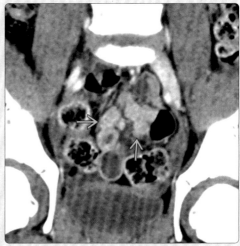

(Left) Transverse ultrasound of the right lower quadrant in a 10 year old with abdominal pain & fever shows a cluster of 3 lymph nodes ➡, each measuring > 5 mm in short axis, at the site of tenderness. Additional enlarged lymph nodes were also present. The appendix was not visualized. (Right) Coronal CECT in the same patient shows a cluster of lymph nodes ➡, each measuring > 5 mm in size. The appendix was normal (not shown). This patient was diagnosed with mesenteric lymphadenitis & treated conservatively.

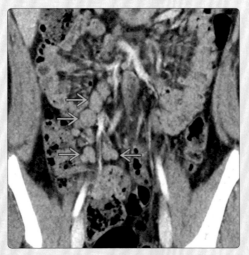

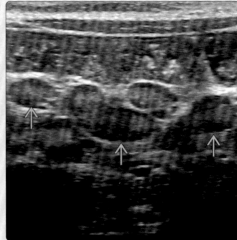

(Left) Coronal CECT from a 10 year old with abdominal pain shows numerous mildly enlarged lymph nodes ➡ in the right abdomen. The appendix was normal (not shown). These findings are consistent with mesenteric adenitis in the absence of other pathology. (Right) Longitudinal ultrasound in a 2 year old with abdominal pain shows mildly enlarged lymph nodes ➡ in the right abdomen. No other pathology was identified. The patient's symptoms resolved with conservative therapy, typical of mesenteric adenitis.

KEY FACTS

TERMINOLOGY

- Benign self-limited cause of acute abdominal pain due to vascular occlusion → segmental omental infarction

IMAGING

- General features
  - Well-demarcated triangular/wedge-shaped or oval focus of ↑ attenuation/echogenicity within omental fat
  - Right mid to upper abdomen, deep to anterior wall
  - ± thickening of overlying peritoneal membrane
  - ± free intraperitoneal fluid &/or pleural effusion
  - No adjacent inflammatory etiologies (e.g., appendicitis)
- US: Echogenic focus with no internal color Doppler flow; painful to direct sonographic palpation
- CT: Focal fat stranding ± hyperattenuating streaky densities due to fibrous bands or thrombosed vessels
  - ± peripheral enhancement
  - ± whirl or vascular pedicle sign with torsion
- Recommendations

  - Ultrasound: Acceptable 1st-line modality despite lower sensitivity for this diagnosis compared to CECT
    - ↑ sensitivity for surgical diagnoses (e.g., appendicitis)

TOP DIFFERENTIAL DIAGNOSES

- Epiploic appendagitis, appendicitis, slow flow vascular malformation, mesenteric contusion, fat-containing masses

PATHOLOGY

- Etiologies: Anatomic vascular variation, hypercoagulability, torsion, systemic states prone to vascular congestion
- Majority of patients obese

CLINICAL ISSUES

- Abdominal pain & tenderness (typically right-sided), nausea, vomiting, fever, ↑ CRP & WBC
- Conservative treatment (analgesia & antibiotics) typically adequate
- Occasional surgical excision if pain intractable, symptoms worsen, or imaging equivocal

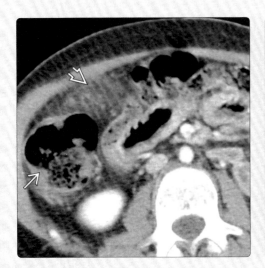

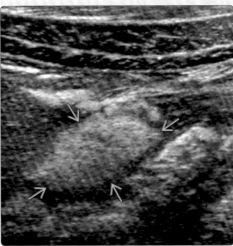

(Left) Axial CECT in an 11 year old with right abdominal pain depicts a focus of inflammatory stranding ⇨ immediately deep to the abdominal wall & anterior to the ascending colon ➡, typical of an omental infarction. (Right) Transverse ultrasound of a 7 year old with abdominal pain shows a well-demarcated, ovoid, hyperechoic focus ➡ deep to the right anterior abdominal wall. A normal appendix was not visualized. An omental infarction was confirmed at surgery.

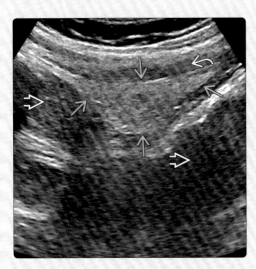

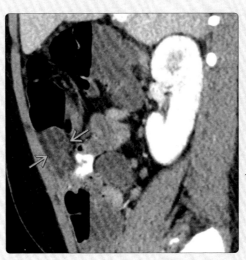

(Left) Longitudinal ultrasound from a 9 year old with right abdominal pain & fever depicts a hyperechoic focus ➡ in the omentum between the ascending colon ⇨ & abdominal wall ➡, consistent with an omental infarction. (Right) Right sagittal CECT in the same patient shows a corresponding focus of omental hyperattenuation ➡ just deep to the anterior abdominal wall, consistent with an omental infarction.

KEY FACTS

IMAGING

- Gold standard exam for blunt abdominal trauma: CECT
  - Abdominal US only 51% sensitive for liver injury
- Parenchymal laceration: Irregular, linear, branching foci of fluid attenuation
- Hematoma: Intraperitoneal, retroperitoneal, subcapsular, or intraparenchymal
  - Fluid attenuation if hematoma fresh & unclotted
  - ↑ attenuation may represent clot, implicate site of injury
  - ± hematocrit level of settling peritoneal blood in pelvis
    - ↑ density of dependent-most fluid component due to layering cellular blood elements
- Active hemorrhage or extravasation: Irregular, nonanatomic focus of high attenuation near vessel; accumulates on delayed images
  - Collection isodense to aorta with arterial injury
  - ± ↑ risk of delayed hemorrhage & nonoperative management failure

- Generalized periportal edema: Frequent finding of resuscitation due to distended intrahepatic lymphatics from vigorous hydration
- Complications: Biliary injury with leak, pseudoaneurysm, arteriovenous fistula, delayed hemorrhage, abscess

PATHOLOGY

- Blunt vs. penetrating trauma: 90% vs. 10%
  - Motor vehicle-related injuries most common: 69%
  - Falls & recreational accidents: 30%
  - Nonaccidental trauma: 1%
- Concomitant splenic injury: 45%

CLINICAL ISSUES

- Presentations: RUQ pain, guarding, rebound tenderness, hypotension, lap-belt ecchymosis (seat belt sign)
- American Association for the Surgery of Trauma grading scale not predictive of need for surgery or outcome
- Nonoperative management of hemodynamically stable patients > 90% successful

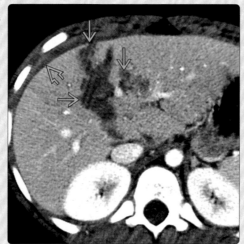
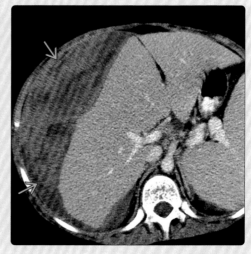

(Left) *Axial CECT in an 11 year old who sustained a handlebar injury to the upper abdomen demonstrates a jagged hypodense laceration ➡ > 3 cm in depth, consistent with a grade III injury. The laceration extends into both the right & left hepatic lobes. A small subcapsular hematoma ➡ is also present.* (Right) *Axial CECT in a 12-year-old boy 1 day after liver biopsy shows a mixed attenuation, > 50% surface area subcapsular hematoma ➡, consistent with a grade III injury. Higher density in the hematoma represents clot.*

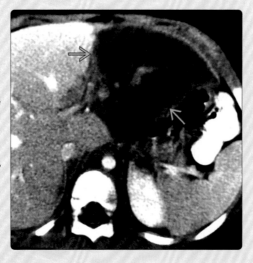
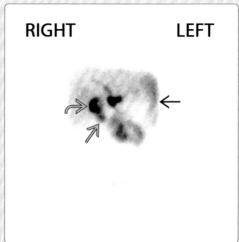

(Left) *Axial CECT shows a large, wedge-shaped, low-density region of the left hepatic lobe ➡, consistent with devascularization or infarction in this patient with trauma.* (Right) *Anterior hepatobiliary scintigraphy in a child after trauma shows accumulation of the radiotracer inferior ➡ to the gallbladder ➡. The radiotracer also collects in the left lateral peritoneum ➡, consistent with a biliary leak.*

RIGHT   LEFT

Splenic Trauma

IMAGING

- CECT: Gold standard for blunt abdominal trauma (accuracy 98%, sensitivity 95%)
  - FAST ultrasound exam: 37-85% sensitivity
- Laceration: Irregular, linear, branching foci of fluid density
- Hematoma: Intraperitoneal, retroperitoneal, subcapsular, &/or intraparenchymal collection(s)
  - Fluid attenuation if fresh, unclotted blood; higher attenuation suggests clotted blood, may implicate site of injury by proximity (sentinel clot)
- Active extravasation: Irregular, nonanatomic focus of ↑ density (isodense to adjacent artery); accumulates on delayed images

PATHOLOGY

- Typical etiologies: Blunt trauma from motor vehicle or bicycle accident, fall, sports, child abuse
- Preexisting splenic enlargement (EBV, hematologic disorders) predisposes to injury

- Associated injuries: Left lower rib fractures, other viscera

CLINICAL ISSUES

- Presentations: LUQ pain & tenderness, hypotension
  - Kehr sign: Pain radiating to left shoulder, phrenic nerve
  - Not clinically apparent (10-20%)
- Treatment: Nonoperative management of isolated blunt splenic injury in stable patients: > 95% success rate
  - American Association for Surgery of Trauma grading scale not predictive of outcomes in pediatrics
    - Injury grade assists with management decisions
- Complications: Pseudocyst, pseudoaneurysm, arteriovenous fistula, delayed rupture (hemorrhage > 48 hours after trauma), venous thrombosis, abscess
  - Routine follow-up CECT does not change outcome or management of asymptomatic patients
- Functional asplenia requires vaccinations (pneumococcal, *Haemophilus influenzae* type b, meningococcal, influenza) + prophylactic antibiotics (if < 5 years old)

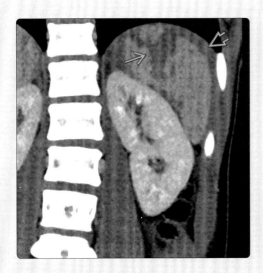
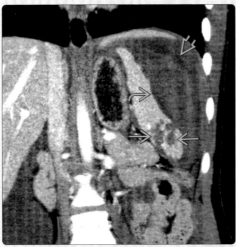

(Left) Coronal CECT in a 14-year-old boy injured while skiing shows a grade III splenic injury. Branching linear hypodensities > 3 cm in depth ➡ that extend to the splenic capsule are consistent with lacerations. A small perisplenic hematoma ➡ is also seen. (Right) Coronal CECT in a patient injured while playing basketball shows a grade III splenic injury with lacerations > 3 cm in depth ➡. A subcapsular hematoma > 50% of the splenic surface area ➡ scallops the splenic margin ➡.

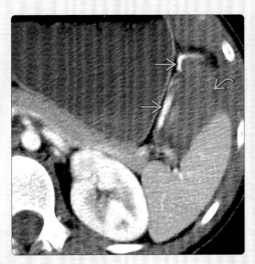
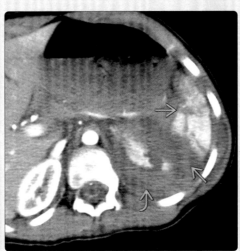

(Left) Axial CECT in a patient with hemophilia & abdominal pain status post fall shows an irregular, nonanatomic collection of dense contrast ➡ tracking medial to a perisplenic hematoma ➡, consistent with active hemorrhage. (Right) Axial CECT shows a fractured spleen ➡ with a perisplenic hematoma ➡.

KEY FACTS

IMAGING

- CECT best imaging tool in acute trauma setting
  - Oral contrast does not significantly improve sensitivity for duodenal injury → delay in imaging & treatment
- Injuries generally classified as hematoma vs. laceration
  - Hematoma: Nonenhancing intraluminal, intramural, &/or paraduodenal collection of ↑ attenuation
  - Duodenal laceration/perforation
    - Interruption of bowel wall, extravasation of intraluminal contents, & free retroperitoneal air: Specific but not sensitive
    - Duodenal wall thickening & ↑ attenuation fluid + stranding in retroperitoneum: Sensitive but not specific
- Associated injuries: Pancreas 42%, liver 29%, spleen 17%
- In cases with persistent clinical symptoms, consider follow-up with ultrasound or UGI every 7 days

PATHOLOGY

- Blunt trauma > 70%, penetrating trauma 20%
  - Motor vehicle collision, fall, handlebar injury, assault
  - Consider nonaccidental trauma in young patients (particularly < 2 years old with delayed presentation)
- Also consider with bleeding disorders, anticoagulation, Henoch-Schönlein purpura, recent endoscopic procedures

CLINICAL ISSUES

- Common symptoms: Abdominal pain, nausea, vomiting
- Overall morbidity 48%, mortality 19%; mortality most commonly due to associated traumatic brain injuries
- Treatment
  - Intramural/intraluminal hematoma: Initial management nonoperative (bowel rest, total parenteral nutrition, nasogastric decompression); drainage in refractory cases
  - Perforation: Primary surgical repair & drainage vs. more complex procedures in severe cases
- Stricture may rarely occur as long-term complication

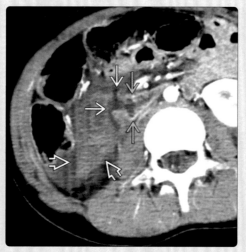

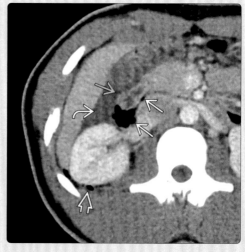

(Left) Axial CECT shows focal disruption ⮕ of the enhancing duodenal wall ⮕ with an adjacent hematoma ⮕. This is a specific but rarely seen finding of traumatic duodenal perforation. (Right) Axial CECT from a 17-year-old boy with abdominal pain, vomiting, & leukocytosis after being kicked shows retroperitoneal air ⮕ posterior to the 2nd & 3rd portions of the duodenum (D2 & D3) ⮕ & posterior to the right kidney ⮕. Adjacent fluid is also noted ⮕. A duodenal laceration was found at surgery.

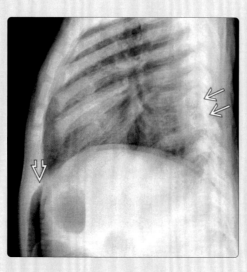

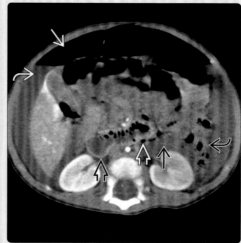

(Left) Cross-table lateral view of the chest in a 9-month-old boy, a victim of nonaccidental trauma, shows free intraperitoneal air ⮕. Healing posterior rib fractures are also present ⮕. (Right) Axial CECT from the same patient shows free intra- ⮕ & retroperitoneal ⮕ air as well as intra- ⮕ & retroperitoneal ⮕ fluid. Mucosal hyperenhancement ⮕ & small bowel wall thickening ⮕ are also noted. Perforations of the duodenum & jejunum were repaired surgically.

Bowel Injury

IMAGING

- Best modality: CECT
- Best clues (but uncommon): Bowel wall discontinuity + extraluminal enteric contents + free intraperitoneal air
- Nonspecific signs: Bowel wall thickening, abnormal bowel wall enhancement, mesenteric fluid/stranding
- Sentinel clot sign: Localized mesenteric hematoma adjacent to bowel (> 70 HU)
- In acute blunt trauma setting, oral contrast does not significantly improve sensitivity & may result in inappropriate delay of diagnosis & treatment

TOP DIFFERENTIAL DIAGNOSES

- Hypoperfusion complex (shock bowel)
- Henoch-Schönlein purpura

PATHOLOGY

- Blunt trauma 77%: Motor vehicle-related, nonaccidental trauma, & bicycle-related most common
  - Associated injuries: Brain (22%), liver (16%), spleen (11%), pancreas (10%), spine (including Chance fracture) (9%), kidney (6%)
- Penetrating trauma 23%
  - With rectal involvement → consider sexual assault

CLINICAL ISSUES

- Signs & symptoms
  - Abdominal pain, peritoneal signs, tachycardia, ↑ WBC
  - Bowel injury in 11% of patients with seat belt sign: Relative risk of 9.4
  - Delayed presentation of symptoms > 24 hours in 6.5%
  - Can be complicated by sepsis, peritonitis, abscess, stenosis/obstruction
- Overall mortality 5%, usually related to associated injuries
- Treatment
  - Perforations: Surgical management
  - Contusion/hematoma: Typically nonoperative
    - Clinical deterioration main indicator for surgery

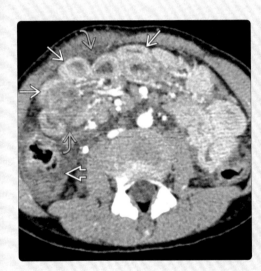
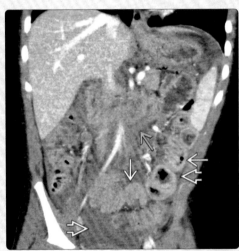

(Left) Axial CECT in a 7 year old shows diffuse small bowel wall thickening ➡, mesenteric hematoma ➡, & right paracolic gutter fluid of increased density ➡. Small bowel devascularization & perforation of the distal ileum were found at surgery. (Right) Coronal CECT in a 2-year-old victim of nonaccidental trauma shows thickened bowel loops, regions of increased ➡ & decreased ➡ bowel wall enhancement, & extensive free fluid ➡. Devascularized jejunum was found at surgery.

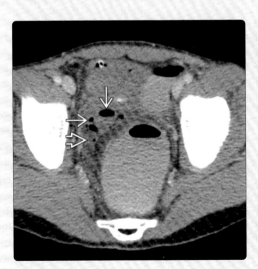
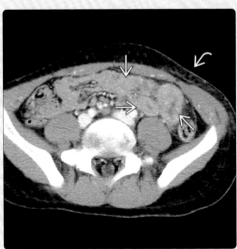

(Left) Axial CECT with rectal contrast in an 11-year-old boy whose rectum was impaled on a metal stake shows gas ➡ & fat stranding ➡ in the perirectal tissues. Extraperitoneal perforation of the rectum was demonstrated at surgery. (Right) Axial CECT in a 12-year-old motor vehicle accident victim shows thick-walled small bowel ➡ in the left abdomen. There is edema of the overlying subcutaneous fat with skin thickening ➡, typical of the seat belt sign. Jejunal perforations were found at surgery.

Pancreatic Trauma

IMAGING

- Modality of choice: CECT
  - Caveat: 20-40% false-negative rate in first 12 hours
- Classic imaging findings
  - Contusion/inflammation: Focal or diffuse ↓ enhancement & ↑ size relative to normal parenchyma
  - Laceration: Linear fluid-attenuation parenchymal defect
    - Usually of short axis; most common at junctions of pancreatic head-neck or body-tail
    - Depth > 50% suggests pancreatic duct disruption
  - Hematoma: Irregular or round fluid collection in/around pancreas; ↑ attenuation if clotted
  - Varying degrees of peripancreatic fluid tracking along/within fascial planes & adjacent compartments
- MRCP or ERCP to assess main pancreatic duct injury

PATHOLOGY

- Mechanisms: Blunt trauma: 93%; penetrating trauma: 7%
- Pancreatic injury in 17% of nonaccidental trauma patients

CLINICAL ISSUES

- Classic triad: Epigastric pain out of proportion to physical findings, ↑ serum amylase (may be normal initially), leukocytosis
- Isolated injuries rare (< 30%); average of 3-4 coexisting injuries per patient
- Management of American Association for Surgery of Trauma grading scale
  - I & II: Typically nonoperative (total parenteral nutrition ± octreotide infusion, percutaneous/endoscopic collection drainage, endoscopic duct stenting)
    - Failure more likely with pancreatic duct injury
  - III-V: No consensus on management strategy
    - Nonoperative: 43% failure rate; ↑ risk of pseudocysts, ERCP failure, & post-ERCP pancreatitis
    - Operative (surgical drainage, partial/distal pancreatectomy): Shorter time to resolution; ↑ rates of fistula formation & leak

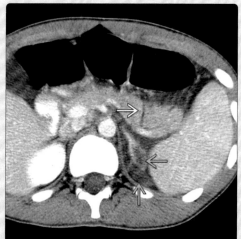
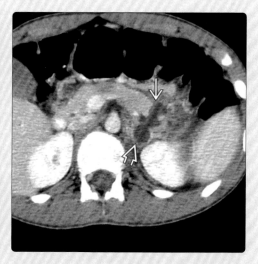

(Left) Axial CECT in a 14 year old who sustained an elbow injury to the abdomen shows a linear, fluid-density laceration ➡ through the pancreatic body near the tail. A left adrenal hematoma ➡ was also noted. (Right) Axial CECT in the same teenager 6 days later shows a pancreatic tail fluid collection ➡ extending into the anterior pararenal space ➡. The patient was treated conservatively. A follow-up US 1 month after the initial injury demonstrated resolution.

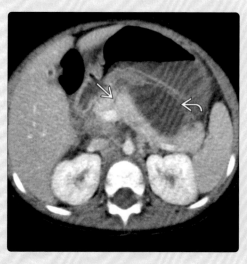
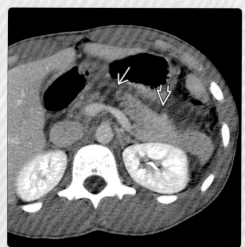

(Left) Axial CECT in a 2-year-old nonaccidental trauma victim with elevated serum amylase shows a laceration at the pancreatic neck-body junction ➡. The > 50% depth of the laceration is concerning for duct injury. A large pancreatic bed fluid collection is seen anteriorly ➡. (Right) Axial CECT in a 15-year-old boy with a football injury shows a grade III laceration involving the neck & body of the pancreas ➡. Poorly defined fluid is seen in the peripancreatic tissues ➡.

Pseudomembranous Colitis

TERMINOLOGY

- Colonic inflammation due to *Clostridium difficile* & its toxins A & B → epithelial necrosis & pseudomembranes

IMAGING

- Classic appearance: Pancolitis with marked wall thickening
- Radiographs
  - "Thumbprinting" ± colonic or small bowel ileus
  - Paucity of colonic gas with luminal narrowing
- CECT
  - Accordion sign: Alternating bands of ↑ & ↓ attenuation of colon due to oral contrast interdigitating between edematous haustra
    - Lumen appears stellate in cross section
  - Target sign: Rings of hyperenhancing mucosa & lower attenuation submucosal/muscular edema
  - Pericolonic stranding usually very mild, ± ascites
- Ultrasound
  - Accordion sign: Echogenic bowel contents between hypoechoic thickened wall; ± ascites
  - Pseudomembranes: Linear hyperechogenicity

PATHOLOGY

- Inflamed colon with discrete or confluent, raised, yellow-white plaque pseudomembranes on endoscopy
- Asymptomatic colonization with *C difficile* common in infants

CLINICAL ISSUES

- Most common symptoms: Watery or bloody diarrhea, dehydration, abdominal pain, leukocytosis, fever
- Primary treatments include: Cessation of inciting antibiotic with addition of metronidazole or vancomycin
- If treated early, full recovery expected
  - 20% recurrence rate despite appropriate therapy
- 3% progress to toxic megacolon; mortality: 38-80%
  - Surgery for severe disease from toxic megacolon or perforation, or if rapidly progressing or refractory

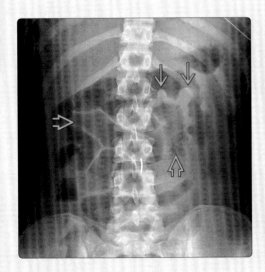

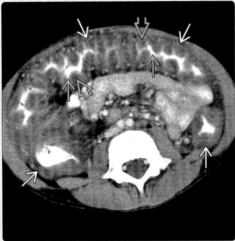

(Left) Supine abdominal radiograph in a 15 year old with known pseudomembranous colitis (PMC) demonstrates "thumbprinting" along the colon due to haustral thickening ➡. A small bowel ileus is also present ➡. (Right) Axial CECT in a 10-year-old child with fever, abdominal pain, & diarrhea demonstrates findings of PMC with pancolonic marked wall thickening ➡. The alternating bands of hyperdense contrast ➡ between the thickened fluid-density haustra ➡ create the accordion sign.

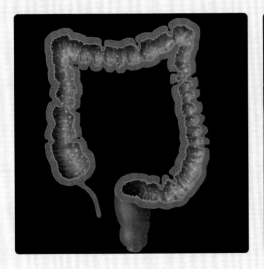

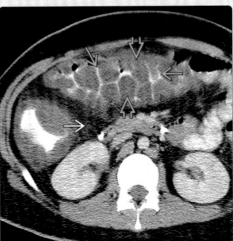

(Left) Graphic of PMC shows pancolitis with marked mural thickening & numerous elevated yellow-white plaques (pseudomembranes). (Right) Axial CECT shows marked pancolitis with enteric contrast ➡ trapped between thickened haustral folds ➡ (the accordion sign). Note the minimal pericolonic fat infiltration ➡, which is typical with PMC.

Crohn Disease

TERMINOLOGY

- Chronic, recurrent, segmental, granulomatous inflammatory bowel disease; etiology unknown

IMAGING

- Small bowel follow-through: Separated/isolated segment of narrowed bowel with irregular mucosa
- US: Thickened bowel wall with loss of gut signature, ↑ perienteric fat echogenicity, ± bowel wall & perienteric hyperemia
- CT/MR enterography
  - Bowel findings: Mucosal hyperenhancement & bowel wall thickening (most sensitive findings), strictures showing upstream effects (dilation & small bowel feces sign), ulcers/fistulas/sinus tracts
  - Mesenteric findings: Engorged vasa recta, fat stranding, fibrofatty proliferation, phlegmon/abscesses
  - Perianal disease: Fistula tract/abscess extending from anus/skin

PATHOLOGY

- Skip lesions of transmural inflammation occur anywhere from mouth to anus: Ileocolic most common

CLINICAL ISSUES

- Annual incidence: 3-15/100,000
- 25% of patients diagnosed in first 2 decades of life
- Children: Pain, diarrhea, & weight loss (presenting feature in 85%)
- Complications
  - Stricturing/penetrating: Fissures, sinus tracts, fistulas, & abscesses, obstruction (20%), perforation (1-2%)
  - Extraintestinal manifestations in up to 30%: Cholelithiasis, sclerosing cholangitis, arthritis, urolithiasis
- Therapies: Bowel rest, steroids, azathioprine, mesalamine, metronidazole, biologic agents (Infliximab); resection of diseased bowel, strictureplasty, & primary fistulotomy
- Recurrence: 30-53% after resection; only 10-20% lead symptom-free lives

(Left) Delayed image from a small bowel follow-through in a patient with Crohn disease shows isolation, narrowing, & irregularity of the terminal ileum ➡ & cecum ➡. It can be inferred that the separated loops are caused by bowel wall thickening & "creeping fat." (Right) Longitudinal ultrasound of the right lower quadrant shows an abnormal segment of bowel ➡ with wall thickening & surrounding echogenic mesenteric fat ➡. Ultrasound may be the 1st modality to suggest Crohn disease in patients being worked up for appendicitis.

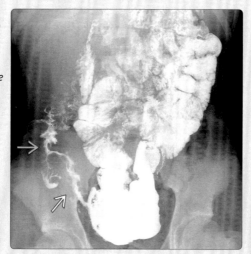

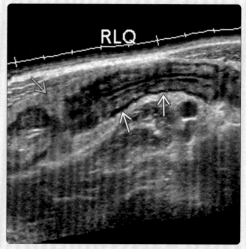

(Left) Coronal T1 C+ FS MR enterography in an adolescent with Crohn disease shows mucosal hyperenhancement & wall thickening of the ileum ➡ & cecum ➡. (Right) Coronal CECT of the abdomen in a patient with Crohn disease shows an abnormal appearance of the terminal ileum ➡ with mucosal hyperenhancement, mild mural stratification, & sacculations. There is a stricture ➡ of the distal-most portion of the terminal ileum with upstream dilation & small bowel feces ➡.

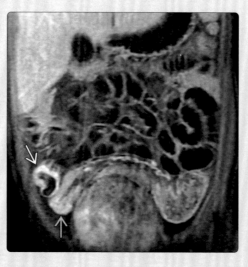

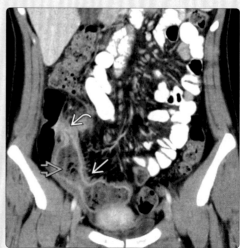

Ulcerative Colitis

KEY FACTS

TERMINOLOGY

- Chronic, idiopathic, diffuse inflammatory disease that primarily involves colorectal mucosa & submucosa
  - Extends retrograde from rectum
  - No skip lesions or transmural involvement

IMAGING

- CT/MR enterography findings
  - Continuous colonic inflammation extending proximally from rectum for variable distance
  - Mucosal hyperenhancement & wall thickening
  - Thickened, edematous haustra (thumbprinting)
  - Luminal narrowing
  - In later disease, dilation or narrowing of colon with loss of haustra

TOP DIFFERENTIAL DIAGNOSES

- Crohn disease
- Pseudomembranous colitis
- Infectious colitis

CLINICAL ISSUES

- Majority of patients diagnosed in 4th-5th decades
  - More common than Crohn disease in preschool age
- Annual incidence: 5-10 cases/100,000 population
- Most common presenting symptom: Bloody diarrhea
  - Anemia, poor growth, perianal symptoms
  - Extraintestinal: Arthralgias, primary sclerosing cholangitis, uveitis
    - Occur in 16-30% of patients
    - ↑ likelihood of colectomy
- Complications
  - Toxic megacolon: 5-10%
  - Stricture: 10%
  - Colorectal cancer risk: ↑ 30x
- Treatment: Sulfasalazine, steroids, azathioprine, methotrexate, LTB4 inhibitors, total colectomy

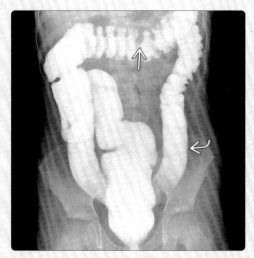

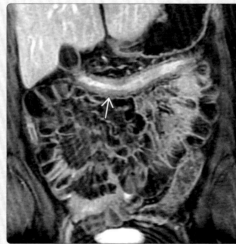

(Left) Supine radiograph from a contrast enema in an adolescent with ulcerative colitis (UC) shows thickening of haustral markings ➡ (thumbprinting) in the transverse colon but loss of haustral markings ➡ in the descending colon. (Right) Coronal T1 C+ FS MR enterography in an adolescent with UC shows diffuse wall thickening ➡ & mucosal hyperenhancement of the transverse colon. The transverse colonic lumen is narrowed without visible haustral markings.

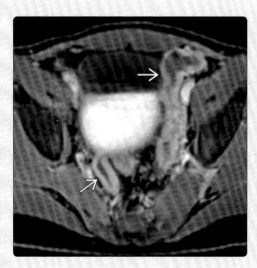

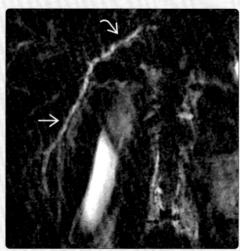

(Left) Axial T1 C+ FS MR of the pelvis in an adolescent with UC shows diffuse wall thickening & enhancement ➡ of the sigmoid colon. (Right) Coronal MRCP of an adolescent with UC shows diffuse irregularity of the right ➡ & left ➡ hepatic ducts. The findings are typical of primary sclerosing cholangitis (PSC). Patients with UC & PSC usually have more extensive colonic disease.

KEY FACTS

TERMINOLOGY

- Acquired narrowing of esophagus, caused by variety of entities; congenital stenosis considered here as well

IMAGING

- Focal or diffuse narrowing of esophagus, associated with proximal dilation & altered peristalsis
- Particular segment affected, as well as length & degree of narrowing, depend on etiology & severity of initial esophageal injury
- Different causes of stricture have different imaging characteristics
- Esophagram findings
  - Esophageal atresia repair: Focal stricture at junction of upper & middle 1/3
  - Peptic stricture: Stricture in distal esophagus
  - Eosinophilic esophagitis: Most commonly normal
  - Caustic strictures: Most common in proximal & mid esophagus

- Multiple strictures can occur
  - Epidermolysis bullosa: Stricture most common in cervical esophagus
  - Infective esophagitis: May progress to strictures
  - Congenital stenosis
    - Membranous web: Upper or middle 1/3
    - Fibromuscular thickening: Middle or distal 1/3
    - Tracheobronchial cartilage remnant/foregut malformation: Distal 1/3

CLINICAL ISSUES

- Infants present with feeding difficulties; food bolus impaction in older children with drooling, vomiting, pain, sensation of food getting stuck
  - ± airway symptoms (e.g., wheezing, recurrent coughing)
- Systemic diseases (such as scleroderma, dermatomyositis, epidermolysis bullosa) have multiorgan involvement
- Balloon dilation used for many conditions; stricture resection or esophageal replacement for refractory cases

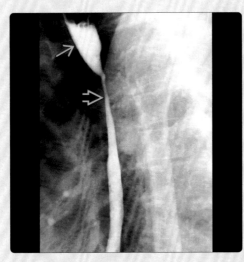

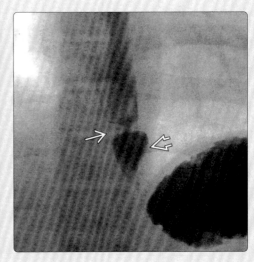

(Left) Lateral esophagram shows distention of the proximal esophagus ➡ with tapering to a long segment of narrowing ⇨ secondary to epidermolysis bullosa in an adolescent child. (Right) Frontal upper GI in an adolescent shows a small hiatal hernia ⇒ with circumferential narrowing ➡ at the gastroesophageal (GE) junction. Rings at the GE junction are termed Schatzki or B rings & are fixed areas of narrowing.

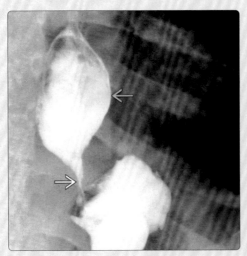

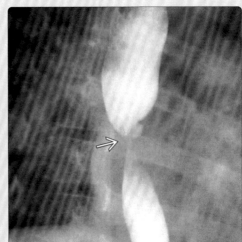

(Left) Oblique esophagram shows dilation of the distal esophagus ➡ with narrowing ➡ at the surgical site of a Nissen fundoplication. This Nissen was too tight & required balloon dilation. (Right) Oblique image from an upper GI series in an adolescent with eosinophilic esophagitis shows a stricture ➡ in the distal esophagus.

Bezoar

KEY FACTS

TERMINOLOGY

- Specific ingested materials accumulate to form indigestible & potentially obstructive mass in GI tract
  - Trichobezoar (hair), lactobezoar (milk & mucous), phytobezoar (indigestible food, typically in adults)

IMAGING

- Radiographs: Round/ovoid/tubular mass with mottled appearance of air in interstices causing distention of affected lumen ± obstruction
  - Rarely diagnosed on radiographs alone
- Upper GI: Filling defect with contrast in interstices; mucosal injuries may be identified
  - Ideally performed after fasting; dynamic study allows evaluation of intraluminal mass mobility
- US: Echogenic arc-like surface & posterior shadowing
  - Low sensitivity for multiple bezoars & gastric bezoars
- CECT: Concentric architecture + air/contrast in mass
  - Up to 97% sensitivity as entire abdomen evaluated

TOP DIFFERENTIAL DIAGNOSES

- Ingested food
- Neoplasm

CLINICAL ISSUES

- Presentation: Palpable abdominal mass, abdominal pain, vomiting, distention, dysphagia, bowel obstruction
- Lamerton sign: Mobile, palpable, & indentable mass in upper abdomen
- Trichobezoar: Children with trichotillomania/trichophagia
  - Treatment: Removal by laparotomy + therapy referral
- Lactobezoar: Premature neonate with dehydration, diarrhea, respiratory distress, weight loss/failure to thrive, feeding intolerance
  - Treatment: NPO, IV fluids, ↓ caloric intake ± gastric lavage & saline dissolution; surgery if necessary
- Complications: Obstruction, mucosal erosion/ulceration, GI bleeding, perforation

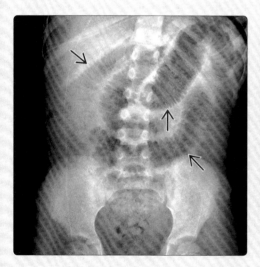

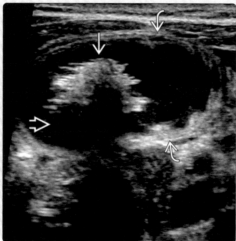

(Left) Frontal supine abdominal radiograph of a 7-year-old girl with pain, emesis, & alopecia shows multiple loops of dilated small bowel ⊒, concerning for a small bowel obstruction. Note the mottled lucencies throughout the dilated loops. (Right) Longitudinal grayscale US from the same patient shows a mass impacted in the distal ileum. The surrounding bowel is dilated & fluid-filled ⊒. The mass has a broad, echogenic, arc-like surface ⊒ with dense posterior acoustic shadowing ⊐. A trichobezoar was removed at surgery.

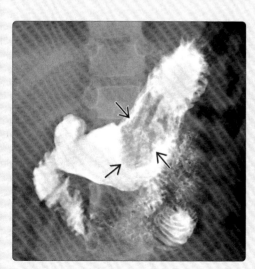

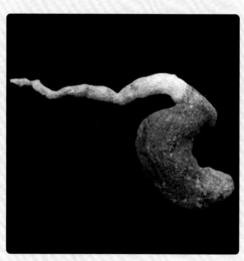

(Left) Frontal image from an upper GI series in a 6-year-old girl with trichotillomania complaining of pain & emesis shows a mobile ovoid filling defect ⊒ with air & barium in its interstices, consistent with a trichobezoar. (Right) Intraoperative photograph from a teenager shows a large trichobezoar that completely filled the stomach & extended through the duodenum to the proximal jejunum.

Gastrointestinal Duplication Cysts

TERMINOLOGY

- GI duplication cysts have 3 defining characteristics
  - Well-developed coat of smooth muscle
  - Epithelial lining representing some part of GI tract
  - Attachment to (± communication with) GI tract
    - Rarely: Isolated cyst with no persistent attachment

IMAGING

- Cystic (80-90%) vs. tubular (10-20%) lesions with well-defined wall
  - Can occur anywhere along GI tract; most frequently associated with jejunum/ileum (53%) & esophagus (18%)
- Contiguous (but not necessarily communicating) with adjacent GI tract
- Ultrasound best modality to visualize key features, though findings with highest specificity have lowest sensitivity
  - Gut signature: Trilaminar appearance of wall; less specific than 5-layered wall

- Y sign: Hypoechoic muscularis propria divided at point of attachment between cyst & adjacent bowel
- Peristalsis of cyst wall pathognomonic (when visualized)

TOP DIFFERENTIAL DIAGNOSES

- Mesenteric lymphatic malformation, ovarian cyst, choledochal cyst, urachal cyst, Meckel diverticulum

CLINICAL ISSUES

- Congenital lesions, most often presenting < 2 years of age
  - Pain, mass, rectal bleeding; may be incidental or detected on prenatal sonography
  - Small bowel obstruction or intussusception most frequent presentation for ileal duplications
  - Complications include ulceration, perforation, hemorrhage, volvulus, intussusception
- Complete surgical resection ideal
- Very good prognosis overall

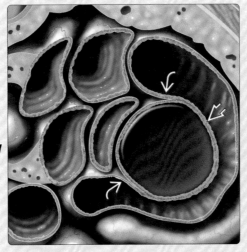

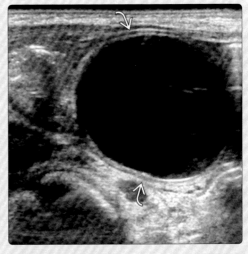

(Left) *Axial graphic shows an enteric duplication cyst* ⤳ *between sectioned bowel loops. Note that the muscular layer of the bowel is continuous with that of the duplication cyst, creating a Y* ⤳ *as the muscle splits.* (Right) *Transverse ultrasound shows a right lower quadrant duplication cyst with a characteristic gut signature* ⤳ *(i.e., echogenic inner mucosal layer, hypoechoic muscular layer, & echogenic outer serosal layer).*

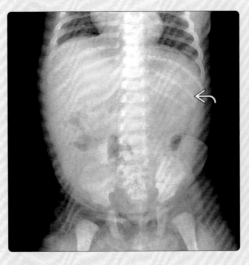

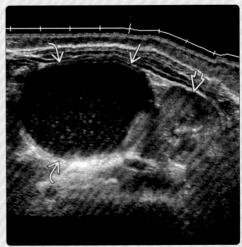

(Left) *AP radiograph in a 5 month old with a palpable mass in the abdominal left upper quadrant shows displacement of gas in the region of concern* ⤳ *that prompted an ultrasound.* (Right) *Transverse panoramic ultrasound in the same patient shows a cystic mass* ⤳ *with internal debris adjacent to the spleen & left kidney* ⤳. *The cyst wall shows alternating layers of echogenicity* ⤳, *typical of gut signature (but not 100% specific for bowel wall). A GI duplication cyst was confirmed at surgery.*

Small Bowel Intussusception

KEY FACTS

TERMINOLOGY

- Telescoping of proximal small bowel segment (intussusceptum) into contiguous distal small bowel segment (intussuscipiens)

IMAGING

- Bowel-within-bowel appearance: Alternating layers of bowel wall & mesenteric fat
  - Target appearance in cross section on CT & US
- Small bowel intussusception (SBI) features that differentiate it from ileocolic intussusception
  - Smaller diameter (mean of 1.5 vs. 2.6 cm)
  - Entrapped lymph nodes less common
  - More common in periumbilical or left abdomen
- Sonographic findings that may indicate need for surgery
  - Length > 3.5 cm
  - Findings of small bowel obstruction (SBO) & ascites
  - Pathologic lead point (but US has low sensitivity)

PATHOLOGY

- Lead points (uncommon): Lymphoid hyperplasia, Meckel diverticulum, duplication cyst, adhesions, polyps, intramural hematoma, foreign body, enteric tubes
- Associated pathology: Henoch-Schönlein purpura, malabsorption syndromes (celiac), cystic fibrosis

CLINICAL ISSUES

- Majority self-limited & spontaneously reduce
- 65% asymptomatic in 1 study; less commonly with abdominal pain, distension, vomiting, blood in stool
- Complications more likely if presentation/diagnosis delayed: SBO, ischemia, necrosis
- If patient asymptomatic without concerning imaging features → conservative management (often spontaneously reduces during study)
- If patient symptomatic or imaging features concerning → surgical consult ± CECT/follow-up US
- Postoperative SBI typically surgically reduced

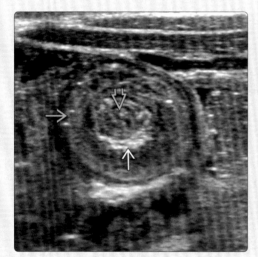

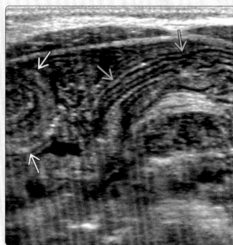

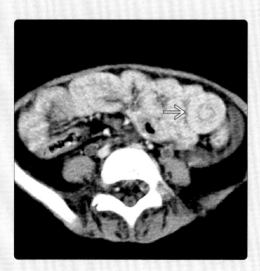

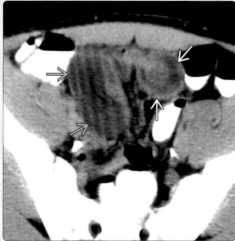

(Left) Periumbilical US from a 14 month old with pain & vomiting shows a cross section of bowel having a target appearance consistent with an intussusception. A crescent of hyperechoic mesenteric fat ➡ is interposed between the intussuscipiens ⊡ & intussusceptum ⊡. The location & diameter are typical of a small bowel intussusception (SBI). (Right) US from the same patient demonstrates an SBI > 3 cm in length in both the longitudinal ⊡ & axial ➡ planes.

(Left) Axial CECT in a child with pancreatitis shows an incidental left lower quadrant SBI ➡. Note the presence of dense oral contrast in the SBI & adjacent loops. Most SBIs are asymptomatic, of short length, & resolve without intervention. (Right) Axial CECT shows a long (> 3.5 cm length) SBI in both axial ➡ & longitudinal ⊡ planes. No oral contrast is seen in the obstructed segment. An underlying large Meckel diverticulum was found at surgery.

Henoch-Schönlein Purpura

TERMINOLOGY

- Immune complex-mediated small vessel vasculitis commonly affecting skin, GI tract, urologic system, joints

IMAGING

- GI features (up to 75%)
  - Circumferential bowel wall thickening of discontinuous segments of variable lengths
    - "Thumbprinting" on radiographs
    - Due to intramural hemorrhage &/or edema
  - Intussusception, commonly ileoileal
- Urologic features (up to 60%)
  - Henoch-Schönlein purpura (HSP) nephritis
    - Normal or bilaterally enlarged & echogenic kidneys
  - Stenosing ureteritis
    - Hydroureteronephrosis & thick urothelium
  - Scrotal wall thickening, edema, & hyperemia
- Arthritis (up to 82%)
- Neurologic features (up to 2%)

- Cerebral edema, intracranial hemorrhage, cerebral vein thrombosis, posterior reversible encephalopathy syndrome
- Pulmonary features (up to 5%)
  - Diffuse alveolar hemorrhage (DAH)
    - Alveolar infiltrates & ground-glass opacities
    - Pleural effusions, often large & requiring chest tube

CLINICAL ISSUES

- Most common primary pediatric vasculitis at 49%
- Purpura or petechiae ultimately in 100%
- Peak age: 7 years
- Typically self-limited, resolves in 3-4 weeks
  - Treatment largely conservative & directed to specific systems involved
  - Recurrence in up to 1/3 of cases
  - HSP nephritis: 20% develop nephritic/nephrotic syndrome
  - DAH: Up to 28% mortality

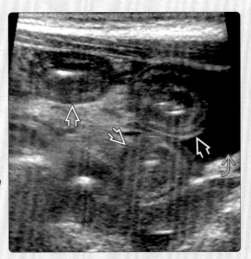
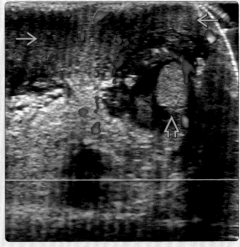

(Left) Transverse US through the right lower quadrant in an 8 year old with Henoch-Schönlein purpura (HSP) demonstrates multiple thick-walled loops of small bowel ⮕ & a small amount of free fluid ⮕. (Right) Transverse color Doppler US of the scrotum shows marked thickening, edema, & hyperemia of the scrotal wall ⮕ in a 6 year old with HSP. A normal left testicle is also seen ⮕.

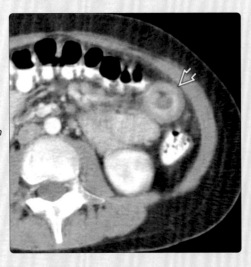
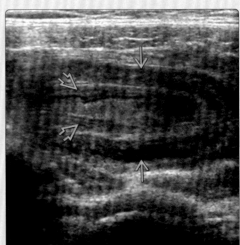

(Left) Axial CECT in a 9 year old with HSP, vomiting, & abdominal pain demonstrates a thick-walled loop of the small bowel ⮕ with mucosal hyperenhancement & mild surrounding mesenteric inflammation. (Right) Longitudinal US from a 4 year old with HSP & abdominal pain shows a small bowel intussusception with well-delineated intussuscipiens ⮕ & intussusceptum ⮕. This intussusception was > 5 cm long & required surgical reduction.

Cystic Fibrosis, Gastrointestinal Tract

TERMINOLOGY

- Cystic fibrosis (CF): Autosomal recessive multisystem disorder caused by dysfunctional chloride ion transport across epithelial surfaces

IMAGING

- Pancreas: Abdominal organ most commonly involved in CF
  - Pancreatic insufficiency: Present in > 70% of patients with CF at initial diagnosis
  - Pancreatitis: Can be acute or chronic
- Intestinal
  - Gastroesophageal reflux disease: Prevalence 6-8x higher than general population
  - Meconium ileus: Congenital bowel obstruction caused by tenacious meconium occluding terminal ileum
  - Distal intestinal obstruction syndrome: Meconium ileus equivalent in older children
  - Constipation: Excess stool throughout colon
  - Intussusception: 10x higher than general population

- Appendix: Enlarged without inflammation
  - Appendicitis rates actually lower in CF patients
- Hepatobiliary: Most common cause of CF mortality after pulmonary complications
  - Hepatic fibrosis/cirrhosis: Occurs in 5-15% of children/adolescents with CF
  - Microgallbladder: Due to atresia/stenosis of cystic duct

PATHOLOGY

- CF most common lethal genetic defect in Caucasians
- > 1,500 genetic defects can result in CF; ΔF508 most common

CLINICAL ISSUES

- Most now detected on newborn screening
- Patients may not manifest until later in childhood
- Median survival: 41.1 years

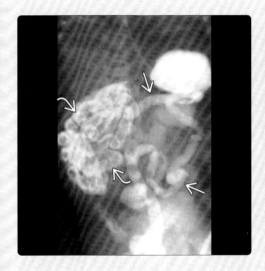

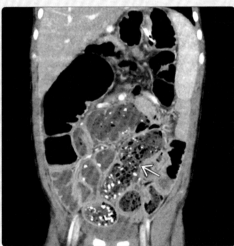

(Left) Neonatal contrast enema shows a microcolon ➡ typical of a congenital distal bowel obstruction. Contrast refluxes into the terminal ileum, outlining filling defects ⇨ of tenacious meconium. Meconium ileus is almost always due to cystic fibrosis (CF). (Right) Coronal CECT in the same patient 9 years later shows stool ➡ in the ileum. The proximal small bowel was dilated & fluid-filled (not shown). Distal intestinal obstruction syndrome occurs more commonly in CF patients that have a history of meconium ileus in infancy.

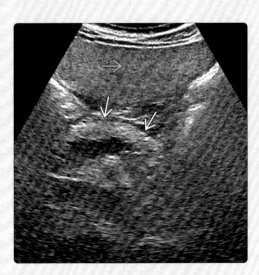

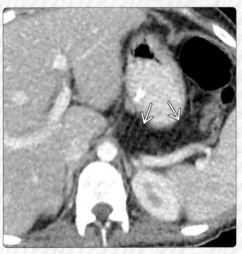

(Left) Ultrasound of the abdomen shows the pancreas ➡ to be hyperechoic & atrophied, typical of fatty replacement in this CF patient. There is also loss of the normal echogenic portal triads in the liver ➡, suggesting hepatic steatosis. (Right) Axial CECT in a child with CF shows fatty replacement ➡ of the pancreas. CF is the most common cause of pancreatic lipomatosis. Patients with CF can also get acute or chronic pancreatitis, though acute pancreatitis is more common in patients with normal pancreatic exocrine function.

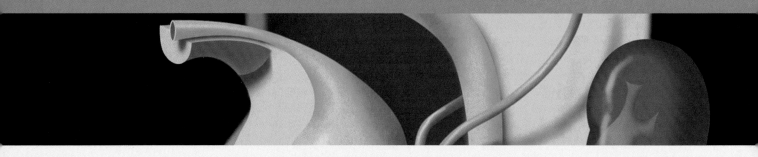

SECTION 5
Genitourinary

Introduction & Normals

Congenital Urinary Tract Abnormalities

Multicystic Renal Disease

Renal Masses

Miscellaneous Renal Conditions

Bladder Abnormalities

Adrenal Abnormalities

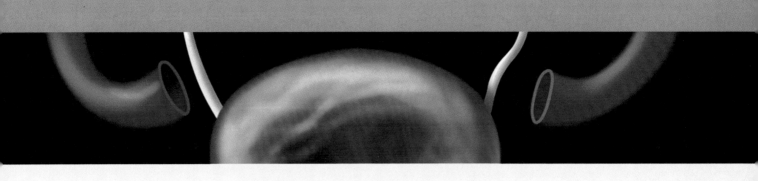

Uterine/Ovarian Abnormalities

Scrotal/Testicular Abnormalities

Genitourinary Tract Imaging Modalities

Radiographs

Plain radiographs are rarely utilized in the evaluation of the pediatric GU tract due to their low sensitivity for GU pathology. Associated pathologic calcifications may be incidentally detected, including urinary tract calculi, teratomas (which may resemble a tooth), & remote adrenal hemorrhages. Ultrasound is typically the next step in each of these scenarios.

Ultrasound

In most pediatric patients (except for those who are obese or have significant deformities of body habitus due to underlying spinal abnormalities), sonography provides excellent visualization of the kidneys, urinary bladder, & reproductive organs. Therefore, in conjunction with its ready availability, lack of ionizing radiation, & noninvasive nature, it generally serves as the study of choice for the initial investigation of suspected pediatric GU pathology.

Ultrasound excels at detecting hydronephrosis as well as renal parenchymal cysts & masses. However, its characterization of most medical diseases of the kidney is quite limited, rarely progressing beyond descriptions of increased echogenicity, abnormal intrarenal Doppler flow, or abnormal volume as nonspecific secondary indicators of renal disease. Stones are often sonographically detectable in the kidney, though tiny nonobstructing stones may be difficult to distinguish from vessels or fat.

The proximal & distal ureters may be visualized in the setting of dilation. However, most of the ureter will not be visualized due to overlying bowel gas. This can limit visualization of mid ureteral stones. With meticulous technique, stones lodged at the ureterovesical junction (UVJ) will often be visualized, even if they are nonobstructing. Ultrasound can also confirm the lack of ureteral obstruction by demonstrating urine passing intermittently through the UVJ into the urinary bladder (a.k.a. a ureteral jet).

Pediatricians should be aware of the limitations of ultrasound in working up urinary tract infections &/or vesicoureteral reflux (VUR). A core concern is that a normal sonographic appearance of the urinary tract does not exclude significant VUR. Additionally, some congenital anomalies that predispose to VUR (such as ureteral duplication) may be difficult to visualize in the absence of urinary tract dilation. Furthermore, ultrasound has limited sensitivity for detecting renal scarring compared to other modalities, which is particularly important to recognize as this finding drives the need for further imaging evaluation in some clinical protocols. In the acute setting, ultrasound also has limited sensitivity for the detection of uncomplicated pyelonephritis compared to CECT, MR, & nuclear medicine renal cortical scans.

Ultrasound does remain the best initial imaging choice for a palpable abdominal mass in a child. Even large masses can typically be localized to the organ of origin, & the imaging features (in conjunction with the patient age) often predict the type of tumor (though not the exact histology). Ultrasound may even visualize some types of local invasion (such as vascular involvement), though establishing the exact size & extent are critical to therapy planning & are best done with CECT (or preferably MR).

The urinary bladder is best visualized on ultrasound when it is well distended, allowing a noninvasive assessment of wall thickness & contour as well as volumes before & after voiding. However, obstructing lesions of the bladder outlet (e.g., posterior urethral valves, small masses, & rarely stones) may be poorly visualized unless attention is specifically directed to that region.

A well-distended urinary bladder also plays a critical role in the assessment of the female reproductive organs, providing a necessary acoustic window through which to visualize the uterus & ovaries. If adequate bladder distention is lacking in the acute setting, instillation of fluid via a Foley catheter may be required if oral &/or intravenous hydration do not quickly fill the bladder. In teenagers who are sexually active or undergoing routine manual pelvic exams, a transvaginal ultrasound probe can be used to assess the uterus & ovaries; this technique is most commonly employed for concerns of ovarian torsion or ectopic pregnancy & does not require bladder distention.

Ultrasound also serves as the primary modality for imaging the scrotum. The evaluation of scrotal masses (including hernias, hydroceles, varicoceles, cysts, & neoplasms) & scrotal pain (due to testicular torsion, appendix torsion, epididymoorchitis, or trauma) is essentially served entirely by sonography.

Doppler is a critical component of assessing pain localized to the male & female reproductive organs. It is particularly important for testicular assessment, where absent (or even asymmetric) blood flow is a key component of diagnosing testicular torsion. It is recognized, however, that Doppler findings are less accurate in detecting ovarian torsion, where a reliable diagnosis must be coupled with the grayscale ultrasound findings (particularly ovarian size) & the clinical assessment.

Renal Doppler is infrequently employed in children and is typically reserved for suspected renal hypertension where a treatable arterial stenosis is of concern. Such assessments can be quite limited in patients that are obese or are unable to hold still. Even in a technically adequate study, Doppler is not sensitive for isolated intrarenal arterial stenoses, though the best screening tool (CT or MR angiography, nuclear medicine, or conventional arteriogram) remains debated.

With the recent FDA approval of ultrasound contrast agents in the USA, ultrasound may find expanded utility in the evaluations of VUR, pyelonephritis, & trauma.

Fluoroscopy

VCUG has long been a mainstay in the evaluation of VUR, though it is less commonly ordered these days due to clinical algorithms favoring "top down" assessments of the GU tract. While the nuclear cystogram remains more sensitive for the detection of VUR, patients with suspected anatomic abnormalities (based on a preceding ultrasound) are typically referred for a fluoroscopic exam due to better definition of relevant anatomy. It should be noted that both studies do require catheterization of the urinary bladder & employ small amounts of ionizing radiation. Some centers will sedate patients for this study while others do not.

Intravenous pyelograms (IVPs) are now rarely used to assess the urinary tract (as other modalities generally provide superior anatomic & physiologic information). They may occasionally be ordered by urologists in patients with suspected ureteral obstructions due to strictures or known stone disease.

Specific types of trauma, particularly straddle injuries & motor vehicle collisions causing pelvic fractures, may require a retrograde urethrogram to look for urethral injury.

Computed Tomography
NECT is the most sensitive & specific test for the detection of urinary tract calculi & may reveal findings of associated obstruction. However, CECT typically does not preclude the visualization of significant stones & can be used when other diagnoses are being entertained (such as appendicitis), particularly if ultrasound is not able to adequately address these concerns (as may occur in the obese patient). CT should not be routinely ordered in a patient with known stone disease as the primary acute concern (i.e., new obstruction) can usually be assessed by ultrasound, even if the stone is not sonographically visible.

CECT remains the modality of choice when renal trauma is suspected, & the radiologist may obtain 10- to 15-minute delayed images of the urinary tract to look for urine extravasation if a renal injury is confirmed on the routine images. Dedicated bladder evaluation may also be performed after trauma if there is hematuria in the setting of pelvic fractures; this typically involves filling the bladder via a Foley catheter for a targeted scan after the initial trauma CT of the abdomen & pelvis has been performed.

CECT can be used to further characterize a newly detected renal, adrenal, or ovarian mass. Depending on the availability, MR is preferred for this assessment at some centers due to the lack of ionizing radiation & increased soft tissue contrast.

Magnetic Resonance
MR is rarely used to evaluate the urinary tract in the absence of known complex anomalies, in which case the urologist (typically after having obtained multiple other exams) may order an MR urogram. This test provides not only excellent anatomic visualization of the entire urinary tract but can provide physiologic information that has previously only been available with nuclear medicine studies. It is gaining interest as a "one stop" GU imaging exam though its optimal utilization is still being established.

Renal & adrenal masses are perhaps best characterized by MR, which also allows for excellent delineation of adenopathy & local spread (including tumor rupture & invasion of the spine, vasculature, or adjacent viscera). Bone metastases are also frequently detected on MR.

MR is quite useful for evaluating anomalies of the female genital tract, particularly congenital anomalies of the uterus that may be difficult to fully discern by ultrasound. It can also be used for further characterizing ovarian masses detected on ultrasound.

Nuclear Medicine
Nuclear studies have a variety of uses in evaluating pediatric urinary tract anomalies.

Most studies will require intravenous injection of a nuclear radiotracer that is then tracked by dedicated cameras through the anatomy of interest over time. Renal cortical scans (where radiotracer is taken up by the kidney but not excreted during the time of imaging) are highly sensitive for acute pyelonephritis & chronic scarring. Renograms (where radiotracer is taken up & excreted by the kidney during imaging) provide a variety of renal function assessments. Diuretic renograms in particular remain a critical exam for urologists planning treatment for chronic obstructions at the

ureteropelvic junction or UVJ levels as these exams follow the flow of radiotracer through the collecting systems, ureters, & bladder before & after a dose of Lasix.

Nuclear cystograms are more sensitive than fluoroscopic studies at detecting VUR but lack the anatomic detail. They may be used as a 1st-line study in some cases of suspected VUR but more frequently will be used to follow low-grade VUR once the lack of an underlying anatomic abnormality has been confirmed.

Selected References

1. ACR Appropriateness Criteria: Hematuria—Child. https://acsearch.acr.org/docs/69440/Narrative/. Published 1999. Reviewed 2012. Accessed March 11, 2017
2. ACR Appropriateness Criteria: Urinary Tract Infection—Child. https://acsearch.acr.org/docs/69444/Narrative/. Published 2016. Accessed March 11, 2017
3. Morrison JC et al: Use of ultrasound in pediatric renal stone diagnosis and surgery. Curr Urol Rep. 18(3):22, 2017
4. Mattoo TK et al: Renal scarring in the randomized intervention for children with vesicoureteral reflux (RIVUR) trial. Clin J Am Soc Nephrol. 11(1):54-61, 2016
5. Ramanathan S et al: Multi-modality imaging review of congenital abnormalities of kidney and upper urinary tract. World J Radiol. 8(2):132-41, 2016
6. Van Batavia JP et al: Clinical effectiveness in the diagnosis and acute management of pediatric nephrolithiasis. Int J Surg. 36(Pt D):698-704, 2016
7. Bush NC et al: Renal damage detected by DMSA, despite normal renal ultrasound, in children with febrile UTI. J Pediatr Urol. 11(3):126.e1-7, 2015
8. Chevalier RL: Congenital urinary tract obstruction: the long view. Adv Chronic Kidney Dis. 22(4):312-9, 2015
9. Dickerson EC et al: Pediatric MR urography: indications, techniques, and approach to review. Radiographics. 35(4):1208-30, 2015
10. Malkan AD et al: An approach to renal masses in pediatrics. Pediatrics. 135(1):142-58, 2015
11. Mattoo TK et al: The RIVUR trial: a factual interpretation of our data. Pediatr Nephrol. 30(5):707-12, 2015
12. Narchi H et al: Renal tract abnormalities missed in a historical cohort of young children with UTI if the NICE and AAP imaging guidelines were applied. J Pediatr Urol. 11(5):252.e1-7, 2015
13. Stein R et al: Urinary tract infections in children: EAU/ESPU guidelines. Eur Urol. 67(3):546-58, 2015
14. Botta S et al: To V(CUG) or not to V(CUG) in infants with prenatal hydronephrosis? J Urol. 192(3):640-1, 2014
15. Downs SM: UTI and watchful waiting: the courage to do nothing. Pediatrics. 133(3):535-6, 2014
16. Ristola MT et al: NICE guidelines cannot be recommended for imaging studies in children younger than 3 years with urinary tract infection. Eur J Pediatr Surg. ePub, 2014
17. RIVUR Trial Investigators et al: Antimicrobial prophylaxis for children with vesicoureteral reflux. N Engl J Med. 370(25):2367-76, 2014
18. Suson KD et al: Evaluation of children with urinary tract infection–impact of the 2011 AAP guidelines on the diagnosis of vesicoureteral reflux using a historical series. J Pediatr Urol. 10(1):182-5, 2014
19. La Scola C et al: Different guidelines for imaging after first UTI in febrile infants: yield, cost, and radiation. Pediatrics. 131(3):e665-71, 2013
20. Renkema KY et al: Novel perspectives for investigating congenital anomalies of the kidney and urinary tract (CAKUT). Nephrol Dial Transplant. 26(12):3843-51, 2011

(Left) *Prone longitudinal US in a 4 year old shows a normal left kidney* ➡️ *with no dilation of the renal collecting system* ➡️. *Posterior acoustic shadowing from an overlying rib* ➡️ *partially obscures the upper pole.* **(Right)** *Transverse pelvic US shows the normal uterus* ➡️ *& ovaries* ➡️ *of a 16-year-old girl. Note the normal small follicles* ➡️ *in each ovary as well as the normal small volume of physiologic free fluid* ➡️. *The distended urinary bladder* ➡️ *is a necessary acoustic window for this type of scan.*

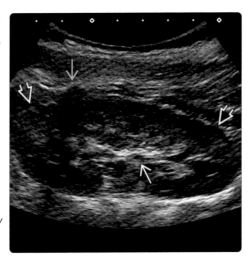
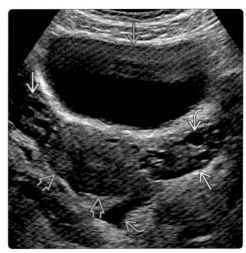

(Left) *Longitudinal US in a newborn shows accentuated corticomedullary differentiation of the kidney* ➡️, *a normal finding for this age. Very mild distention of the renal collecting system* ➡️ *is noted. A normal adrenal gland is also seen* ➡️ *(but will gradually become less visible over the following weeks).* **(Right)** *Frontal view of a fluoroscopic VCUG in a 5 month old shows left grade IV* ➡️ *& right grade II* ➡️ *vesicoureteral reflux. Note the partially visualized urinary bladder* ➡️.

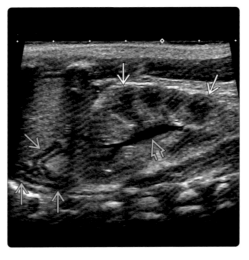
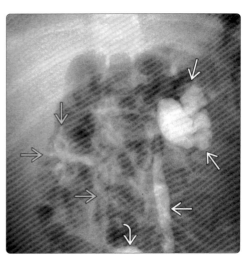

(Left) *Longitudinal US in a 10 day old shows marked dilation of right renal calyces* ➡️ *& renal pelvis* ➡️. *No hydroureter was seen, typical of a ureteropelvic junction (UPJ) obstruction.* **(Right)** *Posterior renogram in the same patient shows centrally decreased radiotracer accumulation of the right kidney* ➡️. *The time-activity curve shows normal uptake & excretion on the left* ➡️ *but prolonged accumulation on the right* ➡️. *No drainage occured after giving Lasix, typical of a UPJ obstruction*

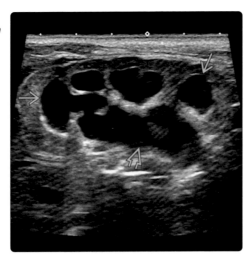
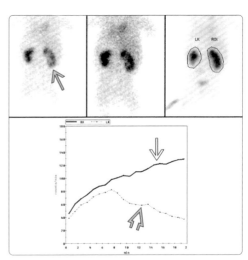

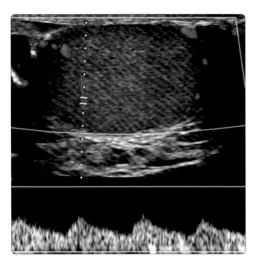

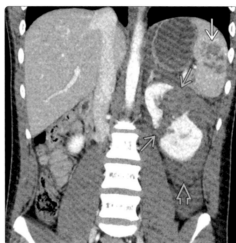

(Left) *Longitudinal color Doppler US shows normal blood flow in the right testicle of a 13-year-old boy with right scrotal pain. This flow was symmetric compared to the left (not shown). These findings exclude testicular torsion.* (Right) *Coronal CECT in a teenager after a dirt bike accident demonstrates a "through & through" grade IV left renal laceration ⇨ & large perinephric hematoma ⇨. Splenic lacerations are also noted ➡.*

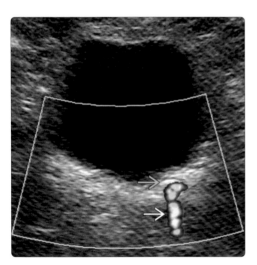

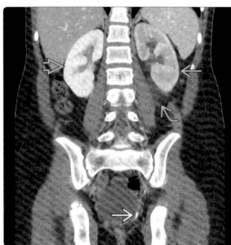

(Left) *Transverse color Doppler US of the urinary bladder in an 11 year old shows an echogenic focus ⇨ at the left ureterovesical junction (UVJ) with associated twinkle artifact ➡, typical of a UVJ stone.* (Right) *Coronal CECT in a different 11 year old shows a left UVJ stone ➡. Obstruction is suggested by the delayed enhancement of the left kidney ⇨ (compared to the right ⇨) as well as the left perinephric fluid ⇨. Note that CT scans performed for urinary tract calculi are typically done without contrast.*

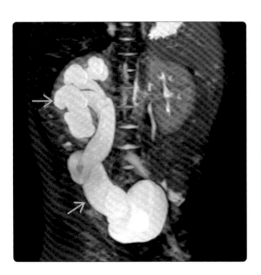

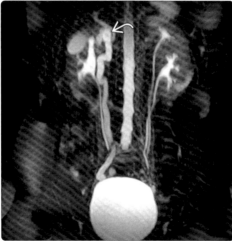

(Left) *Coronal MR urogram MIP in a 6 month old with known right hydroureteronephrosis ⇨ confirmed a primary megaureter with distal UVJ obstruction on delayed contrast-enhanced images (not shown).* (Right) *Coronal MR urogram MIP shows bilateral duplicated collecting systems & ureters in a teenager with flank pain & "giggle incontinence," likely related to the dilated right upper pole moiety ➡ inserting ectopically in the vagina (not shown).*

Ureteropelvic Junction Obstruction

IMAGING

- Marked pelvocaliectasis that ends abruptly at ureteropelvic junction (UPJ) with normal caliber ureter downstream
- Dilated calyces relatively uniform in size & distribution; all connect centrally to disproportionately dilated pelvis
- Thinned but otherwise intact renal parenchyma
- Severity of delayed nephrogram, excretion, & collecting system drainage (on IVP, CECT, MRU, or nuclear renal scan) depends on degree of obstruction
- Contrast entering dilated collecting system (by excretion, retrograde injection, or vesicoureteral reflux during VCUG) may be very dilute due to mixing with retained urine
- ± crossing vessel at obstruction site on CECT, MRU, or US
- Nuclear medicine renal scan well-established for initial assessment & follow-up of renal function & obstruction
- MR urography may provide optimal combination of anatomic & physiologic assessment

CLINICAL ISSUES

- UPJ obstruction most common form of urinary tract obstruction in children
- Due to abnormal smooth muscle arrangement at UPJ, abnormal innervation of proximal ureter, crossing vessel, or fibrous scar at UPJ
- May be diagnosed antenatally or in infancy/childhood with urinary tract infection, intermittent flank pain, or hematuria
- Associated with contralateral MCDK: Requires prompt intervention as MCDK has no function & UPJ may compromise remaining function
- Treatment: Pyeloplasty, ureteroureterostomy (narrowed segment resected or crossing vessel rerouted), or endoureteral balloon plasty/stenting
  - Following successful surgery, pelvocaliectasis persists
  - Appropriate renal growth & adequate drainage on nuclear scans help measure surgical success
- Prognosis: Excellent if renal function has not been compromised by longstanding high-grade obstruction

(Left) Coronal CECT shows a markedly hydronephrotic right kidney ➡. On adjacent images (not shown), the renal pelvis appeared dilated, but no ureter was visualized, consistent with ureteropelvic junction (UPJ) obstruction. (Right) Frontal fluoroscopic image in the OR during cystoscopy & retrograde ureterography shows a dilated right renal collecting system & abrupt caliber change at the UPJ ➡. Intraoperative imaging may be performed to exclude an intraluminal polyp or stone & determine the best surgical approach.

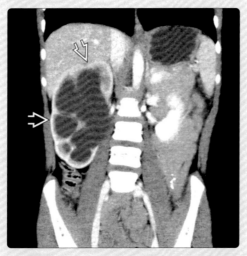
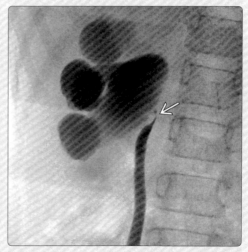

(Left) Longitudinal US of the kidney ➡ in an infant with prenatal hydronephrosis shows dilated calyces ➡ & a large renal pelvis ➡, subsequently diagnosed as a UPJ obstruction. Hypoechoic renal pyramids ➡ are normal in infants. (Right) Posterior images of a Tc-99m MAG3 diuretic renal scintigraphy show minimal uptake in a dilated right kidney ➡. The time activity curve for the right kidney shows progressive accumulation of counts ➡ with no washout during the exam, typical of a UPJ obstruction.

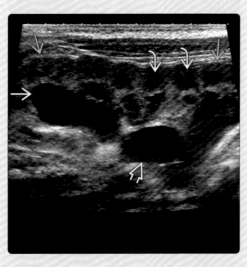
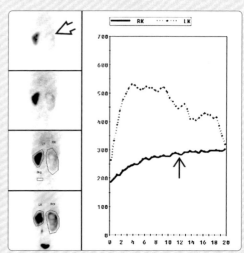

TERMINOLOGY

Definitions

- Variable degrees of blockage to urine flow at level of ureteropelvic junction (UPJ)

IMAGING

General Features

- Best diagnostic clue
  - Marked pelvocaliectasis that ends abruptly at UPJ with normal caliber ureter
  - Severity of delayed renal enhancement, excretion, & collecting system drainage depends on degree of obstruction
  - Obstruction often partial, can improve or worsen

Radiographic Findings

- May see mass effect from enlarged hydronephrotic kidney

Ultrasonographic Findings

- Grayscale ultrasound
  - Moderate to severe pelvocaliectasis without hydroureter
  - Dilated calyces relatively uniform in size & distribution; all connect centrally to disproportionately dilated pelvis
  - Abrupt tapering of pelvis at UPJ
  - Thinned but otherwise intact renal parenchyma
- Color Doppler
  - Search for crossing aberrant vessel at site of obstruction
  - Ureteral jets (in urinary bladder) useful in excluding complete obstruction

Fluoroscopic Findings

- Voiding cystourethrogram
  - Assess for ipsilateral or contralateral vesicoureteral reflux (VUR): Found in up to 8.2% of UPJ obstructions
- Intraoperative retrograde ureterogram
  - Variably used to confirm focal narrowing & search for intraluminal polyp or stone
  - Shows abrupt transition of normal caliber ureter to dilated renal pelvis
  - Contrast entering renal pelvis becomes very dilute by retained volume of urine

CT Findings

- CECT: Delayed nephrogram in enlarged kidney
  - Marked renal pelvic > calyceal dilation with normal or nonvisualized ureter
  - Delayed contrast excretion into collecting system
  - May see crossing vessel at UPJ

MR Findings

- Similar to CECT findings
- MR urography drainage curves & differential function can be used to guide timing of surgery

Nuclear Medicine Findings

- Delayed uptake, excretion, & drainage of radiotracer

Imaging Recommendations

- Best imaging tool
  - Sonography usually performed 1st
  - Nuclear renal scan then used to grade degree of obstruction & determine if surgical intervention or percutaneous drainage required
  - MR urography may be viable single test alternative, optimizing anatomic & physiologic assessment
- Protocol advice
  - Serial exams every 6-12 months (if patient remains asymptomatic) to determine when to intervene

DIFFERENTIAL DIAGNOSIS

Multicystic Dysplastic Kidney (MCDK)

- No discernible normal renal parenchyma
- Cysts do not interconnect

Ureteral Fibroepithelial Polyp

- Found in 5% of UPJ obstructions

Hydronephrosis of Other Etiologies

- VUR, renal stone, ureterovesical junction obstruction, ureterocele: All show some degree of hydroureter

PATHOLOGY

General Features

- Theoretical etiologies of obstruction at UPJ
  - Abnormal smooth muscle impairs distensibility
  - Abnormal innervation of proximal ureter
  - Crossing vessel or fibrous scar at UPJ
    - Vessel in 25% of infants or 50% of older children
- Associated abnormalities
  - Contralateral MCDK in 30-40% of UPJ obstructions
    - Requires prompt intervention as MCDK has no function & UPJ may compromise remaining function

CLINICAL ISSUES

Presentation

- Most common signs/symptoms
  - Prenatal: Often detected on fetal sonogram or MR
  - Infants & children: Urinary tract infection, intermittent abdominal pain, flank pain, vomiting, or hematuria

Natural History & Prognosis

- May improve or deteriorate spontaneously
- Prognosis excellent if renal function has not been compromised by longstanding high-grade obstruction
- Following successful surgery, pelvocaliectasis persists for years on sonography
- Appropriate renal growth & adequate drainage on nuclear scans help measure surgical success

Treatment

- Pyeloplasty (open or laparoscopic surgery)
  - Narrowed segment resected or crossing vessel rerouted

SELECTED REFERENCES

1. Chua ME et al: Magnetic resonance urography in the pediatric population: a clinical perspective. Pediatr Radiol. 46(6):791-5, 2016
2. Weitz M et al: To screen or not to screen for vesicoureteral reflux in children with ureteropelvic junction obstruction: a systematic review. Eur J Pediatr. ePub, 2016
3. Parikh KR et al: Pediatric ureteropelvic junction obstruction: can magnetic resonance urography identify crossing vessels? Pediatr Radiol. 45(12):1788-95, 2015

Vesicoureteral Reflux

TERMINOLOGY

- Retrograde flow of urine from bladder toward 1 or both kidneys

IMAGING

- International Reflux Study Committee grading system of vesicoureteral reflux (VUR)
  o I: Reflux into ureter but not reaching renal pelvis
  o II: Reflux reaching pelvis without blunting of calyces
  o III: Mild calyceal blunting
  o IV: Progressive calyceal & ureteral dilation
  o V: Very dilated & tortuous collecting system
  o ± intrarenal reflux as modifier to grade II+
- Voiding cystourethrogram preferred whenever anatomic detail of upper tracts & urethra needed
- Nuclear cystogram preferred when anatomy is known (e.g., renal ultrasound normal) &/or for follow-up studies
- Use of renal US alone for screening controversial: Variable sensitivity & specificity for scar as compared to DMSA

CLINICAL ISSUES

- Usually discovered during work-up of febrile UTI
- Affects up to 2% of general population
  o Risk factors: Family history, sex (F > M), age at presentation, duplication, & other voiding dysfunctions
    - Caucasian children much more commonly affected than African American children
  o Occurs in 25-40% of children with acute pyelonephritis & 5-50% of asymptomatic siblings of children with VUR
- 80% outgrow VUR before puberty
- ↑ grade or longer standing VUR, more numerous UTIs, & subsequent renal scarring → ↑ incidence of renal insufficiency, hypertension, & end-stage renal disease
- Treatment options
  o Prophylactic antibiotic therapy (medical management): Reduces febrile UTI recurrences, not scarring
  o Ureteral reimplantation surgery (surgical management)
  o Endoscopic periureteral injections (minimally invasive endoscopic management)

(Left) Coronal graphic depicts the International Reflux Study Committee grading system. Note the progressive level of reflux, dilation, calyceal blunting, & ureteral tortuosity from grade I on the left to grade V on the right. (Right) VCUG in an infant shows bilateral vesicoureteral reflux (VUR). The calyces are sharp ➡ on the right (grade II). On the left, the calyces are slightly blunted ➡ & the ureter is mildly dilated & tortuous, making this grade III VUR.

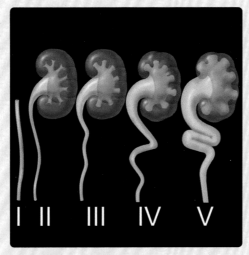

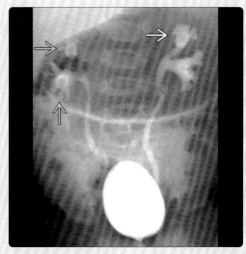

(Left) Posterior nuclear cystogram images show radiotracer extending into the right ureter & reaching the intrarenal collecting system ➡, likely corresponding to fluoroscopic grade II VUR. Note that reflux occurs only during voiding & drains well on the post void image ➡. (Right) Frontal VCUG shows high-grade VUR into the right kidney with a dilated tortuous ureter ➡, blunted calyces ➡, & intrarenal reflux into the tubules ➡. These findings constitute grade V VUR with intrarenal reflux.

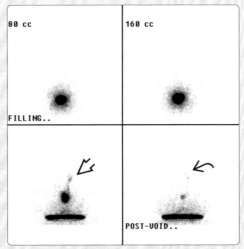

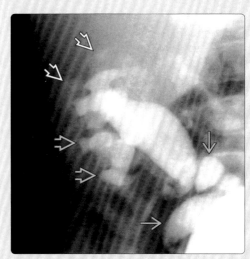

TERMINOLOGY

Definitions

- Vesicoureteral reflux (VUR): Retrograde flow of urine from bladder toward 1 or both kidneys

IMAGING

Ultrasonographic Findings

- Varying degrees of renal collecting system &/or ureteral dilation ± urothelial thickening
  - Normal US does not exclude significant VUR
- Look for signs of scarring: Globally small kidney or polar foci of cortical thinning subtended by dilated calyces
- US contrast agent can be instilled into bladder for sonographic cystogram; requires catheterization

Fluoroscopic Findings

- Voiding cystourethrogram
  - VCUG preferred for anatomic detail of upper tracts or urethra
  - Requires bladder catheterization for contrast installation
  - Contrast seen in ureter &/or renal collecting system confirms VUR; may be transient
  - Ectopic ureters may not be visualized unless they are inadvertently catheterized
  - Voiding images of urethra performed to exclude distal pathology, which may contribute to back pressure

Nuclear Medicine Findings

- Nuclear cystogram
  - Radiotracer instilled into bladder via catheter
  - Continuous posterior imaging performed throughout bladder filling & voiding
    - ↑ detection of transient VUR so that nuclear cystogram is more sensitive for VUR than fluoroscopic VCUG
  - Nuclear cystogram preferred when anatomy is known &/or for follow-up studies
    - Gives no information about urethral abnormalities
- Renal cortical scan (DMSA)
  - Posterior imaging after IV radiotracer injection
  - Photopenic renal cortical foci due to acute pyelonephritis or chronic scarring

Imaging Recommendations

- Best tool controversial
- Historic "bottom-up" approach to UTI work-up: VCUG + renal US; DMSA if 1st-line studies abnormal or febrile UTI
- Current "top-down" approach to UTI work-up: Renal US ± DMSA; VCUG if 1st-line studies abnormal
- **Use of renal US alone for screening controversial due to variable sensitivity (37-100%) & specificity (65-99%) for scar as compared to DMSA**
- DMSA therefore advocated by some as better test for scarring, which serves as surrogate for high-grade VUR requiring treatment (with scarring in 50% of grades IV-V but < 10% of grades I-III VUR)
  - RIVUR trial showed no difference in progressive scarring on antibiotic prophylaxis vs. placebo
  - ↑ scars in older patients, higher grade VUR, & those with recurrent febrile UTI

PATHOLOGY

General Features

- Etiology: Shortened or abnormally angulated insertion of ureter into bladder theorized to result in primary VUR
  - VUR may also be secondary to periureteral (Hutch) diverticulum, ureterocele, bladder outlet obstruction, voiding dysfunction, or neurogenic bladder
  - Risk factors: Family history, sex (F > M), age at presentation, duplication, & other voiding dysfunctions
- Probable association of sterile reflux with renal scarring
  - Antibiotic prophylaxis after 1st UTI reduces febrile UTI recurrences, not scarring
- Associated abnormalities: Duplications, UPJ obstruction, or contralateral multicystic dysplastic kidney

CLINICAL ISSUES

Presentation

- Usually discovered during work-up of febrile UTI

Demographics

- VUR most common in children < 2 years old
- Affects up to 2% of general population
  - VUR in 25-40% of children with acute pyelonephritis
  - VUR in 5-50% of asymptomatic siblings of children with documented reflux

Natural History & Prognosis

- 80% outgrow VUR before puberty
- With higher grade or longer standing VUR, more numerous UTIs, & subsequent renal scarring → ↑ incidence of renal insufficiency, hypertension, & end-stage renal disease

Treatment

- Prophylactic antibiotic therapy (medical management)
  - Reduces febrile UTI recurrences, not scarring
- Ureteral reimplantation surgery (surgical management)
- Endoscopic periureteral injections (minimally invasive endoscopic management) utilizing inert material to alter shape of abnormal/refluxing ureterovesical junction

SELECTED REFERENCES

1. Mattoo TK et al: Renal scarring in the randomized intervention for children with vesicoureteral reflux (RIVUR) Trial. Clin J Am Soc Nephrol. 11(1):54-61, 2016
2. Bush NC et al: Renal damage detected by DMSA, despite normal renal ultrasound, in children with febrile UTI. J Pediatr Urol. 11(3):126.e1-7, 2015
3. Mattoo TK et al: The RIVUR trial: a factual interpretation of our data. Pediatr Nephrol. 30(5):707-12, 2015
4. Narchi H et al: Renal tract abnormalities missed in a historical cohort of young children with UTI if the NICE and AAP imaging guidelines were applied. J Pediatr Urol. 11(5):252.e1-7, 2015
5. Stein R et al: Urinary tract infections in children: EAU/ESPU guidelines. Eur Urol. 67(3):546-58, 2015
6. Botta S et al: To V(CUG) or not to V(CUG) in infants with prenatal hydronephrosis? J Urol. 192(3):640-1, 2014
7. Downs SM: UTI and watchful waiting: the courage to do nothing. Pediatrics. 133(3):535-6, 2014
8. Hoberman A et al: Antimicrobial prophylaxis for children with vesicoureteral reflux. N Engl J Med. 371(11):1072-3, 2014
9. Ristola MT et al: NICE guidelines cannot be recommended for imaging studies in children younger than 3 years with urinary tract infection. Eur J Pediatr Surg. 25(5):414-20, 2014
10. RIVUR Trial Investigators et al: Antimicrobial prophylaxis for children with vesicoureteral reflux. N Engl J Med. 370(25):2367-76, 2014

Ureteropelvic Duplications

TERMINOLOGY

- Presence of 2 separate collecting systems in 1 kidney; 2 ureters draining 1 kidney may join above bladder (partial duplication) or insert into bladder separately (complete)

IMAGING

- Duplicated kidneys tend to be larger than nonduplex kidneys, even without hydronephrosis
- With complete duplication, ureter draining upper pole of kidney inserts in bladder inferior & medial to ureter draining lower pole of kidney (Weigert-Meyer rule)
  - Lower pole ureter inserts orthotopically in trigone
  - Upper pole ureteral orifice ectopic in location & often associated with ureterocele
- Corollary to Weigert-Meyer rule
  - Upper pole tends to obstruct
  - Lower pole tends to have vesicoureteral reflux (VUR)
    - Lack of dilation of ureter & collecting system in no way excludes VUR

- Drooping lily sign: Classic appearance of opacified lower pole collecting system on IVP or VCUG, displaced by mass-like upper pole hydronephrosis
  - Correlation with US critical to confirm upper pole obstruction rather than other mass lesion

CLINICAL ISSUES

- Incidence: 12-15% in general population
- Most often discovered antenatally or incidentally on imaging studies performed for other reasons
- Symptomatic duplications may lead to infection, obstruction, calculi, scarring, hematuria, abdominal or flank pain, voiding dysfunction, urinary retention
- Treatment depends on extent of anomalies & complications
- Prognosis varies with type of duplication & severity of complications
  - Chronic obstruction or VUR, infection, &/or scarring may lead to secondary hypertension & renal insufficiency

(Left) Coronal graphic shows a normal right kidney & a completely duplicated left kidney. There is a poorly draining left upper pole ectopic ureterocele ➡ in the bladder medial & inferior to the lower pole ureteral orifice ➡. The left lower pole ureter inserts into the bladder orthotopically at the trigone. (Right) Longitudinal US in a 1 year old being evaluated for fever shows an uncomplicated duplicated right kidney with a band of cortex ➡ obliquely crossing the central sinus structures.

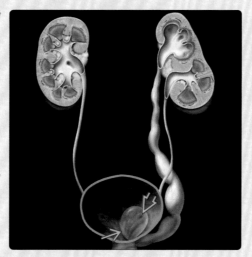
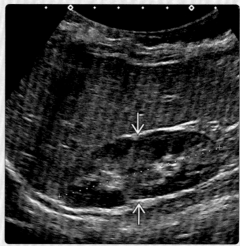

(Left) Frontal VCUG image in a patient with a duplicated right kidney shows grade IV vesicoureteral reflux into the lower pole moiety ➡. Upper pole moieties tend to obstruct while lower poles tend to reflux. When the obstructed nonopacified upper moiety is larger & more severely rotates the lower moiety than seen here, the appearance is often called a drooping lily. (Right) Coronal T2 MR in a 4 month old shows a duplicated right kidney with moderate pelvocaliectasis affecting only the lower pole ➡. The left kidney is not duplicated.

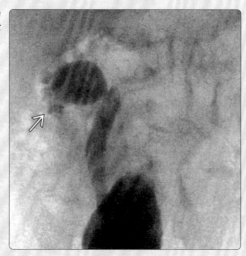
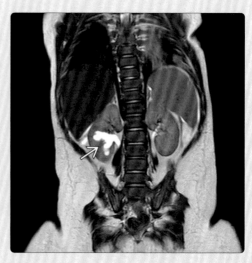

Ureterocele

TERMINOLOGY

- Congenital cystic dilation of distal submucosal portion of 1 or both ureters within urinary bladder
- Categorized according to ureterocele insertion
  - Orthotopic (simple): Orifice located in normal anatomic position in bladder trigone
  - Ectopic: Orifice located anywhere else
- Categorized according to type of kidney drained
  - Single system vs. duplicated system with 2 ureters
    - 1 ureter of duplicated system must be ectopic
- Weigert-Meyer rule: Ureter from upper pole (UP) moiety of duplicated kidney inserts inferior & medial to normal lower pole (LP) moiety insertion site at trigone

IMAGING

- Round/ovoid filling defect in urinary bladder
  - Thin-walled & cystic-appearing on US, MRU
    - Wall appears thicker, collapsed after surgery
- ± visualization of associated dilated distal ureter

- In duplicated system, UP moiety (associated with ureterocele) typically obstructs & LP moiety typically refluxes
  - Varying degrees of hydronephrosis & parenchymal dysplasia of UP moiety
  - Vesicoureteral reflux into LP moiety classically shows drooping lily sign
    - Due to rotation of LP system by obstructed UP

CLINICAL ISSUES

- Prenatal detection: Hydronephrosis typical
- Postnatal presentation: Febrile UTI most common
- Ectopic, extravesical variety > orthotopic, simple, intravesical variety by 3:1 ratio
- Typical treatment: Endoscopic incision of ureterocele, especially if infected or obstructed in neonate
- Prognosis: Excellent if nonobstructing & nonrefluxing; variable if prolonged obstruction or high-grade vesicoureteral reflux has compromised renal function

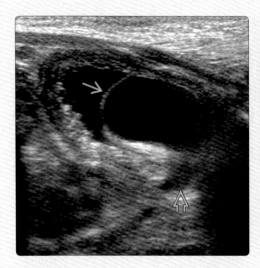
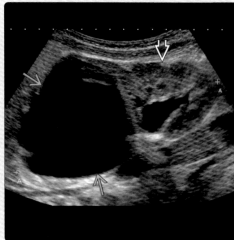

(Left) Longitudinal ultrasound of the urinary bladder in an 18 day old with prenatally detected hydronephrosis shows a large thin-walled cyst ➡ filling much of the bladder lumen, typical of a ureterocele. The cyst connects to a dilated distal left ureter ➡. (Right) Longitudinal ultrasound of the duplicated left kidney in the same patient shows severe pelvocaliectasis & parenchymal thinning of the left upper pole (UP) moiety ➡. The lower pole (LP) moiety shows mild pelvocaliectasis with more normal-appearing renal parenchyma ➡.

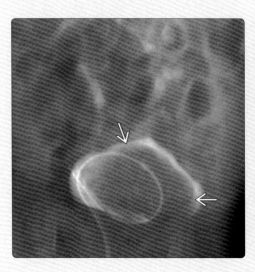
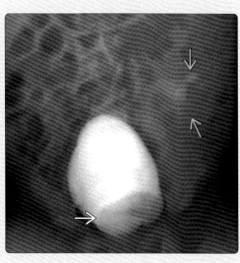

(Left) Frontal early filling image from a VCUG in the same patient shows the ureterocele as a large ovoid filling defect ➡ partially outlined by contrast in the urinary bladder. (Right) Postvoid VCUG in the same patient shows grade II-III vesicoureteral reflux into the LP collecting system ➡. The drooping lily configuration of contrast within the LP strongly suggests obstruction of an UP moiety (as confirmed on the ultrasound). The UP ureterocele ➡ remains visible in the contrast-filled bladder.

KEY FACTS

TERMINOLOGY

- Megaureter: General term for ureteral dilation
  - Can be due to vesicoureteral reflux (VUR), obstruction, both, or neither
- Primary obstructive megaureter: Functional obstruction at juxtavesical segment of ureter due to absent peristalsis

IMAGING

- Variable degree of hydroureteronephrosis with transition to nondilated distal ureter
  - Nondilated aperistaltic terminal ureteral segment
  - Most commonly unilateral: 67% on left
- VUR: Ipsilateral in 5%, contralateral in < 10%
- ± debris, calculi in dilated ureter
- Long-term obstruction can lead to parenchymal thinning & lack of renal growth
- Best imaging modalities
  - Ultrasound best screening exam for urinary tract anomalies (pre- or postnatally)

- Diagnostic & treatment considerations refined with
  - Fluoroscopic VCUG (to assess for VUR &/or bladder outlet obstruction)
  - Nuclear medicine diuretic renography to assess for renal function & delayed ureteral drainage
  - MR urography can assess anatomy & physiology

CLINICAL ISSUES

- Diagnosed prenatally in nearly 50%; remaining cases present over wide range of ages
- May be asymptomatic but can present with UTI, abdominal/flank pain, hematuria ± calculi, renal failure
- 70% regress spontaneously by 7 years of age
  - Initial ureteral diameter < 8.5 mm: Likely to resolve
  - Initial ureteral diameter > 15 mm: Likely to persist
- Surgery for worsening renal function or recurrent UTIs

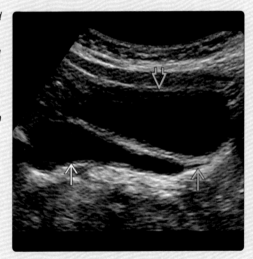
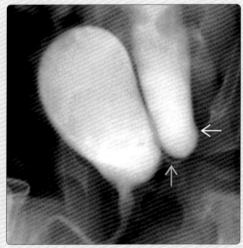

(Left) *Longitudinal ultrasound at the left ureterovesical junction of a male infant shows a dilated left ureter* ⇒ *tapering distally to a normal caliber aperistaltic juxtavesical segment* ⇒ *that shows urothelial thickening. The urinary bladder* ⇒ *is seen anteriorly.* (Right) *Oblique fluoroscopic image from a VCUG in the same patient shows vesicoureteral reflux into the normal caliber juxtavesical segment* ⇒ *with transition to the proximally dilated ureter* ⇒.

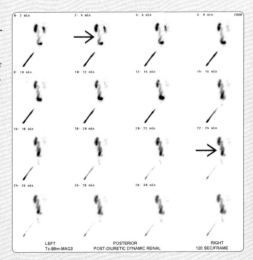
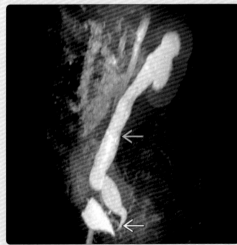

(Left) *Dynamic posterior view postdiuretic images from a Tc-99m MAG3 renogram in the same patient show qualitatively slow drainage of the left dilated ureter* ⇒. *The T1/2 for drainage of the left ureter was > 20 minutes on the quantitative evaluation, consistent with obstruction.* (Right) *Oblique MIP from an MR urogram in a patient with a primary obstructive megaureter shows a narrow juxtavesical segment of the left ureter* ⇒ *with proximal hydroureteronephrosis* ⇒.

Posterior Urethral Valves

TERMINOLOGY

- Varying degrees of chronic urethral obstruction due to fusion &/or prominence of plicae colliculi (which are normal concentric folds within male posterior urethra)

IMAGING

- VCUG
  - Abrupt transition from dilated posterior urethra to small bulbar urethra at level of valvular tissue; actual valve tissue may not be visible
  - Bladder dilation, wall trabeculation, muscular hypertrophy, diverticula, ± patent urachus
  - Vesicoureteral reflux (50-70%)
- Ultrasound
  - Bilateral hydroureteronephrosis
  - Echogenic, dysplastic kidneys with poor corticomedullary differentiation ± cortical cysts, urinomas, ascites
  - Lobular bladder with thickened, irregular wall ± diverticula

- Diagnosis made on VCUG, cystoscopy, or cystosonography

CLINICAL ISSUES

- Severity & duration of obstruction determines age of presentation & clinical symptoms, which include
  - Perinatally: Oligohydramnios, hydronephrosis, anuria, urinary ascites, urinoma, pulmonary hypoplasia
  - In infancy: Urinary tract infection, sepsis, urinary retention, poor urinary stream, failure to thrive
  - In childhood: Abnormal voiding patterns, hesitancy, straining, poor stream, large postvoid residual, renal insufficiency/failure
- Catheterization at birth to relieve obstruction, followed by urgent endoscopic valve ablation; long-term follow-up necessary to monitor renal function & bladder compliance
  - 30-40% will eventually develop end-stage renal disease
  - 75% have long-term urinary bladder dysfunction
  - Fertility issues common in long-term survivors

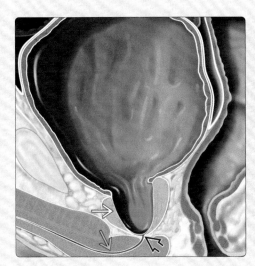

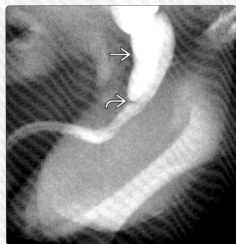

(Left) Sagittal graphic shows an enlarged posterior urethra ➜ extending through the prostate with valve tissue ⊡ at the site of transition to a much smaller anterior urethra ⊡. (Right) Lateral oblique VCUG in a newborn with posterior urethral valves (PUV) shows the same anatomy from the previous graphic. There is a dilated posterior urethra ➜ with an abrupt change in urethral caliber just distal to the valve tissue ⊿.

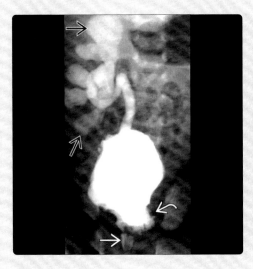

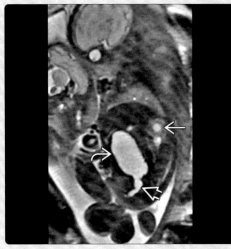

(Left) Frontal VCUG in a newborn shows high-grade vesicoureteral reflux (VUR) into the right kidney ⊡ with irregular bladder wall thickening ⊿ & a dilated posterior urethra ➜. High-grade unilateral VUR can be protective of the contralateral renal function in PUV. (Right) Sagittal SSFSE T2 MR in a 3rd-trimester twin gestation shows a fetus with an elongated mildly thick-walled urinary bladder ⊿, hydronephrosis ➜, & a dilated posterior urethra ⊿, typical of PUV.

Urachal Abnormalities

TERMINOLOGY

- Persistence of all or portion of connection between bladder dome & umbilicus; remnant of fetal allantoic stalk

IMAGING

- Patent urachus or urachal fistula: Open channel from bladder to umbilicus through which urine can leak
- Urachal sinus: Persistence of superficial segment of channel opening onto skin surface
- Urachal diverticulum: Persistence of deep segment of tract, creating diverticulum off of anterior-superior bladder wall
- Urachal cyst: Persistence of intermediary segment with fibrous attachments to bladder & umbilicus
- Size & shape depend on type of remnant, location, & presence of inflammation
- Ultrasound defines static anatomy well
- VCUG useful to show flow dynamics & confirm patency

CLINICAL ISSUES

- Patent urachus presents with umbilical drainage, urinary tract infection, & relapsing periumbilical inflammation
  - Occasionally, urachus remains patent in response to bladder outlet obstruction (posterior urethral valves, pelvic mass, etc.) & will close when outlet repaired
- Urachal sinus presents with periumbilical tenderness, wet umbilicus, or nonhealing granulation of umbilicus
- Urachal diverticula are often asymptomatic & discovered incidentally; rarely they enlarge, fail to drain during urination, & become predisposed to infection or stones
- Urachal cyst presents in childhood or adolescence with suprapubic mass, fever, pain, & irritative voiding symptoms
- Generally, prognosis excellent
  - Urachal tract resected; no further follow-up needed
    - Open surgery previously, now laparoscopic
- Risk of malignancy in adults if not resected
  - Urachal malignancies < 1% of all bladder cancers

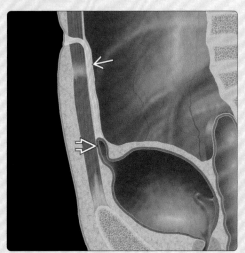
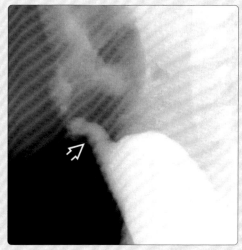

(Left) *Sagittal graphic shows a urachal diverticulum* ➡ *& fibrotic tract* ➡ *to the umbilicus. When the entire tract remains open, it is called a patent urachus. The urachal sinus & urachal cyst are additional variations along this spectrum.* (Right) *Lateral VCUG image in an infant with a history of umbilical drainage shows a tubular contrast-filled connection* ➡ *between the bladder dome & the umbilicus, consistent with a patent urachus.*

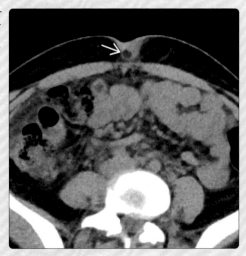
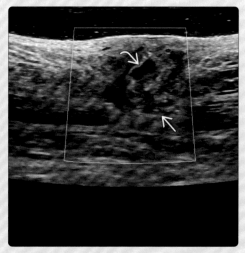

(Left) *Axial NECT in a teenager shows a low-density cyst* ➡ *at the base of the umbilicus with thickening of the periumbilical tissues.* (Right) *Longitudinal US of the same patient shows mild hyperemia* ➡ *& heterogeneity of the periumbilical tissues with a small fluid collection centrally* ➡. *A small urachal cyst was resected. Additional considerations for this appearance could include an evolving hematoma, abscess, inflamed dermoid, or other lesions.*

Renal Ectopia and Fusion

TERMINOLOGY

- Normal renal tissue in abnormal location: Horseshoe or pancake kidney; crossed fused ectopia; pelvic, iliac/pelvic (ptotic/mobile), & thoracic kidneys

IMAGING

- Found anywhere from presacral to intrathoracic; may be bilateral or unilateral; may cross midline
- US typically sufficient to document location & gross morphology of ectopic & fused kidneys
  - Accurate lengths difficult to obtain due to more globular/less reniform shape & poor definition of margin with contralateral kidney
- Other modalities used to answer specific questions (as needed): Drainage, stones, vascular supply, ureteral course
- Ureteral insertion site in bladder provides clue to site where kidney initially formed (i.e., lower pole ureter of crossed fused ectopia inserts into trigone on contralateral side)
- Colon typically occupies empty renal fossa

PATHOLOGY

- Results from abnormal ascent & rotation of fetal kidney
- Malpositioned kidneys more susceptible to trauma, iatrogenic injury, obstruction, infection, & stones
- Isthmus of horseshoe kidney may contain functioning renal tissue or fibrotic nonfunctional tissue
- Associations: Vesicoureteral reflux (20-30%), contralateral renal dysplasia (4%), cryptorchidism (5%), hypospadias (5%)
- Horseshoe kidneys associated with genital anomalies, VACTERL, Turner, & other syndromes
- Adrenal ectopia reported in association with renal ectopia

CLINICAL ISSUES

- Horseshoe kidney most common: 1 in 400 births
- All types of ectopia more common in boys than girls
- Primary concern: Avoidance of iatrogenic injury to renal parenchyma & supplying vessels during routine surgery
- Treat complications of obstruction, reflux, & stones

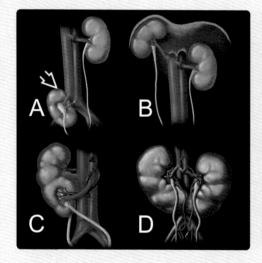

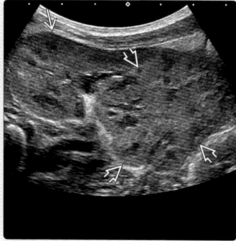

(Left) Graphic shows variations of renal ectopia & fusion: (A) Pelvic kidney ➡, (B) subdiaphragmatic/thoracic kidney, (C) crossed fused renal ectopia, & (D) horseshoe kidney. (Right) Longitudinal US shows a crossed fused renal ectopia in the left abdomen with a relatively normal upper moiety ➡ & a malrotated, globular lower moiety ➡. Note that the long axis of each moiety is different, which helps distinguish this entity from a duplication. Also, no renal tissue will be seen in the contralateral renal fossa in this setting.

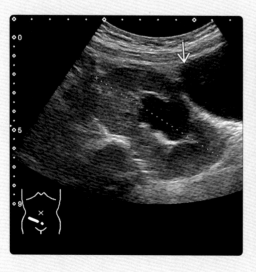

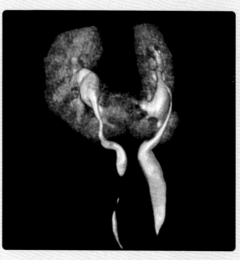

(Left) Longitudinal US shows a pelvic kidney (between cursors) abutting the bladder dome ➡ in the right lower quadrant. It is easy to imagine this kidney being injured during a laparoscopic appendectomy. (Right) 3D reformation from a CECT scan in a patient with multiple congenital anomalies shows a horseshoe kidney with fused lower poles & anteriorly directed renal pelves.

Multicystic Dysplastic Kidney

TERMINOLOGY

- Multicystic dysplastic kidney (MCDK): Congenital nonfunctional kidney replaced by multiple cysts & dysplastic tissue
- MCDKs usually involute with time: Cysts shrink & residual tissue may lose reniform shape

IMAGING

- Reniform-shaped multicystic mass occupying renal fossa
  - ± lobulated outer contour (due to cysts of variable size)
  - Wide range of sizes: Up to 15 cm in length in newborn period; may be only 1-2 cm after years of involution
- Cysts of varying size do not connect
  - Largest cyst typically peripheral, not central
- Poorly defined intervening echogenic parenchyma without normal corticomedullary architecture
- Can be segmental in duplicated kidneys
- Nuclear scintigraphy documents lack of renal function in MCDK

CLINICAL ISSUES

- MCDK 2nd most common abdominal mass in neonate (after hydronephrosis)
- > 50% discovered antenatally or in infancy as palpable mass
- Unilateral MCDK with normal contralateral kidney: Excellent prognosis
  - Vast majority involute with time & remain asymptomatic
  - Rare reports of Wilms tumor developing in MCDK
- Unilateral MCDK with abnormal contralateral kidney (up to 40%, typically ureteropelvic junction obstruction or vesicoureteral reflux): May develop renal insufficiency
- Bilateral MCDK: Incompatible with life
- Nonurologic abnormalities: Cardiac & musculoskeletal most common
- Associated syndromes: Turner syndrome, trisomy 21, chromosome 22 deletions, Waardenburg syndrome, others

(Left) Frontal graphic of the right kidney shows multiple cysts of varying size replacing the renal parenchyma. There is minimal intervening dysplastic renal tissue. A ureter may or may not be recognizable at the renal hilum on imaging studies. (Right) Coronal SSFSE T2 fetal MR shows a multicystic mass in the left renal fossa ⟹ with no discernible normal left renal tissue, most consistent with a left multicystic dysplastic kidney (MCDK). The right kidney ⟹ & volume of amniotic fluid appear normal.

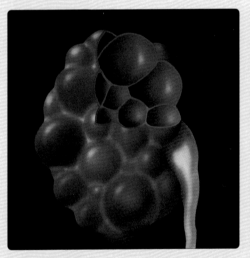
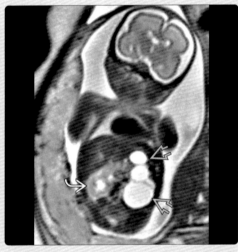

(Left) Prone postnatal US of the left flank in the same patient shows multiple cysts ⟹ of varying size replacing the left kidney. A reniform shape is retained, but no normal left renal parenchyma is seen. (Right) Posterior images of the same infant during a Tc-99m MAG3 renal scan show normal function of the right kidney ⟹ but no function on the left side ⟹, confirming a left MCDK. Early transient activity in MCDK on nuclear scans merely reflects that the tissue is being perfused, but continued images show no function.

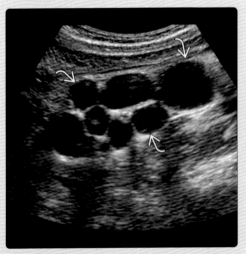
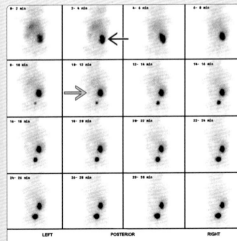

Polycystic Kidney Disease, Autosomal Recessive

KEY FACTS

TERMINOLOGY

- Autosomal recessive polycystic kidney disease: Single gene ciliopathy with marked bilateral renal enlargement due to dilated distal tubules & collecting ducts

IMAGING

- Radiographs: Bilateral flank "masses" bulging lateral abdominal contours & displacing bowel gas centrally
  - Lack of urine production in utero → oligohydramnios → pulmonary hypoplasia
    - Bell-shaped thorax ± pneumothorax, pneumomediastinum
- US: Bilaterally enlarged echogenic kidneys in newborn with loss of corticomedullary differentiation
  - 2-6 standard deviations above mean size for age
  - Dilated, radially arranged tubules on high-resolution linear transducers ± small cysts (< 1 cm)
  - Tiny, punctate hyperechoic foci (likely calcium deposits) develop with time & correlate with renal failure
  - Macroscopic cysts infrequent
- MR: Large kidneys of diffusely high T2 signal intensity
- Variable degrees of liver disease

CLINICAL ISSUES

- Perinatal form: More severe renal disease with pulmonary hypoplasia, less hepatic disease
  - Renal insufficiency → renal replacement therapy (dialysis or transplant)
  - Pulmonary hypoplasia → respiratory distress, may be life-limiting
  - Enlarged palpable kidneys → may require nephrectomies
- Juvenile form: Less renal disease, more hepatic disease
  - Portal hypertension & fibrosis develop in 50%
  - Liver transplant when associated with progressive hepatic fibrosis
- Severity & outcomes vary within affected families
  - Survival rate for milder forms up to 82% at age 3 years & 79% at 15 years

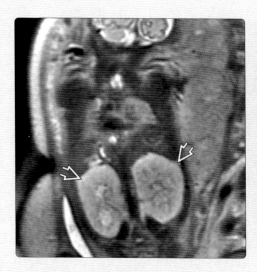
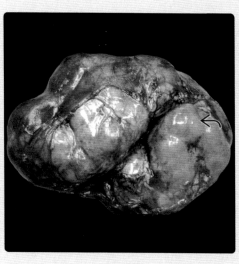

(Left) *Coronal SSFSE T2 fetal MR shows marked enlargement & increased signal of both kidneys* ➡ *without discrete cysts. Note the lack of amniotic fluid, reflecting poor renal function from autosomal recessive polycystic kidney disease (ARPKD).* **(Right)** *Frontal view of a newborn with a history of oligohydramnios shows bowel loops displaced centrally by bilateral flank "masses"* ➡ *(due to massively enlarged kidneys). Note the bell-shaped thorax & left pneumothorax* ➡ *from pulmonary hypoplasia.*

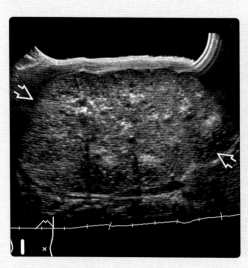
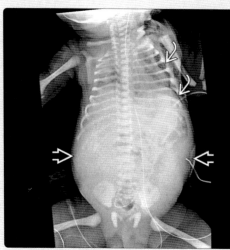

(Left) *Extended field of view US shows a newborn kidney measuring >10 cm in length* ➡*. There is loss of corticomedullary differentiation with replacement of the renal parenchyma by microscopic cysts & dilated tubules with hyperechoic walls.* **(Right)** *Gross pathology shows a kidney removed from an infant with ARPKD in order to relieve mass effect & permit peritoneal dialysis. Macroscopic cysts* ➡ *are visible along the surface of this kidney, which is > 14 cm long.*

KEY FACTS

TERMINOLOGY

- Autosomal dominant polycystic kidney disease (ADPKD): Hereditary ciliopathy characterized by multiple renal cysts & various other systemic manifestations
  - Cystic organ involvement: Kidneys (100%), liver (50%), pancreas (9%), brain/ovaries/testis (1%)
  - Cerebral "berry" aneurysms (5-10% in adults)

IMAGING

- Renal size within 2 standard deviations above normal at time of diagnosis in 1/2 of pediatric patients
- Scattered renal cysts of variable number & size
  - ↑ throughout life: 54% of ADPKD cysts appear in 1st decade; 72% occur within 2nd decade
  - May be complicated by hemorrhage, infection, or rupture
- Renal parenchyma often otherwise normal

PATHOLOGY

- 90% autosomal dominant; 10% spontaneous mutations
- Family history lacking in almost 1/2 of patients due to variable expressivity & spontaneous mutations

CLINICAL ISSUES

- Typically asymptomatic with excellent prognosis in childhood
  - Discovered incidentally or upon screening children of affected adults
  - Flank pain, hematuria, hypertension, & renal failure also reported in children
- Prognosis in adulthood variable
  - Hemorrhage, infection, rupture of cysts; renal failure; hypertension; rarely malignancy
  - 4th leading cause of chronic renal failure in world
- Treat symptoms & complications: Hypertension, pain, renal infection; ultimately requires renal transplant

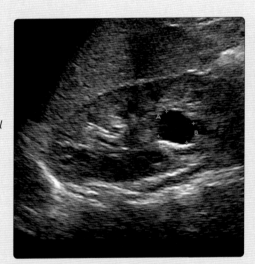
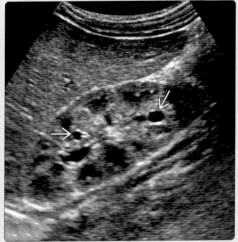

(Left) Longitudinal US in a 5 year old being screened for cysts due to a relevant family history shows a solitary central cyst between the cursors, likely due to autosomal dominant polycystic kidney disease (ADPKD). (Right) Longitudinal oblique US in a 9 month old with a family history of renal failure shows several small cysts ➡ in the medullary portion of the right kidney.

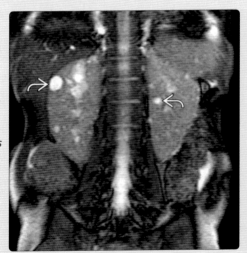
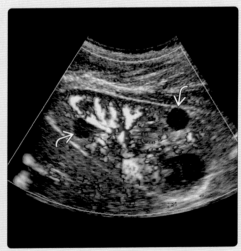

(Left) Coronal SSFP MR in the same 9 month old shows numerous cysts ➡ of varying size scattered through both kidneys in this patient with ADPKD. (Right) Longitudinal power Doppler US shows normal blood flow in the renal parenchyma between the cysts ➡. Vascular compression by enlarging cysts is one theory to explain progressive renal insufficiency in ADPKD.

Mesoblastic Nephroma

KEY FACTS

TERMINOLOGY

- Mesoblastic nephroma (MN): Hamartomatous renal tumor of young infants
- Classic benign vs. more aggressive cellular variants
  - Studies vary on which type more common

IMAGING

- Solitary renal mass in fetus or infant
- Well-defined oval/round mass
  - Classic type usually solid, smaller
  - Cellular type usually larger with cystic/necrotic/hemorrhagic foci

PATHOLOGY

- Classic type similar to infantile myofibroma
- Cellular type similar to infantile fibrosarcoma
  - Local recurrence, metastases

CLINICAL ISSUES

- 3-6% of childhood renal tumors
- Presentations include
  - Palpable abdominal mass in young infant
  - Hypertension, hypercalcemia, hematuria
  - Prenatally detected renal mass with polyhydramnios (70%), preterm labor
- Most MN diagnosed before 3 months of age
  - Classic type more common in this timeframe
- After 3 months
  - Wilms tumor becomes more common
  - Remaining MN more likely to be cellular
- Nephrectomy with wide margins usually curative

DIAGNOSTIC CHECKLIST

- Preoperative feature for best differentiating solid renal masses in children: Age

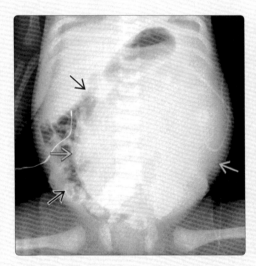
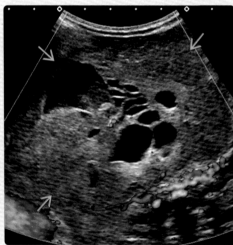
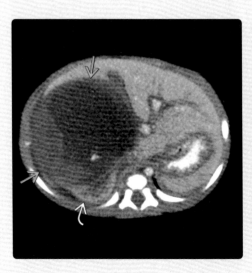
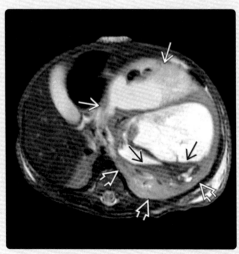

(Left) AP radiograph of the abdomen in a neonate with a prenatally detected abdominal mass shows displacement of gas-filled bowel loops ➡ into the right abdomen by a large round mass ➡. (Right) Longitudinal color Doppler ultrasound of the abdomen in the same patient shows the 11-cm mixed cystic & solid mass ➡ with little detectable internal vascularity. The cellular subtype of mesoblastic nephroma was confirmed upon resection.

(Left) Axial CECT in a patient with cellular mesoblastic nephroma shows a crescent of residual right kidney ➡ splayed along the posterior margin of the heterogeneous mass ➡. This claw sign helps to identify the kidney as the organ of origin for the tumor. (Right) Axial T2 FS MR in a patient with a mesoblastic nephroma shows a heterogeneous mass ➡ in the left flank. The layering fluid-fluid levels ➡ are typical of hemorrhage within cysts. A "claw" of the splayed residual left kidney is seen posteriorly ➡.

IMAGING

- Ultrasound frequently 1st study performed; CECT & MR better characterize tumor & local extent
  - Large, heterogeneous but predominantly solid hypoechoic (US)/hypoenhancing (CT/MR) renal mass
  - Must carefully evaluate
    - Adjacent soft tissues for tumor rupture, adenopathy
    - Renal vein & inferior vena cava for tumor thrombus
    - Contralateral kidney for synchronous tumor or nephrogenic rests
- Chest radiograph or CT: Lung metastases in 10-20%

TOP DIFFERENTIAL DIAGNOSES

- Neuroblastoma: Extrarenal, more often calcified
- Congenital mesoblastic nephroma: < 3-12 months old
- Clear cell sarcoma: Look for skeletal metastases
- Renal cell carcinoma: Equal incidence > 12 years old
- Pyelonephritis: Renal abscess usually more infiltrative & cystic; ± fever, positive urinalysis

PATHOLOGY

- Arises from primitive metanephric blastemal tissue
  - Persistence after 34 weeks gestation termed "nephroblastomatosis" → 30-40% develop Wilms tumor

CLINICAL ISSUES

- Most common abdominal tumor in children 1-8 years old
  - 80% of cases < 5 years old
- Typical presentation: Incidentally discovered palpable mass
  - ± hematuria, failure to thrive, hypertension, fever, anemia
- Predisposing syndromes in 10% of cases: Obtain quarterly screening renal ultrasounds until 8 years old
- Preferred treatment: Upfront complete surgical resection
  - Preoperative chemotherapy for unresectable or bilateral tumors or tumor thrombus above hepatic veins
  - Postoperative chemotherapy ± radiation
- Prognosis based on stage, tumor size, histology
  - 90% 5-year-survival for localized abdominal disease

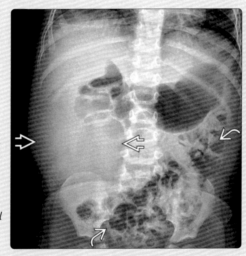
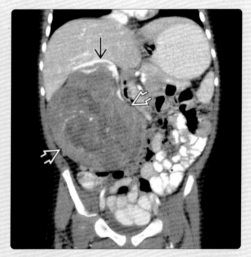

(Left) *AP abdominal radiograph of a 3-year-old child with a firm, palpable mass shows leftward displacement of bowel loops ➡ by a right-sided soft tissue mass ➡. CT was performed next in this child due to suspicion for a neoplasm.* (Right) *Coronal CECT in the same patient confirms a large, heterogeneous, solid mass ➡ arising from the right kidney. A residual "claw" of normal renal tissue ➡ is splayed along the upper pole of this Wilms tumor. No contralateral lesions or venous invasion were identified.*

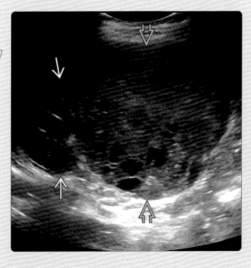
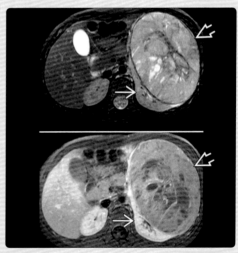

(Left) *Longitudinal US in a 5 year old with hypertension & abdominal fullness shows a round heterogeneous mass ➡ extending out of the lower pole of the left kidney ➡. Wilms tumor was confirmed upon surgery.* (Right) *Axial T2 (top) & T1 C+ (bottom) FS MR images show a large, well-defined, heterogeneous mass ➡ arising from a splayed "claw" of the left kidney ➡ in a 6 year old with a Wilms tumor.*

Wilms Tumor

TERMINOLOGY

Definitions

- Malignant tumor of primitive metanephric blastema

IMAGING

General Features

- Location: > 90% unilateral, 5-10% bilateral
- Size: Typically large (mean diameter: 5-10 cm)
- Morphology: Usually spherical with smooth contours; may be lobulated, multicentric, or have local extension

Radiographic Findings

- Mass displacing adjacent bowel

Ultrasonographic Findings

- Large, hypoechoic, heterogeneous mass
- May see local invasion & adenopathy
- Color Doppler can be useful to detect tumor thrombus vs. compression of veins by bulky mass

CT Findings

- Large, poorly enhancing, heterogeneous mass replacing most of kidney; "claw" of residual kidney along tumor margin
- Displaces adjacent organs, especially bowel
- ± adjacent adenopathy
- Predilection for invasion of renal vein & inferior vena cava
- May have local extension into perirenal fat or gross tumor rupture with distant ascites
- Lung metastases in 10-20% at time of diagnosis
  - Well-defined solid nodules

MR Findings

- Generally follows CECT characteristics
- MR venography useful in detecting vascular invasion

Imaging Recommendations

- Best imaging tool
  - Ultrasound often performed initially for palpable mass
  - CECT or MR to further characterize tumor, local extent, adenopathy
    - MR better for detection of contralateral lesions
  - Chest radiograph or CT for staging

DIFFERENTIAL DIAGNOSIS

Neuroblastoma

- Suprarenal (adrenal gland) or paraspinal (sympathetic chain)
  - Typically displaces rather than invades kidney
- Much more likely than Wilms to contain Ca^{2+}, cross midline, & engulf or "lift" adjacent vessels

Congenital Mesoblastic Nephroma

- Solid or mixed solid & cystic tumor of infants
  - > 90% diagnosed in 1st year of life
  - Most common renal tumor < 3 months old

Renal Cell Carcinoma

- Solid renal mass typically seen in 2nd decade of life
- Incidence equal to Wilms after 12 years old

Clear Cell Sarcoma

- Solid renal mass with skeletal metastases at diagnosis

Pyelonephritis

- Renal abscess usually more infiltrative than neoplasm
- Clinical & laboratory features of upper UTI often present

PATHOLOGY

General Features

- Etiology
  - Primitive metanephric blastema differentiates by 34 weeks gestation; may persist as nephrogenic rests (nephroblastomatosis)
    - Found in 1% of infant autopsies
    - Wilms tumor develops in 30-44%
- Associated abnormalities
  - Overgrowth syndromes (Beckwith-Wiedemann, isolated hemihypertrophy)
  - WAGR syndrome: Wilms tumor, aniridia, genitourinary anomalies, mental retardation
  - Sporadic aniridia, Denys-Drash syndrome, Trisomy 18, Sotos syndrome, Bloom syndrome

CLINICAL ISSUES

Presentation

- Asymptomatic flank mass, hematuria, failure to thrive
- Less common: Hypertension, fever, anemia

Demographics

- Most common abdominal neoplasm ages 1-8 years old
- 80% occur < 5 years old; peak at 3.6 years old

Natural History & Prognosis

- Prognosis based on stage, tumor size, histology
- 5-year survival for localized abdominal disease > 90%

Treatment

- Upfront complete resection (nephrectomy) preferred
  - Limited uses of renal-sparing resection
- Preoperative chemotherapy for unresectable or bilateral tumors or tumor thrombus extending above hepatic veins
- Postoperative chemotherapy ± radiation

DIAGNOSTIC CHECKLIST

Consider

- Children with predisposing syndromes require ultrasound screening every 3 months until 8 years of age

SELECTED REFERENCES

1. Chung EM et al: Renal tumors of childhood: radiologic-pathologic correlation part 1. The 1st decade: from the Radiologic Pathology Archives. Radiographics. 36(2):499-522, 2016
2. Kieran K et al: Current surgical standards of care in Wilms tumor. Urol Oncol. 34(1):13-23, 2016
3. Servaes S et al: Comparison of diagnostic performance of CT and MRI for abdominal staging of pediatric renal tumors: a report from the Children's Oncology Group. Pediatr Radiol. 45(2):166-72, 2015

Pyelonephritis

TERMINOLOGY

- Acute infection of renal parenchyma; often difficult to clinically distinguish from lower UTI

IMAGING

- Imaging work-up of UTI controversial
  - See professional society guidelines
- With pyelonephritis, marked inflammatory response to renal parenchymal infection causes swelling that alters normal tissue properties & effectively ↓ radiologic contrast agent delivery to site, which results in
  - ↓ uptake on nuclear cortical scan
  - ↓ perfusion on Doppler imaging with altered echotexture on grayscale US
  - Striated or wedge-shaped foci of ↓ enhancement on CECT/MR
- US with Doppler least invasive & readily available but less sensitive than nuclear renal cortical scans, CT, & MR

- US frequently performed to search for associated complications (abscess, stones, scarring), congenital anomalies, & hydronephrosis

CLINICAL ISSUES

- Symptoms nonspecific: Malaise, irritability, fever, abdominal/flank pain, vomiting, hematuria, dysuria, change in urinary habits/enuresis, strong-smelling urine
- Treatment: 7- to 14-day course of antimicrobial therapy; may be started IV & changed to oral
  - Obtain work-up for vesicoureteral reflux (VUR) & congenital anomalies
    - Pyelonephritis associated with VUR in ~ 25-40%
- Complications: Perirenal abscess, necrotizing papillitis, pyonephrosis (obstruction), & cortical scarring
  - Permanent scarring more likely < 2 years old
  - Recurrent infections & scarring can lead to hypertension &/or end-stage renal disease

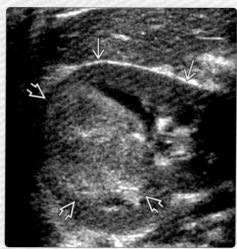

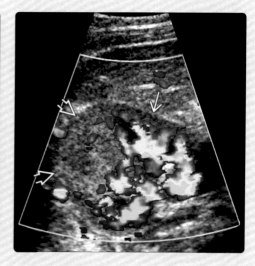

(Left) Transverse US of the mid right kidney ➡ shows a focus of increased echogenicity ⇒ with loss of normal corticomedullary differentiation, typical of pyelonephritis. (Right) Transverse color Doppler US of the same right kidney ➡ shows decreased perfusion ⇒ in the area of pyelonephritis due to marked swelling & inflammatory response.

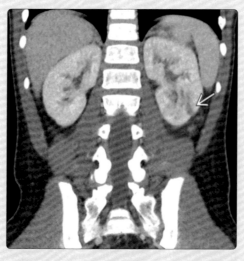

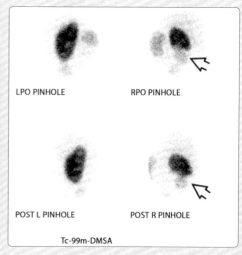

(Left) Coronal CECT image in a 13 year old scanned for possible appendicitis shows focal decreased enhancement ➡ in the left renal lower pole with adjacent fat stranding, consistent with pyelonephritis. (Right) Posterior pinhole images from Tc-99m DMSA renal cortical scintigraphy show absent radiotracer in the lower pole of the right kidney ⇒ in a patient with acute pyelonephritis. Large, wedge-shaped photopenic areas suggest pyelonephritis, while smaller, crescent-shaped cortical defects suggest scarring.

LPO PINHOLE   RPO PINHOLE

POST L PINHOLE   POST R PINHOLE

Tc-99m-DMSA

TERMINOLOGY

Synonyms

- Acute lobar nephronia, focal bacterial nephritis

Definitions

- Acute infection of renal parenchyma

IMAGING

General Features

- Best diagnostic clue
  - Inflammatory response to renal parenchymal infection causes swelling with focal ↓ in blood flow & delivery of radiologic contrast agents

Ultrasonographic Findings

- Grayscale ultrasound
  - Localized or generalized swelling; unilateral renal enlargement may be only clue to pyelonephritis
  - Poor corticomedullary differentiation with focal areas of ↑ or ↓ echogenicity
  - Occasionally, rounded or mass-like areas of altered echotexture noted
- Color Doppler
  - ↓ perfusion noted in areas of pyelonephritis
    - Power Doppler US improves accuracy & sensitivity
  - ↑ resistive indices (not specific)

CT Findings

- CECT
  - Wedge-shaped areas of poor enhancement
    - Enhancement may be striated
  - Inflamed parenchyma can be mass-like
    - Can distort normal renal contour & appear as partially cystic neoplasm during abscess development
  - Inflammatory changes in perirenal fat

Nuclear Medicine Findings

- Tc-99m DMSA or glucoheptonate for renal cortical scan
  - ↓ accumulation of agent, typically in wedge-shaped distribution that points toward renal hilum
    - Findings persist for up to 6 weeks
    - No volume loss until scarring ensues

Imaging Recommendations

- Best imaging tool
  - US with Doppler readily available & least invasive but less sensitive than nuclear renal cortical scans, CECT, & MR
  - US frequently performed to search for associated complications (abscess, stones, scarring), congenital anomalies, & hydronephrosis

DIFFERENTIAL DIAGNOSIS

Renal Infarction

- Wedge-shaped pattern of ↓ perfusion
- Retained thin rim of capsular enhancement
- May see abnormalities of vessels

Renal Scarring

- Associated cortical volume loss & dilated calyx

Renal Neoplasm

- Well-circumscribed mass, typically round & large

PATHOLOGY

General Features

- Etiology
  - Renal infection may occur via ascending route from vesicoureteral reflux (VUR) or by hematogenous spread
    - Associated with VUR in ~ 25-40%

CLINICAL ISSUES

Presentation

- Most common signs/symptoms
  - Malaise, irritability, fever, abdominal/flank pain, vomiting, hematuria, dysuria, change in urinary habits/enuresis
- Other signs/symptoms
  - Strong-smelling urine in any age
- Laboratory studies
  - Urine dipstick for nitrite, leukocyte esterase; both associated with higher likelihood of positive urine culture
  - Urine for Gram stain; *Escherichia coli* causative in > 80% of 1st-time UTIs, *Klebsiella* 2nd most common
    - Urine specimen for culture: Catheter specimen, clean-catch midstream, or suprapubic aspirate
    - Urine culture considered positive when single organism grows as follows
      - □ > 1,000 colony-forming units (cfu)/mL for suprapubic aspirate
      - □ Or > 10,000 cfu/mL for catheter specimen
      - □ Or > 100,000 cfu/mL for clean-catch midstream specimen
  - Bloodwork: Leukocytosis, occasionally positive blood cultures as well
- Complications
  - Renal or perirenal abscess, necrotizing papillitis, pyonephrosis (obstruction), & cortical scarring
    - Recent study found that 1/2 of all patients with acute pyelonephritis went on to develop scarring
    - Scarring may be greater in younger patients

Natural History & Prognosis

- Excellent (in absence of complications or recurrence)
  - Renal scarring from recurrent infections may lead to hypertension & chronic renal failure

Treatment

- 7- to 14-day course of antimicrobial therapy; may be started IV & changed to oral
- Imaging work-up for VUR & congenital anomalies
- Prophylactic antibiotics for VUR & other predisposing conditions controversial

SELECTED REFERENCES

1. de Bessa J Jr et al: Antibiotic prophylaxis for prevention of febrile urinary tract infections in children with vesicoureteral reflux: a meta-analysis of randomized, controlled trials comparing dilated to nondilated vesicoureteral reflux. J Urol. 193(5 Suppl):1772-7, 2015
2. Morello W et al: Acute pyelonephritis in children. Pediatr Nephrol. 31(8):1253-65, 2015
3. Narchi H et al: Renal tract abnormalities missed in a historical cohort of young children with UTI if the NICE and AAP imaging guidelines were applied. J Pediatr Urol. 11(5):252.e1-7, 2015

TERMINOLOGY

- Definition: Concretion in urinary system

IMAGING

- Most stones seen in kidneys & upper urinary tract
- Range in size from 1-2 mm to > 1 cm
- NECT most sensitive modality to detect stones
  - Calcified density in urinary system
- Ultrasound shows hyperechoic urinary tract focus with posterior acoustic shadowing &/or twinkle artifact
- Signs of obstruction (US/CT/MR)
  - Hydroureteronephrosis
  - Nephromegaly
  - Perinephric/periureteral edema
  - Lack of ureteral jet in urinary bladder on Doppler ultrasound
  - High-resistance renal artery flow on Doppler ultrasound
  - Delayed renal enhancement & excretion after IV contrast administration

TOP DIFFERENTIAL DIAGNOSES

- Phleboliths
- Nephrocalcinosis
- Ureteropelvic junction obstruction

CLINICAL ISSUES

- Presentations: 94% of adolescents have colicky flank pain; younger children have nonspecific symptoms (abdominal pain, nausea, vomiting, & irritability)
  - Hematuria microscopic in up to 90%, gross in up to 32%
  - Concomitant urinary tract infection in 8-20%
- Treatment: Depends on stone size, location, presence of obstruction, & underlying etiology
  - Analgesia, ↑ fluid intake
    - Up to 60% of stones < 5 mm pass spontaneously
  - Surgical management required in 22%: Extracorporeal shock wave lithotripsy, ureteroscopy, or percutaneous nephrolithotomy

(Left) Transverse ultrasounds of the left kidney in an adolescent with left flank pain show an echogenic focus ➡ within the renal collecting system. With color Doppler ultrasound, there is considerable twinkle artifact ➡ posterior to the echogenic focus, typical of a calculus. (Right) Coronal NECT in the same patient shows a small nonobstructing calcified stone ➡ in the lower pole of the left kidney. Approximately 75% of pediatric patients with renal stones have an identifiable predisposition to stone formation.

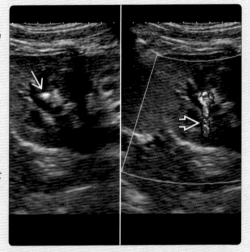
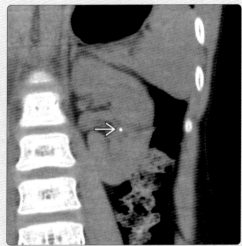

(Left) AP radiograph of the abdomen in an adolescent shows a small calcified stone ➡ inferior & medial to the right renal shadow ➡, likely in the proximal ureter. (Right) Retrograde pyelogram in the same patient shows a small filling defect ➡ in the midportion of the right ureter at the level of the nonobstructing stone.

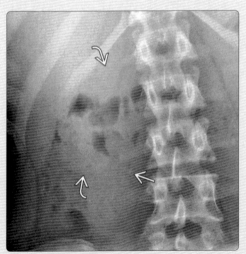
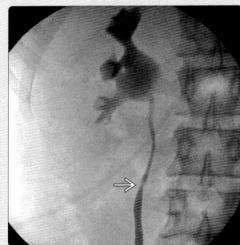

TERMINOLOGY

Synonyms

- Nephrolithiasis, nephrolith, urolithiasis, urolith, urinary stone, kidney stone, renal calculi

Definitions

- Concretion in urinary system

IMAGING

Radiographic Findings

- Radiography
  - Focal Ca^{2+} over kidneys, ureters, or bladder
  - Can be used to follow radiographically visible stones
- IVP
  - Identifies obstructive calculi in known stone formers

CT Findings

- NECT
  - Focal Ca^{2+} in renal collecting system, ureters, or bladder
  - Stones can obstruct urinary system; most do not
    - Signs of obstruction: Hydronephrosis, hydroureter, perinephric or periureteral stranding, enlarged kidney, loss of slightly hyperattenuating renal pyramids
- CECT
  - Not primarily used for stone work-up
  - Obstructed kidney shows delayed enhancement

Ultrasonographic Findings

- Grayscale ultrasound
  - Hyperechoic focus ± posterior acoustic shadowing
  - Stones usually visible in kidney, proximal or distal ureter, or urinary bladder
    - Midureteral stones difficult to find due to bowel gas
  - Signs of obstruction: Hydronephrosis, hydroureter to level of urinary stone, enlarged kidney
- Color Doppler
  - Twinkle artifact: Color in/posterior to stone
  - Signs of obstruction: High-resistance renal artery flow, lack of ureteral jet in urinary bladder

Imaging Recommendations

- Best imaging tool
  - NECT most sensitive modality to detect stones
    - Often initial study in 1st-time stone disease
    - Beware multiple CTs due to radiation dose
  - In known stone formers, presence or absence of obstruction may be only imaging question
    - US detects urinary obstruction without radiation

DIFFERENTIAL DIAGNOSIS

Phleboliths

- Round Ca^{2+} with lucent center in abnormal stagnant vein
- Most common in pelvis, near bladder

Nephrocalcinosis

- Symmetric Ca^{2+} within bilateral renal parenchyma
  - Cortical, medullary, or diffuse

Ureteropelvic Junction Obstruction

- Chronically dilated renal collecting system due to intrinsic or extrinsic process; no visible stone

PATHOLOGY

General Features

- Etiology
  - 75% of children with stones have identifiable predisposition
    - Metabolic cause of stones in 40-50% of patients
    - Structural urinary tract anomalies in 30% of patients
    - Infection in 4% of patients
- Metabolic causes of pediatric stone disease
  - Calcium stones
    - Hypercalciuria: Most common metabolic abnormality causing pediatric stones
      - Accounts for 34-50% of children with identifiable metabolic cause of stones
    - Hyperuricosuria: Can be caused by excess purine production or ingestion, renal tubular disorders, medications, or juvenile gout
      - Present in 2-20% of children with stones
    - Hypocitruria: Can be caused by renal tubular acidosis
      - 10% of children with stones
    - Hyperoxaluria: Can be caused by primary hyperoxaluria or ↑ intestinal absorption due to bowel disease
      - Found in 10-20% of children with stones
  - Uric acid stones: Seen with excessively acidic urine such as in diarrheal states or diet high in animal protein
    - Radiolucent stones
  - Struvite stones: Caused by urease-splitting bacteria
    - Often appear as staghorn calculi

CLINICAL ISSUES

Presentation

- Most common signs/symptoms
  - Depends on age
    - 94% of adolescents present with colicky flank pain
    - Nonspecific symptoms (abdominal pain, nausea, vomiting, & irritability) in younger children
  - Microscopic hematuria in up to 90% of patients
- Other signs/symptoms
  - Gross hematuria in up to 32%
  - Concomitant urinary tract infection in 8-20%

Treatment

- Analgesia, ↑ fluid intake
  - Up to 60% of stones < 5 mm pass spontaneously
- Medical treatment depends on underlying cause
- Surgical management required in 22%
  - Extracorporeal shock wave lithotripsy, ureteroscopy, or percutaneous nephrolithotomy

SELECTED REFERENCES

1. Chen TT et al: Radiation exposure during the evaluation and management of nephrolithiasis. J Urol. 194(4):878-85, 2015
2. Hernandez JD et al: Current trends, evaluation, and management of pediatric nephrolithiasis. JAMA Pediatr. 169(10):964-70, 2015

KEY FACTS

IMAGING

- CECT for abdominal trauma typically done in late cortical or early nephrographic phase
  - Delayed images for collecting system injury if renal laceration or perinephric fluid found on initial images
- CECT findings include
  - Renal parenchymal contusion, laceration
  - Subcapsular or perinephric/perirenal hematoma
  - Collecting system/ureteropelvic junction (UPJ) laceration
  - Active hemorrhage: High attenuation (isodense to vessel) nonanatomic collection on initial images; accumulates on delayed images
  - Vascular thrombosis or avulsion: Delayed or persistent renal enhancement vs. subtotal or global nonenhancement
- US sensitivity varies widely (23-100%) across studies; contrast-enhanced US may have future role

CLINICAL ISSUES

- Etiology: Blunt trauma 90% (motor vehicle-related > falls > sports-related, abuse & assault > bicycle accidents), penetrating trauma 10%
  - Renal injuries found in up to 19% of abdominal trauma from child abuse
  - Rapid deceleration: ↑ risk of vascular pedicle & UPJ injury
- Presentation: Flank pain, hematuria, ecchymosis
- Nonoperative management in stable patients: 85%
- Early complications (< 4 weeks): Urinoma (most common but most reabsorb), delayed bleeding, perinephric abscess, sepsis, infected urinoma
- Late complications (> 4 weeks): Page kidney (hypertension due to renal compression by subcapsular hematoma → ↓ renal perfusion → activates renin-angiotensin system), hydronephrosis, calculi, chronic pyelonephritis

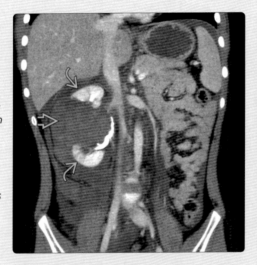
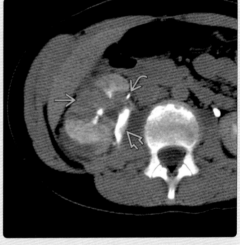

(Left) Coronal CECT shows a transected right kidney with separation of the renal poles ⬈ by a hematoma ⬊ along the fracture plane. (Right) Delayed axial CECT in a 15-year-old boy after a snowmobile accident shows a right renal grade IV laceration ⬊ that extends to the UPJ. Extravasation of contrast-opacified urine is noted ⬊. The ureter distal to the injury is opacified with contrast ⬈, indicating that the UPJ tear is incomplete.

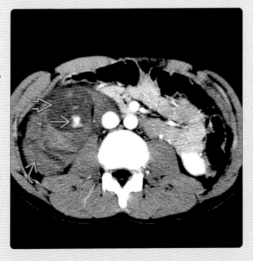
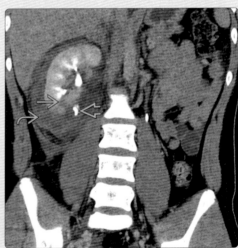

(Left) Axial CECT of a 15 year old after a football injury shows active arterial extravasation ⬊ along a devascularized right renal lower pole ⬊. There is a large perinephric hematoma ⬊. (Right) Delayed coronal CECT on a follow-up exam in a 14-year-old boy after a skiing accident shows a grade IV laceration ⬊ with urinary contrast extravasation ⬊ from the lower pole collecting system. The perinephric urinoma ⬊ had increased in size compared to the initial study, requiring a ureteral stent.

Renal Vein Thrombosis

KEY FACTS

TERMINOLOGY

- Obstruction of renal vein(s) by thrombus

IMAGING

- Ultrasound with Doppler
  - Enlarged, echogenic kidney with ↓ corticomedullary differentiation
  - ± visualization of main renal vein thrombus
  - High-resistance renal arterial waveforms (RI > 0.9)
    - May see complete diastolic flow reversal
- CECT/MR
  - Heterogeneous or delayed renal enhancement
  - ± filling defect in renal vein with inferior vena cava extension
- Chronic appearance: Renal atrophy ± Ca^{2+}
- Associated adrenal hemorrhage or Ca^{2+} may be present

TOP DIFFERENTIAL DIAGNOSES

- Acute tubular necrosis
- Pyelonephritis
- Transient neonatal renal medullary hyperechogenicity
- Tumor thrombus

PATHOLOGY

- In neonates, thrombosis begins in small intrarenal veins → proximal extension to main renal vein
  - ↑ renal venous pressure & ↓ arterial flow
- Etiologies: Dehydration, sepsis/infection, iatrogenic

CLINICAL ISSUES

- Most commonly diagnosed in neonatal period
  - Renal dysfunction, oliguria, hypertension
  - Classic triad of palpable flank mass, hematuria, & thrombocytopenia usually absent
- Irreversible damage occurs in 70%
  - Up to 20% will have persistent hypertension
- Treatment controversial & may depend upon comorbidities
  - Supportive, ± anticoagulation, rarely thrombolysis

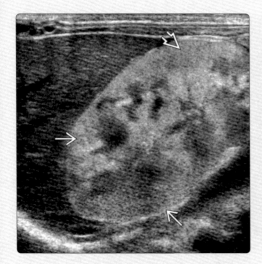
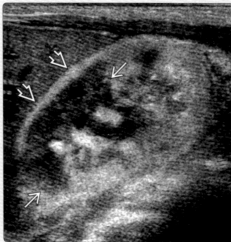

(Left) Longitudinal oblique US in a newborn shows an enlarged, hyperechoic right kidney with poorly defined hypoechoic medullary pyramids in the upper pole ➡. Corticomedullary differentiation is lost in the lower pole ➡. (Right) Longitudinal US obtained 2 days later shows progressive ischemia in the upper pole with a new large hypoechoic focus involving the medulla & cortex ➡. A thin rim of echogenic peripheral cortex ➡ remains.

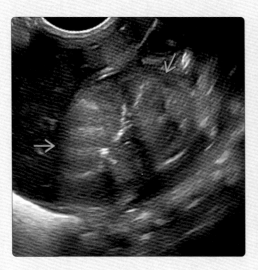
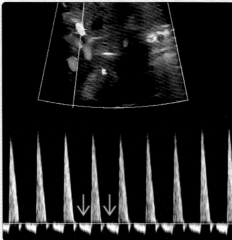

(Left) Longitudinal US in a newborn with oliguria shows diffusely increased echogenicity of the right kidney ➡ with diminished corticomedullary differentiation due to renal vein thrombosis. Scattered echogenic striations are noted. (Right) Pulsed Doppler US in the same newborn with renal vein thrombosis shows a high-resistance renal arterial waveform with complete reversal of diastolic flow ➡, a typical finding with renal vein thrombosis.

TERMINOLOGY

- Bladder dysfunction secondary to neurologic disorder
- Classification: Contractile bladders (hyperreflexive detrusor), intermediate (mixed) bladders, acontractile bladders (detrusor areflexia)

IMAGING

- Voiding cystourethrogram &/or US
  - Towering bladder with thickened trabeculations
  - Bladder volume variable, ranging from small & contracted to large & atonic
  - Involuntary, uninhibited detrusor contractions
  - High filling pressure resulting in ↓ rate of filling or spontaneous cessation of contrast infusion
  - Voiding dysfunction from inhibited micturition reflex
  - ↑ postvoid residual
  - Secondary bladder & upper tract abnormalities
    - Vesicoureteral reflux, functional obstruction, scarring

PATHOLOGY

- Etiologies: Myelodysplasia, sacral agenesis, cerebral palsy, traumatic spinal cord lesions
- Associated abnormalities: Anorectal malformations, lipomeningocele, caudal regression, occult congenital spinal dysraphism, spinal cord tethering

CLINICAL ISSUES

- Presentation: Failure to empty bladder, frequency, nocturia, urgency, retention, incontinence, lower & upper UTI, bladder stones, hematuria
- Complications: Pyelonephritis, hydronephrosis, urolithiasis, epididymitis, sexual dysfunction, autonomic dysreflexia
- Without intervention, 50% show upper urinary tract deterioration in first 5 years of life
- Therapeutic maneuvers: Clean intermittent catheterization, medications (antibiotics, anticholinergics), surgical procedures (operation for continence, bladder augmentation, artificial sphincters)

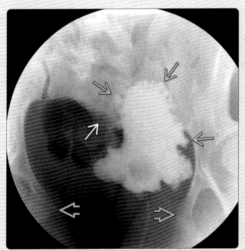
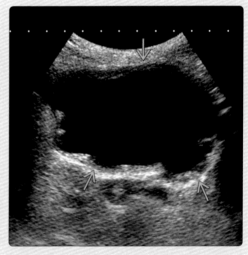

(Left) Voiding cystourethrogram in a teenage girl with a cloacal exstrophy variant & a neurogenic bladder (NGB) who catheterizes 4x/day shows a small hypertonic bladder with trabeculation & multiple diverticula/pseudodiverticula ➡. Note the pubic symphysis diastasis ➡ & sacral truncation ➡ of cloacal exstrophy. (Right) Transverse US in the same patient with a cloacal exstrophy variant shows a trabeculated, lobulated, & thickened urinary bladder ➡.

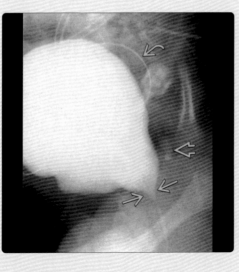
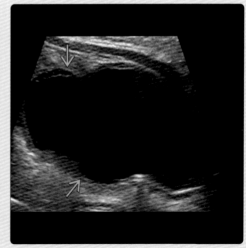

(Left) Oblique cystogram in a 7 day old status post myelomeningocele (MMC) repair shows an atonic, mildly lobular, large capacity bladder with no wall thickening, an open bladder neck ➡, left vesicoureteral reflux ➡, & no significant bladder emptying due to an atonic detrusor, consistent with NGB. Note the ventriculoperitoneal shunt catheter ➡. (Right) Transverse US in the same patient after MMC repair shows a large, mildly lobular bladder ➡ with mild wall thickening in this atonic-type NGB.

Bladder Diverticula

KEY FACTS

TERMINOLOGY

- Herniation of urinary bladder mucosa through bladder detrusor muscle
  - Primary (congenital, 10%): Poor muscular backing near ureterovesical junction (UVJ)
    - Periureteral (Hutch) type most common
  - Secondary (acquired, 90%): Chronically elevated bladder pressures, weak bladder wall in connective tissue disorders, iatrogenic/traumatic causes (prior surgery/catheter)

IMAGING

- Best diagnostic clues
  - Round cystic focus directly adjacent to bladder
    - Changes size with bladder filling &/or voiding
    - Anechoic on ultrasound; ± jet of urine into bladder
    - Fills with contrast on VCUG/CECT/MR
- Diverticula with narrow neck may be small or absent during bladder filling & only seen with voiding

- Contrast may remain after bladder emptying
- Vesicoureteral reflux (VUR) in 50%
  - Large diverticulum incorporates & distorts UVJ → VUR
- Without history of neurogenic bladder or bladder outlet obstruction, multiple diverticula should suggest syndromes
  - Williams, Menkes, Ehlers-Danlos, cutis laxa

TOP DIFFERENTIAL DIAGNOSES

- Everting ureterocele, ureteral stump, ovarian/paraovarian cyst, gastrointestinal duplication cyst

CLINICAL ISSUES

- Presentation: Most commonly asymptomatic
  - May also have urinary tract infection, hematuria, voiding dysfunction, pain
- Complications of stagnant urine (infection, hematuria, calculi) &/or deformed UVJ (VUR or obstruction) determine need for operative treatment
  - Resection of diverticulum ± ureteral reimplantation

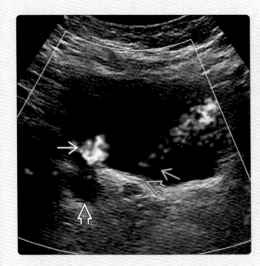

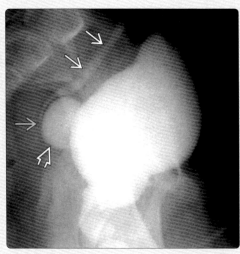

(Left) Transverse color Doppler ultrasound of the urinary bladder shows not only a jet of urine ➡ draining from a diverticulum ➡ but also a jet of urine ➡ emanating from the adjacent ureteral orifice ➡ in this patient with a periureteral (Hutch) diverticulum. (Right) Lateral fluoroscopic VCUG shows VUR ➡ accompanying a periureteral diverticulum ➡. In this case, the ureter inserts directly into the diverticulum ➡, which is important information for the urologist making management decisions.

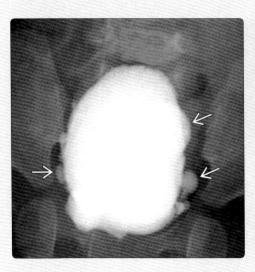

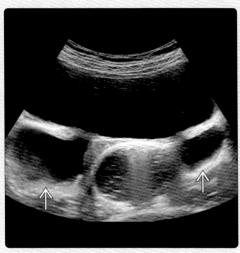

(Left) Frontal fluoroscopic VCUG of an infant girl's bladder at capacity shows multiple diverticula ➡. If there are no clinical findings of neurogenic bladder or bladder outlet obstruction, considerations should include Williams, Menkes, Ehlers-Danlos, or cutis laxa syndromes. (Right) Transverse ultrasound in a patient with Menkes syndrome shows 2 posterior diverticula ➡ with a small amount of debris in the larger right diverticulum. Multiple other diverticula were also present (not shown).

TERMINOLOGY

- Malignant tumor of striated muscle originating from any pelvic organ

IMAGING

- Best clue: Large, heterogeneous, predominantly solid pelvic mass in child with symptoms of urinary tract obstruction
  - Variable cystic components
  - Botryoid variety resembles "bunch of grapes" with cysts protruding into lumen of vagina or urinary bladder
- May originate from bladder, vagina, cervix, uterus, prostate, & paratesticular tissues
  - May also occur in adjacent non-GU soft tissues
- Tumors spread by local extension plus lymphatic & hematogenous routes (to lungs, liver, & bone)
  - 15-20% have metastases at diagnosis
- Work-up typically includes
  - US for initial investigation of urinary tract symptoms or palpable mass

- CECT or MR for tumor characterization & localization
- Staging with chest CT & PET

PATHOLOGY

- Small round blue cell tumor of primitive muscle cells
- Major histologic types: Embryonal (majority, especially in GU sites), alveolar, & undifferentiated (adults)

CLINICAL ISSUES

- Peak incidence: 2-6 years old; 75% < 5 years old
- ↑ incidence in certain syndromes: Neurofibromatosis type 1, Li-Fraumeni, Rubinstein-Taybi, Beckwith-Wiedemann
- Presents with palpable mass, dysuria, hematuria, frequency, urinary retention, vaginal discharge, &/or constipation
- Treated with surgery, chemotherapy, & radiation
- 5-year survival: Stage I (93%) vs. stage IV (~ 30%)
  - Embryonal type has better prognosis than alveolar
  - Bladder & prostate unfavorable, automatically ≥ stage II

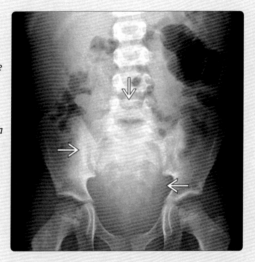

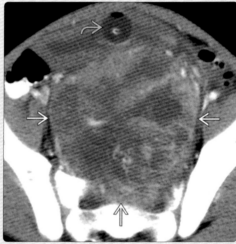

(Left) AP radiograph of a 6-year-old boy shows displacement of bowel by a soft tissue mass ➡ in the pelvis, initially suspected to be due to urinary retention but not relieved by bladder catheterization. (Right) Axial CECT in the same 6 year old with urinary retention shows a large, heterogeneously enhancing mass ➡ displacing the urinary bladder (with Foley balloon in place ➡) anteriorly. This mass was a prostatic origin rhabdomyosarcoma (RMS).

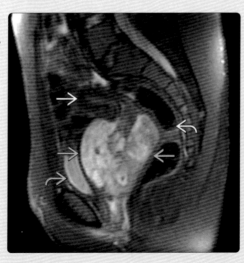

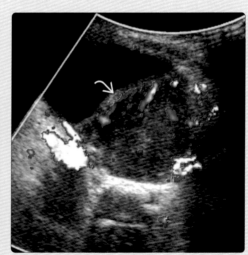

(Left) Sagittal T2 FS MR in a 14-year-old girl shows a heterogeneous mass filling the vagina ➡. The mass displaces the uterus superiorly ➡, the bladder anteriorly ➡, & the rectum posteriorly ➡. RMS was confirmed on biopsy. (Right) Transverse color Doppler US of a patient with hematuria shows blood flow ➡ within a bladder mass, making benign entities such as a clot or fungus ball unlikely. RMS was confirmed on biopsy.

Neonatal Adrenal Hemorrhage

KEY FACTS

TERMINOLOGY

- Perinatal bleeding into normal adrenal gland
  - Associated with many perinatal stressors: Asphyxia, sepsis, birth trauma, coagulopathies
  - ↑ frequency in full-term & large infants

IMAGING

- Right > left; bilateral in 5-10%
- US: Echogenic avascular mass replacing or expanding newborn adrenal gland
  - Appearance varies with timing of imaging
    - Acute: Hemorrhage appears echogenic & mass-like
    - Subacute: Blood products liquefy & contract, creating mixed echotexture mass
    - Chronic: Adrenal resumes normal size, ± Ca²⁺ or cyst
- CT, MR: Nonenhancing ± rim of enhancing adrenal
  - MR may show characteristic features of blood products
- Radiographs (months to years later): Small unilateral or bilateral adreniform Ca²⁺

TOP DIFFERENTIAL DIAGNOSES

- Neuroblastoma
- Congenital adrenal hyperplasia
- Extralobar bronchopulmonary sequestration

CLINICAL ISSUES

- Newborns may present with anemia, dropping hematocrit, jaundice, palpable mass, or adrenal insufficiency
- Observation in most cases: Blood gradually liquefies & retracts
- Medical therapy for adrenal insufficiency rarely needed

DIAGNOSTIC CHECKLIST

- In neonate: Follow-up US in 2-6 weeks to confirm expected evolution with ↓ size; if larger or more solid, work-up for neuroblastoma
- In older child with incidental radiographic paraspinal Ca²⁺: If morphology & extent unclear, start with abdominal US to exclude neuroblastoma

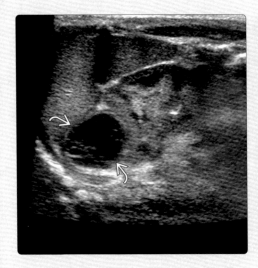
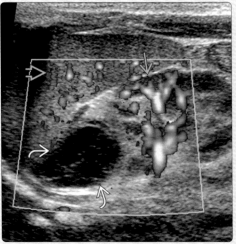

(Left) Longitudinal US shows a complex cystic lesion ➰ in the adrenal gland of a neonate. There are many thin internal septations in this case of subacute neonatal adrenal hemorrhage. Adrenal hemorrhages are fairly common in neonates who are stressed by congenital heart disease, surgery, ECMO, sepsis, etc. (Right) Longitudinal power Doppler US of the same adrenal hemorrhage shows absence of blood flow in the lesion ➰ with normal perfusion of the adjacent kidney ➡ & spleen ➡. Gradual resolution was noted.

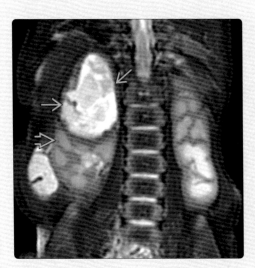
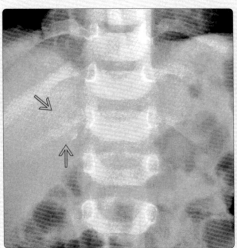

(Left) Coronal T2 FS MR in a 20 day old with left prenatal hydronephrosis shows a heterogeneous right suprarenal mass ➡ deforming the right kidney ➡. Serial US scans showed progressive decrease in the size of the mass over the next 5 weeks. (Right) AP radiograph in the same patient 18 months later shows a small residual suprarenal Ca²⁺ ➡, consistent with a remote adrenal hemorrhage.

TERMINOLOGY

- Malignant tumor of sympathetic chain primitive neural crest cells
- Increasing degrees of cellular differentiation/benignity along spectrum: Neuroblastoma (malignant) → ganglioneuroblastoma → ganglioneuroma (benign)

IMAGING

- Location
  - Adrenal (35-48%)
  - Extraadrenal retroperitoneum (25-35%)
  - Posterior mediastinum (16-20%)
- Small round solitary mass vs. large multilobulated lesion
- Aggressive tumor with tendency to invade adjacent tissues
- Frequently engulfs & displaces adjacent vascular structures (rather than just displacing)
- Ca²⁺ in up to 90% by CT
- Metastases in 50-60% at diagnosis, most commonly to bone, lymph nodes, liver, soft tissues

TOP DIFFERENTIAL DIAGNOSES

- Wilms tumor
- Neonatal adrenal hemorrhage
- Less common adrenal tumors
- Other cystic/solid suprarenal lesions

CLINICAL ISSUES

- Most common extracranial solid malignancy in children
- Median age at diagnosis: 15-17 months
- Wide variety of clinical presentations: Most commonly presents as palpable abdominal mass
- Features associated with better prognosis
  - Age at diagnosis < 18 months
  - Stage 4S/MS
  - Localized tumor not involving vital structures
  - Absent *MYCN* (*N-myc*) oncogene amplification

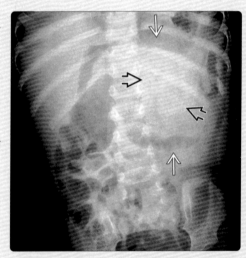
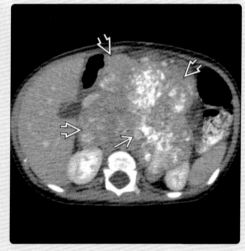

(Left) *Supine AP abdominal radiograph in a 1-year-old boy with a palpable abdominal mass shows displacement of bowel loops ➡ by a large, heterogeneously calcified mass ➡ in the left abdomen.* (Right) *Axial CECT in the same patient shows the large, lobulated, calcified mass ➡ crossing the midline. The mass encases & lifts the aorta ➡ off of the spine. These features are typical of neuroblastoma (NBL).*

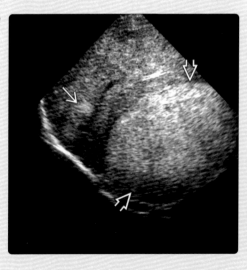
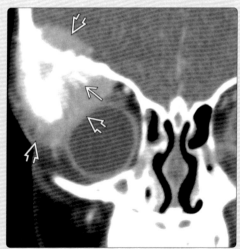

(Left) *Sagittal abdominal US in a young child shows a large, ovoid, right suprarenal mass ➡ with diffusely increased echogenicity. The liver also shows scattered foci of increased echogenicity ➡, which proved to be NBL metastases.* (Right) *Coronal CECT in a 2-year-old patient presenting with eye swelling shows an enhancing mass ➡ arising from the superolateral right orbital wall & extending circumferentially into the adjacent soft tissues. The aggressive periosteal reaction ➡ is typical of NBL metastases in the skull.*

TERMINOLOGY

Definitions

- Malignant tumor of sympathetic chain primitive neural crest cells
- Increasing degrees of cellular differentiation/benignity along spectrum: Neuroblastoma [(NBL), malignant] → ganglioneuroblastoma → ganglioneuroma (benign)

IMAGING

General Features

- Location
  - Anywhere along sympathetic chain from neck to pelvis
    - Adrenal (35-48%), extraadrenal retroperitoneum (25-35%), posterior mediastinum (16-20%), pelvis (2-3%), neck (1-5%), metastatic disease with no primary identified (1%)
- General imaging features
  - Small, round, solitary suprarenal/paraspinal mass vs. large, lobulated lesion crossing midline
  - Aggressive tumor, may invade adjacent tissues
    - Intraspinal invasion via neural foramina
    - Kidney, muscle
  - Frequently engulfs & displaces adjacent vascular structures (rather than just displacing/compressing)
  - Ca^{2+} in up to 90% by CT, only 30% by radiographs
  - Metastases in 50-60% at diagnosis, most commonly to bone, lymph nodes, liver, soft tissues

Radiographic Findings

- Often occult or subtle by radiographs
- Displacement of bowel by soft tissue mass
- Widening of inferior thoracic paraspinal soft tissues
- Bone metastasis
  - May be extensive with little radiographic presence (especially marrow disease)
  - May be only presenting clinical/imaging finding

Imaging Recommendations

- Best imaging tool
  - US excellent 1st-line modality for palpable abdominal mass in child
  - MR increasingly used over CT for characterizing tumor & defining extent at diagnosis & follow-up
  - MIBG remains favored nuclear medicine study for diagnosis, staging, follow-up

DIFFERENTIAL DIAGNOSIS

Wilms Tumor

- Mean age: 3 years
- Ca^{2+} uncommon
- Grows like ball, displacing vessels
- Arises from kidney: Claw sign of residual renal parenchyma

Neonatal Adrenal Hemorrhage

- Cystic &/or solid-appearing avascular suprarenal mass
- Serial US show gradual ↓ in size with ↑ Ca^{2+}

Less Common Adrenal Tumors

- Pheochromocytoma (uncommon in young children)
- Adrenal cortical neoplasms (usually hormonally active)

Other Cystic/Solid Suprarenal Lesions

- Extralobar bronchopulmonary sequestration
- Foregut duplication cyst

PATHOLOGY

Staging, Grading, & Classification

- International NBL Staging System
  - Original 1-4S system based on resection, pathology
  - Used for risk groups by Children's Oncology Group (COG)
- International NBL Risk Group Staging System
  - More comprehensive, imaging-based system
  - Used to stratify as very low, low, intermediate, or high risk in conjunction with age, genetics, histology
    - May replace COG risk stratification

CLINICAL ISSUES

Presentation

- Most common signs/symptoms
  - Painless abdominal mass
- Other signs/symptoms
  - Malaise, irritability, weight loss, limping, opsoclonus-myoclonus, Horner syndrome, cerebellar ataxia, neurologic symptoms related to compression, hypertension, watery diarrhea with hypokalemia
  - Classic presentations
    - Skin metastases: Blueberry muffin syndrome
    - Skull base metastases: "Raccoon eyes"
    - Massive liver metastases: Pepper syndrome
  - 90-95% of NBL patients have elevated levels of catecholamines/metabolites (VMA, HVA) in urine

Demographics

- Median age at presentation: 15-17 months
- 95% diagnosed by 7 years

Natural History & Prognosis

- COG risk stratification
  - Low risk (30% of all NBL, 70% of neonatal NBL): 5-year survival > 95% with observation (select cases) or surgery
    - Spontaneous regression most likely in
      - Newborns with small adrenal lesions
      - Non-*MYCN*-amplified infants with localized disease or asymptomatic 4S/MS disease
  - Intermediate risk (20% of all NBL): 5-year survival > 90% with surgery + chemotherapy
  - High risk (50% of all NBL): 5-year survival of 30-40% with intensive multimodality therapy
    - May include myeloablative therapy with stem cell rescue, biologic agents, I-131 MIBG therapy, especially for refractory/recurrent disease

SELECTED REFERENCES

1. Irwin MS et al: Neuroblastoma: paradigm for precision medicine. Pediatr Clin North Am. 62(1):225-56, 2015
2. Maki E et al: Imaging and differential diagnosis of suprarenal masses in the fetus. J Ultrasound Med. 33(5):895-904, 2014
3. Fisher JP et al: Neonatal neuroblastoma. Semin Fetal Neonatal Med. 17(4):207-15, 2012
4. Brisse HJ et al: Guidelines for imaging and staging of neuroblastic tumors: consensus report from the International Neuroblastoma Risk Group Project. Radiology. 261(1):243-57, 2011

KEY FACTS

TERMINOLOGY

- Dilation of vagina ± uterus secondary to distal stenosis, atresia, transverse vaginal septum, or imperforate hymen
  - Prefix: Hydro meaning fluid, hemato meaning blood
  - Suffix: Metra meaning uterine cavity
  - Suffix: Metrocolpos meaning uterus & vagina

IMAGING

- Well-defined cystic or debris-filled mass in female pelvis between urinary bladder & rectum
- Vertically oriented in sagittal plane, round in axial plane
- Uterus frequently visible arising from dome of collection; may be normal or mildly distended (much less than vagina)
- US may show trilaminar appearance of vaginal wall, swirling internal debris, lack of internal vascularity
- MR often shows aging blood product signal intensities (↑ T1, ↓ T2); can help discern uterine & vaginal anomalies
- Urinary bladder or ureters may be obstructed
- Primary imaging modality for female GU anomalies: US

- MR used when uterine & complex GU anomalies cannot be clearly defined with US

PATHOLOGY

- Imperforate hymen more common cause than vaginal septum
- ± associated anal, renal, vertebral, & cardiac anomalies

CLINICAL ISSUES

- Bimodal age of presentation
  - Infants (due to maternal hormonal stimulation): Pelvic mass, sepsis, or urinary tract obstruction
  - Adolescent girls (pubertal onset): Delayed menarche, cyclic pelvic pain, mass, &/or urinary tract obstruction
- Typically drained with septum or stenotic segment excised from inferior approach with minimal tissue resected
- Immediate prognosis excellent though compromised fertility & endometriosis can be long-term complications

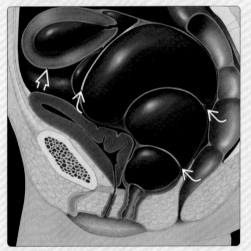
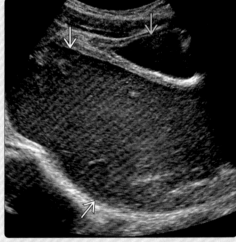

(Left) *Graphic shows potential levels of vaginal septa ➡ causing obstruction & hydro-/hematometrocolpos. Note that the vagina distends with trapped secretions & blood to a much greater degree than the uterus ➡. (Right) Longitudinal US through the pelvis of a 15-year-old girl with urinary retention, cramping, & no history of menses shows a large well-defined, vertically oriented, heterogeneous collection ➡ posterior to the urinary bladder ➡, suggestive of hematometrocolpos.*

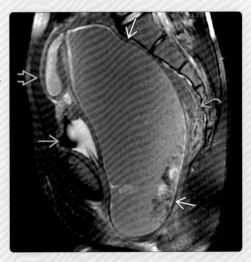
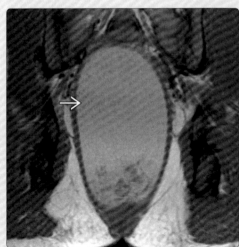

(Left) *Sagittal T2 FS MR in the same patient shows a markedly distended vagina ➡ containing heterogeneous fluid & layering debris. The uterus ➡ projects anteriorly & is much less distended than the vagina, findings typical of hematometrocolpos. Note the mass effect on the urinary bladder ➡ & rectum ➡. (Right) Coronal T1 MR in the same patient shows that the fluid in the vagina is predominantly hyperintense ➡, typical of blood products. A vaginal septum was resected, relieving the obstruction.*

Müllerian Duct Anomalies

TERMINOLOGY

- Abnormal development, improper fusion, or failure of resorption of müllerian (paramesonephric) duct structures
- Müllerian agenesis or hypoplasia (class I in American Fertility Society classification system): Complete or segmental agenesis or variable degrees of uterovaginal hypoplasia
- Unicornuate uterus (class II): Partial or complete unilateral hypoplasia
- Uterus didelphys (class III): Duplication of uterus
- Bicornuate uterus (class IV): Incomplete fusion of superior uterovaginal canal
- Septate uterus (class V): Incomplete resorption of uterine septum
- Arcuate uterus (class VI): Near complete resorption of uterine septum

IMAGING

- Abnormal contour of uterus &/or structural abnormality of endometrial cavity or vagina

- Septate uterus most common (55%)
- US initial tool for evaluating GU pathology
- MR best for definitive diagnosis
- Always image kidneys to look for renal anomaly

PATHOLOGY

- Renal anomaly present in ~ 30%
- Renal agenesis most common (~ 2/3)

CLINICAL ISSUES

- Incidence estimated at 1%
- May be asymptomatic vs. symptoms at menarche
  o Primary amenorrhea, dysmenorrhea, cyclic pain
- Natural history: Fertility issues, spontaneous abortions, ectopic pregnancy
- Treatment surgical: Remove rudimentary horn, resect septum, or relieve obstruction

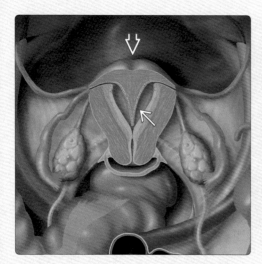

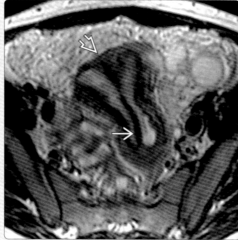

(Left) Graphic of a septate uterus shows minimal indentation of the uterine fundus ➡. There is myometrium in the superior aspect of the septum, though normal zonal anatomy is not present in this portion ➡. (Right) Axial T2 MR of a septate uterus shows that the outer fundal contour is smooth ➡ & the intercornual angle is < 75°. There is a low-signal fibrous septum extending along the length of the endometrial cavity ➡ to a single cervix.

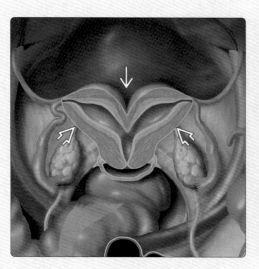

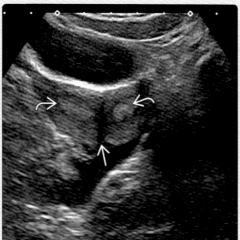

(Left) Graphic of a bicornuate uterus demonstrates a deep external fundal cleft ➡ & 2 symmetric cornua ➡ that are fused inferiorly. (Right) Transverse US shows the outer contour/notch ➡ of this bicornuate uterus due to a small amount of free fluid in the pelvis. The 2 endometrial cavities ➡ are separated by the myometrium.

Ovarian Teratoma

TERMINOLOGY

- Synonyms
  - Dermoid tumor, dermoid cyst, mature cystic teratoma
- Definition
  - Teratomas made up of variety of parenchymal cell types from > 1 germ cell layer, usually all 3

IMAGING

- Best clue: Heterogeneous pelvic mass containing Ca^{2+}, hair, fat, & cystic components
  - Bilateral in up to 15%
- Typically well-defined margins without surrounding inflammatory changes
- US 1st-line modality for female pelvic pain &/or mass
  - Multiple classic signs described for teratoma
    - Dermoid plug: Echogenic nodule protruding into cyst
    - Dermoid mesh: Linear/punctate echogenic foci of hair
    - Tip of iceberg: Echogenic superficial interfaces obscure deeper components of mass

- Radiographs showing tooth-like Ca^2 strongly suggestive
- MR & CT best demonstrate fat, confirming teratoma

CLINICAL ISSUES

- Most common ovarian germ cell tumor
- Most common ovarian neoplasm < 20 years old
- Often incidental finding on physical exam or during imaging for unrelated symptoms
  - With torsion or rupture, acute onset of pain typical
  - If large, may cause palpable mass, swelling, or urinary or gastrointestinal complaints
- Treatment: Surgical resection, ovary-sparing surgery
  - Laparoscopic surgery preferred
- Prognosis generally excellent following resection
- Complications: Ovarian torsion, rupture causing chemical peritonitis (which can lead to severe adhesions), malignancy (2%), paraneoplastic encephalitis

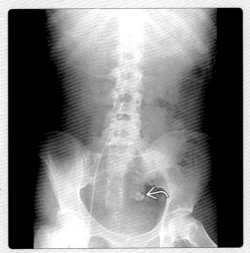
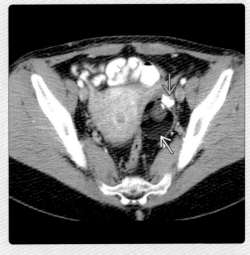

(Left) AP radiograph of the abdomen shows several Ca^{2+} resembling teeth ➡ in the pelvis of a 22-year-old woman with no current abdominal complaints. The right groin central venous catheter is for treatment of an unrelated chronic health condition.
(Right) Axial CECT in the same patient shows the well-encapsulated, mixed density mass in the left adnexa between the iliac vessels & the uterus. This combination of fat ➡ & Ca^{2+} ➡ in the adnexal region is typical of an ovarian teratoma.

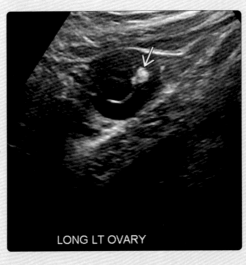
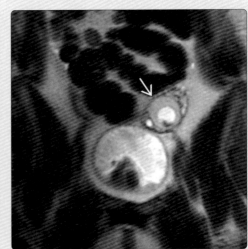

(Left) Longitudinal US of the left ovary in a 14-year-old girl shows a mixed cystic & solid mass with hyperechoic foci ➡ & curvilinear septations.
(Right) Coronal SSFSE T2 MR in the same patient (performed for other medical issues) shows the heterogenous lesion centrally ➡ within the left ovary. It was subsequently surgically shelled out of the ovary (i.e., an ovarian-sparing resection) & found to be a mature teratoma.

LONG LT OVARY

TERMINOLOGY

Definitions

- Teratomas are made up of various parenchymal cell types from > 1 germ layer, usually all 3
  - Cells differentiate along various germ lines, essentially recapitulating any tissue of body
- Term dermoid comes from skin-like lining found in many of these tumors

IMAGING

Radiographic Findings

- May be occult
- $\pm$ Ca^{2+}; those resembling teeth or bone strongly suggest teratoma

Ultrasonographic Findings

- Grayscale ultrasound
  - Heterogeneous mass with cystic & solid components
  - Ca^{2+} may show posterior shadowing
  - Fat & hair appear echogenic; hair may appear reticular
  - $\pm$ fluid-fat-debris levels &/or floating debris within cysts
  - Dermoid mesh sign: Linear & punctate hyperechoic foci (due to hair) within cystic mass
  - Dermoid plug (Rokitansky nodule): Echogenic solid focus bulging into lesion from cyst wall
  - Tip of iceberg sign: Strong echogenic interfaces at leading edge of teratoma obscure deeper components

CT Findings

- Exquisite for identifying fat & Ca^{2+}
- Residual ovary tissue giving rise to teratoma may be difficult to identify if tumor large

MR Findings

- Heterogeneous signal due to mix of elements
- Exquisite for identifying fat

Imaging Recommendations

- Best imaging tool
  - US primary investigative tool for female pelvic pain or palpable mass
  - MR reserved for complex cases or patients ill-suited to sonography
  - CT minimized due to radiation concerns

DIFFERENTIAL DIAGNOSIS

Other Ovarian Lesions

- Benign: Simple/follicular cysts, hemorrhagic cysts, cystadenomas
- Malignant: Germ cell tumors, sex cord-stromal tumors, epithelial tumors, malignant teratomas

Ovarian Torsion

- May require surgical exploration to distinguish
- May coexist with ovarian teratoma

Ectopic Pregnancy

- Correlate with β-hCG

Bladder Calculi

- Ca^2 in pelvis could reside in urinary bladder

PATHOLOGY

General Features

- Associated abnormalities
  - Complications of ovarian teratoma include
    - Ovarian torsion
    - Rupture, causing chemical peritonitis
      □ Severe adhesions can result
    - Malignancy in ~ 2%
- 3 types of ovarian teratomas
  - Mature cystic teratoma (dermoid cyst)
  - Monodermal teratomas (struma ovarii, carcinoid tumors, & neural tumors)
  - Immature teratomas

Gross Pathologic & Surgical Features

- Cyst contents may be oily, milky, or have serous fluid, hair, teeth, cartilage, etc.

CLINICAL ISSUES

Presentation

- Most common signs/symptoms
  - Often incidental finding on physical exam or during imaging for unrelated symptoms
  - With torsion or rupture, acute onset of pain typical
- Other signs/symptoms
  - Abdominal pain, mass, or swelling; urinary or gastrointestinal complaints
  - Elevated α-fetoprotein or hCG more likely with germ cell tumors/immature teratomas
  - Rarely associated with anti-NMDA encephalitis

Demographics

- Most common ovarian neoplasm in patients < 20 years old
- Bilateral in up to 15%

Natural History & Prognosis

- Teratomas enlarge, spontaneously hemorrhage, or twist & come to medical attention
- Prognosis generally excellent following resection
  - Prognosis poor in small minority with malignant foci
- Fertility issues may arise when entire ovary is removed or when chemical peritonitis impairs ovulatory function

Treatment

- Surgical resection, ovary-sparing surgery
- Malignant teratomas treated with surgery, hyperthermic intraperitoneal chemotherapy, neoadjuvant chemotherapy

SELECTED REFERENCES

1. Kelleher CM et al: Adnexal masses in children and adolescents. Clin Obstet Gynecol. 58(1):76-92, 2015
2. Cribb B et al: Paediatric ovarian lesions–the experience at Starship Children's Hospital, New Zealand. N Z Med J. 127(1395):41-51, 2014
3. Papic JC et al: Predictors of ovarian malignancy in children: overcoming clinical barriers of ovarian preservation. J Pediatr Surg. 49(1):144-7; discussion 147-8, 2014
4. Salvucci A et al: Pediatric anti-NMDA (N-methyl D-aspartate) receptor encephalitis. Pediatr Neurol. 50(5):507-10, 2014
5. Anthony EY et al: Adnexal masses in female pediatric patients. AJR Am J Roentgenol. 198(5):W426-31, 2012
6. Epelman M et al: Imaging of pediatric ovarian neoplasms. Pediatr Radiol. 41(9):1085-99, 2011

Ovarian Cyst

TERMINOLOGY

- Follicle: Normal physiologic cyst < 1 cm in diameter
  - Dominant follicle may measure up to 3 cm
- Functional cysts: Can measure up to 3-10 cm
  - Corpus luteal cyst: Dominant follicle after ovulation
  - Follicular cyst: Normal mature follicle fails to involute
- Hemorrhagic cyst: Hemorrhage into functional cyst

IMAGING

- US mainstay of ovarian imaging; MR in limited circumstances
- Well-marginated round or ovoid structure within borders of ovary & having no solid component
  - Thin wall (< 3 mm)
  - No internal septa, nodule, fat, Ca²⁺, or vascularity
  - ↑ heterogeneity with hemorrhage: Internal reticulations (or lace-like pattern) of clot mixed with tiny cystic spaces vs. layering debris

CLINICAL ISSUES

- Usually asymptomatic; pain if large or complicated by rupture, hemorrhage, or torsion
- Treatment/prognosis
  - > 90% of all functional cysts resolve spontaneously
  - Cysts < 3 cm should be considered physiologic in pre- & postmenarchal children
  - Cysts up to 4-5 cm usually monitored with surveillance US
  - Surgery vs. further imaging considered in larger cysts due to risk of torsion or neoplasm
    - For resection, ovarian-sparing approach preferred if benign etiology suspected

DIAGNOSTIC CHECKLIST

- With complex ovarian cystic lesion in child, must consider: Could this be torsion, neoplasm, or other pathology
- Low threshold for follow-up US of asymptomatic cyst in 4-6 weeks if initial study unclear (due to size or mild complexity)

(Left) Transverse color Doppler US of a patient with a simple cyst ➡ shows eccentric but otherwise normal-appearing ovarian tissue ➡ splayed along the cyst. Despite the unalarming sonographic appearance, the patient's symptoms warranted laparoscopy, where the ovary was found to be torsed. (Right) Grayscale endovaginal US shows a large, hemorrhagic ovarian cyst ➡ with internal lace-like echoes & tiny cystic spaces, stretching the ovarian capsule & causing pain. No flow was seen within this lesion to suggest a tumor.

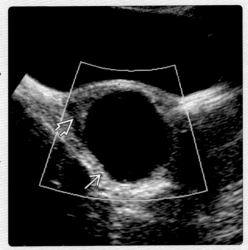

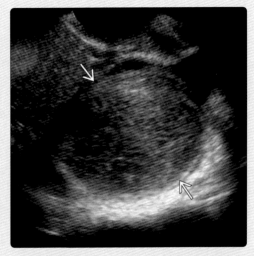

(Left) Transverse endovaginal color Doppler US shows a hypoechoic structure within the right ovary ➡ that has an irregular contour, a hyperechoic rim, & a small amount of echogenic material centrally ➡. There is mild adjacent hyperemia. The findings are characteristic of a corpus luteal cyst. (Right) Coronal CECT of the same patient on the same day shows the typical mildly thickened, irregular, hypervascular wall indicative of a corpus luteal cyst ➡.

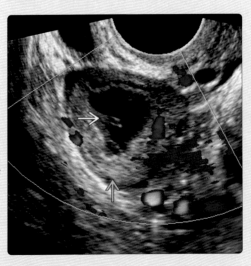

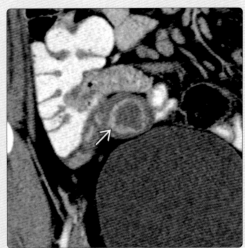

TERMINOLOGY

Definitions

- Definitions of different cyst types & their sizes vary
  - Follicle
    - Generally < 1 cm in diameter
    - Dominant follicle may measure up to 3 cm
  - Functional cysts
    - Corpus luteal cyst
      - After ovulation, dominant follicle becomes corpus luteal cyst
      - Usually < 3 cm, though can be much larger
    - Follicular cyst
      - Occurs when normal mature follicle fails to involute
      - Usually 3-10 cm
  - Hemorrhagic cyst
    - Hemorrhage occurs into 1 of above

IMAGING

Ultrasonographic Findings

- Differentiation of follicle & functional cyst mainly by size
- Follicles & follicular cysts without hemorrhage
  - Unilocular with smooth margin
  - No internal septations, though adjacent follicles can sometimes simulate septations
  - Anechoic with ↑ through transmission
    - May have minimal internal debris
- Corpus luteal cysts
  - Unilocular, though contour may be somewhat irregular
  - Range from anechoic to isoechoic
  - Wall thickness variable due to vascularization
  - Classically have ↑ peripheral vascularity
  - Appearance can be identical to follicular cyst
- Hemorrhagic cysts
  - Contain heterogeneously echogenic debris, which becomes more hypo- or anechoic as clot lysis occurs
  - Reticular or lace-like pattern of internal echoes classic
  - Fluid-debris level sometimes present
  - ↑ through transmission maintained despite echogenicity

MR Findings

- May be performed if US diagnosis unclear
  - Accuracy for MR in characterizing sonographically indeterminate lesions ranges from 83-93%
  - Findings more indicative of neoplasm include
    - Thick, enhancing wall or septations > 3 mm
    - Enhancing mural nodule, papillary projections, or other solid components
    - Size > 5 cm

Imaging Recommendations

- Best imaging tool
  - US mainstay for evaluation of ovaries
    - Characterization of cyst wall & internal components
    - Color Doppler gives additional information, especially in evaluating for presence of solid component
  - MR considered when US indeterminate or if neoplasm suggested but full extent not discernible by US
  - CT use minimized due to radiation concerns

CLINICAL ISSUES

Presentation

- Most common signs/symptoms
  - Usually asymptomatic; pain if large or complicated by rupture, hemorrhage, or torsion
  - Corpus luteal cyst more commonly symptomatic, even without significant hemorrhage

Demographics

- Epidemiology
  - Neonates: Small cysts present in up to 98% at birth
    - ~ 20% ≥ 1 cm
  - Premenarchal: Cysts > 1 cm in 2-5%
  - Postmenarchal: Cysts very common
    - Nonfunctional cysts & malignant ovarian neoplasms also occur at greater rate

Natural History & Prognosis

- Over 90% of all functional cysts resolve spontaneously
  - Larger cysts may take longer to resolve

Treatment

- Cysts < 4-5 cm usually monitored with surveillance US
- Surgery considered in larger cysts due to risk of torsion or neoplasm
  - Options include aspiration, fenestration, & resection
  - For resection, ovarian-sparing approach preferred if benign etiology suspected

DIAGNOSTIC CHECKLIST

Consider

- 3 main concerns for radiologist when cystic ovarian lesion encountered in child
  - Could this be torsed
  - Could this be neoplastic
  - Could this be other pathology (e.g., tuboovarian abscess, ectopic pregnancy, ruptured appendicitis, etc.)

Image Interpretation Pearls

- Superimposed torsion more likely with cysts > 5 cm
- Clinical judgment overrides imaging: Simple or hemorrhagic cyst with otherwise normal-appearing ovarian parenchyma (by grayscale & Doppler US) can still be torsed
  - Simply means that strong clinical suspicion + any ovarian abnormality on imaging may require laparoscopy

Reporting Tips

- Close follow-up if complexity or size of asymptomatic cyst not entirely typical for most simple or hemorrhagic cysts
  - US in 4-6 weeks; subsequent MR &/or gynecology referral if questions persist

SELECTED REFERENCES

1. Bronstein ME et al: A meta-analysis of B-mode ultrasound, Doppler ultrasound, and computed tomography to diagnose pediatric ovarian torsion. Eur J Pediatr Surg. 25(1):82-6, 2015
2. Asävoaie C et al: Ovarian and uterine ultrasonography in pediatric patients. Pictorial essay. Med Ultrason. 16(2):160-7, 2014
3. Papic JC et al: Management of neonatal ovarian cysts and its effect on ovarian preservation. J Pediatr Surg. 49(6):990-3; discussion 993-4, 2014
4. Levine D et al: Management of asymptomatic ovarian and other adnexal cysts imaged at US: Society of Radiologists in Ultrasound Consensus Conference Statement. Radiology. 256(3):943-54, 2010

TERMINOLOGY

- Definition: Twisting of vascular pedicle of ovary, fallopian tube, or both → venous obstruction → edema → arterial compromise → ischemia → hemorrhagic infarction

IMAGING

- Unilaterally enlarged ovary
  - Ovarian volume > 100 mL highly suggestive of torsion
  - Ovarian volume < 20 mL in postpubertal patient never torsed in 1 series
  - Ratio of abnormal to normal ovarian volumes ≥ 5:1 strongly correlated with torsion in same series
- Scattered, predominantly peripheral follicles of 8-12 mm
- Ovary may be displaced to midline or contralateral pelvis or abdomen
- Sonographic whirlpool sign of twisted vascular pedicle
- Variable patterns of Doppler flow within twisted ovary ranging from normal to completely absent
- Pelvic free fluid or hemoperitoneum

CLINICAL ISSUES

- Urgent surgical detorsion required
  - Conservation of ovarian tissue if not frankly necrotic
  - > 90% salvage rate of ovarian function
- Variable rates of retorsion; oophoropexy controversial

DIAGNOSTIC CHECKLIST

- Painful pelvic mass may represent torsed ovary if both normal ovaries not confidently visualized
- Doppler exam of ovarian parenchyma may be normal despite true adnexal torsion
  - Grayscale findings & high clinical suspicion more predictive
- Presence of underlying ovarian cyst/mass can create diagnostic dilemma
  - Experienced clinical evaluation key in these cases
- Normal symmetric grayscale & Doppler US appearance of ovaries makes ovarian torsion highly unlikely

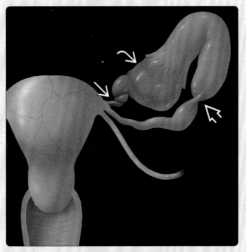
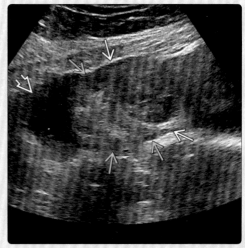

(Left) *Anterior graphic shows torsion of the ovarian vascular pedicle* ➡ *& fallopian tube* ➡, *which results in ischemia of the ovary* ➡ *& distention of the distal segment of the fallopian tube.* (Right) *Transverse pelvic ultrasound for acute pain in a 13-year-old girl shows a large 6- to 7-cm heterogeneous mass* ➡ *in the right pelvis with adjacent free fluid* ➡. *A few follicles* ➡ *are present at the outer margin of the mass.*

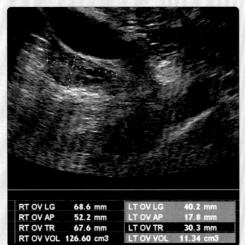
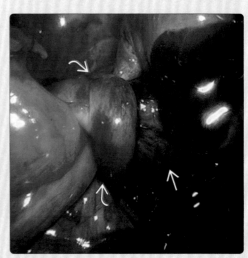

(Left) *Comparison image of the left adnexa in the same 13-year-old girl shows the normal left ovary between the cursors, with a volume of 11 mL. The painful right-sided mass (her right ovary) was over 10x as large & was torsed 3x at laparoscopy.* (Right) *Intraoperative photograph during laparoscopy shows the typical twisting & spiral appearance* ➡ *of adnexal supporting structures. The darker structure deep to the twisted tissue is the torsed ovary* ➡.

RT OV LG	68.6 mm	LT OV LG	40.2 mm
RT OV AP	52.2 mm	LT OV AP	17.8 mm
RT OV TR	67.6 mm	LT OV TR	30.3 mm
RT OV VOL	126.60 cm3	LT OV VOL	11.34 cm3

TERMINOLOGY

Definitions

- Twisting of vascular pedicle of ovary, fallopian tube, or both → venous obstruction → edema → arterial compromise → ischemia → hemorrhagic infarction

IMAGING

General Features

- Best diagnostic clue
  - Unilateral ovarian enlargement with scattered peripheral follicles ± discrete cyst or tumor in setting of acute pain
  - Painful pelvic mass with failure to identify ipsilateral normal ovary also very suspicious
    - Torsed ovary often displaced
  - Doppler exam not sensitive for ovarian torsion
    - Abnormal flow can be useful adjunct to grayscale US
  - Sensitivity: 79-92% by US; 42% by CT

Ultrasonographic Findings

- Grayscale ultrasound
  - Unilateral ovarian enlargement
    - Ovarian volume > 100 mL highly suggestive of torsion
    - Ovarian volume < 20 mL in postpubertal patient never torsed in 1 series
      □ Ratio of abnormal to normal ovarian volumes ≥ 5:1 strongly correlated with torsion in same series
  - Scattered, predominantly peripheral follicles of 8-12 mm in enlarged ovary
  - Variable ovarian parenchymal echotexture due to
    - Edema vs. hemorrhage/infarction
    - Underlying cystic or solid mass
  - Pelvic free fluid or hemoperitoneum
- Color Doppler
  - Sonographic whirlpool sign of twisted vascular pedicle
    - Round, swirling bull's eye or target appearance of hyper- & hypoechoic rings or stripes ± Doppler flow
  - Variable patterns of flow within twisted ovary ranging from normal to completely absent
    - View any asymmetry in flow with suspicion

Imaging Recommendations

- Best imaging tool
  - US: Grayscale findings more reliable (92% sensitive, 96% specific) than Doppler (50% sensitive)
  - Doppler may be normal despite true adnexal torsion
- Protocol advice
  - Endovaginal scanning in patients who are sexually active
  - Transabdominal scanning via well-distended urinary bladder in patients who are not sexually active
    - May need to fill bladder via Foley

DIFFERENTIAL DIAGNOSIS

Appendicitis

- Noncompressible blind-ending tubular structure in right lower quadrant originating from cecum & measuring > 6 mm in diameter with surrounding fat induration
- Appendix more difficult to define with perforation

Ovarian Cyst

- Simple or hemorrhagic cyst may cause pain without torsion
- Avascular internally by Doppler
- Hemorrhagic cyst with septations, debris, nodular clot
- Cyst > 5 cm more likely to be associated with torsion

Isolated Fallopian Tube Torsion

- Dilated fluid-filled tube or paraovarian cystic mass

Ovarian Tumor

- Discrete heterogeneous cystic &/or solid mass
- Painful rarely from rupture or necrosis vs. true torsion

CLINICAL ISSUES

Presentation

- Most common signs/symptoms
  - Acute, severe unilateral lower abdominal/pelvic pain, constant or intermittent
  - Nausea & vomiting (often synchronous with pain)

Demographics

- 50% of cases occur in premenarchal girls
  - ~ 10% occur in perinatal period

Natural History & Prognosis

- Infarction → nonfunctioning ovary → infertility risk
- Variable retorsion rate after detorsion

Treatment

- Urgent surgical detorsion
  - Conservation of ovarian tissue increasingly adopted
  - Oophoropexy (to prevent retorsion) controversial
- > 90% salvage rate for ovarian function
  - Length of symptoms does not always predict viability

DIAGNOSTIC CHECKLIST

Consider

- Painful pelvic mass may represent torsed ovary if 2 normal ovaries are not confidently visualized

Image Interpretation Pearls

- Documenting normal arterial & venous flow in adnexa does not exclude torsion
  - Grayscale US & high clinical suspicion more predictive
- Presence of underlying ovarian cyst/mass can create diagnostic dilemma
  - Hemorrhagic cyst may be painful in absence of torsion despite causing overall ↑ ovarian volume
  - However, cyst/mass also predisposes to torsion & may obscure other classic imaging findings of torsion
  - Experienced clinical evaluation key in these cases
- Completely normal & symmetric grayscale & Doppler appearance of ovaries makes ovarian torsion highly unlikely

SELECTED REFERENCES

1. Rey-Bellet Gasser C et al: Is it ovarian torsion? A systematic literature review and evaluation of prediction signs. Pediatr Emerg Care. 32(4):256-61, 2016
2. Bronstein ME et al: A meta-analysis of B-mode ultrasound, doppler ultrasound, and computed tomography to diagnose pediatric ovarian torsion. Eur J Pediatr Surg. 25(1):82-6, 2015
3. Oskaylı MÇ et al: Surgical approach to ovarian torsion in children. J Pediatr Adolesc Gynecol. 28(5):343-7, 2015

Epididymoorchitis

TERMINOLOGY

- Infectious inflammation of epididymis, testicle, or both
  - Orchitis much less common than epididymoorchitis

IMAGING

- Enlargement of affected tissues (i.e., testicle, epididymis, or both) with accompanying ↑ blood flow
  - ↑ blood flow best demonstrated on transverse side-by-side comparison view
  - Arterial waveforms typically remain low resistance
- Echotexture may be ↑ or ↓, often heterogeneous
- Reactive hydrocele
- Scrotal wall also thickened

TOP DIFFERENTIAL DIAGNOSES

- Torsion of appendage testis
- Testicular torsion
- Scrotal cellulitis

PATHOLOGY

- Bacterial infections may be due to ascending infection (in sexually active adolescents), direct seeding by infected urine with GU anomalies (especially in young children), or hematogenous seeding
- Can also be viral (typically mumps) or posttraumatic
- Some cases of epididymitis likely due to unrecognized appendage torsion

CLINICAL ISSUES

- Gradual onset of painful scrotum, swelling, erythema ± dysuria, enuresis, frequency
  - Prehn sign: Elevation of affected hemiscrotum relieves pain of epididymitis & exacerbates pain of torsion
- Primary therapy: Antibiotics
- Bedrest, scrotal support & elevation, ice packs, antiinflammatory agents, & analgesics also used
- Consider work-up for GU anomalies in younger children & recurrent cases

(Left) Longitudinal graphic through the testis & epididymis shows a focally enlarged inferior aspect of the epididymis ➡ due to epididymitis. If the testicle ➡ were also enlarged & inflamed, this would be epididymoorchitis. (Right) Longitudinal oblique color Doppler US shows a thickened, hyperemic, & heterogeneous epididymis ➡ in a teenager with several days of pain, consistent with epididymitis.

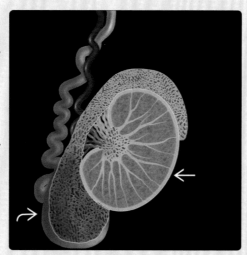
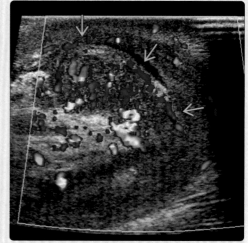

(Left) Grayscale US in a 5-year-old boy with acute left scrotal swelling shows marked enlargement & heterogeneous echotexture of the epididymis ➡. The testicle ➡ has a normal echotexture but was larger than the contralateral side. (Right) Longitudinal color Doppler US of the same 5-year-old boy with left scrotal swelling shows enlargement of the epididymis ➡ & testis ➡ with increased blood flow & a surrounding hydrocele, consistent with epididymoorchitis.

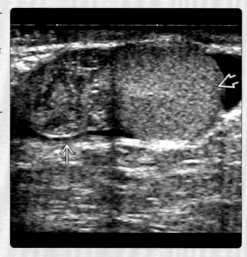
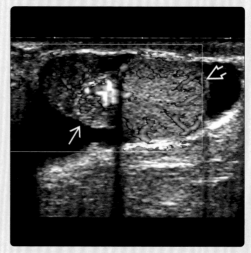

TERMINOLOGY

Definitions

- Infectious inflammation of epididymis, testicle, or both

IMAGING

Ultrasonographic Findings

- Grayscale ultrasound
  - Inflamed epididymis &/or testis typically show ↑ size when compared to asymptomatic side
    - Bilateral in 5-10% of patients
  - Echotexture varies, often heterogeneous
  - Reactive hydrocele common
  - Scrotal wall also thickened
- Color Doppler
  - Hyperemia of involved tissues
    - Flow in testis typically remains low resistance
  - ↑ blood flow often best demonstrated on transverse side-by-side comparison view
- Power Doppler
  - Doppler flow dramatically ↑

Fluoroscopic Findings

- Voiding cystourethrogram
  - May be performed in infants & nonsexually active boys to exclude underlying GU anomaly
    - Ectopic ureter, vesicoureteral reflux
    - Urethral abnormality with reflux into vas deferens
    - Voiding dysfunction/high-pressure voiding pattern

MR Findings

- MR urography if complex GU anomalies suspected & not fully elucidated by US & VCUG

Imaging Recommendations

- Best imaging tool
  - US with Doppler

DIFFERENTIAL DIAGNOSIS

Torsion of Appendage Testis

- Nodular hypo- or hyperechoic avascular mass adjacent to testis with surrounding hyperemia
- May be most common cause of acute scrotum in childhood
  - Some cases of epididymitis likely due to unrecognized appendage torsion

Testicular Torsion

- Unilateral testicular blood flow diminished or absent
- May see twist or knot of spermatic cord above testis

Scrotal Cellulitis

- Generalized wall thickening & hyperemia
- Normal testicle & epididymis
- May be infectious, allergic, related to insect bite, or sign of Henoch-Schönlein purpura

PATHOLOGY

General Features

- Etiology
  - Ascending GU tract infection in sexually active patients

- In males ages 14-35 years, most frequently caused by *Neisseria gonorrhoeae* & *Chlamydia trachomatis*
  - Retrograde passage of infected urine from prostatic urethra to epididymis via ejaculatory ducts & vas deferens
- Bacterial seeding may also occur (*Staphylococcus aureus*, *Escherichia coli*)
  - Directly (from GU anomaly) or hematogenously
- Often caused by viruses, especially mumps
  - Mumps orchitis often has fever, malaise, & myalgia
  - Parotiditis precedes onset of orchitis by 3-5 days
  - Subclinical infections occur in 30-40% of patients
  - Outbreaks of mumps reported in school age children, despite mumps, measles, & rubella (MMR) vaccination

CLINICAL ISSUES

Presentation

- Most common signs/symptoms
  - Gradual onset of painful scrotum, swelling, erythema
  - Systemic symptoms of fever, nausea, vomiting
  - Urinary symptoms of dysuria, enuresis, frequency
- Other signs/symptoms
  - Prehn sign: Elevation of affected hemiscrotum relieves pain of epididymitis & exacerbates pain of torsion
  - Instrumentation & indwelling catheters common risk factors for acute epididymitis

Demographics

- Age
  - Adolescents beginning sexual activity
  - In infants & children, consider work-up for underlying urinary tract anomalies
- Epidemiology
  - 1 in 1,000 men affected yearly; ↓ frequency in children
    - Epididymoorchitis & torsion of testicular appendage more common than testicular torsion
  - MMR vaccine has ↓ incidence of mumps orchitis

Natural History & Prognosis

- Prognosis generally excellent
- Can lead to abscess if not treated
- Can recur in ~ 25%
  - Can lead to long-term fertility problems

Treatment

- Antibiotics mainstay of therapy
  - Reserved for culture positive cases
  - Bedrest, scrotal support & elevation, ice packs, antiinflammatory agents, & analgesics also used
  - Follow-up scans to exclude abscess if not improving
- Work-up GU anomalies in young children & recurrent cases

SELECTED REFERENCES

1. Cordeiro E et al: Mumps outbreak among highly vaccinated teenagers and children in the central region of Portugal, 2012-2013. Acta Med Port. 28(4):435-41, 2015
2. Park SJ et al: Distribution of epididymal involvement in mumps epididymoorchitis. J Ultrasound Med. 34(6):1083-9, 2015
3. Gkentzis A et al: The aetiology and current management of prepubertal epididymitis. Ann R Coll Surg Engl. 96(3):181-3, 2014
4. Redshaw JD et al: Epididymitis: a 21-year retrospective review of presentations to an outpatient urology clinic. J Urol. 192(4):1203-7, 2014
5. Baldisserotto M: Scrotal emergencies. Pediatr Radiol. 39(5):516-21, 2009

Testicular Torsion

TERMINOLOGY

- Spontaneous or traumatic twisting of testis & spermatic cord within scrotum → vascular occlusion/infarction

IMAGING

- ↓ or absent blood flow in testicle on Doppler US
  - Transverse side-by-side comparison image of asymptomatic & symptomatic testicles very helpful
- Spiral twist of spermatic cord just above testis
- ± abnormal lie of testicle within scrotal sac
- Enlarged testis ± altered echotexture
- May see hyperemia after detorsion

TOP DIFFERENTIAL DIAGNOSES

- Epididymoorchitis, torsion of testicular appendage or appendix epididymis, testicular trauma, hernia

PATHOLOGY

- Intravaginal torsion of spermatic cord

- Abnormally high attachment of tunica vaginalis → bell clapper deformity that predisposes to torsion
- Extravaginal torsion of spermatic cord
  - Occurs proximal to attachments of tunica vaginalis
  - More common in neonates; rarely salvageable

CLINICAL ISSUES

- Acute scrotal &/or inguinal pain, swollen erythematous hemiscrotum without trauma, absence of cremasteric reflex, elevation or transverse lie of affected testicle
  - Nausea & vomiting common
  - Low-grade torsion may be tolerated for long periods
- Surgical emergency to prevent testicular infarction
  - Exploration with detorsion & bilateral orchiopexy if testicle viable; nonviable testicle typically removed
    - Testicle twists medially in 2/3 of cases, so manual detorsion laterally can be temporarily effective
  - Salvage rates: 80-100% within 6 hours of pain onset; virtually 0% after 12 hours

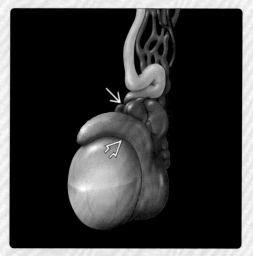
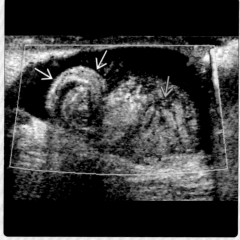

(Left) Anatomic drawing of testicular torsion shows a twisted cord (resembling a snail shell) ➡ & an enlarged epididymis ➡. (Right) Longitudinal power Doppler US at the inguinal-scrotal junction shows a twisted spermatic cord ➡ surrounded by a hydrocele in a teenager with several hours of left-sided scrotal pain. The epididymis is enlarged & heterogeneous ➡, & no flow was seen in the testicle (not shown), consistent with torsion.

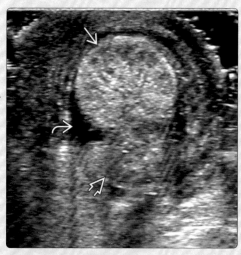
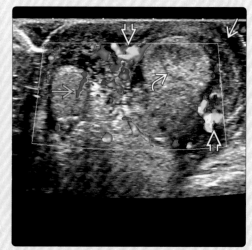

(Left) Transverse US of the left scrotum in a 3-year-old boy with swelling & pain shows a heterogeneous echotexture of the left testicle ➡ with an enlarged epididymis ➡ & a small hydrocele ➡. (Right) Transverse color Doppler US of both testes in the same 3-year-old boy shows scrotal wall thickening ➡ & surrounding hyperemia ➡ with no left testicular blood flow ➡, confirming left testicular torsion. Flow is seen in the right testicle ➡.

TERMINOLOGY

Definitions

- Spontaneous or traumatic twisting of testis & spermatic cord within scrotum → vascular occlusion/infarction

IMAGING

Ultrasonographic Findings

- Grayscale ultrasound
  - Testicular parenchyma may be normal early
    - Gradual development of hypoechoic &/or heterogeneous testicular parenchyma
    - Intratesticular necrosis, hemorrhage, or fragmentation seen if diagnosis delayed
  - Enlarged testicle & epididymis
    - Remote torsion shows small testicle ± Ca²⁺
  - Testicle may lie in abnormal plane
  - Spiral, whirlpool, or knot: Twist of spermatic cord just above testicle (below inguinal canal)
    - Snail shell-shaped mass measuring 11-33 mm
  - Reactive or secondary hydrocele
  - Scrotal wall thickening
- Color Doppler
  - Absent or ↓ blood flow throughout testicle
    - Compare side-by-side with asymptomatic testicle
    - Small percentage of patients with early or partial torsion have normal exam
  - Peripheral capsular & scrotal wall hyperemia
  - Hyperemia may be seen in testicle after detorsion
    - ± high-resistance residual flow in partially or intermittently torsed testicle
- Sensitivity of 86%, specificity of 100%, accuracy of 97% in diagnosis of testicular torsion when presence of intratesticular flow is sole criterion for diagnosis

DIFFERENTIAL DIAGNOSIS

Epididymoorchitis or Orchitis

- Enlarged hypoechoic hyperemic epididymis

Torsion of Epididymal or Testicular Appendage

- Round, devascularized, enlarged, heterogeneous appendix with surrounding hyperemia

Testicular Tumor

- Focal intratesticular mass with abnormal flow in tumor

Testicular Trauma

- Hematocele, irregular contours, heterogeneous parenchymal echogenicity, ± interruption of capsule

Inguinal Hernia

- Incarcerated/strangulated hernia can mimic torsion

PATHOLOGY

General Features

- Embryology/anatomy
  - Intravaginal torsion of spermatic cord (95%)
    - Abnormally high attachment of tunica vaginalis → bell clapper deformity
    - Testicle rotates freely in scrotum → spermatic cord twists → occlusion of venous then arterial flow
    - Present in 12% of male population at autopsy
      - Much higher incidence than testicular torsion
  - Extravaginal torsion of spermatic cord (5%)
    - Occurs proximal to attachments of tunica vaginalis
    - More common in neonates
    - Bilateral in 20%

CLINICAL ISSUES

Presentation

- Most common signs/symptoms
  - Acute scrotal &/or inguinal pain
  - Swollen erythematous hemiscrotum without trauma
  - Physical exam findings predictive of testicular torsion
    - Elevation or transverse lie of affected testicle
    - Anterior rotation of epididymis
    - Absence of cremasteric reflex
    - Pain relief with successful manual detorsion
    - Hard testicle
  - In neonates, purple discoloration of swollen scrotum may indicate extravaginal testicular torsion
- Other signs/symptoms
  - Nausea & vomiting common
  - Low-grade torsion may be tolerated for long periods
  - Almost 1/2 of patients have history of similar symptoms previously that resolved spontaneously
    - Indicates spontaneous torsion & detorsion

Demographics

- Bimodal age peak (teenagers during puberty vs. neonates)
- Much less common than epididymoorchitis & torsion of testicular appendage

Natural History & Prognosis

- Surgical emergency: Infarction if not treated promptly
- Unilateral testicular loss typically does not lead to infertility

Treatment

- Testicle twists medially in 2/3 of cases, so manual detorsion laterally more likely to be effective
  - Manual detorsion described as "opening book"
- Surgical exploration + detorsion + bilateral orchiopexy if viable testicle
  - Nonviable testicle usually removed (due to antisperm antibody theory)
  - Higher risk of subsequent torsion on contralateral side justifies contralateral pexy
- Salvage rates
  - 80-100% within 6 hours of pain onset
  - Virtually 0% after 12 hours
  - Only 9% salvage rate in neonates

SELECTED REFERENCES

1. Sheth KR et al: Diagnosing testicular torsion before urological consultation and imaging: validation of the TWIST score. J Urol. 195(6):1870-6 2016
2. Dajusta DG et al: Contemporary review of testicular torsion: new concepts, emerging technologies and potential therapeutics. J Pediatr Urol. 9(6 Pt A):723-30, 2012
3. Waldert M et al: Color Doppler sonography reliably identifies testicular torsion in boys. Urology. 75(5):1170-4, 2010
4. Baldisserotto M: Scrotal emergencies. Pediatr Radiol. 39(5):516-21, 2009

Torsion of Testicular Appendage

TERMINOLOGY

- Definition
  - Spontaneous twisting of pedunculated vestigial remnant along testicle or epididymis causing ischemia & pain
- Synonyms
  - Twisted appendage, torsed appendix testis, torsion of appendix epididymis, appendiceal torsion

IMAGING

- US with Doppler best imaging modality
- Appendage size best indicator of torsion (> 5-6 mm acutely)
- Spherical shape suggests swelling (normally vermiform)
- Duration of symptoms determines echogenicity
  - < 24 hours: Hypoechoic with salt & pepper pattern
  - > 24 hours: Hypo-, iso-, or hyperechoic
- Classically ↓ or absent internal vascularity of torsed appendix with periappendiceal hyperemia
- Reactive hydrocele & scrotal wall edema common

TOP DIFFERENTIAL DIAGNOSES

- Testicular torsion
- Epididymoorchitis or orchitis
- Isolated scrotal wall edema (from insect bite, trauma, etc.)

CLINICAL ISSUES

- Acute scrotal pain, swelling
  - Most common cause (35-67%)
- ± small, tender, mobile lump at upper pole of testis
- ± blue dot sign (ischemic appendage seen through scrotal wall) in < 30% of patients
- 80% of cases 7-14 years old; mean age: 9 years (vs. mean age of 14 years for testicular torsion, epididymoorchitis)
- Self-limited illness, excellent prognosis
- Analgesics & antiinflammatory agents for symptom relief
- Consider repeat imaging if symptoms persist: Rare reports of secondary infection in infarcted, necrotic tissue

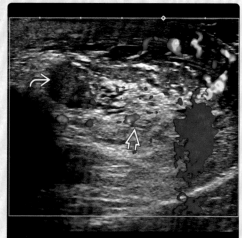

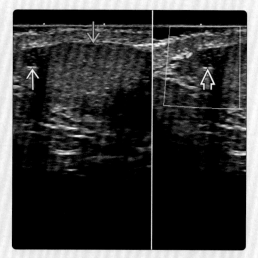

(Left) *Longitudinal color Doppler US in a 7 year old with scrotal pain & swelling shows a lack of blood flow in a small round nodule ➡ adjacent to an inflamed epididymis ➡. Testicular blood flow (not shown) was normal. The findings are consistent with a torsed appendage.* (Right) *Longitudinal ultrasounds of the epididymis in a 6 year old show a hypoechoic nodule ➡ (superior to the testis ➡), which is avascular on Doppler ➡. This was the point of maximal discomfort & likely represented a torsed appendage.*

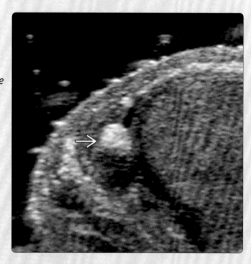

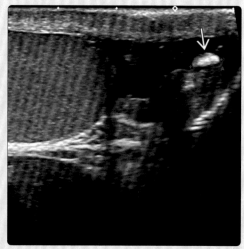

(Left) *Oblique scrotal US shows an echogenic appendage ➡ in a patient with a subacute history of pain. The increased echogenicity may reflect acute hemorrhage vs. more chronic fibrotic change or Ca²⁺ in a torsed appendage.* (Right) *Longitudinal US shows a hyperechoic ovoid focus ➡ surrounded by a small hydrocele, consistent with a partially calcified, chronically torsed appendage. At this point in time, the patient was asymptomatic.*

TERMINOLOGY

Synonyms

- Twisted appendage, torsed appendix testis, torsion of appendix epididymis, appendiceal torsion

Definitions

- Spontaneous twisting of pedunculated vestigial remnant along testicle or epididymis causing ischemia & pain

IMAGING

General Features

- Best diagnostic clue
  - Enlarged, spherical, hypoechoic, avascular nodule along testis or epididymis at site of patient pain + hyperemia of surrounding tissues
- Location
  - Can be difficult to differentiate testicular vs. epididymal appendage (not clinically relevant)

Ultrasonographic Findings

- Grayscale ultrasound
  - Size best indicator of torsion (> 5-6 mm acutely)
  - Spherical shape suggests swelling (normally vermiform)
  - Duration of symptoms determines echogenicity
  - Reactive hydrocele
  - Scrotal wall edema
  - Epididymal head enlargement
- Color Doppler
  - Classically, ↓ or absent internal vascularity of torsed appendix with periappendiceal hyperemia
    - Findings can be variable
  - Testicular blood flow may be normal or ↑

Imaging Recommendations

- Best imaging tool
  - US with Doppler
    - More sensitive & specific for diagnosing appendage torsion than
      - Clinical signs alone
      - Imaging in other causes of acute scrotal pain (i.e., testicular torsion or epididymoorchitis)

DIFFERENTIAL DIAGNOSIS

Testicular Torsion

- Abnormal Doppler (absent, diminished, or high-resistance flow) in painful testis compared to asymptomatic side
- Whirlpool or knot sign of twisted spermatic cord above testis
- Normal grayscale appearance of testicular parenchyma early with subsequent changes of frank infarction

Epididymoorchitis/Orchitis

- Hyperemia & enlargement of affected side ± tissue heterogeneity
- Global tenderness on physical exam

Isolated Scrotal Wall Edema

- Thickening, heterogeneity, & hyperemia of scrotal wall
- May be isolated & self-limited or due to cellulitis, insect bite, allergic reaction, or Henoch-Schönlein purpura

PATHOLOGY

General Features

- Etiology
  - Spontaneous twisting of appendage most common, occasionally associated with trauma or tumor

CLINICAL ISSUES

Presentation

- Most common signs/symptoms
  - Acute scrotal pain & swelling
  - ± small, tender, mobile lump at upper pole of testis
  - ± blue dot sign of ischemic appendage seen through scrotal wall in minority of patients (< 30%)
- Other signs/symptoms
  - Metachronous & bilaterally synchronous cases of appendiceal torsion rarely reported

Demographics

- Age
  - 80% of cases occur between ages 7-14 years
  - Mean age: 9 years
    - Younger than testicular torsion & epididymoorchitis
- Epidemiology
  - Most common cause (35-67%) of acute scrotal pain
    - Appendix torsion 2.5x more common than testicular/spermatic cord torsion

Natural History & Prognosis

- Self-limited illness, excellent prognosis
- Pain usually resolves within 1 week
- Consider repeat imaging if symptoms persist
  - Rare reports of secondary infection in infarcted, necrotic tissue

Treatment

- Analgesics & antiinflammatory agents for symptom relief
  - Antibiotics not indicated in routine cases
- Reports of manual detorsion with US guidance
  - Reduction by pulling or squeezing appendage
  - Success if pain relieved, appendix size ↓, Doppler flow restored
- Resection of torsed appendage if scrotum explored due to concern for testicular/spermatic cord torsion
  - Surgery not indicated if torsed appendix diagnosis clear

DIAGNOSTIC CHECKLIST

Image Interpretation Pearls

- Can be difficult to distinguish from epididymitis if no discrete nodule visualized
  - Appendage torsion more common, especially in prepubertal population

SELECTED REFERENCES

1. Lev M et al: Sonographic appearances of torsion of the appendix testis and appendix epididymis in children. J Clin Ultrasound. 43(8):485-9, 2015
2. Boettcher M et al: Differentiation of epididymitis and appendix testis torsion by clinical and ultrasound signs in children. Urology. 82(4):899-904, 2013
3. Yusuf GT et al: A review of ultrasound imaging in scrotal emergencies. J Ultrasound. 16(4):171-8, 2013
4. Sung EK et al: Sonography of the pediatric scrotum: emphasis on the Ts–torsion, trauma, and tumors. AJR Am J Roentgenol. 198(5):996-1003, 2012

TERMINOLOGY

- Divided into germ cell & nongerm cell tumors
  - Germ cell tumors (GCTs) ~ 2/3 of pediatric tumors (yolk sac tumors, teratoma, embryonal carcinoma, choriocarcinoma, mixed type, seminoma)
  - Nongerm cell tumors (NGCTs) ~ 1/3 of pediatric tumors (Leydig cell, Sertoli cell, juvenile granulosa cell)
  - Lymphoma & leukemia can also involve testes

IMAGING

- Intratesticular mass of variable echogenicity & vascularity
- Vary widely in size, from imperceptible to testis-replacing
- Teratomas characteristically have extremely complex appearance with cystic areas, Ca^{2+}, solid components, & punctate or linear echogenic hairs
- Epidermoids (true cysts, not neoplasms) appear solid, targetoid, or have "onion skin" from laminations of keratinizing stratified squamous epithelium

- Regressed mixed GCTs may appear as subtle architectural distortion with ill-defined microcalcification
- NGCTs often small & well defined

CLINICAL ISSUES

- 2 age peaks: < 2 years vs. late adolescence
- Presentations: Asymptomatic or painless mass most common; mild discomfort or pain in abdomen, groin, or testicle; perceived scrotal heaviness
- 10% associated with cryptorchidism (orchiopexy before puberty→ relative risk 2x; post puberty → relative risk 5x)
- Most prepubertal testicular masses benign (teratoma, epidermoid) but yolk sac tumors (YSTs) 2nd most common
  - YSTs: 90% have ↑ AFP, used as tumor marker
- Most postpubertal intratesticular masses malignant: Embryonal carcinoma & mixed GCT most common
- Standard of care: Orchiectomy; testis-sparing enucleation increasingly performed in prepubertal boys without ↑ AFP; ± adjuvant chemo depending on tumor type & stage

(Left) *Longitudinal US of a juvenile granulosa cell tumor in a newborn with firm testicular enlargement shows a heterogeneous mass replacing the testis* ➡. *There are numerous hypoechoic foci* ➡ *separated by thin septations* ➡, *a classic appearance for this rare tumor.* (Right) *Gross pathological photograph status post orchiectomy in the same patient shows complete replacement of the testis by a gray-white tumor* ➡ *with scattered cystic spaces* ➡ *& foci of hemorrhagic staining* ➡.

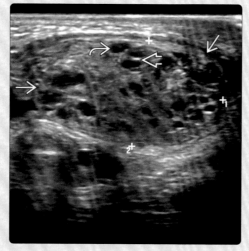
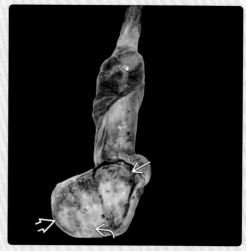

(Left) *Longitudinal color Doppler US shows a well-defined, spherical, avascular intratesticular mass with a multilamellar onion skin appearance, characteristic of an epidermoid* ➡. *The mass was treated in this case by enucleation rather than orchiectomy because of the confident imaging diagnosis.* (Right) *PA chest radiograph in a patient with a testicular mixed germ cell tumor demonstrates numerous, well-defined, 2- to 4-cm "cannonball" lesions* ➡ *in the lungs due to metastases.*

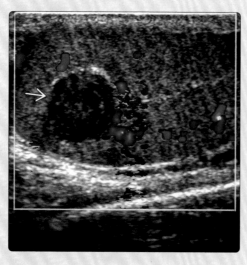
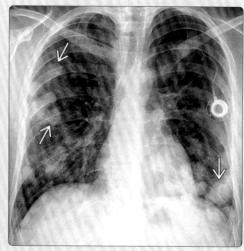

Testicular Trauma

TERMINOLOGY

- Hydrocele: Simple fluid between layers of tunica vaginalis
- Hematocele: Blood between tunica vaginalis layers
- Hematoma: Contained collection of blood products within testis, epididymis, or scrotal wall; may involve ≥ 1 site
- Testicular fracture: Disruption of testicular parenchyma
- Testicular rupture: Disruption of tunica albuginea, often with extrusion of testicular parenchyma
- Devascularization: Vascular pedicle injury causing absent or diminished blood flow without true torsion (twisting)
- Traumatic epididymitis: Epididymal contusion causing inflammation, enlargement, & hypervascularity
- Traumatic testicular ectopia: Traumatic dislocation of testis into inguinal canal, abdominal cavity, or perineum

IMAGING

- US with Doppler to look for alteration of normal testicular echotexture, disruption of tunica albuginea, absent or diminished blood flow, & complex hydrocele

TOP DIFFERENTIAL DIAGNOSES

- Viral epididymitis, testicular torsion, torsion of testicular appendage, neoplasm

CLINICAL ISSUES

- Presentations: Intense scrotal pain in setting of recent trauma ± ecchymosis, swelling, skin abrasion, or laceration
  - Physical exam has poor correlation to degree of injury; therefore US important to guide management
- Testicular fracture/rupture → urologic emergency → prompt treatment reduces infection, atrophy, necrosis
  - Testis can usually be repaired to avoid orchiectomy
  - Salvage rate for rupture: 90% → 45% after 72 hours
- Large hematocele or hematoma may require evacuation
- Possible complications: Infarction, infection, atrophy, ↓ sex hormones & spermatogenesis, infertility

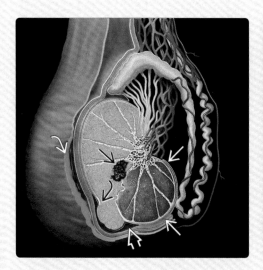

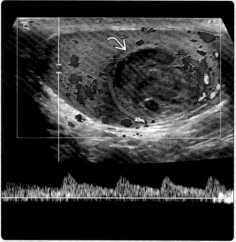

(Left) Sagittal graphic shows various manifestations of testicular trauma, including a scrotal hematoma ⊋, rupture of the tunica albuginea ⊅, segmental testicular infarction ⊨, parenchymal hematoma ⊡ & small hematocele ⊟. (Right) US in a teenager with hemophilia A who hit a tree while skiing shows a well-defined, heterogeneous, avascular intratesticular hematoma ⊋, which was smaller on follow-up US (not shown). Note that a neoplasm would have internal blood flow & would not be smaller on follow-up imaging.

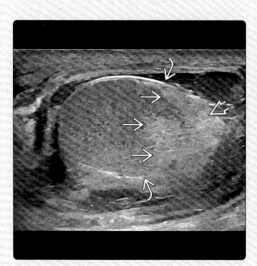

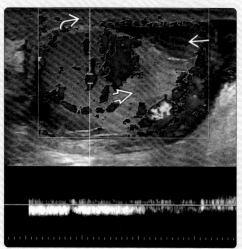

(Left) US in an 11 year old with trauma during basketball shows a jagged demarcation through the parenchyma ⊋, due to a testicular fracture, as well as hyperechogenicity in the lower pole due to segmental infarction ⊨. The echogenic tunica albuginea ⊋ is interrupted. (Right) Doppler US in the same boy shows avascularity in the lower testis due to segmental infarction ⊨ (with reactive hypervascularity of the adjacent parenchyma). There is also a surrounding hematocele ⊋ as well as a scrotal wall hematoma ⊋.

SECTION 6
Musculoskeletal

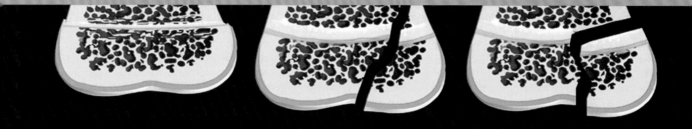

Soft Tissue Masses

Focal, Multifocal, and Diffuse Bone Lesions

Abnormalities of Hip

Constitutional Disorders of Bone

Rheumatologic Diseases

Miscellaneous

Imaging Modalities

Radiography

Although there have been great advances in imaging technology, radiographs (i.e., x-rays or plain films) remain the most important imaging test in most circumstances of suspected musculoskeletal pathology. Most studies will require 2-3 views to adequately image the site of interest. Each of these views is typically obtained with different patient positioning &/or projection of the x-ray beam to analyze different components of the anatomy of interest on each view. With appropriate techniques, the associated radiation exposure is usually minimal, & radiography is less expensive than other more advanced imaging modalities. Most cases of trauma require no imaging beyond radiographs.

Specific circumstances

- Joint effusions: Radiographs show high sensitivity for abnormal volumes of joint fluid at some sites (such as the elbow & the knee). However, the sensitivity is very low at other sites, including the hip & the shoulder; high clinical suspicion of joint effusion at these sites will require further imaging with ultrasound or MR. It should also be noted that radiographs are not specific for the various processes that can cause joint capsule distention, including hemarthrosis, septic arthritis, transient synovitis, & synovitis secondary to juvenile idiopathic arthritis, among others.
- Infection: The earliest radiographic findings of osteomyelitis actually relate to the overlying soft tissues rather than the bones. Thickening & edema of the surrounding soft tissues (with blurring of the normal fat-muscle interfaces) will manifest long before bone findings (which often require 10-14 days to become visible on radiographs).
- Occult fractures: Some particular clinical scenarios are notorious for producing false-negative radiographs in the setting of a fracture, requiring a low threshold for temporary immobilization until confirmatory findings manifest radiographically. Two classic examples include the spiral toddler's fracture of the mid to distal tibial diaphysis & the nondisplaced supracondylar fracture of the distal humerus.
- Nonaccidental trauma: When there is clinical suspicion for child abuse, a full skeletal survey must be obtained. While each institution will differ slightly in exactly how it performs this exam, most will follow a similar protocol of obtaining at least 1 targeted view of every body part. The radiologist involved in the case will then help decide what additional images will be required before the patient leaves the department. In some cases, a follow-up skeletal survey should be performed in 2-3 weeks, mainly to search for healing fractures that were occult on the initial survey.
- Foreign bodies: Some foreign bodies (such as glass & metal) are easily demonstrated by radiographs. Other foreign bodies (such as wood) will typically require ultrasound for detection.
- Tumors: Some bone neoplasms, especially focal lesions involving the cortex, will be easily detected & characterized by radiographs, with the classic example being osteosarcoma. Other lesions, particularly systemic processes involving the marrow (such as leukemia or metastatic neuroblastoma) may only show subtle alterations of mineralization & periosteal reaction,

potentially going undetected until an MR or nuclear medicine bone scan is obtained.

Ultrasound

Ultrasonography has many advantages in evaluating the pediatric musculoskeletal system. It uses no radiation, is relatively inexpensive, requires no sedation, & provides excellent superficial spatial resolution. It also enables dynamic assessments, differentiates cystic vs. solid masses, & characterizes vascular flow. Additionally, comparison to the contralateral normal side does not have the same cost in time, sedation, & radiation as carried by other modalities. The relatively high volume of water-rich cartilage in the infant also provides excellent acoustic windows that will disappear as normal ossification takes place (such that ultrasound can be used in some scenarios for problem solving in infants but not older children). Specific indications include the evaluations of infant hips for developmental dysplasia, retained nonradiopaque foreign bodies, soft tissue masses & fluid collections, & traumatic soft tissue injuries. Disadvantages of ultrasound include that it is limited by gas, bone, & fat; therefore, the deep extent of a lesion may not be determinable sonographically.

Specific circumstances

- Joint effusions: Ultrasound is exquisitely sensitive to fluid, though some joints are easier to interrogate sonographically than others. When an urgent process such as septic arthritis is suspected, ultrasound may be the only imaging modality required to confirm the presence of drainable fluid (though it cannot distinguish infected vs. noninfected fluid).
- Osteocartilaginous relationships: Because of its high fluid content, unossified cartilage (of which there is abundance in young infants) is well visualized & can be used as an acoustic window for deeper structures. The most common such circumstance in which ultrasound is employed is the visualization of the unossified femoral heads in young infants to look for developmental dysplasia of the hips. It can also be used to look for separation of the epiphysis from the physis & metaphysis at fracture sites that, while rare, tend to occur in young children, including the proximal & distal humerus.
- Palpable masses: "Lumps & bumps" in children are most commonly benign, though they can incite anxiety in caregivers for more ominous processes. Ultrasound is an easy way to determine which masses will need further work-up (including MR &/or biopsy/excision) vs. those that will not.
- Infection: Ultrasound is frequently used to look for drainable fluid collections in the setting of cellulitis, suppurative lymph nodes, or adjacent osteomyelitis. Dynamic compression can help reveal truly drainable fluid vs. necrotic phlegmonous collections that are not yet drainable. Ultrasound can also determine the volume of drainable fluid as well as its exact location. Occasionally, periosteal elevation by subperiosteal fluid can suggest osteomyelitis of an adjacent bone (though ultrasound will not be able to determine the extent of intraosseous abnormalities).
- Foreign bodies: Wooden foreign bodies are common & are typically occult radiographically. However, the air within wooden foreign bodies lends itself to excellent sonographic visualization. This is best performed prior to attempts at removal as the gas introduced during

attempted extractions can interfere with detection of the body sonographically.

- Soft tissue trauma: Discrete muscular & ligamentous injuries can be difficult to visualize without heavy sports medicine experience by the technologist &/or radiologist. However, some tendon disruptions are easily demonstrated (particularly in comparison to the normal contralateral side).

Magnetic Resonance

MR imaging uses no ionizing radiation & produces excellent soft tissue contrast in multiple planes, providing a number of methods to interrogate the characteristics of a lesion. It remains the best imaging modality for determining the localized extent/depth of a pathologic process, including its relationship to adjacent critical structures (such as arteries & nerves). MR is also unsurpassed in its depiction of intraarticular pathology. However, MR is costly, has a relatively long exam time, & may require sedation/anesthesia (particularly under the age of 6 years) &/or IV contrast. The bottom line: When there is a high suspicion of pathology at a targeted musculoskeletal site, MR is the ultimate imaging tool for investigation (though it should almost always be preceded by radiographs). Such indications include joint trauma, infection, soft tissue masses, & bone tumors.

A common question that arises when ordering MR is regarding the need for IV contrast. The vast majority of trauma cases do not need IV contrast. However, most cases of suspected infection, inflammation, & tumors will need IV contrast. Contrast is particularly helpful in assessing infection in children as it helps define drainable fluid collections & can help identify sites of infected unossified cartilage in infants.

Whole-body MR for the screening of multifocal processes has gained some acceptance in the last decade in specific circumstances. These types of studies use larger fields of view with less spatial resolution than targeted MR scans, though the anatomic detail still remains superior to nuclear medicine exams. Such indications include multifocal infections, chronic recurrent multifocal osteomyelitis, & tumor screening in genetically predisposed individuals. Variable utility has been demonstrated in the work-ups of Langerhans cell histiocytosis, nonaccidental trauma, & juvenile idiopathic arthritis.

Specific circumstances
- Soft tissue trauma: MR excels at the depiction of injured ligaments, tendons, muscles, menisci, & articular cartilage. However, such evaluations are rarely needed emergently & are typically arranged in conjunction with a referral to orthopedics/sports medicine.
- Stress injuries: Repetitive microtrauma creates characteristic marrow & periosteal patterns on MR prior to being radiographically visible.
- Infection: MR has the highest sensitivity & specificity for musculoskeletal infection, demonstrating characteristic soft tissue & bony changes that may be radiographically occult. The evaluation of musculoskeletal infection is generally considered the most urgent/emergent use of MR in orthopedics.
- Masses: Both bone & soft tissue tumors are well characterized by MR, with MR being most helpful in narrowing the differential diagnosis of soft tissue lesions (as bone lesions are often diagnosed by radiographs). MR is particularly useful in directing biopsy & surgery.

Computed Tomography

CT is fast but utilizes ionizing radiation & must be employed judiciously. It allows multiplanar assessments & provides better soft tissue contrast than radiographs. Cortical bone detail is excellent by CT, though marrow evaluation is limited.

CT is helpful in the detection & characterization of specific fractures that are intraarticular or complex, or for fractures that are often subtle but risk significant consequences if the diagnosis is delayed. Additional CT indications include the evaluations of osteoid osteoma, sequestra of osteomyelitis, tarsal coalitions, & union of complicated fractures. Unlike MR, IV contrast is rarely used in musculoskeletal applications of CT (unless there is a specific question about vascular injury related to a complex fracture).

Nuclear Medicine

In general, nuclear medicine scans have excellent sensitivity (but low specificity) for whole-body screening of bone pathology. Ionizing radiation is used (as administered in an IV injection), but the doses vary according to the type of study being performed, the radiotracer being injected, & the size of the patient.

Traditional bone scan indications include metastatic disease, stress fracture, spondylolysis, osteomyelitis, osteoid osteoma, & avascular necrosis. The sensitivity of bone scans can be further increased by the addition of SPECT imaging, which is essentially equivalent to obtaining cross-sectional slices of the 3D volume sets traditionally displayed in nuclear medicine. Greater specificity can be achieved in combination with simultaneously acquired bone CT (e.g., for the detection of spondylolysis).

FDG PET has seen increasing pediatric use in the last decade, primarily as related to cancer staging. However, it may also be useful in the staging of Langerhans cell histiocytosis & the work-up of discrete musculoskeletal masses.

Selected References

1. ACR Appropriateness Criteria: Developmental Dysplasia of the Hip. https://acsearch.acr.org/docs/69437/Narrative/. Published 1999. Reviewed 2013. Accessed Dec. 2016
2. ACR Appropriateness Criteria: Limping Child Ages 0-5. https://acsearch.acr.org/docs/69361/Narrative/. Published 1995. Reviewed 2012. Accessed Dec. 2016
3. ACR Appropriateness Criteria: Suspected Physical Abuse. https://acsearch.acr.org/docs/69443/Narrative/. Published 2016. Reviewed Dec. 2016
4. Hryhorczuk AL et al: Pediatric musculoskeletal ultrasound: practical imaging approach. AJR Am J Roentgenol. 206(5):W62-72, 2016
5. Winfeld MJ et al: Radiographic assessment of congenital malformations of the upper extremity. Pediatr Radiol. ePub, 2016
6. Montgomery NI et al: Pediatric osteoarticular infection update. J Pediatr Orthop. 35(1):74-81, 2015
7. Little KJ: Elbow fractures and dislocations. Orthop Clin North Am. 45(3):327-40, 2014
8. Morrow MS et al: Imaging of lumps and bumps in pediatric patients: an algorithm for appropriate imaging and pictorial review. Semin Ultrasound CT MR. 35(4):415-29, 2014
9. Pugmire BS et al: Role of MRI in the diagnosis and treatment of osteomyelitis in pediatric patients. World J Radiol. 6(8):530-7, 2014
10. Vanderhave KL et al: Applications of musculoskeletal ultrasonography in pediatric patients. J Am Acad Orthop Surg. 22(11):691-8, 2014
11. Callahan MJ: Musculoskeletal ultrasonography of the lower extremities in infants and children. Pediatr Radiol. 43 Suppl 1:8-22, 2013
12. Pai DR et al: Musculoskeletal ultrasound of the upper extremity in children. Pediatr Radiol. 43 Suppl 1:48-54, 2013
13. Khanna G et al: Pediatric bone lesions: beyond the plain radiographic evaluation. Semin Roentgenol. 47(1):90-9, 2012
14. Karmazyn B: Ultrasound of pediatric musculoskeletal disease: from head to toe. Semin Ultrasound CT MR. 32(2):142-50, 2011

(Left) *AP radiographs in an 18 month old with refusal to bear weight [taken at presentation (left) & 3 weeks later (right)] show a subtle nondisplaced spiral toddler's fracture ➡ of the mid tibia. Note the periosteal reaction ➡ on the follow-up study.* **(Right)** *Coronal US of the left hip in a 2 month old with suspected hip dysplasia shows a normal appearance of the unossified cartilage of the femoral head ➡ & greater trochanter ➡. The a angle ➡ of the acetabular roof is > 60°, within normal limits.*

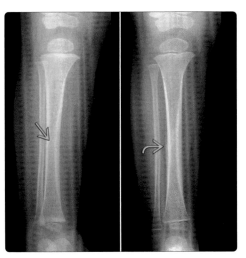
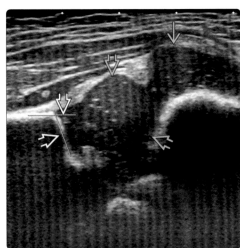

(Left) *AP radiograph of the hips in a 4 year old with left hip pain shows no abnormality, though it must be remembered that radiographs are not sensitive for hip joint effusions.* **(Right)** *Sagittal oblique US of the left hip in the same patient shows distention of the joint capsule by anechoic fluid ➡ along the femoral neck ➡. Note the partial ossification ➡ of the femoral head surrounded by hypoechoic unossified cartilage ➡. The patient was ultimately diagnosed with toxic synovitis.*

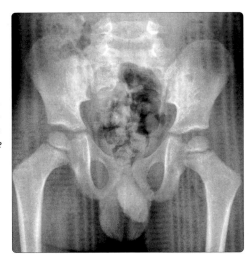
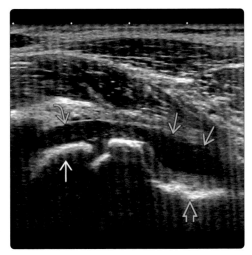

(Left) *Coronal NECT in a 12 year old with bilateral foot pain & flat feet shows bilateral nonosseous middle facet talocalcaneal coalitions ➡. The narrowing, irregularity, & oblique orientations of the articulations are all abnormal.* **(Right)** *Lateral radiograph in a 23 month old who fell down steps & is not weight-bearing on the left leg presents for follow-up imaging 10 days after an initially normal exam. The current image shows a band of sclerosis ➡ from a healing stress fracture within the calcaneus.*

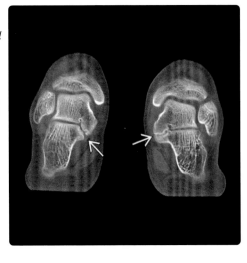
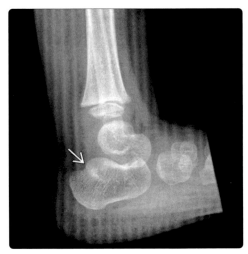

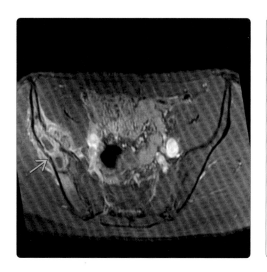

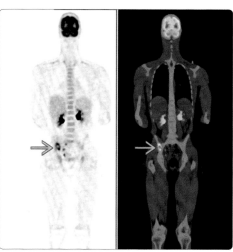

(Left) Axial T1 C+ FS MR in a 16 year old with Langerhans cell histiocytosis (LCH) shows a heterogeneously enhancing lesion ⇒ centered in the right iliac bone & extending into the surrounding soft tissues. (Right) Coronal FDG PET without (left) & with (right) CT superimposition in the same patient shows increased metabolic activity ⇒ within the LCH lesion. No additional lesions were identified. PET is highly sensitive for LCH.

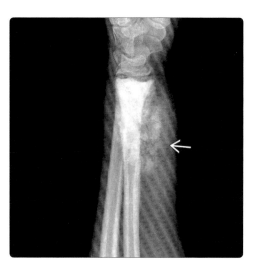

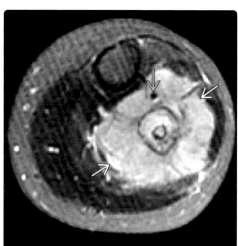

(Left) Lateral radiograph in a 13 year old with osteosarcoma shows increased sclerosis of the distal radius with cloud-like Ca²⁺ (or osteoid) ⇒ about the bone. (Right) Axial T2 FS MR in a 9 year old with a mass in the lower leg shows a hyperintense T2 fibular lesion with a large soft tissue component ⇒. The anterior neurovascular bundle ⇒ was completely encased by the mass. This lesion was a biopsy-proven Ewing sarcoma.

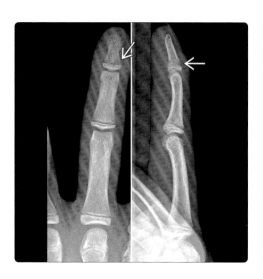

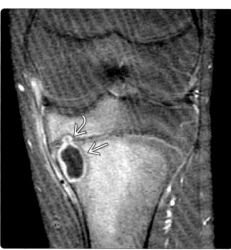

(Left) Frontal & lateral radiographs of the middle finger in a 14 year old after a basketball injury 2 weeks prior show increased lucency ⇒ of the metaphysis of the distal phalanx. This is a "stubbed finger" fracture complicated by osteomyelitis. (Right) Coronal T1 C+ FS MR in a 14 year old with proximal tibial pain shows a rim-enhancing intraosseous Brodie abscess ⇒ with surrounding marrow edema. The abscess extends across the proximal tibial physis ⇒.

KEY FACTS

TERMINOLOGY

- Primary (1°) growth center = 1° ossification center
  - Where majority of bone formation occurs
    - Predominately at long bone physes in childhood
- Secondary (2°) growth center = 2° ossification center
  - Ossification centers that do not significantly contribute to longitudinal growth
    - Surrounded by growth plate & unossified cartilage
    - Found at long bone articulations (epiphyses) & equivalents (apophyses, carpals, tarsals)
- Endochondral ossification: Bone formation on preexisting cartilage model at 1° & 2° growth centers

IMAGING

- Radiographs: Multiple &/or irregular growth centers normal at some locations but can be confused with pathology
  - Upper extremity: Trochlea, pisiform
  - Lower extremity: Femoral condyles, tibial tubercle, medial malleolus, calcaneal apophysis, cuneiforms

- MR: Normal ossification centers (± normal surrounding cartilage) without abnormal edema/fluid signal

TOP DIFFERENTIAL DIAGNOSES

- Osteochondroses
- Osteochondritis dissecans
- Osteomyelitis
- Osteonecrosis

CLINICAL ISSUES

- 1° & 2° growth centers normally asymptomatic
- Pathology can occur at growth centers (e.g., acute/chronic trauma, infection, & osteonecrosis)

DIAGNOSTIC CHECKLIST

- Familiarity with normal irregular ossification prevents mistaking multiple/irregular growth centers with pathology
- Comparison with contralateral side can be helpful
- MR useful in difficult cases

(Left) Coronal T1 MR shows changes of the humeral head at 3 ages. The secondary growth center of the epiphysis ➡ is intermediate signal (red marrow) at 7 months & ↑ signal (yellow marrow) at 13 months. Note the greater tuberosity center at 13 months ➡. Epiphyseal cartilage ➡ surrounds these centers. (Right) Radiograph shows multiple medial malleolar ossification centers ➡. SPGR MR shows the ossified centers as low signal ➡ within bright epiphyseal cartilage ➡. No edema is seen on the T2 FS MR ➡.

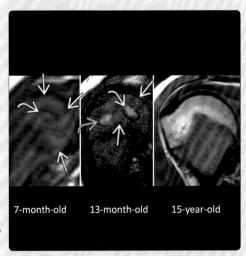

7-month-old   13-month-old   15-year-old

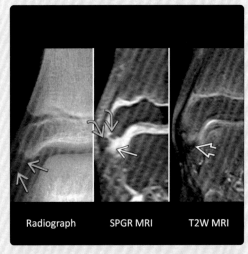

Radiograph   SPGR MRI   T2W MRI

(Left) Note the left elbow secondary growth centers: Capitellum ➡, radial head ➡, internal (medial) epicondyle ➡, trochlea ➡, olecranon ➡, & external (lateral) epicondyle ➡. The trochlear irregular ossification & the multiple olecranon growth centers are normal findings. (Right) Right elbow dislocation in a 7 year old shows a growth center ➡ at the expected location of the trochlea but with no medial epicondylar (ME) growth center ➡, which should form 1st. This pattern indicates that the ME has been avulsed & resides in the joint.

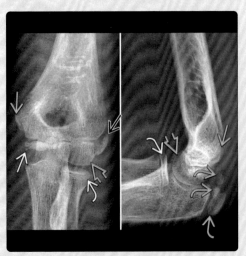

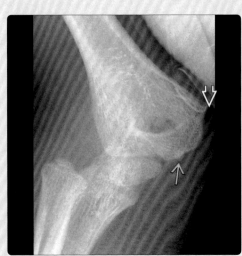

Normal Developmental Variants Confused With Disease

KEY FACTS

IMAGING

- Growing skeleton demonstrates range of normal age-related radiographic appearances due to
  - Abundant radiolucent growth cartilages
  - Gradual endochondral ossification of such cartilages
- Normal developmental variants have
  - Typical orientation, site, & patient age
  - No overlying swelling or point tenderness
    - May be clouded by isolated soft tissue injury
- MR useful when source of symptoms unclear (e.g., is fragmented growth center incidental normal variant or pathologic due to fracture, infarction, or infection)
  - Marrow edema on T2 FS/STIR MR favors pathology
  - ± soft tissue edema &/or joint effusion

TOP DIFFERENTIAL DIAGNOSES

- Physeal fractures
- Incomplete fractures
- Remote trauma
- Child abuse
- Ligamentous disruption
- Avascular necrosis

CLINICAL ISSUES

- Normal variants usually asymptomatic; come to attention incidentally on imaging (often with history of regional trauma)

DIAGNOSTIC CHECKLIST

- If unclear whether or not bony appearance is abnormal vs. incidental normal developmental variant in regionally symptomatic child
  - Review prior radiographs
  - Determine exact site of tenderness
  - Consider
    - Contralateral radiographs of asymptomatic side
    - Splinting with follow-up radiographs in 10-14 days to assess for healing changes

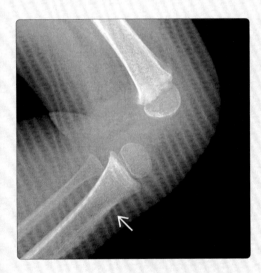

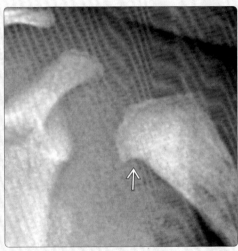

(Left) *Lateral radiograph of the knee in a 2-year-old patient shows a normal anterior tibial metadiaphyseal concavity* ➔ *at the site of the unossified tibial tubercle. Transversely oriented fractures may be seen at this level but show focal buckling or cortical interruption.* **(Right)** *AP radiograph in a 6-day-old boy shows an accentuated metaphyseal curvature* ➔ *in the medial proximal humerus, a normal finding in a young child at this level. The curve still flows smoothly with the diaphyseal cortex (passing the "marble test").*

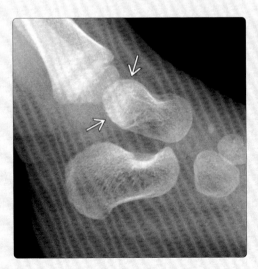

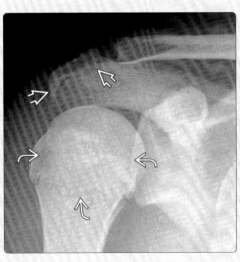

(Left) *Lateral radiograph in a 2-year-old girl shows poorly defined sclerosis in the posterior talus* ➔*, a commonly seen normal finding at this age. Linear sclerosis in the posterior calcaneus or cuboid (not present here) would suggest a fracture in this age group.* **(Right)** *AP internal rotation radiograph of the right shoulder in a 15-year-old boy shows an unfused acromion ossification center* ➔*. The obliquity of the proximal humeral physis* ➔ *is viewed at different heights from this perspective (a common fracture mimic).*

VACTERL Association

TERMINOLOGY

- Nonrandom association of anomalies involving multiple organ systems
  - **V**ertebral/vascular
  - **A**nal atresia/auricular
  - **C**ardiac
  - **T**racheoesophageal fistula
  - **E**sophageal atresia
  - **R**enal/radial ray/rib
  - **L**imb
- VACTERL association diagnosed when ≥ 3 of above malformations present; causative gene unknown

IMAGING

- Actively seek other features of VACTERL association when 1-2 components present
- Initial imaging in suspected cases: Radiographs & US
  - Radiographs: Spine & limbs (if limb anomaly present on physical exam)
  - US: Head, spine, renal/bladder, echocardiography
- Further imaging depends on clinical exam & initial imaging findings

CLINICAL ISSUES

- Incidence of VACTERL: 1/10,000 to 40,000 liveborns
- Children with VACTERL: 72% have 3 anomalies, 24% have 4 anomalies, 8% have 5 anomalies
  - Cardiac: 40-80%
  - Renal: 50-80%
  - Anal: 55-90%
  - Tracheoesophageal: 50-80%
  - Vertebral: 60-80%
  - Limb: 40-50%

DIAGNOSTIC CHECKLIST

- Consider VACTERL in child with vertebral & other anomalies

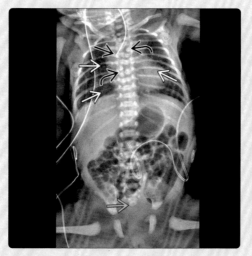
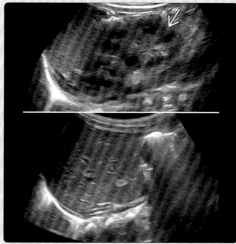

(Left) Frontal radiograph in a newborn shows vertebral segmentation anomalies ⊅. The nasogastric tube (NG) could not be advanced beyond the upper esophagus ⊅ due to esophageal atresia (with the bowel gas indicating an associated tracheoesophageal fistula). Mild central pulmonary vascular congestion ⊅ is secondary to a VSD. There is partial sacral agenesis ⊅ in this child with an ARM. (Right) Longitudinal US images of the left (top) & right (bottom) renal fossae in the same patient show a solitary left kidney ⊅.

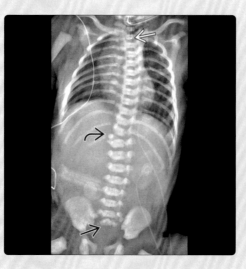
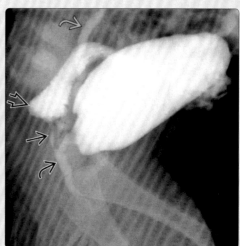

(Left) Frontal radiograph in a newborn shows vertebral segmentation anomalies ⊅ & partial agenesis of the sacrum ⊅. The NG tube could not be passed beyond the upper esophagus due to esophageal atresia ⊅ (with the lack of abdominal gas indicating the absence of a tracheoesophageal fistula). (Right) Lateral view from a VCUG in the same child shows a rectourethral fistula ⊅ from the rectal pouch ⊅ to the posterior urethra ⊅. Left vesicoureteral reflux ⊅ is also seen in this child with an ARM.

TERMINOLOGY

Synonyms

- VATER, VACTER, VACTEL association, TREACLE, ARTICLE

Definitions

- Nonrandom association of anomalies involving multiple organ systems (except brain)
  o **V**ertebral/vascular
  o **A**norectal malformation (ARM)/auricular
  o **C**ardiac
  o **T**racheoesophageal fistula (TEF)
  o **E**sophageal atresia (EA)
  o **R**enal/radial ray/rib
  o **L**imb
- VACTERL association diagnosed when ≥ 3 of above malformations present
  o Clubfoot & hip dysplasia excluded if no other limb anomalies present
- No clinical or laboratory evidence of alternative diagnosis

IMAGING

Radiographic Findings

- Axial skeleton
  o Vertebral anomalies
    – Cleft, block, butterfly vertebrae; hemivertebrae; hypersegmentation; vertebral bars; caudal regression
    – Secondary scoliosis, kyphosis
  o Other spine issues: Cord tethering (8-78%)
  o Ribs: Fused; bifid; hypoplastic; supernumerary/cervical
- Limbs or extremities
  o Radial ray: Dysplastic or absent radius; radioulnar synostosis; thumb hypoplasia; radial polydactyly; absent scaphoid; radial artery hypoplasia
  o Hands: Polydactyly most common (20%); syndactyly
  o Reduction deformities (34%): Aplasia/hypoplasia of humerus, radius, femur, tibia, or fibula
- Head & neck
  o Choanal atresia, cleft lip/palate, auricular defects
- Chest
  o Congenital heart disease: Ventricular septal defect (30%); patent ductus arteriosus (26%); atrial septal defect (20%)
  o EA/TEF
  o Lung agenesis, horseshoe lung (posterior lung fusion), ectopic bronchus
- Abdomen & pelvis
  o Imperforate anus ± fistula
  o Microgastria, duodenal atresia, malrotation, Meckel diverticulum

Ultrasonographic Findings

- Prenatal US may suggest diagnosis
- Prenatal detection rates of VACTERL anomalies
  o Renal malformations: 45%; TEF: 44%; cardiac malformations: 20%; vertebral: 13%; limb: 11%
- Neonatal head US to evaluate for findings suggestive of other diagnoses (e.g., hydrocephalus)
- Spinal US to evaluate for tethered cord
- Renal/bladder US to evaluate for renal/GU anomalies

  o Renal agenesis most common (bilateral in ~ 13%); multicystic dysplasia; horseshoe kidney; ectopia; hydronephrosis
  o Persistent urachus; cryptorchidism

Imaging Recommendations

- Consider specific work-up for VACTERL in
  o All infants with 2 features of VACTERL association
  o All infants with TEF/EA
  o All infants with ARM
- Radiographs & US used initially in suspected cases
  o Radiographs: Spine & limbs (if limb anomaly present on physical exam)
  o US: Head, spine, renal/bladder, echocardiography
  o Additional & advanced imaging depending on initial radiographic & clinical exam findings

PATHOLOGY

General Features

- Etiology
  o No unifying causative gene identified

CLINICAL ISSUES

Presentation

- Most common signs/symptoms
  o Neonatal: Depends on anomaly constellation
- Other signs/symptoms
  o Prenatal imaging
    – Polyhydramnios (EA), kyphoscoliosis, absent radius, cardiac &/or renal anomalies, single umbilical artery
  o Prematurity: ~ 1/3
  o Stillborn: 12%

Demographics

- Epidemiology
  o 1/10,000 to 40,000 liveborn infants
  o Frequency of anomalies in VACTERL
    – Cardiac: 40-80%
    – Renal: 50-80%
    – Anal: 55-90%
    – Tracheoesophageal: 50-80%
    – Vertebral: 60-80%
    – Limb: 40-50%
  o Children with VACTERL: 72% have 3 anomalies, 24% have 4 anomalies, 8% have 5 anomalies
    – Most common 3-anomaly combinations: Cardiac-renal-limb & cardiac-renal-anal

Natural History & Prognosis

- Mortality (not due to any specific defect)
  o 28% neonatal mortality
  o 48% mortality in 1st year
- Intelligence usually normal

SELECTED REFERENCES

1. Solomon BD et al: An approach to the identification of anomalies and etiologies in neonates with identified or suspected VACTERL (vertebral defects, anal atresia, tracheo-esophageal fistula with esophageal atresia, cardiac anomalies, renal anomalies, and limb anomalies) association. J Pediatr. 164(3):451-7.e1, 2014
2. Solomon BD: VACTERL/VATER association. Orphanet J Rare Dis. 6:56, 2011

Polydactyly

TERMINOLOGY

- Polydactyly: Extra digits of hands or feet
  - Preaxial: Radial side of hand, tibial side of foot
  - Postaxial: Ulnar side of hand, fibular side of foot
  - Central (mesoaxial): Involves central digits
  - Mirror-image polydactyly: Central thumb/great toe-like digit with variable duplication of 2nd-5th digits
- Syndactyly: Fusion of digits
  - Simple (soft tissue fusion) vs. complex (osseous fusion)
  - Complete (entire digit) vs. incomplete (spares distal digit)
- Polysyndactyly: Polydactyly + syndactyly (soft tissue ± osseous fusion of digits)

IMAGING

- Radiographs of affected hand/foot done primarily to detect skeletal elements within extra digit(s)
- Extra digit can range from small entirely soft tissue skin tag → rudimentary digit with hypoplastic bones → fully developed extra digit

- Affected phalanges, metacarpals/metatarsals may be bifurcated or duplicated
- Skeletal survey indicated if syndromic association suspected

PATHOLOGY

- Most cases sporadic & isolated
- However, ~ 300 syndromes associated with polydactyly
  - Trisomies (13, 18, 21), Meckel-Gruber, VACTERL, etc.
- If polydactyly discovered on prenatal US or MR, other anomalies must be sought

CLINICAL ISSUES

- Widely heterogeneous phenotypes of polydactyly
- Prognosis depends on complexity of duplication & associated anomalies
- Surgery directed at creating functional, aesthetic hand or foot: Excision of extra digit; partial excision/reshaping of bifid or broad metacarpals/metatarsals; tendon, ligament, capsule repair/reconstruction

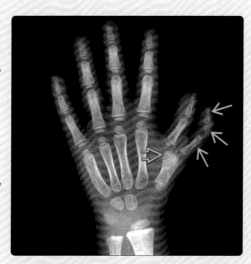
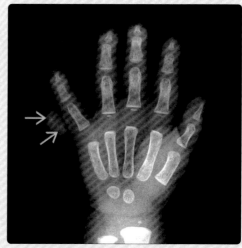

(Left) PA radiograph shows the left hand of a 2-year-old girl with preaxial polydactyly. The duplicated thumb is triphalangeal ➡ (Wassel type VII). The distal end of the 1st metacarpal is broad ➡ but not duplicated. (Right) PA radiograph shows the left hand of a 2-year-old boy with postaxial polydactyly (type B). There is an incompletely formed 6th digit, which contains 2 small, incompletely formed phalanges ➡.

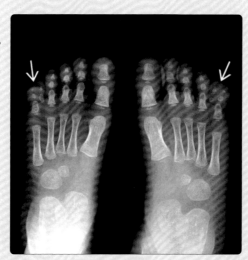
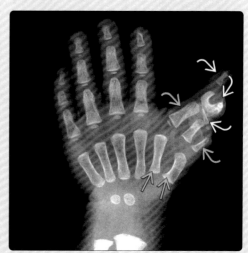

(Left) AP radiograph of both feet in a 2-year-old girl shows bilateral postaxial polydactyly (type B) with duplication of the 5th middle & distal phalanges ➡. (Right) PA radiograph of the left hand in a girl with multiple limb anomalies shows a complex preaxial polydactyly with 2 metacarpals ➡, 3 proximal phalanges ➡, & a complex array of middle & distal phalanges ➡ with soft tissue & osseous fusion.

Clubfoot

TERMINOLOGY

- Plantarflexion of calcaneus relative to tibia (equinus) + hindfoot inversion (varus) + forefoot adduction (varus)
- Synonyms: Talipes equinovarus, CAVE (**C**avus, forefoot **a**dductus, hindfoot **v**arus & **e**quinus)

IMAGING

- Talus: Lateral rotation within ankle joint
  - Talus point of reference for hindfoot
- Calcaneus: Relative medial rotation + equinus
- Navicular: Medial subluxation on talus
- Cuboid: Medial subluxation on calcaneus
- Metatarsals: Inverted, appear parallel on lateral view
- AP view: "Laterally pointing" hindfoot + adducted forefoot
  - Long axis of talus very lateral to 1st metatarsal
  - Long axis of calcaneus lateral to 5th metatarsal
- Measurements made on weightbearing views
  - ↑ tibiocalcaneal angle on lateral view (> 90° = calcaneal equinus)
  - ↓ talocalcaneal angle on lateral & AP views (hindfoot varus)
  - ↑ talus-1st metatarsal angle (forefoot varus)
- Frequently detected on screening 2nd-trimester ultrasound
- Prenatal MR performed for other abnormalities (e.g., myelomeningocele) may detect clubfoot

PATHOLOGY

- Isolated, idiopathic, congenital form most common
- Additional anomalies in 24-50%
  - Myelomeningocele, arthrogryposis, myotonic dystrophy
  - Various syndromes (trisomies 18, 21)
- Association with intrauterine "packing disorders" (e.g., oligohydramnios, twinning)

CLINICAL ISSUES

- 50% bilateral
- Treatment primarily conservative with manipulation & casting; selective use of surgery

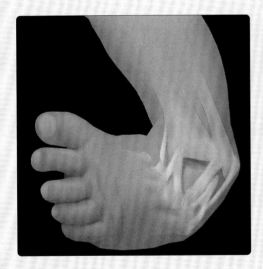

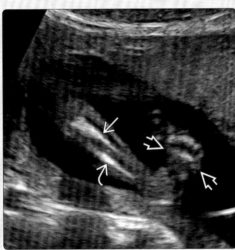

(Left) Oblique graphic shows a clubfoot with equinus, inversion, & forefoot adduction. (Right) Sagittal US through the lower leg of a 27-week gestation fetus with amniotic band syndrome shows abnormal positioning of the foot relative to the foreleg with the tibia ➡, fibula ➡, & all metatarsals ➡ visible in their long axes on a single image (consistent with clubfoot).

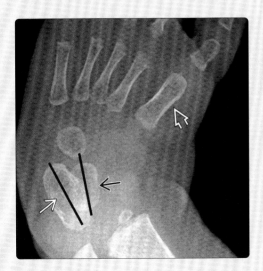

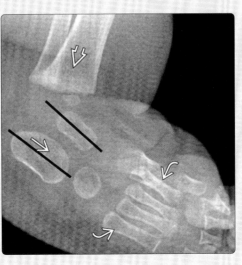

(Left) AP radiograph in a 9 month old with clubfoot shows hindfoot varus with a reduced talocalcaneal angle (black lines). There is varus angulation of the forefoot ➡ with the long axis of the talus ➡ far lateral to the 1st metatarsal & the long axis of the calcaneus ➡ lateral to the 5th metatarsal. (Right) Lateral view shows hindfoot varus with a reduced talocalcaneal angle (black lines). The angle between the long axes of the tibia ➡ & calcaneus ➡ is > 90° (hindfoot equinus). The metatarsals ➡ appear parallel.

KEY FACTS

TERMINOLOGY

- Fracture of immature skeleton involving cartilaginous primary growth plate (physis)

IMAGING

- Most fractures detected & managed by radiographs alone
  - Widening or interruption of normally uniform undulating lucent physis
  - Translation &/or angulation of bony fragment adjacent to physis with overlying soft tissue swelling
  - Persistent physeal widening > 3 mm post reduction suggests tissue entrapment requiring open reduction
- CT: Helps evaluate comminution, displacement, articular surface "step-off," loose intraarticular fragment(s)
- MR: Can detect nondisplaced fractures, assess cartilaginous & soft tissue injury or entrapment

TOP DIFFERENTIAL DIAGNOSES

- Incomplete fracture

- Chronic physeal stress injury
- Rickets

CLINICAL ISSUES

- Peak age: 11-12 years
- 6-30% of childhood fractures involve physis
- Overall complication rate: ~ 14% (but varies by site)
  - Premature physeal closure with limb shortening or angulation; risk highest in distal femur, tibia
  - Joint incongruity due to intraarticular extension with > 2-mm articular surface gap → degenerative arthritis
  - Osteomyelitis (particularly with nailbed injury)

DIAGNOSTIC CHECKLIST

- Always evaluate involved growth plate for premature closure on follow-up studies

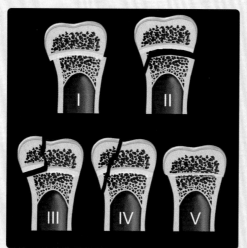
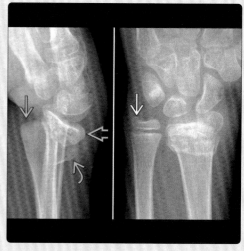

(Left) Graphic shows the relationship of the epiphyseal, physeal, & metaphyseal components of the 5 main types of Salter-Harris (SH) fractures. (Right) Lateral (left) & PA (right) radiographs of the wrist in a 9 year old show a SH II fracture of the distal radius with ~ 60% dorsal translation of the epiphyseal ⇨ & metaphyseal ⇨ fracture fragments with ~ 45° apex volar angulation. Note the uncovering of the volar metaphysis ⇨. A nondisplaced ulnar styloid fracture ⇨ is noted.

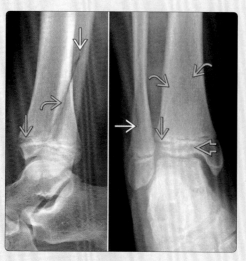
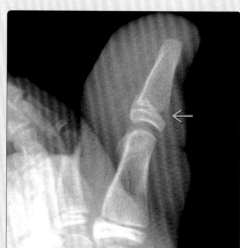

(Left) Lateral (left) & AP (right) radiographs of the ankle in a 15 year old show a classic SH IV triplane fracture with sagittal epiphyseal ⇨, horizontal physeal ⇨, & coronal metaphyseal & diaphyseal ⇨ components. A fibular fracture ⇨ is also present. (Right) Lateral radiograph in a 10 year old after a toe stubbing injury shows a subtle, nondisplaced SH II fracture ⇨ of the great toe distal phalanx. If there is a nailbed injury, the patient should be given prophylactic antibiotics to prevent osteomyelitis.

TERMINOLOGY

Synonyms

- Salter-Harris (SH) fractures 1-5 (I-V)

Definitions

- Fracture of immature skeleton involving cartilaginous primary growth plate (physis)

IMAGING

General Features

- Relative frequency of extremity involvement
  - Upper: Distal radius > phalanges > distal humerus, others
  - Lower: Distal tibia > phalanges > others

Radiographic Findings

- Upon presentation
  - Partial or complete physeal widening with metaphyseal &/or epiphyseal fracture lines
  - Varying degrees of fragment translation &/or angulation
  - Overlying soft tissue edema
- Immediately after reduction
  - Persistent physeal widening > 3 mm suggests tissue entrapment requiring open reduction
    - Displaced periosteum > ligament or tendon
- Long-term follow-up
  - Evaluate affected physis for premature closure

CT Findings

- Helps evaluate comminution, displacement, articular surface "step-off," loose intraarticular fragment(s)
  - ≥ 2-mm articular surface "step-off" generally requires open reduction + internal fixation

MR Findings

- May alter clinical management in acute setting by
  - Detecting nondisplaced fractures
  - Visualizing fracture relationship to radiolucent cartilage (changing fracture classification)
  - Visualizing entrapped structures (requiring open reduction)
  - Visualizing adjacent neurovascular injury
- May alter management of long-term complications by
  - Detecting & quantifying bony bridges
  - Detecting degenerative changes

Ultrasonographic Findings

- May visualize displacement of cartilaginous epiphyses, physeal &/or cortical interruption, subperiosteal fluid
  - Particularly useful in neonates/infants/toddlers with limited ossification of epiphyses

Imaging Recommendations

- Best imaging tool
  - Typically detected & managed by radiographs alone
  - CT, MR, & US have limited indications

DIFFERENTIAL DIAGNOSIS

Incomplete Fracture

- Cortical buckle deformity of metadiaphysis shows no fracture line extension to physis

Chronic Physeal Stress Injury

- Chronic pain in adolescent high-level athletes
- Widened physis mimics nondisplaced SH I fracture

Rickets

- Variety of metabolic abnormalities can inhibit endochondral ossification → metaphyseal fraying & cupping + widening of physis with loss of zone of provisional calcification
- Multiple physes symmetrically involved

PATHOLOGY

General Features

- ± associated injuries of neurovascular bundle, ligaments, cartilage, other bones

Staging, Grading, & Classification

- Type I (~ 8.5%): Involves only physis
- Type II (~ 73%): Involves physis & metaphysis
- Type III (~ 6.5%): Involves physis & epiphysis
- Type IV (~ 12%): Involves physis, metaphysis, & epiphysis
- Type V (< 1%): Crush fracture involving physis

CLINICAL ISSUES

Presentation

- Most common signs/symptoms
  - Pain, swelling, point tenderness, limited range of motion, inability to bear weight

Demographics

- Peak age: 11-12 years
- 6-30% of childhood fractures involve physis

Natural History & Prognosis

- Overall complication rate ~ 15%
  - Early physeal closure → limb shortening or angulation
    - Much more common in lower extremities
      - Follow knee & ankle fractures for ≥ 1 year or until skeletal maturity due to risk of growth disturbances
    - 2x as likely in displaced vs. nondisplaced fractures
  - Joint incongruity due to articular surface involvement → degenerative arthritis
  - Osteomyelitis with adjacent nailbed trauma ("stubbed toe osteomyelitis") or penetrating injury

Treatment

- Closed reduction & casting for low SH categories (unless unstable post reduction)
  - < 2-mm displacement → ↓ risk of growth arrest
  - Follow-up at 5-7 days to ensure stability
- Open reduction & internal fixation often required with higher categories (due to articular surface involvement)
- Subsequent growth arrest (with bone bridge across physis) resulting in angular deformity or limb length discrepancy → bone bridge resection vs. contralateral epiphysiodesis

SELECTED REFERENCES

1. Chen J et al: Imaging appearance of entrapped periosteum within a distal femoral Salter-Harris II fracture. Skeletal Radiol. 44(10):1547-51, 2015
2. Mayer S et al: Pediatric knee dislocations and physeal fractures about the knee. J Am Acad Orthop Surg. 23(9):571-80, 2015
3. Little JT et al: Pediatric distal forearm and wrist injury: an imaging review. Radiographics. 34(2):472-90, 2014

Apophyseal Injuries

TERMINOLOGY

- Apophysis: Nonarticular secondary center of ossification that serves as attachment site for muscle or tendon
- Acute injury: Avulsion fracture of osseous &/or cartilaginous apophysis through subjacent physis
- Chronic injury: Repetitive submaximal tensile forces (avulsive microtrauma) exceed rate of repair, leading to local growth plate disturbance (± symptoms)

IMAGING

- Acute injury: Displaced apophyseal ossification center
- Chronic injury: Mild soft tissue swelling with ossific irregularity &/or physeal widening at tendon attachment site
- Radiographs usually diagnostic of acute avulsion
- Further imaging may be required if fragment nondisplaced, ossification center not yet present, or chronic apophysitis suspected
  - MR more sensitive & specific than US

TOP DIFFERENTIAL DIAGNOSES

- Osteomyelitis
- Osteosarcoma
- Muscle injury
- Stress injury of bone

CLINICAL ISSUES

- Acute injury: Sudden onset of pain with sensation of "pop" & instant ↓ of muscle function during athletic activity
- Chronic injury: Insidious onset of pain & swelling without specific event or associated bruising
- Most acute pelvic avulsions occur from ages 12-18 years
  - Most occur during kicking or sprinting
    - Soccer, gymnastics, rugby, track & field
  - AIIS, ASIS, ischial tuberosity > iliac crest, pubic symphysis
- Conservative (nonsurgical) therapy: Highly successful
- Surgical fixation reserved for displacement > 1.5-2.0 cm

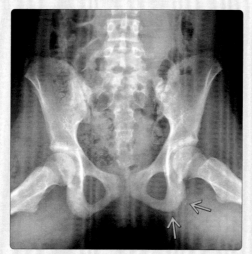

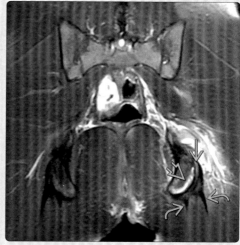

(Left) Frog leg lateral radiograph in a 13-year-old girl with acute onset of left hip pain & the sensation of a "pop" during cheerleading shows displaced bony fragments ➡ adjacent to the left ischial tuberosity. (Right) Coronal T2 FS MR in the same patient shows the attachments of the hamstring tendons ➡ to the displaced curvilinear osteocartilaginous apophysis ➡ at the ischial tuberosity. Fluid ➡ undercuts the displaced fragment, typical of an acute avulsion injury.

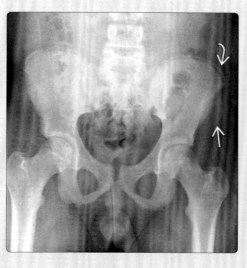

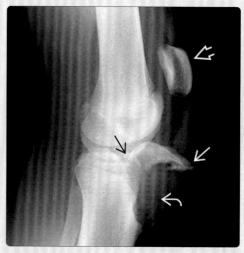

(Left) AP radiograph in a 16-year-old boy with a history of pain & a "pop" while kicking a ball shows an inferiorly displaced bony fragment ➡ avulsed from the anterior superior iliac spine. The lateral left iliac wing apophysis ➡ also shows fragmentation & growth plate widening, suggesting avulsion. (Right) Lateral radiograph in a 13 year old shows a tibial tubercle avulsion ➡ with the fracture line extending superiorly through the epiphysis ➡. Note the marked soft tissue edema ➡ & high-riding patella ➡.

TERMINOLOGY

Definitions

- Apophysis: Nonarticular secondary center of ossification that serves as attachment site for muscle or tendon
- Acute injury: Avulsion fracture of osseous &/or cartilaginous apophysis through subjacent physis
- Chronic injury: Repetitive submaximal tensile forces (avulsive microtrauma) exceed rate of repair, leading to local growth plate disturbance (± symptoms)

IMAGING

General Features

- Best diagnostic clue
  - Acute injury: Displaced apophyseal ossification center
  - Chronic injury: Soft tissue swelling with ossific irregularity at tendon attachment site
- Location
  - Acute avulsion injury
    - Pelvis/hips: High concentration of muscle attachments
      - Ischial tuberosity (hamstrings: Biceps femoris, semimembranosus, semitendinosus)
      - Anterior inferior iliac spine (AIIS) (rectus femoris)
      - Anterior superior iliac spine (ASIS) (sartorius)
      - Iliac crest (tensor fascia lata, abdominal wall muscles)
      - Pubic symphysis (adductors)
      - Greater trochanter (gluteus medius & minimus)
      - Lesser trochanter (iliopsoas)
    - Tibial tubercle (patellar tendon)
    - Medial epicondyle of humerus (flexor group & ulnar collateral ligament)
  - Chronic stress injury
    - Tibial tuberosity: Osgood-Schlatter disease
    - Humeral medial epicondyle: Little leaguer elbow
    - Calcaneal apophysis: Sever disease

Radiographic Findings

- Acute avulsion injury
  - Displacement of apophyseal ossification center
    - Tangential view: Crescentic, triangular, or irregular bone fragment
    - En face view: Poorly defined or ovoid fragment
  - Moderate to marked soft tissue edema
- Healed/remote acute avulsion fracture
  - Bony remodeling from prior injury
  - ± heterotopic ossification of soft tissues
- Chronic stress injury
  - Ossific irregularity/fragmentation at tendon attachment
  - Underlying physeal widening without true fragment displacement
  - Mild overlying soft tissue swelling

MR Findings

- Fluid-sensitive sequences (T2WI FS or STIR)
  - Acute injury: Bright fluid deep to displaced apophysis + edema of surrounding soft tissues & subjacent marrow
  - Chronic injury: Mild ↑ signal, widening, & irregularity of physis without discrete fluid

Imaging Recommendations

- Best imaging tool
  - Radiographs usually diagnostic of acute avulsion
  - MR useful in some settings
    - Acute injury: Nondisplaced fragment or purely cartilaginous fragment (prior to ossification)
    - Chronic apophysitis

PATHOLOGY

General Features

- Etiology
  - Osteochondral junction: Weakest point of immature musculoskeletal system
  - ↑ muscle strength of adolescence causes ↑ forces on relatively weak sites of muscle/tendon attachments
  - Acute apophyseal avulsions: Essentially Salter-Harris growth plate fractures
  - Chronic injury (apophysitis): Repetitive submaximal tensile stresses exceed rate of bone repair
    - Physeal widening due to impaired endochondral ossification or chondrocyte hypertrophy
    - Chronic stress injury may weaken physis & predispose to acute avulsion

CLINICAL ISSUES

Presentation

- Most common signs/symptoms
  - Acute: Sudden onset of pain with sensation of "pop" & instant ↓ of muscle function during athletic activity
  - Chronic: Insidious onset of pain & swelling without specific event or associated bruising

Demographics

- Age
  - Acute pelvic avulsions: Typically 12-18 years
  - Medial epicondyle avulsions: 9-14 years
  - Tibial tubercle avulsions: 13-16 years
- Epidemiology
  - Acute
    - Pelvic: Most occur with kicking or sprinting
      - Soccer, gymnastics, rugby, track & field
      - AIIS, ASIS, ischial tuberosity most common
    - Tibial tubercle: Common in basketball
    - Medial epicondyle: Throwing or dislocation
  - Chronic
    - Little leaguer: Valgus stress of overhead throwing
    - Osgood-Schlatter: Repetitive traction of jumping
    - Sever disease: Traction by Achilles tendon

Treatment

- Most conservative therapy successful
  - Initial rest followed by physical therapy
- Surgical fixation reserved for higher grade injuries
  - More likely if displacement > 1.5-2.0 cm

SELECTED REFERENCES

1. Schuett DJ et al: Pelvic apophyseal avulsion fractures: a retrospective review of 228 cases. J Pediatr Orthop. 35(6):617-23, 2015
2. Raissaki M et al: Imaging of sports injuries in children and adolescents. Eur J Radiol. 62(1):86-96, 2007

Incomplete Fractures

TERMINOLOGY

- Incomplete fracture: Macroscopic fracture line does not traverse entire bony diameter
  - Pediatric bones more elastic than adult bones
  - Greater propensity to bow or bend before breaking
- Buckle fracture: Focal outward bulge of cortex (without frank interruption) on compression side; cortex usually intact on tension side
- Plastic deformation: Smooth but accentuated bending of shaft without visible fracture line
- Greenstick fracture: Discrete fracture line on tension side does not extend through opposite cortex

IMAGING

- 2 tangential views show at least 1 unbroken cortex
- Occurs in diaphysis or metadiaphysis
- Typically diagnosed & managed by radiographs alone
- Contralateral comparison views may be helpful
  - Especially in plastic deformation

TOP DIFFERENTIAL DIAGNOSES

- Bowing due to underlying skeletal disease
  - Systemic or localized bony dysplasias
  - Metabolic bone diseases
- Normal developmental variants
- Salter-Harris type II fracture

CLINICAL ISSUES

- Pain, swelling, tenderness, disuse of limb after fall
- Greenstick type refractures in 7-20%

DIAGNOSTIC CHECKLIST

- Imaginary marble should smoothly roll down diaphyseal & metaphyseal cortex on radiograph: If it dips or bounces, strongly consider incomplete fracture
- Look carefully for metaphyseal fracture line extending to physis (implying Salter-Harris type II fracture): Complications & follow-up different from buckle

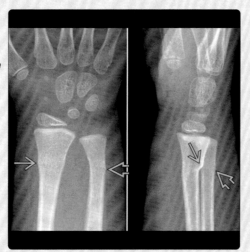
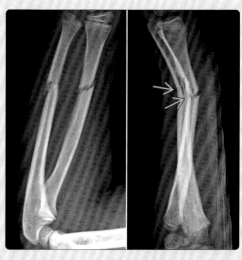

(Left) PA & lateral radiographs of the wrist in a 5 year old after a fall show a buckle deformity ➡ of the distal radial metadiaphyseal junction as well as an incomplete fracture (with cortical interruption) of the distal ulna ➡. (Right) AP & lateral radiographs of the forearm in a 5 year old after a fall show incomplete fractures of the distal radial & ulnar diaphyses. Note the intact "bent but not broken" posterior cortex of each bone ➡, typical of greenstick fractures.

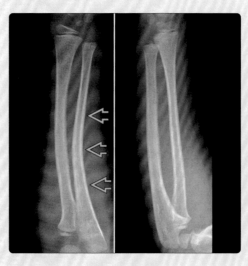
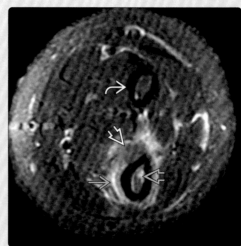

(Left) AP radiograph of the forearm in a 5 year old after a fall shows a plastic (bowing) deformity of the ulnar diaphysis ➡. The radial curvature is within normal limits. The ulnar deformity is not readily visible on the lateral view. (Right) Axial T2 FS MR in the same patient 4 days later (performed for specific elbow complaints) shows marrow ➡, periosteal ➡, & soft tissue edema in/about the ulnar diaphysis with no cortical break. Subperiosteal hemorrhage ➡ is noted. The radius ➡ is normal.

TERMINOLOGY

Definitions

- Incomplete fracture: Macroscopic fracture line does not traverse entire bony diameter
  - Pediatric bones more elastic than adult bones
    - Greater propensity to bow or bend before breaking
- Greenstick fracture: Discrete fracture line on tension side does not extend through opposite cortex
  - Appearance of bent immature tree branch ("green stick")
- Plastic deformation: Smooth but accentuated bending of shaft without visible fracture line
  - "Bowing fracture"
- Buckle fracture: Focal outward bulge of cortex (without frank interruption) on compression side; cortex usually intact on tension side
  - "Torus" term no longer in favor (as it implies circumferential bulging)
- Incomplete fracture with cortical disruption: Frank cortical disruption/angulation on compression side

IMAGING

General Features

- Best diagnostic clue
  - Cortical bump or angulation at site of pain + overlying soft tissue swelling after fall
- Location
  - Buckle fractures: Most often at distal metadiaphysis of radius & ulna or proximal tibia
  - Plastic deformation: Most common in diaphysis of ulna, fibula, or radius
  - Greenstick fractures: Most common in forearm diaphyses

Radiographic Findings

- Buckle fracture
  - Focal protuberance of cortex on compression side
- Plastic deformation
  - Subtle increased curvature of long bone diaphysis
  - Adjacent bone of forearm or lower leg often fractured
    - May be different type or dislocation
  - Periosteal reaction may be limited during healing
- Greenstick fracture
  - Visible hairline (or larger) fracture on convex tension side of cortex

Ultrasonographic Findings

- Focal interruption/bulging of echogenic cortex ± subperiosteal hemorrhage, soft tissue edema

Imaging Recommendations

- Typically diagnosed & managed by radiographs alone
- Contralateral comparison views may be helpful

DIFFERENTIAL DIAGNOSIS

Bowing due to Underlying Skeletal Disease

- Systemic or localized bony dysplasias
- Metabolic bone diseases

Normal Developmental Variants

- Few sites of normal cortical angulation/protuberance

- Comparison views of contralateral side may be helpful

Salter-Harris Type II Fracture

- Fracture line extends to physis

CLINICAL ISSUES

Presentation

- Most common signs/symptoms
  - Pain, swelling, tenderness, disuse of limb, or limp; typically after fall

Natural History & Prognosis

- Buckle fracture: Complete healing typical
- Plastic deformation: Does not typically remodel
- Greenstick fracture
  - Refracture in 7-20%
  - Rare median nerve entrapment or transection
  - Rare development of small subperiosteal cortical "cyst" during healing (due to entrapped medullary fat)

Treatment

- Buckle fracture
  - 3-week immobilization with splint
  - Follow-up not required in some circumstances
- Greenstick fracture
  - Depending on angulation, may require closed reduction & casting
  - Some advocate completing fracture for improved alignment
  - Prolonged immobilization may reduce refractures
- Plastic deformation
  - ± closed reduction
    - Requires significant force, adequate sedation
    - Prevents limitations of pronation-supination
    - Correction of rotational component may be required

DIAGNOSTIC CHECKLIST

Image Interpretation Pearls

- Imaginary marble should smoothly roll down diaphyseal & metaphyseal cortex on radiograph
  - If it dips or bounces, strongly consider incomplete fracture (especially with overlying swelling)
- Look carefully for metaphyseal fracture line extending to physis (implying Salter-Harris type II fracture)
  - Complications & follow-up different from buckle

SELECTED REFERENCES

1. Herren C et al: Ultrasound-guided diagnosis of fractures of the distal forearm in children. Orthop Traumatol Surg Res. 101(4):501-5, 2015
2. Pountos I et al: Diagnosis and treatment of greenstick and torus fractures of the distal radius in children: a prospective randomised single blind study. J Child Orthop. 4(4):321-6, 2010
3. Schmuck T et al: Greenstick fractures of the middle third of the forearm. A prospective multi-centre study. Eur J Pediatr Surg. 20(5):316-20, 2010
4. Carson S et al: Pediatric upper extremity injuries. Pediatr Clin North Am. 53(1):41-67, v, 2006
5. Swischuk LE et al: Frequently missed fractures in children (value of comparative views). Emerg Radiol. 11(1):22-8, 2004

Child Abuse, Metaphyseal Fractures

TERMINOLOGY

- Classic metaphyseal lesion (CML) or metaphyseal corner fracture: Transverse fracture of subphyseal metaphysis that undercuts subperiosteal bone collar peripherally
  - Fracture of infants with high specificity for child abuse

IMAGING

- Most common at distal femur, proximal & distal tibia
- Radiographic appearance
  - Acute fractures subtle, often difficult to identify initially
    - Triangular fragment at metaphyseal corner when x-ray beam perpendicular to bone long axis
    - Bucket-handle fragment adjacent to metaphysis when x-ray beam angled caudal or cranial relative to physis
  - Healing fractures more conspicuous
    - Subperiosteal new bone formation & callus require 7-14 days to appear radiographically

PATHOLOGY

- Due to tensile & torsional forces from twisting or pulling extremity or from acceleration/deceleration of shaking
  - 95% of cases with CML have ≥ 1 additional injury
- No established evidence that rickets/metabolic bone disease can cause CML

CLINICAL ISSUES

- Wide range of clinical presentations for nonaccidental trauma (NAT)
  - Injury inconsistent with history or stage of development
  - Multiple injuries in various stages of healing
  - Bruising in nonmobile infant
- Initial skeletal survey obtained for
  - < 2 years old with suspicion of NAT
  - < 5 years old with suspicious fracture
  - Concern for NAT in any child unable to communicate
- Obtain follow-up skeletal survey in 2 weeks: Healing increases fracture conspicuity

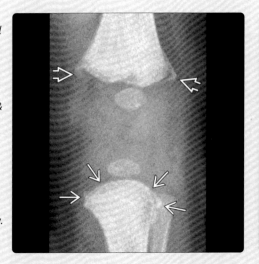

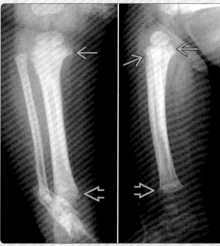

(Left) AP radiograph in a 1-month-old girl shows a typical metaphyseal corner fracture at the distal femoral metaphysis ➡ with a bucket-handle appearance of a proximal tibial metaphyseal fracture ➡. (Right) AP (left) & lateral (right) radiographs of the right lower leg in a 6 month old with bruising show lucent irregularities of the subphyseal tibial metaphyses proximally ➡ & distally ➡. A corner fragment is best appreciated anteriorly at the distal tibia on the lateral view.

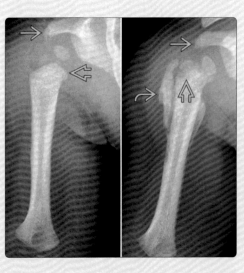

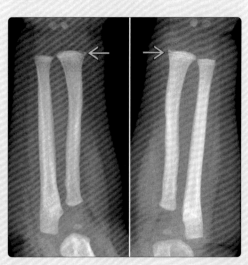

(Left) AP radiographs of the right humerus in the same patient at the time of presentation (left) & 2 weeks later (right) show an evolving acromion fracture ➡ (which has a high specificity for nonaccidental trauma). Initial image shows minimal proximal humeral metaphyseal abnormality ➡ that becomes much more conspicuous on the follow-up study with abundant periosteal reaction ➡. (Right) AP radiographs in the same patient (at presentation) show bilateral corner fractures of the distal radial metaphyses ➡.

TERMINOLOGY

Synonyms

- Nonaccidental trauma (NAT), battered child syndrome
- Metaphyseal corner fracture, classic metaphyseal lesion (CML), bucket-handle fracture

Definitions

- Fracture of infants that extends though subphyseal metaphysis & undercuts subperiosteal bone collar peripherally; highly specific for child abuse

IMAGING

Radiographic Findings

- Involves long bone metaphyses, most commonly distal femur, proximal & distal tibia, proximal humerus
- Acute fractures subtle, often difficult to identify initially
- Appearance depends on radiographic projection
  - Triangular fragment at metaphyseal corner when x-ray beam perpendicular to metaphysis long axis
  - Bucket-handle fragment adjacent to metaphysis when x-ray beam angled caudal or cranial relative to physis
- Healing fractures more conspicuous
  - Callus & subperiosteal new bone formation require 7-14 days to appear

Nuclear Medicine Findings

- Tc-99m MDP skeletal scintigraphy or 18F-NaF PET complementary to initial skeletal survey
  - Focal ↑ in radionuclide activity with 24 hours, normalizing within 6 months
  - Overall, sensitivity of scintigraphy for detecting fractures > initial skeletal survey, with exception of CML, skull & scapular fractures, remote injuries
  - Scintigraphy specificity lower than initial skeletal survey

Imaging Recommendations

- Initial skeletal survey
  - Indications
    - < 2 years old with suspicion of NAT
    - < 5 years old with suspicious fracture
    - Concern for NAT in any child unable to communicate
  - Images include: AP & lateral skull, lateral cervical & lumbar spine, AP & lateral & both obliques thorax, AP pelvis, AP humeri, AP forearms, PA hands, AP femurs, AP lower legs, AP feet
  - Additional views based on clinical & imaging findings
- Follow-up skeletal survey
  - Typically 2 weeks from initial evaluation
  - Indications
    - Concerning fractures on initial study
    - Normal initial study with persistent suspicion
  - Used to confirm suspected fractures & identify additional fractures
  - In 1 study, clarified questionable fractures or identified new fractures in 48% of cases
- Tc-99m MDP skeletal scintigraphy or 18F-NaF PET as complementary or problem-solving tools
- NECT for suspected intracranial injury; CECT for suspected intrathoracic or intraabdominal injury

DIFFERENTIAL DIAGNOSIS

Osteogenesis Imperfecta

- Multiple fractures ± Wormian bones, blue sclera
- ± osteoporosis

Rickets

- Metaphyseal fraying, cupping, widening ± fractures
- Demineralization

Leukemia

- Metaphyseal lucent bands ± fractures, more aggressive permeative lesions

Menkes Syndrome

- Osteoporosis, metaphyseal corner spurs, Wormian bones, tortuous intracranial arteries, & brittle hair

PATHOLOGY

General Features

- Due to tensile & torsional forces from twisting or pulling extremity or from acceleration/deceleration of shaking
- No established evidence that rickets/metabolic bone disease can cause CML

CLINICAL ISSUES

Presentation

- Wide range of clinical presentations for NAT
  - Injury inconsistent with history or stage of development
  - Multiple injuries in various stages of healing
  - Bruising in nonmobile infant
  - Retinal hemorrhages
- 1 study evaluating bruising as indicator for CML
  - 25% had bruising at sites other than fracture site
  - Only 13% had bruising at/near fracture site
- Another study found that 95% of cases with CML had at least 1 additional injury
  - 84% had additional non-CML fractures, most commonly long bone & rib
  - 43% had cutaneous injuries (bruising or burns)
  - 28% had traumatic brain injury

Demographics

- CML most common fracture in fatal NAT cases in 1 study
- Present in 50% of infants at high risk for NAT compared to 0% in infants at low risk for NAT

Treatment

- Multidisciplinary investigation of maltreatment allegation
- Ensure "at risk" child & siblings placed in safe environment

SELECTED REFERENCES

1. Servaes S et al: The etiology and significance of fractures in infants and young children: a critical multidisciplinary review. Pediatr Radiol. 46(5):591-600, 2016
2. Thackeray JD et al: The classic metaphyseal lesion and traumatic injury. Pediatr Radiol. ePub, 2016
3. Barber I et al: The yield of high-detail radiographic skeletal surveys in suspected infant abuse. Pediatr Radiol. 45(1):69-80, 2015
4. Kleinman, PK. Diagnostic imaging of child abuse. Cambridge, United Kingdom New York: Cambridge University Press, 2015
5. Perez-Rossello JM et al: Absence of rickets in infants with fatal abusive head trauma and classic metaphyseal lesions. Radiology. 141784, 2015

Other Fractures of Child Abuse

IMAGING

- High specificity for child abuse
  - Classic metaphyseal lesions, posterior rib fractures
  - Scapular fractures
    - Transverse or oblique fractures of mid acromion process most common
    - Acromion tip fracture mimics ossification center
  - Sternal fractures
    - Linear lucency or buckling of anterior cortex
    - Widened sternal synchondrosis or malalignment of sternal segments
  - Spinous process fractures
    - Cartilage/bone avulsion at interspinous ligamentous attachment due to hyperflexion & shaking
    - Ossific density adjacent to spinous process may represent acute or remote injury
- Moderate specificity for child abuse
  - Vertebral body fractures
    - Compression deformity &/or anterosuperior endplate fracture
  - Vertebral fracture-dislocations
    - Neurocentral synchondrosis fracture extending through endplate apophyses with retropulsion of vertebral centrum
    - Facet dislocation ± fracture
  - Transphyseal fracture/distal humeral epiphyseal separation
    - Capitellar ossification center, radius, & ulna displaced posteriorly & medially relative to distal humerus
    - Distal humeral cartilage maintains alignment with radius & ulna (not true dislocation)
  - Complex skull fractures, hand & foot fractures, pelvic fractures
- Low specificity for child abuse
  - Clavicle, long bone shaft, & linear skull fractures common but have low specificity for nonaccidental trauma

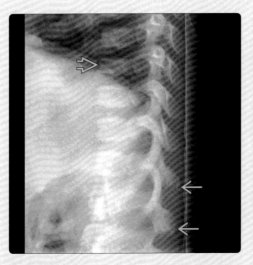
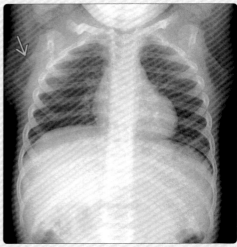

(Left) Lateral radiograph of the spine in an 8 month old with bruising & a subdural hematoma shows irregularity, lucency, & sclerosis of the T12 & L1 spinous processes ➡ as well as compression of the T9 vertebral body ➡. Spinous process fractures are highly suggestive of child abuse. (Right) AP chest radiograph in a 2 year old with bruising shows a fracture of the right scapular body ➡.

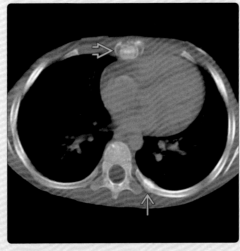
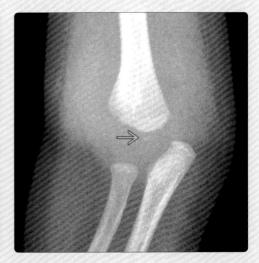

(Left) Axial CECT (in bone windows) in a young child with abdominal pain shows healing fractures of the sternum ➡ & a posterior left rib ➡. Both of these fractures are highly suggestive of child abuse. (Right) External oblique elbow radiograph in a 1 month old not using his arm shows medial translation of the capitellar ossification center ➡, radius, & ulna relative to the distal humerus, typical of a distal humeral epiphyseal separation fracture that is highly associated with child abuse.

TERMINOLOGY

Synonyms

- Nonaccidental trauma (NAT)

IMAGING

General Features

- Best diagnostic clue
  - Classic metaphyseal lesions (CML) & posterior rib fractures: High specificity for NAT
    - Other high-specificity injuries include scapular, spinous process, & sternal fractures
  - Multiple fractures, bilateral fractures, & fractures of varying ages: Moderate specificity for NAT
    - Other moderate-specificity injuries include epiphyseal separation, vertebral body, digital, complex skull, & pelvic fractures
  - Any injury incompatible with age & history → suspect NAT
- Distribution of fractures due to NAT
  - Skull 27%, ribs/sternum 18%, vertebra 2%, pelvis < 1%
  - Clavicle 4%, humerus 11%, forearm 7%, hand < 1%
  - Femur 18%, tibia & fibula & ankle 12%, tarsal & metatarsal < 1%

High-Specificity Fractures

- Scapular fractures
  - Acromion most commonly involved
- Sternal fractures
  - Rare, result from direct force to sternum
  - Linear lucency or buckling of anterior cortex
  - May require dedicated views or CT for evaluation
- Spinous process fractures
  - Avulsion of cartilage &/or bone at interspinous ligamentous attachments due to shaking, hyperflexion
  - ± vertebral body compression deformity

Moderate-Specificity Fractures

- Vertebral body fractures
  - Compression deformity &/or anterosuperior endplate fracture
- Vertebral fracture-dislocations
  - Neurocentral synchondrosis injury
    - Fracture extending through superior & inferior endplate apophyses & neurocentral synchondrosis posteriorly due to hyperflexion
  - Facet dislocation ± fracture
    - Widened interspinous distance on AP & lateral views
    - Retrolisthesis on lateral view
- Epiphyseal separations
  - Transphyseal fracture of distal humerus
    - Largely unossified capitellar ossification center translated posteriorly & medially relative to distal humerus but maintains alignment with radius
    - Mimics dislocation (rare in infants); most dislocations occur laterally
    - MR, US, or arthrogram helpful to confirm diagnosis & evaluate degree of displacement
    - Up to 50% due to NAT but can occur with birth or accidental trauma
  - Proximal femoral epiphyseal separation
    - Proximal femoral diaphysis translated laterally & proximally relative to femoral head
    - Birth trauma may appear identical
- Complex skull fractures
  - > 1 fracture line, stellate or branching, comminuted
- Digital fractures of hands & feet
- Pelvic fractures
  - Subtle, typically involve superior pubic ramus in infants
  - ± association with sexual assault in older children

Low-Specificity Fractures

- Clavicle, long bone shaft, & linear skull fractures common

Dating Fractures

- Soft tissue swelling only in first 1-2 days, ↓ by 7 days; seen again (less pronounced) from 15-35 days
- Subperiosteal new bone formation after 7-10 days, ↑ thickness until 25 days
- Soft callus usually by 15 days, ↓ by 35 days
- Bridging & remodeling by 14-21 days
- Hard callus by > 35 days

PATHOLOGY

General Features

- Hyperextension/hyperflexion with acceleration-deceleration forces from shaking account for many NAT-related fractures, including CML, posterior rib fractures, spinal fractures, avulsion-type injuries of scapula
- Grabbing & twisting/torsional forces: Transcondylar & digital fractures
- Direct impact mechanism: Sternal, skull, & scapular body fractures

CLINICAL ISSUES

Presentation

- Wide range of clinical presentations for NAT
  - Injury inconsistent with history or stage of development
  - Multiple injuries in various stages of healing
  - Bruising in nonmobile infant
  - Burns, retinal hemorrhages
- Majority of spinal fractures clinically inapparent
  - Severe & undiagnosed may result in cord injury
  - Significant association with intracranial injury

Treatment

- Multidisciplinary investigation of maltreatment allegations must involve physicians, social worker, legal authorities
- Ensure "at risk" child & siblings given safe environment

SELECTED REFERENCES

1. Kleinman PK: Diagnostic imaging of child abuse. Cambridge, United Kingdom New York: Cambridge University Press, 2015
2. Supakul N et al: Distal humeral epiphyseal separation in young children: an often-missed fracture-radiographic signs and ultrasound confirmatory diagnosis. AJR Am J Roentgenol. 204(2):W192-8, 2015
3. Barber I et al: Prevalence and relevance of pediatric spinal fractures in suspected child abuse. Pediatr Radiol. 43(11):1507-15, 2013
4. Kleinman PK et al: Yield of radiographic skeletal surveys for detection of hand, foot, and spine fractures in suspected child abuse. AJR Am J Roentgenol. 200(3):641-4, 2013

TERMINOLOGY

- Fatigue fracture: Fracture due to abnormal stresses applied (over time) to normal bone
- Insufficiency fracture: Fracture due to normal stresses applied to abnormal bone
- Stress response/reaction: Result of stresses upon bone prior to development of macroscopic fracture
- Chronic physeal stress injury: Repetitive stress to growth plate interrupts normal endochondral ossification

IMAGING

- Stress injury of formed bone
  - Periosteal new bone ± transversely oriented lucent cortical fracture or band of sclerosis on radiographs
  - Transverse linear focus of ↓ signal (fracture line) + poorly defined marrow edema on MR = stress fracture
  - Limited marrow, periosteal, & soft tissue abnormalities without discrete fracture line = stress response
- Chronic physeal stress injury

  - Asymmetric lengthening ("widening") of lucent growth plate with metaphyseal irregularity on radiographs

TOP DIFFERENTIAL DIAGNOSES

- Stress fracture of bone: Osteomyelitis, osteoid osteoma, bone malignancy, bone infarct
- Stress injury of physis: Rickets, leukemia

CLINICAL ISSUES

- Fatigue fractures occur in
  - Athletes with overuse or recent change in routine
  - Newly ambulating children
  - Children with malalignment or altered weight-bearing
  - Preadolescent children with no recognized ↑ activity
- Insufficiency fractures occur in children with focal or systemic processes leading to bone weakening
- Treatment includes cessation of stresses with adequate time for bone repair & recovery of normal ossification

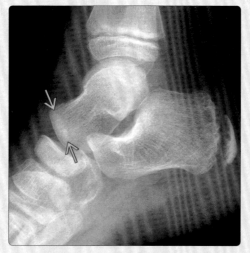
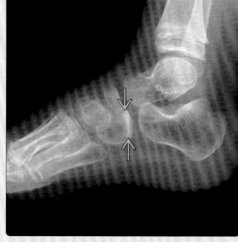

(Left) *Lateral radiograph of the ankle in an 8 year old with limping shows a band of vertically oriented sclerosis in the talar head ➡, typical of a stress injury.* (Right) *Lateral radiograph of the foot in a 3 year old shows a band of vertically oriented sclerosis in the posterior aspect of the cuboid ➡, a common location for a stress injury.*

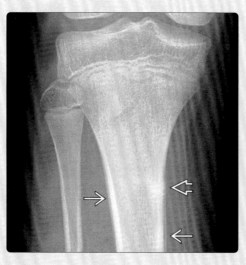
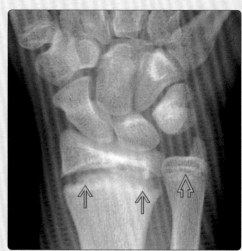

(Left) *AP radiograph shows circumferential benign periosteal reaction ➡ & a focus of medial cortical sclerosis ➡ in the tibia of a 12 year old, consistent with a stress fracture.* (Right) *PA wrist radiograph in a 13-year-old female gymnast with pain shows abnormal lengthening of the cartilaginous distal radial physis with metaphyseal irregularity ➡ & loss of the normal thin dense zone of provisional calcification. Note the normal distal ulnar physis ➡. This is a classic pattern for a chronic physeal stress injury ("gymnast wrist").*

TERMINOLOGY

Definitions

- Fatigue fracture: Fracture due to abnormal stresses applied (over time) to normal bone
- Insufficiency fracture: Fracture due to normal stresses applied to abnormal bone
  - Demineralized or otherwise weakened bone from focal or systemic process
- Stress response/reaction: Result of stresses upon bone prior to development of macroscopic fracture
- Chronic physeal stress injury: Repetitive stress to metaphyseal vasculature & cartilaginous growth plate interrupts normal endochondral ossification

IMAGING

Radiographic Findings

- Stress fracture
  - Poor cortical definition with varying degrees of cortical thickening/periosteal new bone
  - ± transversely oriented
    - Hairline fracture lucency extending centrally from involved cortex
    - Sclerotic band of medullary cavity
- Chronic physeal stress injury
  - Broad or focal lengthening ("widening") of lucent physis
  - Metaphyseal irregularity with loss of normal thin radiodense zone of provisional calcification

CT Findings

- Hairline transversely oriented unicortical lucency extending centrally with adjacent solid smooth periosteal reaction

MR Findings

- T1WI
  - Transverse hypointense stress fracture line extending from cortex into medullary cavity
  - Varying degrees of surrounding poorly defined hypointense marrow edema
- T2WI FS
  - Poorly defined hyperintense signal of marrow, periosteum, & soft tissues without discrete fracture line: Stress response
  - Transverse linear hypointense focus of medullary signal: Stress fracture
  - Metaphyseal extension of cartilaginous physeal signal intensity: Chronic physeal stress injury
    - Broad vs. small "tongue" of unossified cartilage
- T1WI C+ FS
  - Enhancing marrow, periosteal, & soft tissue edema

Nuclear Medicine Findings

- Bone scan: Intense cortical uptake; sensitivity ~ 100%
- SPECT/CT: ↑ specificity for location & etiology
  - May help separate fracture from osteoid osteoma
  - Excellent for pars interarticularis stress fracture

DIFFERENTIAL DIAGNOSIS

Focal Periosteal Reaction, Marrow Edema

- Osteoid osteoma
- Osteomyelitis
- Bone malignancy
  - Ewing sarcoma, metastatic neuroblastoma, leukemia

Linear Sclerosis Within Bone

- Infarction

Lucent & Irregular Physes/Metaphyses

- Rickets
- Epiphysiodesis (drill type)
- Leukemia

CLINICAL ISSUES

Presentation

- Most common signs/symptoms
  - Stress fracture: Pain, swelling with appropriate history
  - Chronic physeal stress injury: Pain; rarely asymptomatic
  - Symptoms typically for weeks prior to presentation
- Other signs/symptoms
  - Stress fracture
    - Bone percussion → pain
    - Palpable periosteal thickening, warmth
- Clinical profile
  - Fatigue fractures in
    - Athletes with recent changes in routine
      - Medial tibial stress syndrome: Overuse or repetitive stress injury to shin area; may progress to fracture
    - Newly ambulating children
      - Young child with new refusal to bear weight
    - Children with malalignment or altered weight-bearing
    - Preadolescent children with normal play activities & no elevation of activity intensity
  - Insufficiency fractures in
    - Children with focal or systemic processes leading to bone weakening
      - New stress reaction/insufficiency fracture in osteoporotic hindfoot due to ↑ ambulation after weeks of casting for preceding distal tibial fracture

Treatment

- Stress fracture
  - Prevention paramount: Gradual ↑ in new activity intensity + prompt activity reduction when pain occurs
  - Combination of reduced activity, rest, immobilization, casting, & (rarely) internal fixation
- Chronic physeal stress injury
  - Rest & immobilization typically sufficient for endochondral ossification to resume

SELECTED REFERENCES

1. Boyle MJ et al: Femoral neck stress fractures in children younger than 10 years of age. J Pediatr Orthop. ePub, 2016
2. Bedoya MA et al: Overuse injuries in children. Top Magn Reson Imaging. 24(2):67-81, 2015
3. Swischuk LE et al: Tibial stress phenomena and fractures: imaging evaluation. Emerg Radiol. 21(2):173-7, 2014
4. Rauck RC et al: Pediatric upper extremity stress injuries. Curr Opin Pediatr. 25(1):40-5, 2013
5. Jaimes C et al: Taking the stress out of evaluating stress injuries in children. Radiographics. 32(2):537-55, 2012
6. Galbraith RM et al: Medial tibial stress syndrome: conservative treatment options. Curr Rev Musculoskelet Med. 2(3):127-33, 2009

TERMINOLOGY

- Collection of poorly understood "disorders" of immature skeleton: > 70 entities, many with eponyms
- Many entities reflect symptomatic growth disturbances with elements of idiopathic osteonecrosis &/or overuse injury
- Symptoms range from asymptomatic → pain → growth disturbances
- Outcomes range from resolution of self-limited process → permanent deformity if untreated

IMAGING

- Affect certain sites where bone growth occurs by endochondral ossification (epiphyses, apophyses > metaphyses)
- Radiographs: Fragmentation, sclerosis, flattening
  - Depending on location, symptoms, & patient age, such findings do not necessarily connote disease

- Normal variants of irregular epiphyseal ossification can occur at certain locations
- MR: Marrow & soft tissue edema typically correlate with symptoms
  - Subtracted pre/postcontrast T1 FS images may show ↓ enhancement in setting of ischemia/necrosis

CLINICAL ISSUES

- Presentation is site-dependent: Pain, limp, or limb deformity possible
- Conservative therapy with rest effective for many, though certain entities (e.g., Blount, Legg-Calvé-Perthes) often require surgical intervention to preserve long-term function

DIAGNOSTIC CHECKLIST

- Not every irregular ossification center abnormal
  - Correlate with site, patient age, & symptoms
    - Helpful to know locations where irregular ossification normally occurs vs. never occurs
  - MR useful adjunct for determining source of pain

(Left) Lateral radiograph (left) & sagittal T2 FS MR (right) of a 12-year-old boy with anterior knee pain show fragmentation of the inferior pole of the patella ⮥ with adjacent soft tissue swelling ⮥. The findings are consistent with Sinding-Larsen-Johansson. (Right) Sagittal T2 FS MR shows edema in the calcaneal apophysis ⮥, consistent with Sever disease in this 8-year-old boy with posterior heel pain. Fragmentation & sclerosis may normally be seen at this level but edema should not.

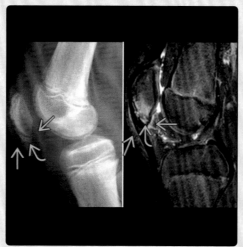

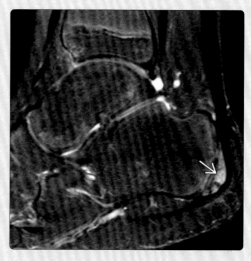

(Left) AP radiograph (left) shows downsloping, beaking, & irregularity of the medial tibial metaphysis ⮥ (Blount disease). Coronal GRE MR (right) shows abnormal ossification of the medial tibial epiphysis & metaphysis with an osseous bridge ⮥ across the tibial physis. (Right) AP radiograph (left) of an 8-year-old girl with Panner disease shows fragmentation & sclerosis of the capitellum ⮥. There is low signal intensity at this level on the T1 (middle) & T2 FS (right) MR images ⮥ with interspersed fluid signal intensity ⮥.

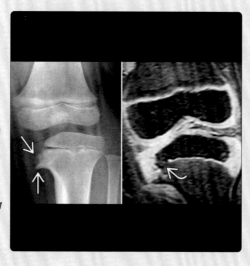

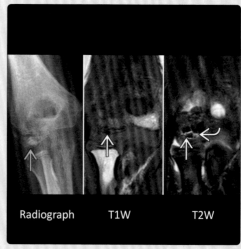

Radiograph   T1W   T2W

Osteochondritis Dissecans

TERMINOLOGY

- Focal joint disorder with progressive changes in subchondral bone & overlying articular cartilage that may lead to early joint degeneration
- Divided into adult osteochondritis dissecans (OCD) & juvenile OCD (JOCD) based on skeletal maturity (with closed or open physes, respectively)

IMAGING

- Locations: Knee most frequently affected
  - Lateral aspect of medial femoral condyle (69%), lateral femoral condyle (15%), patella (5%), femoral trochlea (1%); bilateral in 15-33%
  - Less frequent in elbow, ankle, hip
- Radiographs: Crescentic/ovoid lucent subchondral bone lesion surrounded by sclerotic margin
  - ± intraarticular ossific fragment, joint effusion
- MR visualizes osseous & cartilaginous changes
  - MR findings of instability direct therapy

TOP DIFFERENTIAL DIAGNOSES

- Normal irregular distal femoral epiphyseal ossification, avascular necrosis, acute osteochondral fracture

PATHOLOGY

- Favored mechanism: Repetitive microtrauma
- JOCD may represent growth disturbance of secondary physis; little necrosis or inflammation on histology

CLINICAL ISSUES

- Most common in adolescent athletes
- Symptoms often last > 1 year prior to diagnosis
  - Pain aggravated by activity
  - Mechanical symptoms (clicking, catching, grinding, locking) raise concern for unstable OCD
- Traditional treatment schemes lack strong evidence
  - Stable JOCD may heal conservatively over 6-18 months
  - Variety of surgical treatment options for stable OCD failing conservative therapy or unstable OCD

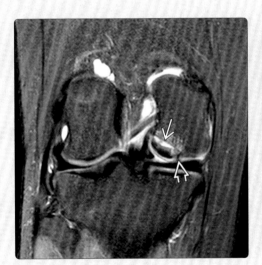
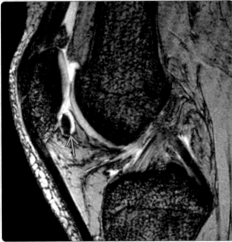

(Left) *Coronal T2 FS MR in a 15-year-old girl shows a complex osteochondral lesion of the medial femoral condyle. Fluid ➡ undercuts the fragment with an overlying T2-hypointense cartilage crack ➡ noted, consistent with an unstable lesion.* (Right) *Sagittal midline T2* GRE MR in the same patient shows a displaced intraarticular osteochondral fragment ➡ along the inferior patellar articular surface.*

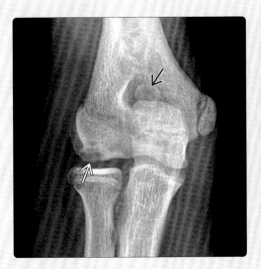
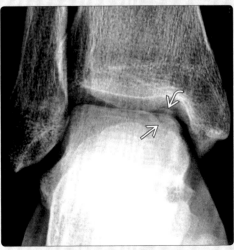

(Left) *AP elbow radiograph in a 13-year-old boy with pain & locking shows an irregular lucent defect ➡ with sclerotic margin in the humeral capitellum, typical of osteochondritis dissecans (OCD). The detached intraarticular fragment ➡ lies in the olecranon fossa.* (Right) *AP ankle radiograph in a 16-year-old boy shows a crescentic lucent lesion in the medial talar dome ➡ with a bony fragment ➡ protruding into the joint space, consistent with OCD.*

Soft Tissue Foreign Bodies

TERMINOLOGY

- Penetrating injury → soft tissue foreign body (FB)
- Chronic FB → granulomatous reaction → soft tissue mass

IMAGING

- Most FBs are not radiopaque (e.g., wood splinters)
- Some FBs are radiopaque (e.g., metal, glass, bone)
- Radiographs assess radiopaque FBs & osseous changes
- US: Excellent detection of superficial FBs
  - Typically echogenic
  - ± posterior shadowing depending on composition
  - Hypoechoic rim of edema/granulomatous reaction
- MR: FB typically of low signal on all sequences
  - Nonanatomic, geographic shape (e.g., linear, triangular)
  - FB may be small or very subtle
  - GRE may show blooming if metallic or Ca^{2+}
  - Adjacent edema or granulomatous reaction
  - Detects associated cellulitis, abscess, osteomyelitis

TOP DIFFERENTIAL DIAGNOSES

- Posttraumatic fat necrosis
- Soft tissue sarcoma
- Benign soft tissue tumors
- Venous malformation

CLINICAL ISSUES

- Erythema, swelling, &/or induration of overlying skin
  - Sinus tract to skin surface may develop
- Acute: Sensation of FB under skin after injury; ± history of skin penetration &/or attempted FB removal
- Chronic: Firm painless soft tissue mass
  - May occur long after injury that introduced FB
  - Often no specific trauma recalled
- Treatment: Surgical or US-guided removal

DIAGNOSTIC CHECKLIST

- If radiolucent superficial FB suspected → US

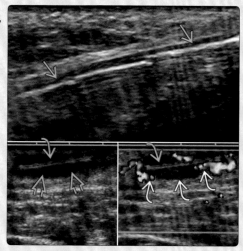

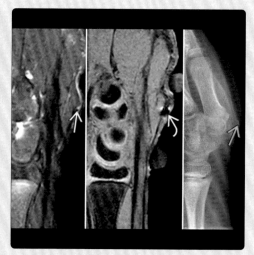

(Left) Initial US (top) of the left buttock in a 5-year-old boy who fell on a plastic toy shows a linear subcutaneous echogenic foreign body (FB) ➡. Removal was performed without imaging guidance. US 6 weeks later (bottom) shows a retained portion of the FB ➡ with adjacent hypoechoic ➡ but hypervascular ➡ granulation tissue. (Right) Sagittal MR images in a 10-year-old girl with a palpable lump show a focus of low signal ➡ on T2 FS (left) that blooms on GRE ➡ (middle). A lateral radiograph confirmed a FB ➡ (right).

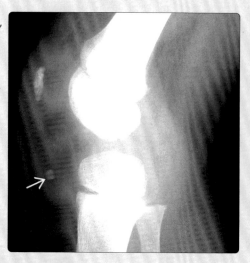

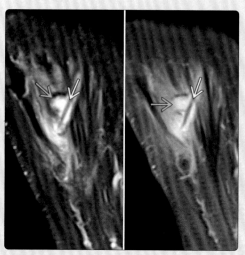

(Left) Lateral radiograph in a patient with a "palpable mass" shows a radiopaque FB ➡ in the infrapatellar soft tissues. The sharp margins, cube-like morphology, & density all suggest that the FB is made of glass. At surgery, a piece of glass with surrounding granulomatous reaction was found. (Right) Coronal long axis T2 FS (left) & T1 C+ FS (right) MR images of the foot show a linear low-signal retained toothpick ➡ surrounded by high-signal granulation tissue ➡.

Supracondylar Fracture

IMAGING

- AP radiograph: Transverse fracture through distal humeral metadiaphyseal junction at coronoid & olecranon fossae
  - Variable degrees of displacement
- Lateral radiograph: Visible posterior fat pad due to joint effusion (may be only finding of nondisplaced fracture)
  - Anterior humeral line fails to bisect capitellum due to dorsal displacement of distal fracture fragment
- Radiocapitellar alignment generally maintained on all views (in contradistinction to true dislocation)

TOP DIFFERENTIAL DIAGNOSES

- Lateral condylar fracture
- Posterior dislocation
- Distal humeral epiphyseal separation/transphyseal fracture

PATHOLOGY

- Accounts for 60% of pediatric elbow fractures
- Most common in children 5-7 years old; rare in adults (< 3%)

- Extension/FOOSH (fall on outstretched hand) mechanism (98%) vs. flexion with direct olecranon trauma (2%)
- Modified Gartland classification (I-IV) to direct treatment
  - Classified by degree of displacement, rotation, instability
  - Treatment ranges from casting to closed reduction with percutaneous fixation to open reduction internal fixation

CLINICAL ISSUES

- Pain, deformity, loss of function, swelling, discoloration
- ↑ risk of associated injuries if fracture displaced
  - Nerves (10-20%): Anterior interosseous/median > ulnar, radial
  - Vessels (3-14%): Spasm, laceration, thrombus, rupture
    - Radial pulse returns in > 50% after closed reduction
- Return of function in > 90% regardless of Gartland type

DIAGNOSTIC CHECKLIST

- Consider follow-up radiographs in 10-14 days to identify healing occult fracture if joint effusion only finding initially

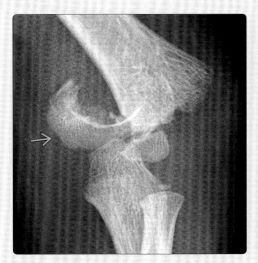

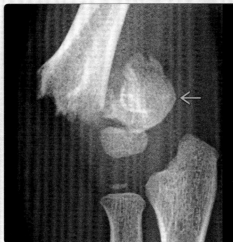

(Left) AP radiograph in a 5 year old after a fall shows a complete, transversely oriented distal humeral fracture through the olecranon & coronoid fossae with > 50% medial translation of the metaphysis ⇒. (Right) Lateral radiograph in the same patient shows no cortical contact of the posteriorly translated distal fragment ⇒ with the proximal fragment (representing a Gartland III or IV supracondylar fracture). The elbow articulations remain intact on both views (i.e., this is not an elbow dislocation).

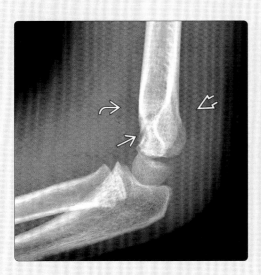

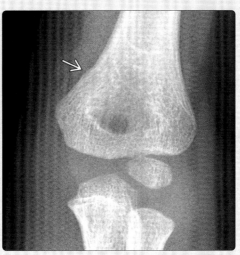

(Left) Lateral radiograph after a fall shows anterior cortical disruption ⇒ in the typical location of a supracondylar fracture. There is mild dorsal angulation of the distal fragment (with hinged but intact posterior cortex) such that an anterior humeral line no longer bisects the capitellum (i.e., Gartland IIA). There is a large elbow joint effusion with elevation of the anterior ⇒ & posterior ⇒ fat pads. (Right) AP radiograph in the same child shows subtle medial cortical buckling ⇒ of the supracondylar humerus.

Lateral Condylar Fracture

TERMINOLOGY

- Posterior oblique fracture through lateral condyle of humeral metaphysis with distal extension through unossified epiphyseal cartilage (Salter-Harris IV)
  - Fracture line may dissipate within epiphyseal cartilage before reaching articular surface

IMAGING

- AP view: Ranges from sliver of nondisplaced metaphyseal fracture fragment to marked translation & rotation of larger triangular metaphyseal fragment + capitellum
- Lateral view: Posterior oblique fracture plane; displacement of lucent anterior & posterior fat pads by joint effusion
- Internal oblique view: Best determines displacement
- Cartilaginous extension not radiographically visible but implied by degree of bone fragment displacement
  - Lack of bone fragment displacement does not ensure cartilage integrity/fracture stability
- Arthrography, MR, or US characterizes extent of cartilaginous articular surface injury

CLINICAL ISSUES

- 10-20% of pediatric elbow fractures (2nd most common)
  - Most common intraarticular pediatric elbow fracture
- Typically 5-10 years old; peak age: 6 years
- Jakob classification used to determine therapy
  - Type I (≤ 2-mm displacement): Typically casted
  - Type II (> 2-mm displacement without rotation): Closed reduction with percutaneous pinning
  - Type III (> 2-mm displacement with rotation): Open reduction & fixation
- Cast maintained for 4-6 weeks with operative or nonoperative treatment
- Complications include stiffness, late displacement, nonunion, delayed union, malunion, prominence or spurring of lateral condyle, capitellar avascular necrosis, tardy ulnar nerve palsy, arthritis

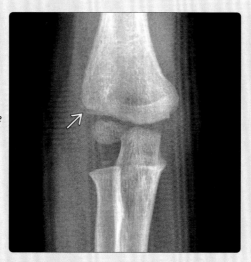
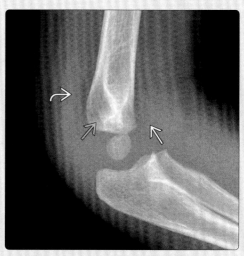

(Left) *AP radiograph in a 2 year old who fell off of a laundry basket shows an oblique fracture line through the lateral condyle with a sliver of a metaphyseal osseous fragment ➡. This is a Jakob type I fracture.* (Right) *Lateral radiograph in the same child shows an elbow joint effusion with elevation of both the anterior ➡ & posterior ➡ fat pads. The fracture line has a posterior oblique course ➡, typical of lateral condylar fractures.*

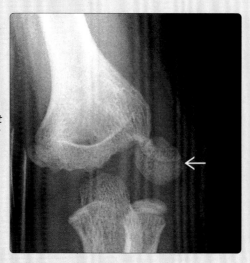
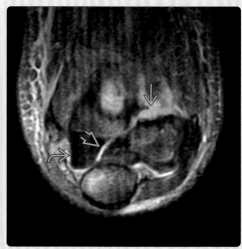

(Left) *AP radiograph in a 7 year old status post fall shows a displaced & rotated Jakob type III lateral condylar fracture fragment ➡. This fracture was treated with open reduction & K-wire fixation.* (Right) *Coronal T2 FS MR in an 8 year old status post fall (obtained with the patient splinted in 90° of flexion) shows hyperintense fluid tracking through the humeral lateral condylar metaphysis ➡. The fracture then extends distally ➡ through the unossified trochlear cartilage ➡.*

Medial Epicondyle Avulsion

TERMINOLOGY

- Acute injury: Avulsion fracture of medial epicondyle (ME) ossification center
- Chronic stress injury: Traction apophysitis, medial epicondylitis, Little Leaguer's elbow

IMAGING

- Acute injury: Distal &/or medial displacement of ME ossification center with moderate soft tissue swelling
  - Remember CRITOE pattern of ossification at elbow
    - Should normally see ME in expected location on AP radiograph if trochlea present
      - Important observation as avulsed, entrapped ME can simulate trochlear ossification center
  - Unreliable fat pad sign: Joint effusion may be absent
    - ME may become extracapsular > 2 years of age
- Chronic injury: Widening & irregularity of cartilaginous physis deep to ME
  - Less pronounced ME separation & soft tissue swelling

- ± fragmentation & edema of ME

PATHOLOGY

- Weakest link of immature musculoskeletal system: Osteocartilaginous interface
  - Acute tensile force → osteocartilaginous avulsion
    - Skeletally mature patients more likely to injure ligaments, tendons, muscles
  - Chronic submaximal valgus forces (repetitive microtrauma) exceed healing capacity of system → irritation & disturbance of normal ossification

CLINICAL ISSUES

- Typical age for acute & chronic ME injuries: 8-14 years
- Acute avulsion fracture: Elbow dislocation in 50%, entrapped ME in 15-20%
- Chronic stress injury: Same mechanism predisposes to capitellar osteochondritis dissecans & olecranon stress injuries
  - Typically overhead throwing athletes (e.g., pitchers)

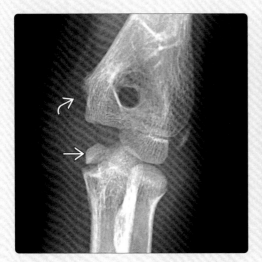

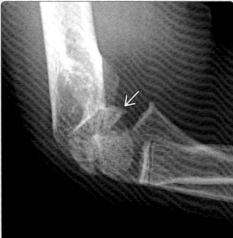

(Left) AP radiograph shows an ossific fragment ➡ adjacent to the medial margin of the olecranon of the ulna. No medial epicondyle (ME) ossification center is identified in its expected location ➘, though soft tissue swelling is noted at this level. (Right) Lateral radiograph in the same child shows that the avulsed ME ossification center ➡ is trapped in the joint. This incarcerated fragment must be reduced prior to casting.

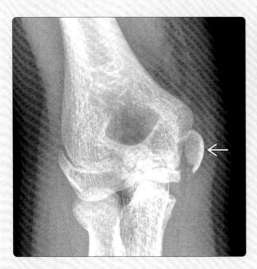

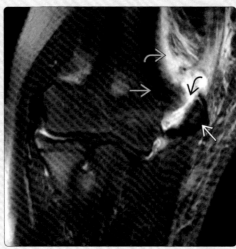

(Left) AP radiograph shows an acute avulsion of the ME ossification center with mild rotation & distal displacement of the fragment ➡. (Right) Coronal T2 FS MR in a 13-year-old pitcher with an acute injury shows a displaced ME ossification center ➡. Hyperintense fluid ➘ is interposed between the fragment & the medial humeral metaphysis ➘. There is moderate adjacent soft tissue edema ➘.

KEY FACTS

TERMINOLOGY

- Complete: Macroscopic fracture line traverses entire bony diameter (both cortices on single view)
  - Also includes physeal (Salter-Harris)
- Incomplete: Macroscopic fracture line does not traverse entire bony diameter (but opposite cortex often deformed)
  - Includes buckle, plastic (bowing) deformity, greenstick

IMAGING

- Focal, abrupt cortical angulation, "buckling," &/or discrete fracture line with overlying soft tissue swelling
  - Few sites of normally occurring cortical angulation/protuberance in children
  - Comparison radiographs helpful if uncertain
- ± physeal extension of fracture with displacement of metaphyseal fragment & epiphysis
- Distal radial metaphysis/metadiaphyseal junction
  - Up to 85% of pediatric forearm fractures

- Buckle (on compression side), complete oblique/transverse, or physeal fractures
  - Distal ulnar injury usually present
- Diaphysis
  - Plastic (bowing) deformity, greenstick (with cortical interruption of tension side), or complete fractures
  - Both shafts usually fractured (unless dislocated)
- Proximal radius & ulna fractures considered with elbow
  - Radial neck & ulnar olecranon most common

CLINICAL ISSUES

- Presentation: Pain, swelling, tenderness, ↓ use after FOOSH (**f**all **o**n **o**ut**s**treched **h**and)
- Treatment ranges from casting to closed reduction to surgery depending on fracture type & degree of displacement
  - Remodeling potential of pediatric fractures > > adults due to residual bone growth

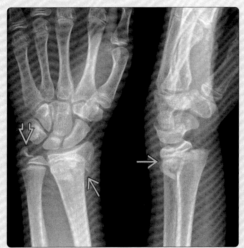
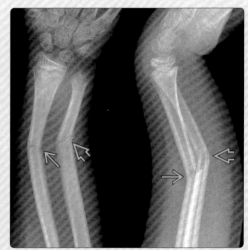

(Left) PA & lateral views of the wrist in a 12 year old show a comminuted Salter-Harris II fracture ➡ of the distal radius with ~ 50% dorsal translation of the distal fracture fragment. An ulnar styloid fracture ➡ is also present. Though not seen in this case, an ulnar metadiaphyseal fracture also frequently occurs in this setting. (Right) AP & lateral forearm radiographs in a 6 year old show a complete ulnar diaphyseal fracture ➡ with an incomplete greenstick radial diaphyseal fracture (note the intact cortex ➡).

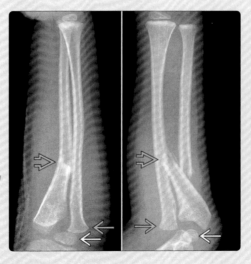
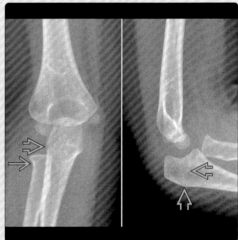

(Left) AP & lateral forearm radiographs in a 4 year old show a complete fracture of the proximal ulnar diaphysis ➡ with dislocation of the proximal radius ➡ relative to the capitellum ➡, consistent with the Monteggia fracture-dislocation complex. The radial head has not yet ossified. (Right) AP & lateral elbow radiographs in a 5 year old show nondisplaced fractures of the radial neck ➡ (with focal angulation of the cortex) & proximal ulna ➡ (with linear lucency & cortical interruption), which often occur together.

ACL Injuries

TERMINOLOGY

- Intrasubstance anterior cruciate ligament (ACL) tears may be complete or partial; differentiation can be difficult
  - Typically in athletes at or near skeletal maturity (F > M)
- Avulsion fractures of tibial eminence at distal ACL attachment more frequent in skeletally immature patients
  - Most common at 8-14 years of age (M > F); ACL intact or partially torn

IMAGING

- Radiographs: Joint effusion most common but nonspecific
  - Less common but more specific secondary findings
    - Deep lateral condylar notch: > 2 mm on lateral view
    - Segond fracture: Vertically oriented avulsion from lateral proximal tibia on frontal view
- MR: ↑ intrasubstance signal of ACL with disrupted fibers
  - "Kissing" contusions (poorly defined edema/hemorrhage in lateral femoral & posterolateral tibial condyles)
  - Additional injuries: Menisci, MCL, posterolateral corner

PATHOLOGY

- Complete ACL tears: Pivot shift injury
- Tibial eminence fractures
  - Hyperextension force ± valgus or rotational stress
  - May occur from direct blow to femur with knee flexed

CLINICAL ISSUES

- Lachman test: Anterior translation force applied to proximal tibia with knee mildly flexed; lack of solid/firm endpoint = positive test
- Anterior drawer test: Anterior translational force applied to proximal tibia with knee flexed at ~ 80-90°; ↑ translation (vs. contralateral side) = positive test

DIAGNOSTIC CHECKLIST

- Absence of effusion following acute injury virtually excludes ACL tear
- ACL tear usually diagnosed clinically; MR to look for associated injuries

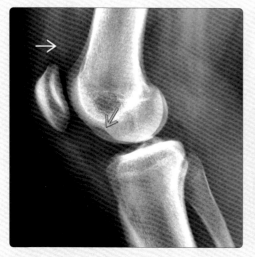

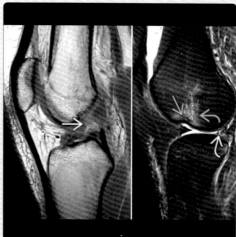

(Left) Lateral radiograph of a 17-year-old girl with a right knee injury during a soccer game shows a joint effusion ➡ & a deep lateral condylar notch ➡ that measures > 3 mm. (Right) Sagittal PD (left) & T2 FS (right) MRs in the same patient show a subchondral fracture of the lateral femoral condyle ➡ (the MR equivalent of the lateral notch sign) with underlying edema ➡ + a complex tear of the lateral meniscus ➡. The more central PD image shows a complete midsubstance ACL tear ➡.

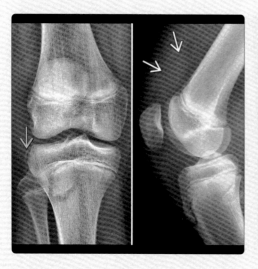

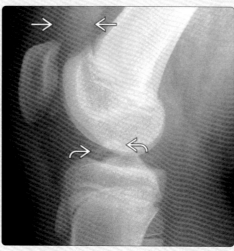

(Left) Frontal (left) & lateral (right) radiographs in a boy with a right knee injury show a joint effusion ➡ & a Segond fracture ➡ of the lateral tibia. Segond fractures are nearly always associated with ACL tears. (Right) Lateral radiograph of a 12-year-old boy following a wrestling injury shows a displaced bone fragment ➡ at the level of the intercondylar eminence, compatible with an ACL avulsion fracture of the tibia. Note the large joint effusion ➡.

TERMINOLOGY

- Transient patellar dislocation (TPD): Lateral dislocation & relocation of patella from direct or indirect injury
  - Shearing, tensile, compressive forces → injuries of medial patella, lateral femur, & soft tissues

IMAGING

- Radiographs show large joint effusion ± osseous fragments (of patella or lateral femoral condyle)
  - Associated patellar injury best seen with additional tangential/axial view (e.g., sunrise view)
- MR shows characteristic medial patella & lateral femoral condyle "kissing" contusions, medial patellofemoral ligament (MPFL) tear, & chondral/osteochondral injuries

PATHOLOGY

- MPFL = condensation of medial retinaculum extending from superomedial patella to medial epicondyle of femur
  - Strongest passive medial stabilizer of patella

CLINICAL ISSUES

- Signs/symptoms: Knee giving way, hemarthrosis/effusion, tenderness along medial retinaculum, sensation of impending dislocation with manual pressure upon patella
- Patellar dislocation clinically occult in 45-73% of cases
  - Due to transient nature of process, patients frequently unaware that patella has dislocated
- Predisposing factors may be congenital or acquired
  - Patella: Alta, lateral subluxation/tilt, dysplasia
  - Trochlear dysplasia
  - Lateralization of tibial tubercle
  - Deficient/absent soft tissue medial stabilizers
  - Generalized ligamentous laxity (e.g., Ehlers-Danlos)
- If managed conservatively, 15-40% have recurrent TPD
  - Surgery for 1st-time TPD with intraarticular bodies, major tear of medial stabilizers, or recurrence
- Recurrent dislocations ↑ risk for persistent symptoms & degenerative changes

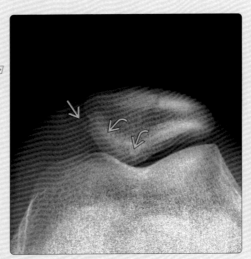
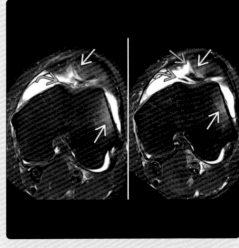

(Left) Axial radiograph of the patella in a 16-year-old boy with a recent transient patellar dislocation (TPD) shows an osseous fragment ⇨ adjacent to the medial patella with irregularity ⇨ of the entire medial facet. (Right) Axial T2 FS MR (superior on the left, inferior on the right) in the same patient shows "kissing" bone contusions ⇨ of the lateral femoral condyle & medial patella. There is also full-thickness articular cartilage loss of the medial patellar facet ⇨ with an associated intraarticular osteochondral body ⇨.

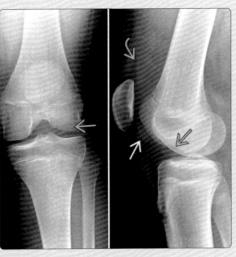
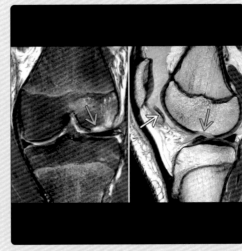

(Left) Frontal & lateral radiographs in a 14-year-old boy with a recent TPD show a large osseous fragment in the anterior knee joint ⇨ with an associated lucency in the lateral femoral condyle ⇨. A lipohemarthrosis is also present ⇨. (Right) Coronal T2 FS (left) & sagittal PD (right) MR images in the same boy confirm a displaced, rotated osteochondral fracture fragment ⇨ in the anterior aspect of the joint with a donor site ⇨ at the lateral femoral condyle.

Tibial Tubercle Avulsion

TERMINOLOGY

- During adolescence, substantial traction force of patellar tendon may acutely avulse tibial tubercle ossification center from underlying physis

IMAGING

- Bone fragment retracted proximally by patellar tendon from expected site of tibial tubercle ossification center
- Many variables, including fragment size & shape, degree of comminution & displacement, pattern of extension

TOP DIFFERENTIAL DIAGNOSES

- Normal ossification variant, Osgood-Schlatter disease, patellar sleeve avulsion fracture, patellar tendon rupture

PATHOLOGY

- Portion of physis deep to tibial tubercle ossification center uniquely composed of strong fibrocartilage
- As patient nears physeal closure, this growth plate converts to weaker hyaline cartilage, predisposing to avulsion

- o Timing coincides with ↑ muscle strength, athletic activity
- Mechanisms of avulsion include forceful quadriceps contraction with extension (i.e., jumping) or passive knee flexion during quadriceps contraction (i.e., landing)
- Prior Osgood-Schlatter disease in 25% of patients
- Associated injuries (< 5%): Tears of patellar tendon, ACL, collateral ligaments, & menisci; compartment syndrome
- o Adjacent soft tissues may become entrapped

CLINICAL ISSUES

- Vast majority: Boys 13-17 years old
- Presentations include swelling, tenderness, knee held in mild flexion with inability to fully extend actively, palpable bone fragment, high-riding patella
- Nonoperative management if minimally displaced & limited to distal tibial tubercle
- o Excellent prognosis with appropriate therapy
- o Complications in 25-30%: Bursitis & tubercle prominence > refracture, genu recurvatum, limb length discrepancy

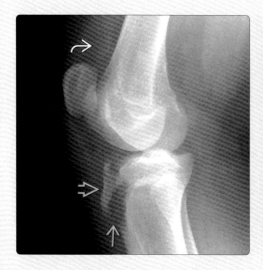
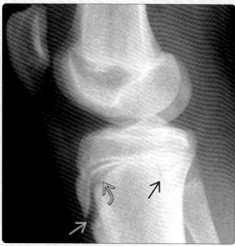

(Left) *Lateral knee radiograph with mild internal rotation in a 17-year-old boy after a football injury shows moderate proximal displacement of a large tibial tubercle fragment ➡️ with widening of the growth plate ➡️. A moderate joint effusion is noted ➡️.* (Right) *Lateral knee radiograph in a 15-year-old boy after a fall shows mild widening & irregularity of the growth plate deep to the tibial tubercle ➡️ with posterior extension to the proximal tibial physis ➡️ & metaphysis ➡️ as a Salter-Harris II fracture.*

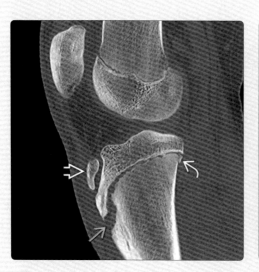
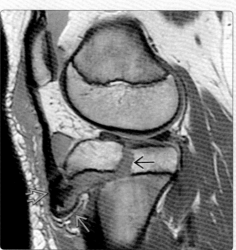

(Left) *Sagittal bone CT in a 14-year-old boy after a basketball injury shows mild widening & irregularity of the growth plate ➡️ deep to the tibial tubercle with posterior extension to the metaphysis ➡️. A well-defined proximal fragment ➡️ is likely chronic.* (Right) *Sagittal PD MR in a 15-year-old boy after a fall shows avulsion of a tibial tubercle fragment by the patellar tendon ➡️. The fracture extends proximally with a Salter-Harris III configuration ➡️. Stripped distal periosteum ➡️ is entrapped in the fracture.*

IMAGING

- Distal tibial fracture in 3 planes; may be true Salter-Harris (SH) IV or combinations of SH II & III
- Classic triplane fracture pattern
  - Coronal fracture plane through distal tibial metaphysis & diaphysis
  - Transverse fracture plane through physis (growth plate)
  - Sagittal fracture plane through epiphysis
- Oblique coronal plane of metaphysis/diaphysis may be hidden on lateral radiograph if nondisplaced & overlapping tibial-fibular interface
- CT more accurate for determining course & comminution of fracture, amount of displacement, & articular surface involvement

PATHOLOGY

- Fracture typically occurs around time of earliest physeal closure, which affects planes of fracture extension
  - Fusion begins in central tibial physis at Kump bump

CLINICAL ISSUES

- 5-10% of pediatric intraarticular ankle fractures
- Typically affects adolescents within 18 months of tibial growth plate closure
  - Girls 13-14 years old
  - Boys 15-16 years old
  - 2-part triplane younger than 3-part triplane fractures
- Mechanism: External rotation
- Presentation: Pain, bruising, swelling, inability to bear weight
  - Associated fibular fracture in 1/2 of patients
- Nonoperative treatment for ≤ 2 mm of displacement & extraarticular fractures
  - Closed reduction with internal rotation of foot
- Operative treatment for > 2 mm of articular step-off
  - Internal fixation with screws, percutaneous K-wires

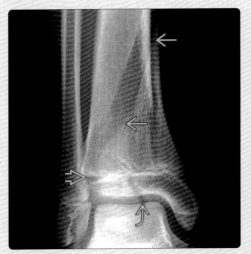
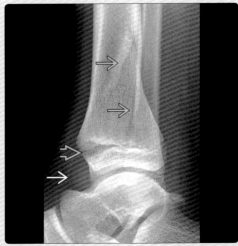

(Left) AP radiograph in a 15-year-old boy after a fall shows a triplane fracture of the distal tibia with the following fracture planes: Coronal oblique of the metaphysis & diaphysis ➡, horizontal of the anterolateral physis ➡, & sagittal of the epiphysis ➡. (Right) Lateral radiograph of the same patient shows the coronal metadiaphyseal ➡ & horizontal anterior physeal ➡ components. Note the moderate tibiotalar joint effusion ➡.

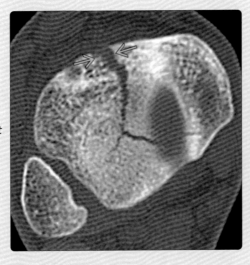
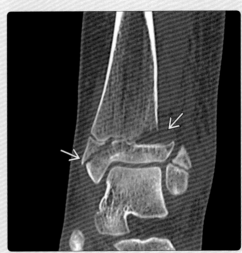

(Left) Axial bone CT in the same patient shows the predominantly sagittal fracture plane through the distal tibial epiphysis. In many cases, the axial plane of imaging allows the most accurate assessment of the articular surface distraction ➡, which is a key determinant for treating with a closed vs. open reduction. (Right) Coronal bone CT in a 13 year old who sustained an ankle injury after falling from a scooter shows an extraarticular intramalleolar triplane fracture ➡ variant.

Transient Synovitis

TERMINOLOGY

- Idiopathic self-limited inflammation of pediatric hip
- Synonyms: Toxic synovitis

IMAGING

- Radiographs: Low sensitivity for hip joint effusion; look for convex gluteal fat pad & medial joint space widening
- US: Highly sensitive for joint fluid
  - Distention of joint capsule by anechoic, hypoechoic, or complex fluid
  - ± synovial thickening, hyperemia
- MR: Nonspecific fluid + synovial enhancement
  - Findings favoring transient synovitis over septic arthritis
    - Absence of adjacent marrow or soft tissue edema
    - Normal enhancement/perfusion of femoral head

TOP DIFFERENTIAL DIAGNOSES

- Septic arthritis
- Juvenile idiopathic arthritis
- Trauma
- Reactive effusion due to adjacent bone pathology (e.g., Legg-Calvé-Perthes)

PATHOLOGY

- Viral etiology considered most likely

CLINICAL ISSUES

- 3-8 years of age; mean: 4.7-5.5 years
- Limping ± pain; typically afebrile (> 90%)
- Kocher criteria: ↑ likelihood for septic arthritis over transient synovitis with ↑ number of positive parameters
  - Fever, non-weight-bearing, ↑ WBC, ↑ ESR
- Transient synovitis self-limited, lasting 7-10 days
- Conservative management with bed rest + NSAIDs
  - Hip aspiration expedites clinical improvement

DIAGNOSTIC CHECKLIST

- Imaging alone cannot exclude infection of detected fluid

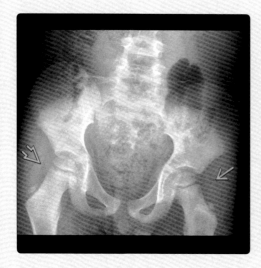
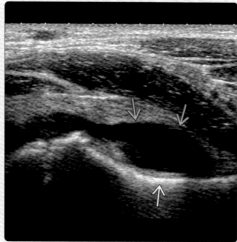

(Left) AP radiograph of the pelvis in an afebrile 5 year old with a new onset of limp & left hip pain shows bowing of the left gluteal fat pad ➡ as compared to the normal right side ➡, suggesting a left hip joint effusion. (Right) Sagittal ultrasound of the left hip in the same patient shows convex bowing of the joint capsule ➡ by hypoechoic fluid that distends the joint at the femoral neck ➡. The patient had normal laboratory markers & was successfully treated conservatively for transient synovitis.

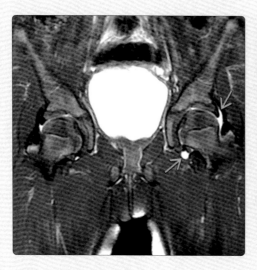
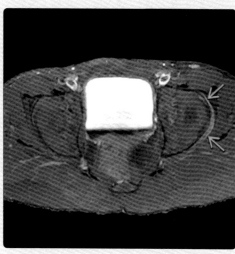

(Left) Coronal T2 FS MR in a 4 year old with several days of left thigh pain & limping shows a small left hip joint effusion ➡ with no adjacent marrow or soft tissue edema. (Right) Axial T1 C+ FS MR in the same patient shows mildly increased synovial enhancement of the left hip joint ➡ as compared to the right. The patient was successfully treated conservatively for transient synovitis given the combination of clinical & imaging features.

Musculoskeletal

TERMINOLOGY

- Septic arthritis: Microbial (typically bacterial) invasion of joint leading to inflammation & purulence

IMAGING

- US: Highly sensitive for fluid distending joint capsule
  - Complexity & volume do not predict/exclude infection
- MR: Nonspecific joint fluid with synovial thickening
  - Findings favoring septic arthritis over transient synovitis
    - Presence of marrow &/or soft tissue edema
    - ↓ enhancement/perfusion of articular epiphysis

TOP DIFFERENTIAL DIAGNOSES

- Transient synovitis, juvenile idiopathic arthritis, trauma, reactive effusion due to adjacent bone pathology

PATHOLOGY

- Mechanism: Hematogenous spread vs. direct spread from adjacent osteomyelitis or puncture wound

- Most common organisms overall: *Staphylococcus aureus* > streptococcal species
  - Neonates: Group B streptococci, gram (-) rods, *Neisseria gonorrhoeae*
  - < 4 years of age: *Kingella kingae* most common
  - Adolescents: *Neisseria gonorrhoeae*

CLINICAL ISSUES

- Best clue: Joint effusion in non-weight-bearing child with fever > 38.5°C + ↑ serum inflammatory markers (i.e., multiple positive Kocher criteria)
- Treatment: Emergent arthroscopy/arthrotomy with joint irrigation + IV antibiotics to prevent long-term sequelae

DIAGNOSTIC CHECKLIST

- Synovitis has many etiologies; always consider infection
  - Imaging alone cannot exclude infection of joint fluid
  - Joint aspiration required for 100% confidence

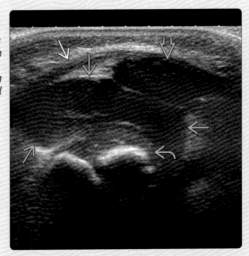
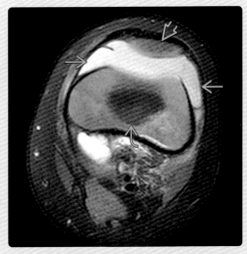

(Left) Longitudinal US of the anterior midline knee in a 1 year old with swelling shows a large hypoechoic joint effusion ➡ deep to the quadriceps tendon ➡ & unossified patella ➡. The partially ossified distal femoral epiphysis ➡ lies deep to the effusion. (Right) Axial T2 FS MR of the same patient shows the effusion ➡ lifting the unossified patellar cartilage ➡ off of the partially ossified distal femoral epiphysis ➡. Septic arthritis was confirmed upon joint drainage.

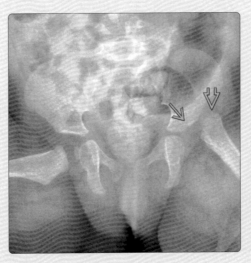
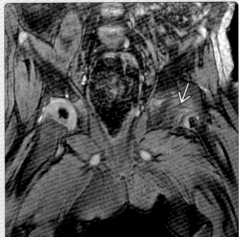

(Left) Frog leg lateral radiograph of the pelvis in a 1 year old with a history of left hip neonatal septic arthritis shows sequelae of delayed treatment: The left acetabulum is dysplastic ➡ with dislocation of the femur ➡ & no visible femoral head ossification center. The right hip is normal. (Right) Coronal T2* GRE MR of the same patient shows complete destruction of the left femoral head ➡ due to prior septic arthritis. This is one of the most feared consequences of septic arthritis, leading to lifelong morbidity.

TERMINOLOGY

Definitions

- Septic arthritis: Microbial (typically bacterial) invasion of joint leading to inflammation & purulence

IMAGING

General Features

- Location
  - Affects lower extremity joints in ≥ 75% of cases
  - Multiple joints in ~ 10-15%

Radiographic Findings

- Sensitivity for fluid distending joint capsule varies on location: Knee, ankle, elbow > > hip, shoulder
  - Displacement of fat pads ± widening of joint space, soft tissue edema with blurred fat-muscle interfaces

Ultrasonographic Findings

- Anechoic to complex fluid distending joint capsule; complexity & volume do not predict sterile vs. infected fluid
- Synovial thickening, ± hyperemia

MR Findings

- Nonspecific synovitis (as with many etiologies)
  - Homogeneously bright T2/STIR fluid in joint
  - Synovial thickening & enhancement
- Findings favoring septic arthritis over transient synovitis
  - Presence of marrow &/or soft tissue edema
  - ↓ enhancement/perfusion of articular epiphysis, especially in tight joint (e.g., femoral head at hip)
- Findings favoring septic arthritis over reactive fluid secondary to adjacent metaphyseal osteomyelitis
  - Epiphyseal marrow edema, surrounding soft tissue edema, epiphyseal nonenhancement

Imaging Recommendations

- Best imaging tool
  - US: Highly sensitive for joint fluid; ~ 5% false-negative rate in first 24 hours
  - MR ± contrast
    - Best tool for detecting adjacent bone & soft tissue infections/collections
    - Can detect other diagnoses

DIFFERENTIAL DIAGNOSIS

Transient Synovitis

- Typically without fever or ↑ serum inflammatory markers
- Nonspecific MR appearance of synovitis
  - Joint fluid + mild synovial thickening & enhancement
  - Lacks surrounding marrow or soft tissue edema

Juvenile Idiopathic Arthritis

- ± "rice bodies": Numerous, tiny low T2 signal intensity bodies of uniform size throughout joint fluid

Trauma

- ± marrow & soft tissue edema, ligament & cartilage injuries

Reactive Effusion Due to Adjacent Bone Pathology

- Osteomyelitis, bone tumor, Legg-Calvé-Perthes

PATHOLOGY

General Features

- Mechanisms of joint seeding
  - Hematogenous spread: Vascularized synovium lacking basement membrane allows bacterial entry
  - Direct spread: Adjacent osteomyelitis, puncture wound
- Causative organisms
  - *Staphylococcus aureus* > streptococcal species overall
  - Neonates: Group B streptococci, gram (-) rods, *Neisseria gonorrhoeae*
  - < 4 years of age: Gram (-) bacteria, *Kingella kingae*
    - *K. kingae* often lacks systemic markers of inflammation
  - Unvaccinated: *Haemophilus influenzae* B
  - Immunosuppressed: *Streptococcus pneumoniae*
  - Sexually active: *N. gonorrhoeae*
- Osteocartilaginous destruction caused by
  - Neutrophil & bacterial proteolytic enzymes → articular & unossified epiphyseal cartilage damage
  - ↑ joint pressure by pus → ↓ perfusion of articular epiphysis → ischemic injury

CLINICAL ISSUES

Presentation

- Fever, pain, swelling, ↓ motion, non-weight-bearing
- Kocher criteria: ↑ likelihood for hip septic arthritis over transient synovitis with ↑ number of predictors
  - Fever > 38.5°C, non-weight-bearing, WBC > 12 x 10⁹ cells/L, ESR ≥ 40 mm/hour; later addition to original criteria: CRP > 20 mg/L
    - With all present, specificity for septic arthritis ~ 60-99%

Demographics

- ~ 6.5% of pediatric arthritis; peak age: ~ 2-3 years

Natural History & Prognosis

- Long-term sequelae in up to 40%
  - Limited motion, dislocation, degeneration, ankylosis, limb length discrepancy, avascular necrosis

Treatment

- Emergent arthroscopy or arthrotomy + joint irrigation
- IV antibiotics for 2-4 days followed by oral antibiotics for 10 days; longer course for concomitant osteomyelitis

SELECTED REFERENCES

1. Rosenfeld S et al: Predicting the presence of adjacent Infections in septic arthritis in children. J Pediatr Orthop. 36(1):70-4, 2016
2. K Schallert E et al: Metaphyseal osteomyelitis in children: how often does MRI-documented joint effusion or epiphyseal extension of edema indicate coexisting septic arthritis? Pediatr Radiol. 45(8):1174-81, 2015
3. Laine JC et al: The use of ultrasound in the management of septic arthritis of the hip. J Pediatr Orthop B. 24(2):95-8, 2015
4. Monsalve J et al: Septic arthritis in children: frequency of coexisting unsuspected osteomyelitis and implications on imaging work-up and management. AJR Am J Roentgenol. 204(6):1289-95, 2015
5. Dodwell ER: Osteomyelitis and septic arthritis in children: current concepts. Curr Opin Pediatr. 25(1):58-63, 2013
6. Sultan J et al: Septic arthritis or transient synovitis of the hip in children: the value of clinical prediction algorithms. J Bone Joint Surg Br. 92(9):1289-93, 2010

Musculoskeletal

IMAGING

- Long bone metaphyses 70% (femur > tibia > humerus), short bones 6%, pelvis 5%, spine 2%
  - Metaphysis or equivalent > epiphysis, diaphysis
  - Multifocal in 10% overall but 22% in neonates
- Absence of radiographic bone findings does not exclude early osteomyelitis
  - Earliest finding: Soft tissue swelling next to bone
  - Bone destruction, periosteal reaction by 7-14 days
- MR: Best advanced imaging choice if diagnosis unclear (but symptoms localized) or with concern for complications
  - T1: Poorly defined metaphyseal marrow abnormality
  - T2 FS/STIR: Bright marrow, periosteal, & soft tissue edema; ± adjacent joint effusion
  - T1 C+ FS: Rim-enhancing abscesses
- Nuclear medicine bone or whole-body MR helpful if site & diagnosis unclear

TOP DIFFERENTIAL DIAGNOSES

- Malignancy (Ewing sarcoma, leukemia, neuroblastoma), Langerhans cell histiocytosis, septic arthritis

PATHOLOGY

- Hematogenous seeding > > penetrating injury or contiguous spread
  - *Staphylococcus aureus* in > 80-90% (> 55% due to MRSA)
  - Children 6 months to 3 years of age: *Kingella kingae*
  - Neonates: Group B *Streptococcus*
  - Sickle cell disease: *Salmonella*
  - Penetrating foot trauma: *Pseudomonas aeruginosa*

CLINICAL ISSUES

- Presents with fever, pain, limp, tenderness, swelling, ↓ range of motion, ↓ weight bearing
  - Presentation often nonspecific, may delay diagnosis
- Labs: ↑ ESR, CRP > ↑ WBC
- Treat with IV then PO antibiotics + abscess drainage

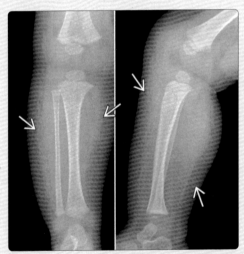
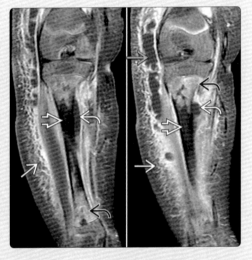

(Left) AP (left) & lateral (right) radiographs of a 9-month-old infant show extensive subcutaneous edema of the lower leg with blurring of soft tissue planes ➡ but no discrete bony abnormality. (Right) Coronal T1 C+ FS MR images show foci of decreased marrow enhancement ➡ from an intraosseous abscess with adjacent increased marrow enhancement ➡ from infected or reactive viable marrow. Subperiosteal ➡ & soft tissue ➡ fluid collections & overlying fat edema ➡ are noted in this patient with MRSA osteomyelitis.

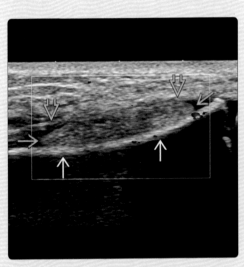
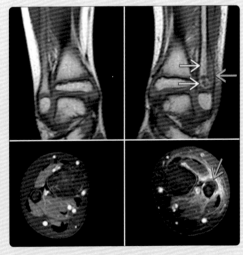

(Left) Longitudinal color Doppler ultrasound in a 6 year old with fever & lower extremity swelling shows an echogenic avascular collection ➡ that is lifting the periosteum ➡ off of the fibular cortex ➡. (Right) Coronal T1 (top) & axial T1 C+ FS (bottom) MR images in the same patient show heterogeneous marrow of the distal left fibula ➡ with a rim-enhancing subperiosteal abscess ➡. Surrounding soft tissue edema is also noted in this patient with MSSA osteomyelitis. Note the normal right leg images.

TERMINOLOGY

Definitions

- Bone infection, most commonly bacterial

IMAGING

General Features

- Best diagnostic clue
  - Radiographs: Nonspecific soft tissue edema in setting of limp, pain, swelling, &/or fever (< 7-10 days)
  - MR: Poorly defined metaphyseal/metadiaphyseal marrow abnormalities + subperiosteal/soft tissue fluid
- Location
  - Long bone metaphyses 70% (femur > tibia > humerus), short bones 6%, pelvis 5%, spine 2%
    - Metaphysis or equivalent > epiphysis, diaphysis
  - Multifocal in 10% overall but 22% in neonates

Radiographic Findings

- Absence of findings does not exclude early osteomyelitis
- Earliest finding: Soft tissue swelling next to bone
  - Displacement or obliteration of fat planes
  - Reticulation of subcutaneous fat
- Lytic bone lesion in 7-14 days (or longer) after onset
  - Vague lucency → permeation → destruction
- Periosteal reaction seen by 7-14 days

Ultrasonographic Findings

- Sensitive for drainable fluid collections

MR Findings

- Poorly defined, heterogeneous dark (T1)/bright (T2 FS or STIR) marrow (due to loss of normal fatty marrow signal)
- Soft tissue changes usually moderate to marked
  - Discrete soft tissue & subperiosteal fluid collections
- ± adjacent joint effusion
  - Septic arthritis more likely than reactive fluid
- T1 C+ FS particularly helpful in
  - Defining rim-enhancing drainable collections
  - Visualizing infection of unossified cartilage of infants

Nuclear Medicine Findings

- Bone scan: ↑ uptake on 3 phases is 80-94% sensitive
  - Positive in 24-72 hours; can demonstrate multiple sites

Imaging Recommendations

- Best imaging tool
  - MR most sensitive & specific modality for early infection with localized symptoms
    - Confirms diagnosis or delineates alternative processes
    - Shows drainable abscesses & intraspinal extension
  - Bone scintigraphy helpful if site & diagnosis unclear

DIFFERENTIAL DIAGNOSIS

Ewing Sarcoma

- Aggressive lytic diaphyseal/metadiaphyseal lesion, most common in patients > 5 years old

Neuroblastoma Metastases or Leukemia

- Aggressive but frequently subtle metaphyseal lytic lesions, most common in patients < 5 years old

Langerhans Cell Histiocytosis

- Punched-out, well-defined lytic lesions + enhancing mass
- Flat bones & spine frequently involved

Septic Arthritis

- Effusion + enhancing thickened synovium

PATHOLOGY

General Features

- Pathophysiology: Hematogenous seeding > > penetrating injury or contiguous spread
  - Slow flow through looping metaphyseal venules
    - Primary sites for bacterial lodging
  - Intramedullary infection → edema, vascular congestion → ↑ pressure → transcortical spread
- Organisms identified in only 35-66% of needle aspirates, 36-55% of blood cultures
  - *Staphylococcus aureus* > 80-90% of cases (> 55% due to methicillin-resistant strains)
  - *Streptococcus* species in ~ 10%
  - Children 6 months to 3 years of age: *Kingella kingae*
    - PCR much more sensitive than culture
  - Neonates: Group B *Streptococcus*
  - Sickle cell disease: *Salmonella*
  - Immunocompromised: *Streptococcus pneumoniae*, tuberculosis
  - Penetrating foot trauma: *Pseudomonas aeruginosa*

CLINICAL ISSUES

Presentation

- Most common signs/symptoms
  - Pain, ↓ range of motion, ↓ weight bearing, tenderness, swelling, fever; minor trauma history in 1/3 of patients
- Labs: ↑ ESR, CRP > ↑ WBC

Demographics

- 50% of cases occur before 5 years of age

Natural History & Prognosis

- Complications include septic arthritis, venous thrombosis, fracture, septic emboli, multisystem failure, growth disturbance; more likely with treatment delay of > 4 days

Treatment

- Identify infectious agent: Image-guided needle aspiration or open surgical biopsy + blood culture
- Antibiotics (IV followed by PO), pain management
- Surgery/intervention: Abscess (intraosseous, subperiosteal, soft tissue) drainage

SELECTED REFERENCES

1. Al-Qwbani M et al: Kingella kingae-associated pediatric osteoarticular infections: an overview of 566 reported cases. Clin Pediatr (Phila). ePub, 2016
2. Ilharreborde B: Sequelae of pediatric osteoarticular infection. Orthop Traumatol Surg Res. 101(1 Suppl):S129-37, 2015
3. K Schallert E et al: Metaphyseal osteomyelitis in children: how often does MRI-documented joint effusion or epiphyseal extension of edema indicate coexisting septic arthritis? Pediatr Radiol. 45(8):1174-81, 2015
4. Dodwell ER: Osteomyelitis and septic arthritis in children: current concepts. Curr Opin Pediatr. 25(1):58-63, 2013
5. Jaramillo D: Infection: musculoskeletal. Pediatr Radiol. 41 Suppl 1:S127-34, 2011

Soft Tissue Abscess

TERMINOLOGY

- Abscess: Walled-off liquefied collection of necrotic tissue, inflammatory cells, & bacteria

IMAGING

- Most commonly affects single site: Typical lymph node location vs. other subcutaneous or intramuscular focus
  - Septic emboli can cause multifocal collections
- Ultrasound: Excellent for detecting superficial collections & defining drainability
  - Thick-walled centrally avascular collection with surrounding edema ± hyperemia
  - Swirling internal debris upon compression
- MR: Clearly defines deep extent, evaluates adjacent bone/cartilage/joint, & helps exclude other diagnoses
  - Centrally nonenhancing fluid collection with thick, enhancing wall & peripheral poorly defined edema
  - Whole-body MR may be useful to screen large territories for drainable collections in setting of systemic infection

TOP DIFFERENTIAL DIAGNOSES

- Soft tissue sarcoma, lymphatic malformation, hematoma

PATHOLOGY

- *Staphylococcus aureus* > > streptococcal species
  - ↑ incidence of methicillin-resistant *S. aureus* (MRSA)
- *Bartonella henselae*: Regional lymphadenitis ± suppuration in cat scratch disease

CLINICAL ISSUES

- Presentation: Swelling, fluctuance, erythema, tenderness, limited motion, fever, sepsis
- Treatment: Drainage procedure ± antibiotics (IV or oral)
  - With adequate drainage of abscess & no cellulitis, antibiotics may not be required
  - Small abscess without drainable fluid collection may be treated with antibiotics & topical care only
  - Trial of oral antibiotics in systemically well person

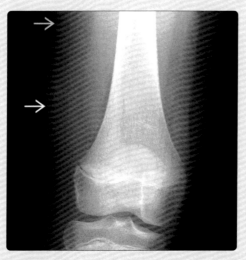
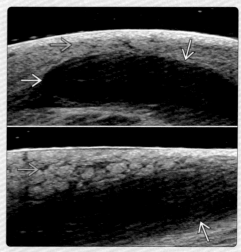

(Left) *AP radiograph of the knee in an 11-year-old patient with lateral swelling & tenderness of the distal thigh shows blurring of the normally sharp interfaces between subcutaneous fat & muscle ➡, typical of edema. There is focal bulging of the soft tissues distally ➡.* (Right) *Longitudinal ultrasound images (top & bottom) of the same patient show thickening & reticular edema of the subcutaneous fat ➡ overlying a heterogeneously hypoechoic ovoid collection ➡.*

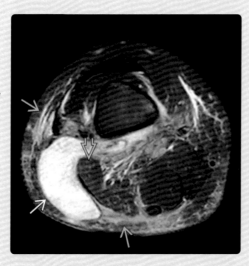
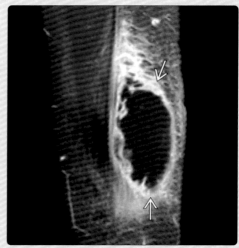

(Left) *Axial T2 FS MR of the same patient shows a well-circumscribed, crescentic, hyperintense collection ➡ overlying the distal biceps femoris muscle ➡. There is surrounding soft tissue edema ➡.* (Right) *Sagittal T1 C+ FS MR in the same patient shows thick, irregular rim enhancement of the fluid collection ➡, typical of an abscess. Pus was encountered upon surgical drainage.*

TERMINOLOGY

Synonyms

- Pyomyositis, suppurative lymphadenitis

Definitions

- Abscess: Walled-off liquefied collection of necrotic tissue, inflammatory cells, & bacteria
- Phlegmon: Poorly defined focus of necrotic & inflammatory tissue ± components of liquefaction
- Cellulitis: Poorly defined inflammatory changes of superficial soft tissue infections
- Suppurative or purulent: Pus forming/containing

IMAGING

General Features

- Best diagnostic clue
  - US: Thick-walled avascular collection with swirling internal echogenicities & overlying edema
  - MR: Centrally nonenhancing fluid collection with thick, enhancing wall & peripheral poorly defined edema
- Location
  - Most commonly affects single site; possibilities include
    - Expected sites of lymph nodes
    - Isolated collection in muscle > tendon sheath, bursa
    - Spread from deep (adjacent osteomyelitis & subperiosteal abscess) or superficial (cellulitis, penetrating wound) source
  - Septic emboli can cause multifocal collections

Radiographic Findings

- Edema: Subcutaneous reticulation with blurring of normally sharp fat-muscle interfaces
- ± focal bulge at site of collection

Ultrasonographic Findings

- Grayscale ultrasound
  - Well-defined collection with thick, irregular wall
  - Contents range from anechoic to isoechoic
    - Internal debris swirls with dynamic compression
- Color Doppler
  - No internal vascularity; ± ↑ peripheral vascularity

MR Findings

- T2 FS/STIR
  - Collection of hyperintense fluid centrally
  - Wall may show hypointense inner rim (minerals, hemorrhage, fibrous tissue) & hyperintense outer rim (granulation tissue)
  - Surrounding edema
- Mildly thickened, irregular, enhancing rim after contrast without substantial nodularity
- Restricted diffusion centrally

Imaging Recommendations

- Best imaging tool
  - US excellent for detecting superficial collections & defining drainability
  - MR more clearly defines collection deep extent & relationships to vital structures, evaluates adjacent bone & cartilage for infection, helps exclude other diagnoses

DIFFERENTIAL DIAGNOSIS

Soft Tissue Sarcoma

- Typically solid, well-circumscribed mass with little (if any) surrounding edema
- Variable enhancement ± foci of necrosis, cysts

Lymphatic Malformation

- Multicystic mass crossing soft tissue compartments
- Fluid-fluid levels due to internal hemorrhage
- Rim & septal enhancement only

Hematoma

- Heterogeneous intramuscular collection after trauma

Myositis Ossificans

- Heterogeneous intramuscular mass with marked surrounding edema on T2 FS/STIR MR
- Peripheral Ca^{2+} within weeks diagnostic
- Occurs after injury but trauma history lacking in 40%

Rhabdomyolysis/Infarction

- Large regions of necrotic muscle after compression/trauma
- Very ↑ serum markers of muscle breakdown

PATHOLOGY

General Features

- Most common organisms
  - *Staphylococcus aureus* > > streptococcal species
  - *Bartonella henselae*: Regional lymphadenitis ± suppuration in cat scratch disease
    - Axillary, epitrochlear > head/neck or inguinal nodes
  - Mycobacterial infections may result in large muscular abscesses (classically psoas with rim Ca^{2+})
- Mechanisms
  - Cellulitis spreading to deeper soft tissues or regional lymph nodes
  - Extension from adjacent deep infection
  - Hematogenous seeding of muscle
  - Puncture wound

CLINICAL ISSUES

Presentation

- Most common signs/symptoms
  - Swelling, erythema, tenderness, limited motion, fever
  - ± fluctuance, spontaneous drainage

Treatment

- Drainage procedure + IV antibiotics
  - Drainage may not be necessary if collection < 2 cm in noncritical location

SELECTED REFERENCES

1. Verma S: Pyomyositis in children. Curr Infect Dis Rep. 18(4):12, 2016
2. Penn EB Jr et al: Pediatric inflammatory adenopathy. Otolaryngol Clin North Am. 48(1):137-51, 2015
3. Pattamapaspong N et al: Pitfalls in imaging of musculoskeletal infections. Semin Musculoskelet Radiol. 18(1):86-100, 2014
4. Soldatos T et al: Magnetic resonance imaging of musculoskeletal infections: systematic diagnostic assessment and key points. Acad Radiol. 19(11):1434-43, 2012
5. Ranson M: Imaging of pediatric musculoskeletal infection. Semin Musculoskelet Radiol. 13(3):277-99, 2009

Infantile Hemangioma, Musculoskeletal

TERMINOLOGY

- Widespread misuse of "hemangioma" in literature
  - True hemangioma: Benign vascular neoplasm
- Infantile hemangioma (IH)
  - Most common soft tissue tumor of childhood
  - Predictable life cycle: Usually absent at birth → rapid growth over 1st few weeks/months of life (proliferating phase) → spontaneous regression over subsequent months to years (involuting phase)

IMAGING

- Elongated, lobulated, well-defined, highly vascular, solitary or multifocal, superficial soft tissue mass(es)
  - Common cutaneous IH not usually imaged due to typical timeline & appearance
  - Deeper subcutaneous IH without typical skin findings likely to be imaged (as diagnosis less clear)
- Doppler should clearly document characteristic internal vascularity throughout proliferating IH
- Imaging features change with involution

CLINICAL ISSUES

- Most IHs require no imaging or therapy
- Complications &/or associated anomalies more likely if IH large, segmental, facial, or multifocal
  - Ulceration (most likely with intertriginous & perioral lesions), bleeding
  - Compression of vital structures (airway, orbit)
  - Heart failure, liver failure, hypothyroidism, &/or compartment syndrome with high liver lesion burden
- Therapy reserved for large or complicated lesions or for significant residua following involution
  - Select β-blockers have replaced steroids as primary therapy due to low side effect profile

DIAGNOSTIC CHECKLIST

- If imaging appearance, timeline, or physical exam findings atypical for IH, exclude other lesions by biopsy
- US liver if ≥ 5 cutaneous IHs (for ↑ risk of hepatic lesions)

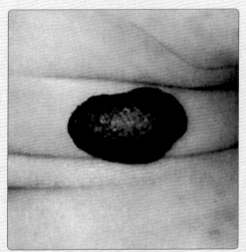
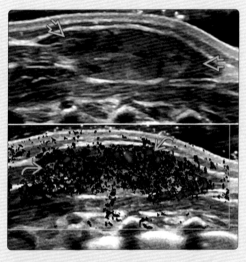

(Left) Photograph of a 4-month-old patient shows a well-defined, raised "strawberry" lesion on the neck that appeared after birth, typical of a proliferating infantile hemangioma (IH). (Right) Longitudinal US images at the site of a palpable back mass in the same patient show a well-defined lentiform subcutaneous lesion ➡ with mildly heterogeneous internal echogenicity. The mass demonstrates a high vessel density ➡ on color Doppler imaging, typical of a proliferating deep IH.

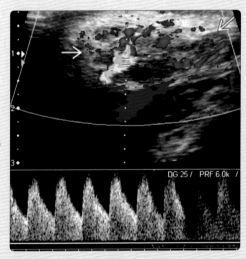
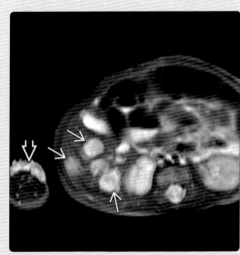

(Left) Pulsed Doppler US through a heterogeneous subcutaneous mass ➡ in an infant shows a high vessel density of low-resistance arterial waveforms, typical of an IH. (Right) Axial T2 FS MR through the abdomen of a 3 month old with > 5 cutaneous IHs shows multiple round, hyperintense hepatic IHs ➡. A lobular superficial hyperintense right forearm IH ➡ is partially visualized as well.

Venous Malformation

KEY FACTS

TERMINOLOGY

- Subtype of congenital slow- or low-flow vascular malformation due to error in vein formation; not neoplastic
  - Differs from hemangioma (benign vascular neoplasm of capillaries) or arteriovenous malformation (high flow)

IMAGING

- Most commonly cutaneous, subcutaneous, &/or intramuscular; may involve bone, synovium, &/or viscera
  - Focal, multifocal, or diffuse throughout region
- Well-circumscribed lobulated mass vs. extensive confluent, infiltrative lesion
  - ± discrete serpentine venous channels of abnormal number, size, shape, & location
- Radiography: Phleboliths in mass essentially diagnostic
- MR: High fluid signal intensity ± layering fluid-fluid levels
  - Phleboliths typically small, round, & dark
  - Diffuse or patchy enhancement of venous malformation
- US: Mass of heterogeneous echotexture
  - Hypoechoic/anechoic tubular channels in clusters
    - Compressible; will slowly refill
  - Phleboliths: Round echogenic foci with posterior acoustic shadowing & twinkle (color) artifact
  - Detectable venous waveforms often sparse

CLINICAL ISSUES

- Soft, compressible mass without thrill
  - Enlarges with Valsalva/crying/dependent positioning
  - Bluish skin discoloration with superficial lesions
  - Episodic pain &/or swelling
- Grow proportional to child but may enlarge suddenly due to hemorrhage, thrombosis, or hormonal changes
- Large varicosities can lead to thromboembolism
- Prognosis depends on lesion size, extent, & location
  - More extensive lesions may cause lifelong morbidity
- Treatments include conservative therapy (compression garments, antiinflammatory medications), percutaneous procedures (sclerotherapy, laser), surgical resection

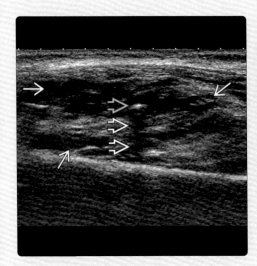

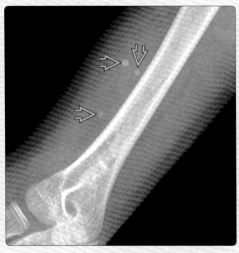

(Left) Longitudinal US of the upper arm in a 9-year-old girl with new pain & swelling shows a multilobulated collection of hypoechoic channels ➡ within the biceps muscle. There is an echogenic focus ➡ in the mass with posterior acoustic shadowing ➡. (Right) AP radiograph of the humerus in the same patient confirms numerous round intralesional calcifications with lucent centers ➡, typical of phleboliths in a venous malformation (VM).

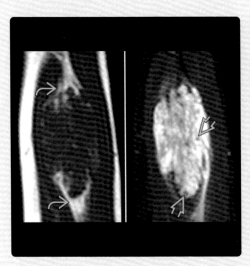

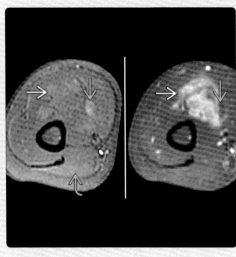

(Left) Coronal T1 (left) & STIR (right) MR images of the same VM show the lobulated soft tissue mass following fluid signal intensity except for the thin septations & phleboliths ➡. Note the fat ➡ along the margins & septations. (Right) Axial T1 FS pre- (left) & post- (right) contrast MR images through the same mass show that the lesion ➡ is largely isointense to muscle ➡ before contrast followed by heterogeneous enhancement. A focal thrombus ➡ shows T1 brightness before contrast & no enhancement after contrast.

KEY FACTS

TERMINOLOGY

- Rhabdomyosarcoma (RMS): Mesenchymal sarcoma arising from rhabdomyoblasts (primitive muscle cells); lacks normal differentiation into skeletal muscle

IMAGING

- Solid, mildly heterogeneous intramuscular mass without significant surrounding soft tissue edema
  - Usually round with well-circumscribed, lobular margins
  - Variable internal vascularity & enhancement, most commonly in low to moderate range
- Radiographs show focal soft tissue fullness, no Ca^{2+}
- US & MR features can strongly suggest sarcoma
  - US excellent choice for initial work-up of palpable mass
  - MR better at defining deep extent & relationships to critical structures (e.g., neurovascular bundle, joints, etc.)
- PET best for staging

CLINICAL ISSUES

- Most common soft tissue sarcoma in children
  - Embryonal: Most common type in patients < 15 years old; commonly of genitourinary, head & neck, or retroperitoneal origin
  - Alveolar: Typically in older children; commonly extremity, paratesticular, & truncal
  - Undifferentiated: Rarely occurs in children
- Typically presents as enlarging, firm, painless mass
- 2 age peaks: 2-6 years, 14-18 years
- Prognosis worse with alveolar subtype, tumor > 5 cm, metastatic disease at presentation (lung, bone marrow, lymph nodes most common), certain tumor sites (extremity & chest worse)
- Treated with neoadjuvant & adjuvant chemotherapy, surgery, radiation

(Left) Transverse US in a 2 year old with a lump on her forearm shows a well-circumscribed, mildly heterogeneous soft tissue mass ➡ at the interface of the subcutaneous fat ➡ & muscle ➡. While not specific, the appearance of a soft tissue "solid ball" in a child is very concerning for a soft tissue sarcoma. This mass proved to be an alveolar RMS. (Right) Sagittal STIR MR shows a well-circumscribed, intermediate signal intensity soft tissue mass ➡ in the posterior right forearm. This mass was a biopsy-proven alveolar RMS.

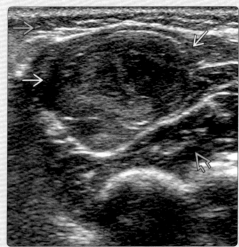
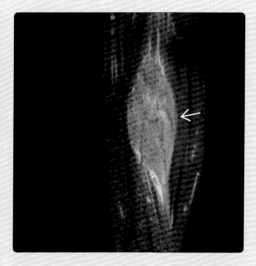

(Left) Axial T1 C+ FS MR in the same patient shows moderate generalized enhancement of the mass ➡ with mild heterogeneity. The enhancement patterns of RMS can be quite variable. (Right) Coronal T2 FS MR in a 10 year old with an intramuscular gluteal mass (not shown) demonstrates numerous hyperintense osseous metastatic foci ➡ within the lower lumbar spine, pelvis, & femurs. Biopsy of the mass showed alveolar RMS.

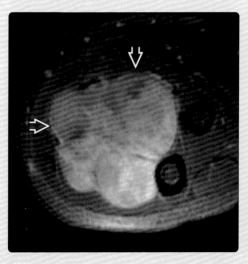
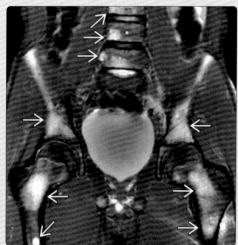

Ewing Sarcoma

TERMINOLOGY

- Ewing sarcoma family of tumors: Aggressive small round blue cell tumors that most commonly arise in bone
  - Includes Ewing sarcoma, primitive neuroectodermal tumor, Askin tumor, extraosseous Ewing sarcoma

IMAGING

- Highly aggressive radiographic appearance
  - Lucent ill-defined intramedullary lesion, poorly marginated; can show mild expansile remodeling
    - Sclerosis (inside bone) in up to 25%
  - Permeative or moth-eaten cortical destruction
  - Aggressive periosteal reaction: Spiculated, sunburst, lamellated onion skin appearance, &/or Codman triangle
  - Associated soft tissue mass often disproportionately larger than amount of bone destruction
- Greater propensity for flat bones (e.g., scapula, pelvis) than other primary bone malignancies

- Diaphyseal involvement of long bones more common than with other bone malignancies
- MR for local evaluation: Intraosseous & soft tissue extent, relationship to joint & neurovascular bundle
- Chest CT + PET/CT for staging

CLINICAL ISSUES

- 2nd most common primary bone malignancy in children after osteosarcoma
  - Median age: 15 years
- Presents with pain, swelling, palpable mass; ± systemic symptoms/signs of leukocytosis, fever, anemia, ↑ ESR
  - Can mimic osteomyelitis
  - Pelvic lesions tend to be larger at presentation & have worse outcome
- 60-70% 5-year survival with localized disease
- 20-30% 2-year survival with metastatic disease
- Primary therapies: Neoadjuvant & adjuvant chemotherapy + surgical resection &/or radiation

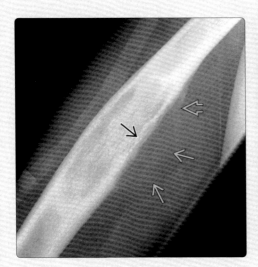
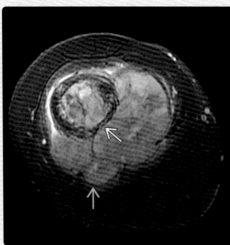

(Left) Lateral radiograph in a 17 year old with pain shows mild expansion of the mid femoral diaphysis. There is an underlying lucent lesion with variable margin definition. The overtly aggressive features include cortical permeation ➡, elevated & interrupted periosteal reaction ➡, & a soft tissue mass ➡. (Right) Axial T2 FS MR in the same patient shows an intramedullary mass permeating the cortex ➡ nearly circumferentially with an overlying solid soft tissue mass ➡. These features are classic for Ewing sarcoma.

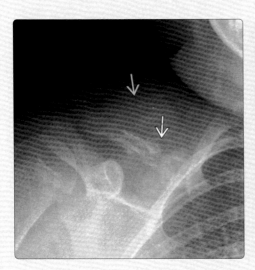
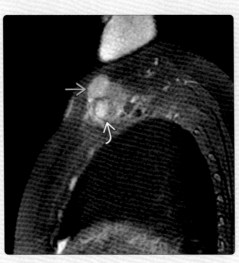

(Left) AP radiograph in a 7 year old who presented with soft tissue swelling about the clavicle shows a destructive, permeative lesion ➡ with aggressive periosteal reaction & a soft tissue mass ➡. (Right) Sagittal T2 FS MR in the same child shows a hyperintense lesion within the clavicle ➡ permeating the cortex & extending into an overlying soft tissue mass ➡. These features are typical for Ewing sarcoma.

TERMINOLOGY

- Osteosarcoma: Malignant tumor with ability to produce osteoid directly from neoplastic cells

IMAGING

- Aggressive metaphyseal/metadiaphyseal lesion with variable mix of bone destruction (lysis) & bone production (sclerotic/blastic cloud-like osteoid)
  - 55-80% around knee; axial skeleton < 20%
- Radiographs often diagnostic or highly suggestive
- MR to characterize tumor + intra- & extraosseous extent
  - Large field of view joint-to-joint imaging
    - Look for skip metastases
    - T1 best sequence for intraosseous tumor margin
  - High-detail focused imaging with surface coils
    - Heterogeneous signal intensity on all sequences
    - Evaluate relationship to physis, joint, neurovascular bundle
- PET for distant metastases; chest CT for small nodules

CLINICAL ISSUES

- Most common malignant primary bone tumor in children/young adults; bimodal age distribution (10-30 years, > 60 years)
  - Predisposition with Li-Fraumeni, hereditary retinoblastoma, Rothmund-Thomson, prior radiation
- Typical presentations include pain, mass
- Treatment
  - Neoadjuvant chemotherapy → surgical resection → adjuvant chemotherapy
    - Improved survival if necrosis > 90% at resection
  - Lung nodule metastasectomy (if low-volume disease)
- Prognosis depends on age, gender, tumor volume, histology, location, & stage
  - 5-year survival 70-80% without metastases, 20-30% with metastases at presentation
- ↑ incidence of secondary malignancies (hematologic > breast, thyroid, respiratory, soft tissue malignancies)

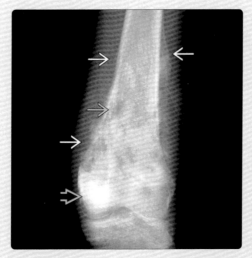

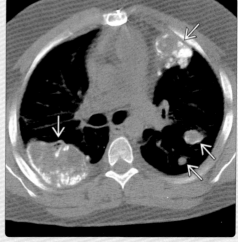

(Left) AP radiograph in a 13-year-old patient with the gradual onset of knee pain shows aggressive forms of periosteal reaction ➡ along the distal femoral metadiaphysis. There is a mix of blastic ➡ & lytic ➡ changes in the distal femur, typical of osteosarcoma. (Right) Axial CECT (in bone windows) shows calcified pleural & parenchymal lung metastases ➡ in a patient with a large pelvic osteosarcoma.

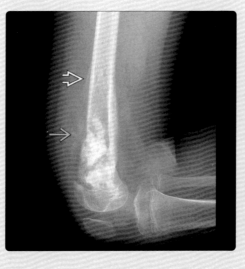

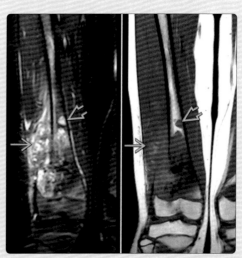

(Left) Lateral radiograph in an 8 year old with thigh pain shows an aggressive mixed lytic & blastic lesion of the distal femoral metadiaphysis with cloud-like osteoid ➡ anteriorly. Note the elevated, interrupted periosteal reaction (Codman triangle) proximally ➡. (Right) Coronal STIR (left) & T1 (right) MR images of the same patient show heterogeneity of the metadiaphyseal mass with extraosseous extension of tumor ➡. A small skip metastasis is noted ➡.

KEY FACTS

TERMINOLOGY

- Leukemia: Malignancy of hematopoietic stem cells diffusely infiltrating or replacing normal bone marrow
- Granulocytic sarcoma or chloroma: Soft tissue mass of leukemic cells typically found with AML

IMAGING

- Radiographs often normal or with subtle findings
  - Diffuse osteoporosis
  - "Leukemic lines": Lucent metaphyseal bands; thin, dense zone of provisional calcification often intact
  - Focal bone destruction: Poorly defined metaphyseal lytic lesions with permeative appearance
  - Aggressive periosteal reaction (lamellated, spiculated, interrupted), even if some components appear smooth
  - Pathologic fracture
  - Soft tissue chloroma (granulocytic sarcoma)
  - Mediastinal mass (from thymic infiltration)
  - ± avascular necrosis in treated patients

- MR: Leukemia may completely replace normal fatty marrow; ± superimposed acute infarction, fracture, or osteomyelitis causing focal symptoms

CLINICAL ISSUES

- Leukemia most common childhood malignancy
  - Subtypes: ALL > 75%, AML 15-20%, CML < 5%
  - ↑ ALL risk in Down syndrome, Li-Fraumeni syndrome, Fanconi anemia, immunodeficiencies
- Most common presentations
  - Bone or joint pain, limp, swelling; may be recurrent
  - Fatigue (from anemia), fever ± infection (from neutropenia), petechiae &/or bleeding (from thrombocytopenia)
  - Hepatosplenomegaly, lymphadenopathy > 60%
  - SVC syndrome, tachypnea, respiratory distress
- Treatment: Chemotherapy with steroids ± radiation, GCSF, stem cell transplant
- ALL: 5-year survival > 85%; 60-80% for others

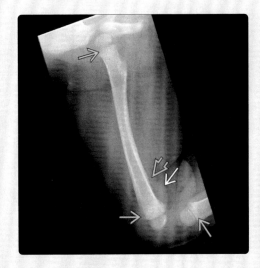

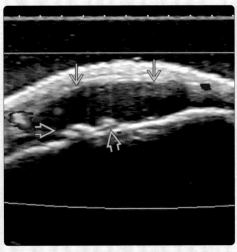

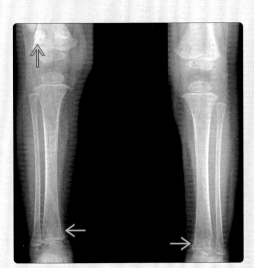

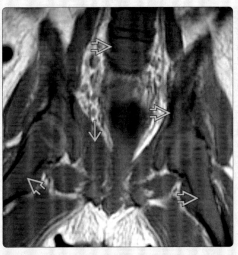

(Left) Lateral radiograph in a 14 month old with anemia, fever, & refusal to bear weight shows subtle metaphyseal lucencies ➡. There is a Codman triangle of aggressive periosteal reaction at the distal femur ➡ in association with a soft tissue mass ➡. (Right) Transverse color Doppler US (same patient) shows a left temporal soft tissue mass ➡ with underlying calvarial permeation & irregular periosteal reaction ➡. The patient was diagnosed with acute myelogenous leukemia (AML) & multifocal granulocytic sarcoma.

(Left) AP radiograph of each lower leg in an 11 month old shows pathologic fractures of the femoral, tibial, & fibular metaphyses ➡ at sites of underlying permeative osteolytic change. This patient was ultimately diagnosed with leukemia. (Right) Coronal T1 MR in a 21 month old with AML shows diffuse loss of normal bright fatty marrow signal throughout all visualized bones ➡, typical of leukemic marrow. An associated intramuscular granulocytic sarcoma ➡ was more clearly seen on other sequences.

KEY FACTS

TERMINOLOGY

- Langerhans cell histiocytosis (LCH): Spectrum of diseases caused by clonal proliferations of specific dendritic cells
- Single system (SS) (unifocal or multifocal) vs. multisystem (MS) disease
  - Bone (80-90%), skin (50%) most frequently involved
  - Risk organ (RO) involvement: Liver, spleen, marrow; confers worse prognosis (high risk)
  - Others: Lymph nodes, lung, pituitary, thymus, GI tract

IMAGING

- Best clue: Well-defined round or lobulated lytic punched-out skull lesion(s) without sclerotic rim
- Variable radiographic appearance of skeletal lesions depending on phase of disease ± therapy
- Monostotic vs. multifocal involvement: 50-75% vs. 10-20%
- Affected sites: Flat bones (50%) vs. long bones (30%)
  - Skull > ribs > femur > pelvis > spine

- FDG PET highly sensitive for active LCH (FDG avid); less sensitive for vertebral disease than whole-body STIR MR

CLINICAL ISSUES

- 90% of LCH cases < 15 years at presentation
  - SS, unifocal (70% of cases); peak age: 5-15 years
  - SS, multifocal (20% of cases); peak age: 1-5 years
  - MS RO+ (10% of cases); peak age: 0-2 years
- Mortality: SS or MS RO- < 5% vs. MS RO+ 10-50%
- Spontaneous regression of unifocal bone disease common
- Chemotherapy, steroids for multifocal SS or MS disease
- Disease reactivation in 25-75% (MS > SS)
- Long-term sequelae in 25-70% (MS > SS)

DIAGNOSTIC CHECKLIST

- LCH almost always reasonable diagnostic consideration for pediatric bone lesion due to variable appearances

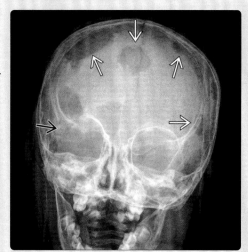

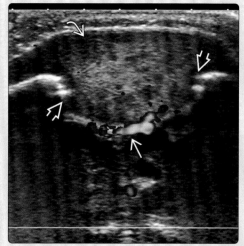

(Left) AP radiograph of the skull in a 1-year-old girl with palpable masses shows multiple punched-out lytic lesions of the calvarium ➡️. The superior & lateral walls of the right orbit are destroyed ➡️. (Right) Coronal color Doppler ultrasound of the midline frontal calvarium in the same patient shows a discrete hypovascular soft tissue mass ➡️ filling a site of complete osteolysis ➡️. The mass is compressing the adjacent superior sagittal sinus ➡️.

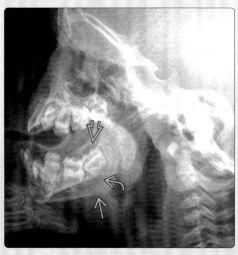

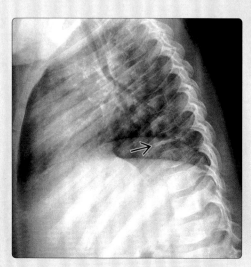

(Left) Lateral radiograph of the face in a 1 year old with jaw pain & a palpable abnormality shows interruption of the mandibular cortex ➡️ with loss of the normal lamina dura ➡️ at an adjacent tooth, creating the appearance of a floating tooth. Note the intact lamina dura (thin, circular, radiodense line) ➡️ around the contralateral tooth. Langerhans cell histiocytosis (LHC) was proven at biopsy. (Right) Lateral radiograph of a 2 year old who presented with multisystem LCH shows typical vertebra plana at T9 ➡️.

Fibroxanthoma

KEY FACTS

TERMINOLOGY

- Very common benign fibrous lesion of pediatric bone
- Term fibroxanthoma includes
  - Nonossifying fibroma
    - \> 2-cm length; encroachment on medullary cavity
  - Fibrous cortical defect
    - < 2-cm length
    - Essentially isolated to cortex

IMAGING

- Eccentric, elongated, bubbly, lucent lesion in long bone metaphysis/diaphysis with well-circumscribed lobular or smooth sclerotic margin & no periosteal reaction
- Expected involution/healing → gradual sclerosis, resolution
- Typical locations
  - Metaphysis of long bone: Up to 93%
    - Distance from physis ↑ with age
  - Located around knee: 55-89%
- Radiographs usually diagnostic

- Atypical features should suggest other lesion or superimposed complication (such as pathologic fracture)

CLINICAL ISSUES

- Benign lesion; no malignant transformation risk
  - More likely developmental defect than neoplasm
- Occurs in up to 35% of children
  - Peak age: 10-15 years (75% in 2nd decade)
- Usually asymptomatic & incidentally discovered
- May develop symptoms (uncommon)
  - Acute pain with pathologic fracture
  - Gradual pain with stress fracture of adjacent bone (very rare)
  - Paraneoplastic rickets/osteomalacia (extremely rare)
- Gradual healing with spontaneous regression of most cases in late adolescence
- Treatment only required if patient at high risk for pathologic fracture

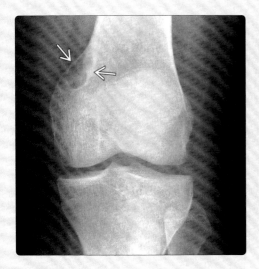
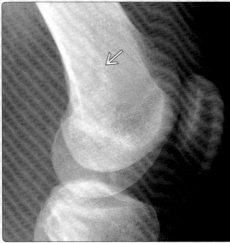

(Left) AP radiograph of the left knee in a 14-year-old boy with pain after an injury shows an incidental eccentric bubbly lucent lesion ➡ in the medial femoral metaphysis with a well-circumscribed sclerotic border, typical of a nonossifying fibroma (NOF) or fibroxanthoma. There is mild expansile remodeling at this level without periosteal reaction. (Right) Lateral radiograph of the knee in the same patient again demonstrates the nonaggressive features of the NOF ➡.

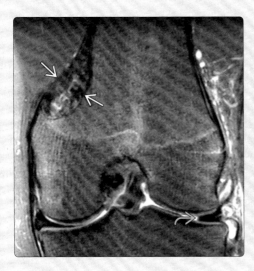
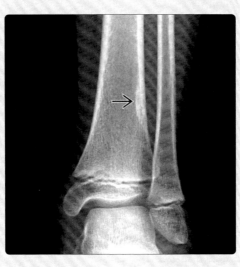

(Left) Coronal T2 FS MR in the same patient shows heterogeneous but largely hypointense signal of the intralesional content ➡ with normal adjacent marrow & soft tissues. (The study was performed for, & confirmed, a suspected meniscal tear ➡.) (Right) AP radiograph in a 9-year-old boy shows an eccentric, smoothly marginated, mixed lucent & sclerotic lesion ➡ in the distal tibial metadiaphysis, typical of a partially healed fibroxanthoma.

Osteoid Osteoma

KEY FACTS

TERMINOLOGY

- Benign osteoblastic lesion characterized by < 2-cm nidus of osteoid/woven bone in fibrovascular stroma

IMAGING

- Best clue: Well-defined small lucent lesion in long bone cortex with surrounding sclerosis & edema
- Locations
  - Cortical: 70-80%
    - Diaphyses > metaphyses of long bones
  - Medullary: 20-30%
    - Epiphyses or equivalents (intraarticular 10%)
    - Spine posterior elements
- Radiographs/CT
  - Small round or ovoid lucent nidus ± central Ca^{2+}
  - Surrounding cortical thickening, solid periosteal reaction
- MR
  - Variable nidus signal on T2 FS MR; may be "target"
  - Surrounding marrow, periosteal, & soft tissue edema

- Joint effusion/synovitis if lesion intraarticular
  - Hyperenhancing nidus on early dynamic T1 C+ FS MR
- Nuclear medicine bone scan: Double density sign

TOP DIFFERENTIAL DIAGNOSES

- Osteomyelitis, Langerhans cell histiocytosis, stress injury, osteoblastoma, osteosarcoma

CLINICAL ISSUES

- 5-35 years old; 50% between ages 10-20 years
- Insidious pain, worse at night & relieved by NSAIDs
- Local swelling, erythema, point tenderness
- Spinal involvement → painful scoliosis
- Long-term growth disturbances can result from hyperemia
- Gradual spontaneous regression in 6-15 years
  - NSAIDs accelerate to 3 years (but not well tolerated)
- Surgery curative if nidus completely resected
- Image-guided percutaneous interventions highly effective due to nidus visualization

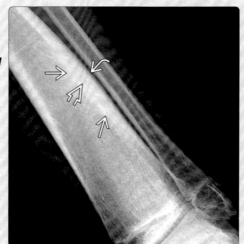

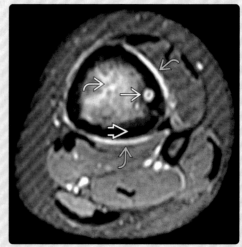

(Left) AP radiograph of the left tibia in a 15-year-old girl with 1 year of lower leg pain shows a region of diaphyseal cortical thickening laterally ➡ with mild overlying solid periosteal reaction ➡ & a subtle lucent focus centrally ➡. (Right) Axial bone CT of the same patient shows calcification within the hypoattenuating nidus ➡ of this osteoid osteoma (OO). The lesion is surrounded by cortical thickening ➡ & medullary sclerosis ➡.

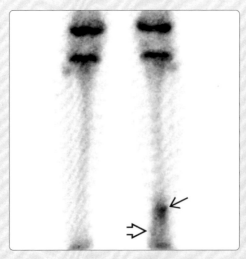

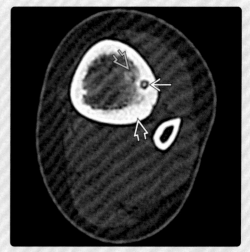

(Left) Tc-99m nuclear medicine bone scan of the same patient shows focally increased uptake at the level of the nidus ➡. This "hot" focus is superimposed on a background of mildly increased radiotracer activity in the distal tibia ➡ (the double density sign typical of OO). (Right) Axial T2 FS MR of the same patient shows a target appearance of the nidus ➡ with adjacent cortical thickening ➡ & surrounding marrow ➡ & periosteal ➡ edema.

Osteochondroma

KEY FACTS

TERMINOLOGY

- Common benign, developmental bony surface lesion resulting from displaced growth cartilage; not neoplastic

IMAGING

- Lobulated sessile or pedunculated bony protuberance
  - Demonstrates flowing corticomedullary continuity with underlying ("parent") bone
  - Covered by cap of hyaline cartilage (MR/US)
- Radiographs usually diagnostic
- MR typically reserved for pain/complications
  - Fracture (± radiographic visibility) may occur at stalk
  - Mass effect may lead to
    - Irritation of overlying soft tissues → bursa formation
    - Compression neuritis → denervation
    - Vascular compression → occlusion, pseudoaneurysm

TOP DIFFERENTIAL DIAGNOSES

- Osteosarcoma, myositis ossificans, periosteal chondroma

PATHOLOGY

- Etiology: Displaced physeal cartilage herniates through periosteal bone cuff; endochondral ossification yields growing bony protuberance
- Solitary much more common than multiple
  - Hereditary multiple exostoses patients
    - Develop characteristic growth disturbances
    - Have 1-5% lifetime risk of malignant degeneration vs. < 1% for solitary osteochondroma
- ↑ osteochondroma incidence with prior radiation

CLINICAL ISSUES

- Most commonly found in patients 10-35 years old
- Typically presents as painless, hard mass; pain most commonly from fracture or soft tissue irritation
- Lesion growth should cease at skeletal maturity
  - Further growth suggests malignant degeneration
- Surgical resection for symptomatic lesions or lesions growing beyond skeletal maturity

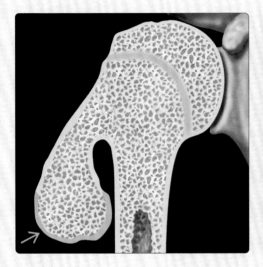

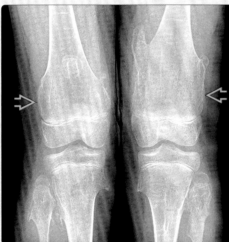

(Left) Graphic of the humerus shows a typical pedunculated osteochondroma (OC). The lesion points away from the joint & has flowing corticomedullary continuity with the parent bone. Note the cartilage cap of the lesion ➡, which allows for continued enlargement until skeletal maturity. (Right) AP radiograph of the knees in a 13 year old with hereditary multiple exostoses (HME) shows numerous OCs ranging from pedunculated to sessile. Note the broadened metadiaphyses ➡ typical of HME.

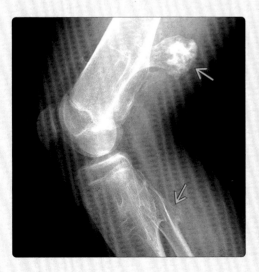

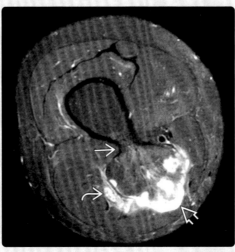

(Left) Lateral radiograph of the right knee in the same HME patient shows that the pedunculated OCs ➡ point away from the joint. Note the characteristic corticomedullary continuity of the OCs with the underlying bones. (Right) Axial T2 FS MR of the right thigh in a 14 year old shows an isolated pedunculated OC with a thin stalk ➡ arising from the posteromedial femur. A thin, high-signal cartilage cap is noted ➡. The sciatic nerve is displaced laterally ➡ & shows abnormal high T2 signal internally.

Developmental Dysplasia of Hip

TERMINOLOGY

- Definition: Spectrum of progressive hip abnormalities developing during infancy, including dysplastic acetabulum & femoral head malpositioning

IMAGING

- Ultrasound is modality of choice for infants 0-4 months old
- Radiographs necessary after 4-5 months
  - Proximal femoral epiphysis & acetabulum ossify, blocking ultrasound beam & limiting evaluation
- CT/MR used in limited circumstances
  - Immediately after operative reduction
  - Evaluation of long-term complications

CLINICAL ISSUES

- Palpable click/clunk upon stress (Ortolani & Barlow), asymmetric skin or gluteal folds, leg length discrepancy
- Much more common in girls, breech positioning, oligohydramnios, Caucasians

- Treatment correlation with ultrasound
  - Normal: α angle ≥ 60°, coverage ≥ 50%, no instability
  - Immature hip (applies only to infants < 3 months of age): α angle 50-59°, coverage 45-50%, no instability
    - Small risk of delayed developmental hip dysplasia (DDH); follow-up recommended to confirm normal development
  - Mild DDH: α angle 50-59°, coverage 40-50%
    - Infants ≥ 3 months usually treated with Pavlik harness to flex, abduct, & externally rotate hips
  - Moderate DDH: α angle ≤ 50°, coverage ≤ 40%, any instability
    - Treated with harness; repeat q4 weeks until normal
  - Severe DDH: Gross acetabular dysplasia, dislocated hip
    - No improvement in harness by 4 weeks → surgical hip reduction & casting required
- Delayed diagnosis/treatment can result in irreversible dysplasia requiring iliac osteotomy/shelving procedure

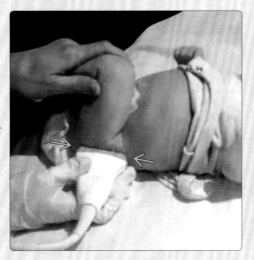
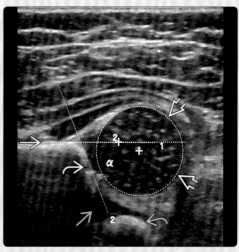

(Left) The US transducer is placed over the lateral hip with slight posterior obliquity ➡ to obtain a coronal flexed image. Note the use of 2 hands (& the foot pedal to save images). (Right) Coronal flexed US in the same patient shows the unossified femoral head ➡, the straight segment of the iliac bone ➡, & a line drawn along the acetabular roof ➡. The α angle is measured between these lines & should be ≥ 60°. The iliac line should cover the femoral head by ≥ 50%. Note the triradiate cartilage ➡ & ischium ➡.

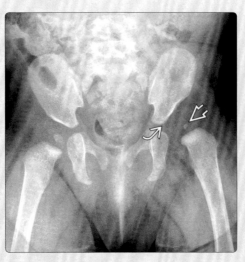
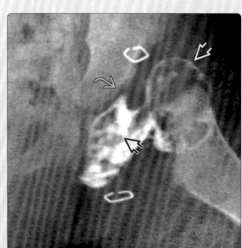

(Left) Frontal radiograph in a 6-month-old boy with a left hip "clunk" reveals severe left developmental dysplasia of the hip. The acetabular roof is quite steep ➡, & the ossified femoral head is small ➡ with superolateral dislocation. (Right) Intraoperative arthrogram shows contrast outlining a dysplastic, mostly unossified left femoral head ➡. Note that the acetabular roof is quite steep ➡. The femur is dislocated from the severely dysplastic & shallow joint space ➡. This child required an osteotomy.

TERMINOLOGY

Definitions

- Developmental dysplasia of hip (DDH): Spectrum of progressive hip abnormalities in infancy resulting in acetabular dysplasia with femoral head malpositioning

IMAGING

General Features

- Best diagnostic clue
  - Abnormal position & delayed ossification of femoral head with abnormally steep & shallow acetabulum

Ultrasonographic Findings

- Sonography directly visualizes cartilaginous & osseous components of hips in early infancy
- Static (anatomic) & stress (dynamic) imaging evaluates
  - Acetabular morphology
  - α angle (normal ≥ 60°)
  - Coverage of femoral head (normal ≥ 50%)
  - Dynamic subluxation during stress maneuvers

Radiographic Findings

- Hilgenreiner (horizontal) line: Drawn through bilateral triradiate cartilages
- Acetabular angle: Angle between line drawn along acetabular roof & Hilgenreiner line
  - Mathematically complementary to α angle of US
  - Decreases as hip matures
    - Normal < 30° in 1st year of life
    - Normal < 24° in 2nd year of life

CT/MR

- Limited CT or MR scans sometimes performed to confirm hip position after open surgical reduction & spica casting
- Either used in evaluation of long-term complications

Imaging Recommendations

- Best imaging tool
  - US modality of choice for infants 0-4 months of age
    - Screening hip US not recommended < 4 weeks of age due to presence of physiologic laxity
    - However, US should be performed if clinical exam suggests dislocation or significant instability
  - Radiographs necessary after 4-5 months
    - Proximal femoral epiphysis & acetabulum ossify, blocking ultrasound beam & limiting evaluation

DIFFERENTIAL DIAGNOSIS

Neuromuscular Disease

- Abnormal muscular tension causes abnormal alignment
- Other findings of neuromuscular disease: Gracile long bones, muscle wasting, coxa valga, "windswept pelvis"

Septic Arthritis

- Acute: Joint fluid may displace femoral head
- Chronic: Abnormal misshapen femoral head & acetabulum

Proximal Focal Femoral Deficiency

- Rare congenital anomaly with varying degrees of proximal femoral hypoplasia/aplasia; acetabulum may be normal

PATHOLOGY

General Features

- Etiology
  - Cartilaginous components on both sides of hip joint must be closely apposed to develop properly
  - DDH likely multifactorial, includes ligamentous laxity
    - Effect of maternal hormones (especially relaxin)
    - Intrinsic acetabular/femoral head deficiency
    - Reduced in utero space: Breech position (extreme hip flexion, knee extension), oligohydramnios, 1st-born

Staging, Grading, & Classification

- Graf staging based on single, static coronal image
- Most recommendations now include description of femoral head coverage & require stress imaging
- **Normal:** α angle ≥ 60°, coverage ≥ 50%
  - Sometimes called Graf type I
  - Requires no treatment
- **Immature hip:** α angle 50-59°, coverage 45-50%
  - Applies only to infants < 3 months of age
  - Sometimes called Graf type IIa
  - Small risk of delayed DDH
    - Follow-up to confirm normal development
    - Requires no treatment
- **Mild DDH:** α angle 50-59°, coverage 40-50%
  - May be observed by orthopedists with repeat US in 1 month, especially if < 2 months of age
  - Older infants usually treated with harness
- **Moderate DDH:** α angle ≤ 50°, coverage ≤ 40%
  - Unstable on stress imaging or clinical exam
  - Treated with Pavlik harness with repeat US q4 weeks
- **Severe DDH:** Gross acetabular dysplasia + dislocated hip
  - If no improvement in Pavlik harness by 4 weeks, continue to operative management

CLINICAL ISSUES

Presentation

- Palpable "click/clunk" upon stress (Ortolani & Barlow), asymmetric skin or gluteal folds, leg length discrepancy
- M:F = 1:5-8

Natural History & Prognosis

- Mild DDH may resolve spontaneously with no problems
- Moderate or severe DDH can cause long-term disability, limb shortening, decreased range of motion, degenerative change, avascular necrosis

Treatment

- Excellent prognosis when diagnosed & treated early
  - Pavlik harness to flex, abduct, & externally rotate hips
    - Increases femoral head engagement with acetabulum
- Delayed diagnosis/treatment can result in irreversible dysplasia requiring iliac osteotomy/shelving procedure

SELECTED REFERENCES

1. Kotlarsky P et al: Developmental dysplasia of the hip: what has changed in the last 20 years? World J Orthop. 6(11):886-901, 2015
2. LeBa TB et al: Ultrasound for infants at risk for developmental dysplasia of the hip. Orthopedics. 38(8):e722-6, 2015
3. Osborn DA: Independent predictors identified for developmental dysplasia of the hip. J Pediatr. 166(5):1322-3, 2015

Musculoskeletal

TERMINOLOGY

- Symptomatic growth disturbance of capital femoral epiphysis due to idiopathic avascular necrosis

IMAGING

- Radiographs: Sclerosis & irregularity with gradual flattening & fragmentation of sclerotic capital femoral epiphysis
  - Do not depict earliest stages of insult or repair
- MR or nuclear medicine bone scan for early changes of ischemia & revascularization
- Femoral head & neck gradually become short & broad with femoral head extrusion, femoroacetabular impingement, labral tears, joint degeneration

TOP DIFFERENTIAL DIAGNOSES

- Septic arthritis, transient synovitis, juvenile idiopathic arthritis, epiphyseal dysplasias

CLINICAL ISSUES

- Limp due to groin, thigh, or referred knee pain

- ↓ range of motion with loss of abduction & internal rotation without history of trauma
- Age: 4-12 years old; peak: 5-7 years old
- M:F = 4-5:1
- 10-20% bilateral, usually asynchronous
- Worse prognosis: > 8 years of age at onset, greater femoral head + lateral pillar involvement, subchondral fracture, metaphyseal changes, physeal arrest, aspherical femoral head with joint incongruence
  - 21-77% with premature physeal closure at hip
    - 3.5 years earlier than unaffected side
    - Many develop limb length discrepancy > 1 cm
- Conservative management: Bed rest, abduction stretching, bracing
  - Best outcomes in patients < 6 years of age
- Surgical interventions: Femoral head containment with joint congruence key to maintaining femoral head shape & preventing accelerated joint degeneration

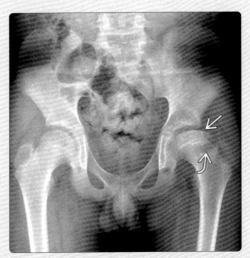
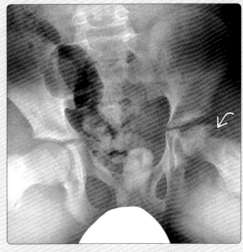

(Left) AP radiograph in a 10-year-old boy with left hip pain shows flattening, broadening, & sclerosis of the left femoral head ➡. The left hip joint is widened, & the acetabular roof is flattened. The femoral neck is short & broad with a lateral metaphyseal lucency ⇥. (Right) Frog leg lateral radiograph in the same patient shows similar left hip findings with better definition of the cystic-appearing femoral neck lucency ⇥. The constellation of findings is typical for Legg-Calvé-Perthes disease.

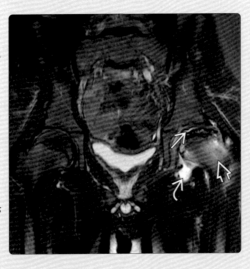
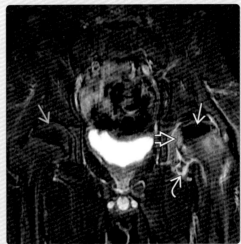

(Left) Coronal T2 FS MR in the same patient shows fluid ➡ within a subchondral fracture of the flattened & hypointense left femoral head. There is hyperintense marrow edema ⇥ in the femoral neck with an adjacent joint effusion ↗. (Right) Subtracted T1 C+ FS MR in the same patient shows no enhancement of ~ 80% of the left femoral head ➡ (as compared to the normal right ⇨) with the medial ~ 20% showing hyperenhancement ⇥. Adjacent reactive synovitis ➚ is noted.

Slipped Capital Femoral Epiphysis

KEY FACTS

TERMINOLOGY

- SCFE: Salter-Harris I fracture of subcapital femoral physis due to chronic stress of weight bearing
  - Femoral head slips posterior & medial to metaphysis

IMAGING

- AP view: Subcapital femoral physis abnormally smooth, lucent, & elongated ("wide")
  - Visible before medial femoral head displacement
- Frog leg lateral view (essential for diagnosis): Posterior displacement of femoral head relative to metaphysis
  - Femoral head-neck angle for severity assessment
- CT/MR more accurately determine severity of slip
- MR more sensitive than radiographs for diagnosis & complications
  - "Preslip" physeal elongation ("widening") on T1
  - ± marrow edema, synovitis with slip on T2 FS/STIR
  - Long-term: Femoroacetabular impingement, labral tear, articular cartilage damage, avascular necrosis (AVN)

- Incidence of bilateral SCFE varies widely: 18-80%
  - At initial presentation: 9-22%
  - Contralateral slip usually within 18 months

CLINICAL ISSUES

- Limp, pain, limited motion; symptoms often mild for weeks with acute worsening
  - Pain in hip, groin, or proximal thigh in 85%
  - Distal thigh or knee pain in 15%
- Girls average 11-12 years, boys average 13-14 years
- Major predisposing factor: Obesity
- Prognosis poorer for unstable (unable to bear weight) SCFE: ↑ AVN risk
- Most common treatments
  - Percutaneous single screw in situ fixation without femoral head manipulation (stable & mild unstable SCFE)
  - Open surgical hip dislocation with capital realignment (increasing use in moderate & severe unstable SCFE)
  - Prophylactic contralateral fixation controversial

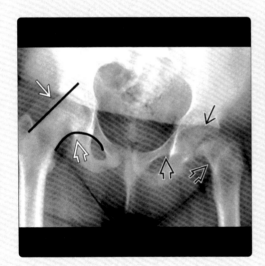
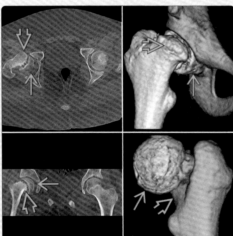

(Left) AP radiograph in an obese 10-year-old girl with left hip pain shows intersection of the lateral right femoral head ➡ by the line of Klein (normal). Such a line would not intersect the slipped left femoral head ➡. A normal continuous Shenton arc can be drawn on the right ➡ but not the left ➡. (Right) Axial (top left) & coronal (bottom left) 2D & posterior (bottom right) & anterior (top right) 3D surface-rendered CT images in a 12 year old show a chronic SCFE with a posteromedial slip of the right femoral head ➡ relative to the neck ➡.

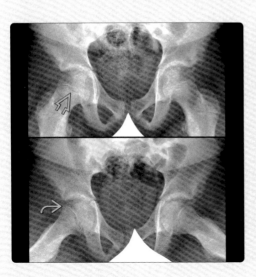
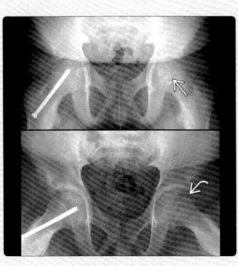

(Left) AP (top) & frog leg lateral (bottom) radiographs in an obese 12-year-old patient with right hip pain show an abnormally smooth & lucent right subcapital physis ➡ with offset of the femoral head-neck junction ➡ consistent with a SCFE. (Right) Follow-up radiographs 1 month later in the same patient status post right SCFE pinning demonstrate interval development of an abnormally smooth & lucent left subcapital physis ➡ with mild head-neck offset on the frog leg lateral view ➡, consistent with a left SCFE.

Achondroplasia

TERMINOLOGY

- Most common nonlethal skeletal dysplasia

IMAGING

- Symmetric shortening of all long bones
  - Proximal most affected (rhizomelic)
- Lower extremity shortening: Femur length similar to tibia
  - Ice cream scoop shape of proximal femurs in infants
  - Chevron shape of epiphyses/metaphyses at knees
  - Relatively elongated fibulae
- Upper extremity shortening: Humerus similar to ulna
  - Short metacarpals & phalanges with trident hand configuration: 3 forks = thumb, digits 2 & 3, digits 4 & 5
- Skull base: Keyhole foramen magnum, narrow jugular foramina → venous hypertension → ventriculomegaly
- Spine: Gibbus deformity of thoracolumbar junction, anterior vertebral body beaking or wedging (bullet-shaped), posterior vertebral body scalloping, progressive narrowing of interpediculate distances from L1-L5

- Pelvis: Squared iliac wings, narrowed sacrosciatic notches, horizontal acetabular roofs, overall coupe-type champagne glass configuration of pelvis

PATHOLOGY

- Autosomal dominant, 80% sporadic
- Mutation at chromosome 4p16.3: Fibroblast growth factor receptor-3 gene (*FGFR3*)

CLINICAL ISSUES

- Incidence: 1:10,000-40,000 live births
- Normal intelligence; lifespan ~ 10 years < unaffected population
- Cervical instability in infancy; progressive lumbar stenosis
- Upper airway obstruction ~ 5%
- Otitis media in 90% during first 2 years
- Obesity common & disabling in older children
- 2-5% risk of sudden death from cervicomedullary compression: Suspect with central hypopnea, ↓ arousal state, hypotonia, hyperreflexia; surgery in 17%

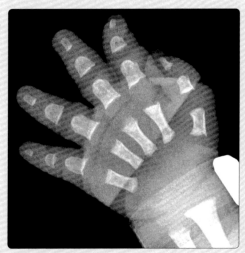
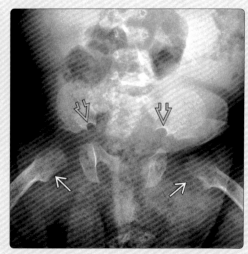

(Left) *PA radiograph shows a trident hand configuration in a newborn with achondroplasia: The fingers are of similar lengths & diverge from one another in 2 pairs plus the thumb. The metacarpals & phalanges are short & broad.* (Right) *AP radiograph in a 4 month old shows an ice cream scoop configuration of the upper femurs* ➡ *in this infant with achondroplasia. Also note the elephant ear configurations of the iliac wings with small sacrosciatic notches* ➡. *The acetabular roofs are horizontal.*

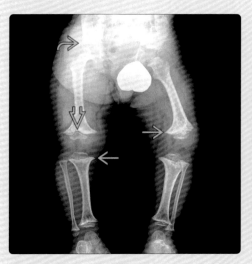
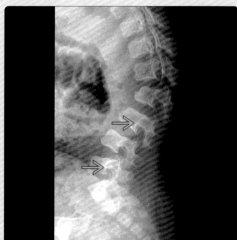

(Left) *AP radiograph in a young patient with achondroplasia shows broad/flared metaphyses* ➡ *with cone- or chevron-shaped distal femoral metaphyses/epiphyses* ➡. *Note the long fibulae & horizontal acetabular roofs* ➡. (Right) *Lateral radiograph shows scalloped posterior vertebral bodies* ➡, *a gibbus kyphotic deformity of the thoracolumbar junction, & exaggerated lumbosacral lordosis, typical of achondroplasia.*

Osteogenesis Imperfecta

TERMINOLOGY

- Group of clinically heterogeneous genetic disorders caused by type I collagen abnormalities
- ↑ bone fragility → frequent fractures → malunion & bowing
  - ↑ likelihood of subsequent fractures

IMAGING

- Numerous in utero or perinatal fractures of short, poorly mineralized bones (type II)
- Other types: Multiple fractures in thin, overtubulated long bones + vertebral fractures + osteoporosis
- Radiographs generally sufficient to suggest diagnosis
- CT or MR for axial skeleton complications

PATHOLOGY

- Modified versions of original (1979) Sillence classification
- Original types I-IV based on clinical, radiologic manifestations, & inheritance

- Types V-IX proposed due to mutations outside type I collagen genes ± different phenotypes, inheritance

CLINICAL ISSUES

- Severity of osteogenesis imperfecta (mild → severe)
  - Type I < IV < VI < VII < III < II
  - Type I: Mild, not deforming
    - Blue sclerae in most; spectrum of fractures from none (in 10%) → numerous (less after puberty)
  - Type II: Lethal in perinatal period
    - Blue sclerae, myriad of prenatal fractures, intracranial hemorrhage, lung hypoplasia → death
  - Type III: Premature death, deformation severe
    - Gray sclerae, triangular face
  - Type IV: Deformation moderate
    - White sclerae, long bone bowing, vertebral fractures
- Associations: Hearing loss (usually as adults), thin skin with subcutaneous hemorrhages, cardiac disease, hernias
- Treatment: Intravenous bisphosphonates, surgery

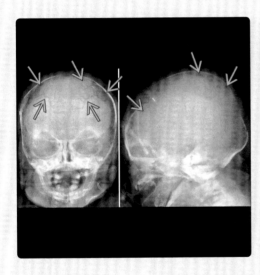

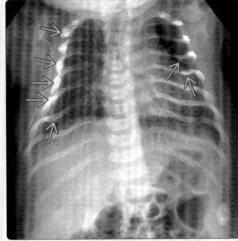

(Left) Frontal & lateral radiographs of the skull in a 1-day-old girl with multiple fractures seen on fetal ultrasound shows multiple (> 10) wormian bones ⮕ throughout the skull. The patient was subsequently diagnosed with type III osteogenesis imperfecta (OI). (Right) Frontal radiograph of the chest in the same patient shows deformities & healing fractures of multiple bilateral ribs ⮕. Intrauterine fractures can be seen in OI, particularly in types II & III.

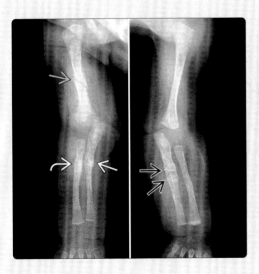

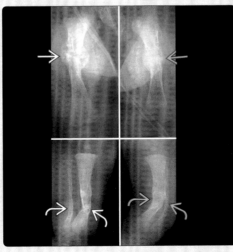

(Left) Frontal radiographs show the right & left upper extremities in the same patient. There are healing fractures of the right humerus ⮕, right radius ⮕, & right ulna ⮕ as well as multiple healing fractures of the left ulna ⮕. (Right) Frontal radiographs show the right & left lower extremities in the same patient with OI type III. There are healing fractures of the right ⮕ & left ⮕ femurs. Bowing deformities of both the right ⮕ & left ⮕ tibias/fibulas (secondary to healing fractures) are also noted.

TERMINOLOGY

- Synovial inflammation of unknown cause
  - Arthritis begins < 16 years of age
  - ≥ 6 weeks of symptoms
- International League of Associations for Rheumatology (ILAR) classification of juvenile idiopathic arthritis
  - Systemic arthritis: Arthritis of ≥ 1 joint + daily spiking fever for ≥ 3 consecutive days
    - Accompanied by ≥ 1 of following: Evanescent rash, hepatomegaly &/or splenomegaly, serositis
  - Oligoarticular arthritis: Arthritis of < 5 joints in first 6 months of disease
  - Polyarticular arthritis: Arthritis of ≥ 5 joints in first 6 months of disease
    - Rheumatoid factor positive or negative
  - Psoriatic arthritis
  - Enthesitis-related arthritis
  - Undifferentiated or unclassified arthritis

IMAGING

- Radiographs: Characteristic findings seen late in disease
  - Early to intermediate: Osteoporosis, joint capsule distention (by effusion &/or synovitis), erosions
  - Late: Joint space loss, ankylosis, growth disturbances
- MR: Joint effusion with synovial thickening & enhancement, bone marrow edema, cartilage loss ± bone erosions
  - Hypointense rice bodies: Detached fragments of necrotic synovium layering in joint effusion
- US: Compressible joint fluid vs. noncompressible synovium
  - Color/power Doppler for active vs. inactive synovitis

CLINICAL ISSUES

- Most common cause of chronic arthritis in children
  - 1-3 years of age (largest peak); 8-10 years (smaller peak)
- Presentations: Joint swelling, stiffness, pain, warmth
- Treatment: NSAIDs, systemic/local corticosteroids, disease-modifying agents (e.g., methotrexate), biologic agents (monoclonal antibodies or soluble receptors)

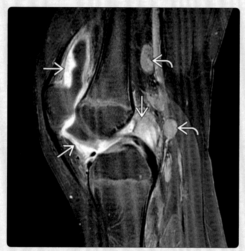
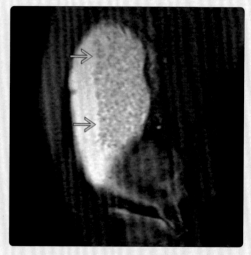

(Left) *Sagittal T1 C+ FS MR in an 8 year old with knee pain for 4-5 months shows markedly thickened, enhancing synovium* ➡ *surrounding a moderate joint effusion. Popliteal lymphadenopathy* ↗ *is also noted. The patient was subsequently diagnosed with juvenile idiopathic arthritis (JIA).* (Right) *Sagittal T2 FS MR in a patient with JIA shows innumerable uniform low-signal nodules (rice bodies)* ➡ *layering dependently within a large knee joint effusion.*

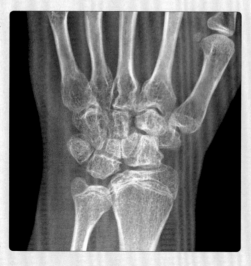
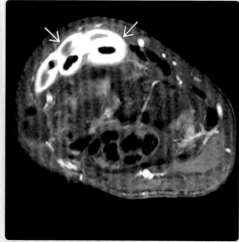

(Left) *PA radiograph of the wrist shows distorted, angular carpal bones with loss of height & diffuse narrowing of the radiocarpal, intercarpal, & MCP joints. This appearance is due to a combination of erosive change & hyperemia in a tight joint.* (Right) *Axial T1 C+ FS MR of the wrist shows thickening & intense synovial enhancement* ➡ *surrounding the extensor pollicis longus & extensor carpi radialis brevis & longus tendons, consistent with tenosynovitis. Nonenhancing fluid is seen within some of the tendon sheaths at these levels as well.*

Dermatomyositis

KEY FACTS

TERMINOLOGY

- Juvenile dermatomyositis: Diffuse nonsuppurative inflammation of striated muscle, subcutaneous fat, & skin
- ~ 85% of juvenile idiopathic inflammatory myopathies

IMAGING

- Patchy to diffusely infiltrative ↑ fluid signal intensity of muscles on STIR or T2 FS MR
  - Symmetric involvement of proximal musculature
    - Thighs > pelvis > shoulders
  - ± chronic muscle atrophy/fatty infiltration
- Subcutaneous fat involvement: High specificity (but low sensitivity) for predicting progression to chronic forms
- Soft tissue Ca^{2+} (30-70%), usually periarticular
  - Develop months to years after disease onset

CLINICAL ISSUES

- Median age of onset: 7-11 years
- Most common signs & symptoms

- Proximal muscle weakness ± tenderness, easy fatigue
- Rash (heliotrope eyelid rash & Gottron papules classic)
- Other cutaneous manifestations: Periungual telangiectasis, scaly alopecia, ulcers, photosensitive rash
  - Shawl sign: Poikilodermatous rash on upper chest or V-shaped rash on upper back
- Other manifestations: Fever, weight loss, arthritis, pericarditis, pulmonary fibrosis, GI ulcers & dysphagia
- Diagnosis classically made by characteristic rash + 3 of 4
  - Symmetric proximal muscle weakness
  - ↑ muscle enzymes in serum
  - Characteristic electromyography
  - Characteristic changes on muscle biopsy
- Diagnosis now more commonly employs characteristic MR findings & autoantibody profiles
- Treatments: Steroids, disease-modifying antirheumatic drugs, IVIg, biologic agents
- Variable disease course: Up to 73% with active disease > 10 years after diagnosis; 3% mortality

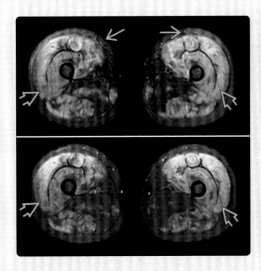

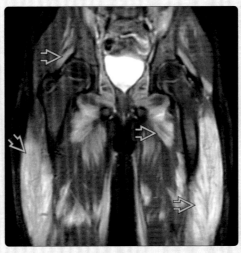

(Left) Axial T2 FS (top) & T1 C+ FS (bottom) MR images of the thighs in a 4-year-old girl with proximal weakness & a rash show extensive, symmetric, infiltrative high T2 signal intensity & enhancement throughout anterior > posterior compartment muscles ➡ with relative sparing medially. Abnormal reticular foci are also seen in subcutaneous fat ➡. (Right) STIR MR in the same patient shows the extent of symmetric muscular edema/inflammation throughout pelvis & thighs ➡, typical of juvenile dermatomyositis.

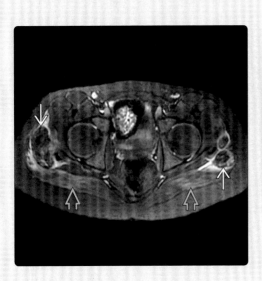

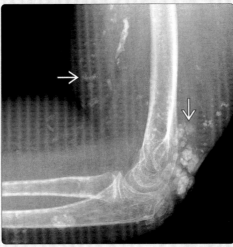

(Left) Axial T2 FS MR (same patient 4 years later) shows the interval development of multiple ovoid, predominantly low signal intensity, intramuscular masses laterally ➡, consistent with calcinosis. Patchy inflammation remains in the gluteus maximus muscles ➡. (Right) Lateral radiograph in a teenager with juvenile dermatomyositis & limited elbow motion shows innumerable soft tissue Ca^{2+} ➡, predominantly in a periarticular location. Note the abundance of Ca^{2+} along the extensor surface of the joint.

Rickets

TERMINOLOGY

- Failure to mineralize cartilage & osteoid at growth plates (physes) of immature skeleton in setting of low ion concentrations (calcium or phosphorous)
  - Lack of phosphate (ultimate problem in all rickets) → failure of chondrocyte apoptosis → disruption of endochondral ossification
- Most common cause: Nutritional vitamin D deficiency

IMAGING

- Loss of normally thin, dense, well-defined zone of provisional Ca²⁺ at interface of physis & metaphysis
- Metaphyseal cupping, splaying, & fraying with lengthening ("widening") of adjacent radiolucent physis
- All sites of endochondral bone formation affected
  - Most pronounced at long bone metaphyses with greatest linear growth
    - Distal femur, proximal tibia, distal radius
- Sites of membranous bone growth less affected

PATHOLOGY

- Fractures due to vitamin D deficiency may occur in mobile patients with radiologic manifestations of rickets (not isolated biochemical abnormalities)
- Findings **not** due to rickets that must suggest child abuse
  - Fractures in nonmobile infants
  - Fractures otherwise typical of child abuse (e.g., classic metaphyseal lesion or corner fracture, etc.)
  - Subdural hematoma or retinal hemorrhage

CLINICAL ISSUES

- Peak age for dietary rickets: 3 months to 2 years
- Most rickets responds to vitamin D therapy ± calcium

DIAGNOSTIC CHECKLIST

- Unexplained physeal widening at 1 site (i.e., without acute or chronic trauma) merits survey at other sites of rapidly growing long bones (knees, wrists)
  - Multisite physeal widening → get metabolic work-up

(Left) *AP radiograph in a young child with rickets shows fraying, cupping, & splaying of the proximal tibial* ⊟ *& fibular* ▰ *metaphyses. There is loss of the normally dense, well-defined zones of provisional calcification (ZPC) that should be seen at the metaphyseal-physeal junctions. The radiolucent tibial physis is lengthened* ⊡. *The epiphyseal ZPC is also lost* ▱ *with poor bony margin definition.* (Right) *AP knee radiograph in a 3 year old with rickets shows typical metaphyseal fraying, cupping, & splaying* ▱, *as well as physeal lengthening* ⊡.

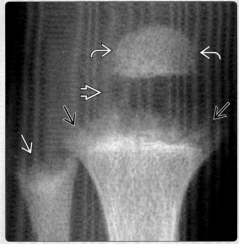
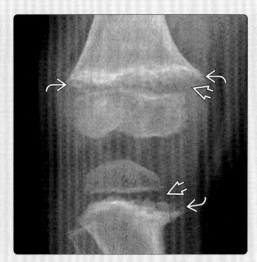

(Left) *PA wrist radiograph in this young child with rickets shows fraying, cupping, & splaying of every visualized metaphysis* ▰. *The normal ZPCs are lost.* (Right) *PA radiograph in the same child 9 weeks after initiation of therapy shows that endochondral ossification has resumed with improved bone formation at all the growth centers. The visualized metaphyses* ▱ *are normalizing in shape & density as compared to the prior study.*

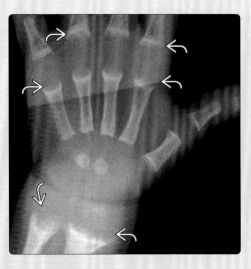
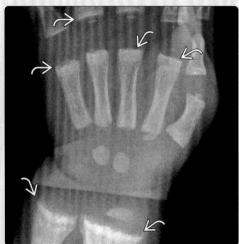

Sickle Cell Disease, Musculoskeletal

IMAGING

- Skull: Widened diploic space
- Vertebrae
  - Infarctions: Central endplate depressions (H-shape or Lincoln log morphology)
  - Bone softening: Biconcave endplates (fish mouth)
- Ribs: Infarction part of acute chest syndrome (chest pain, dyspnea, cough + pulmonary consolidation)
- Long bone infarctions
  - Acute/subacute: Poorly defined marrow, soft tissue, & periosteal edema ± fluid collections
    - Not easily distinguished from osteomyelitis in SCD
      - □ Episodes of vasoocclusion > > osteomyelitis (50:1)
      - □ Cortical disruption & fluid collections (especially larger) favor osteomyelitis
    - Dactylitis (hand-foot syndrome): Hand & foot small tubular bone infarcts, usually at age 6-24 months
  - Chronic: Lucent or sclerotic medullary cavity
    - Diaphysis, metaphysis
    - Epiphyseal infarction most common in humeral & femoral heads: Sclerosis, subchondral collapse

CLINICAL ISSUES

- Typically detected on newborn screening
  - Patients of African descent most frequently affected
- Most common presentations: Pain due to vasoocclusive crisis involving any organ, most commonly bone
  - Painful crisis of bone in 50% by age 5
    - Fever, pain, swelling, ↓ motion, leukocytosis, ↑ inflammatory markers in acute infarction or osteomyelitis
  - Infarction dactylitis often 1st manifestation (infancy); chest/abdominal crises begin at age 2-3 years
    - Acute chest syndrome: Most common cause of death
- Treatment: Hydration, pain management, blood transfusion, prophylactic penicillin, pneumococcal & *Haemophilus influenzae* vaccines to prevent infection

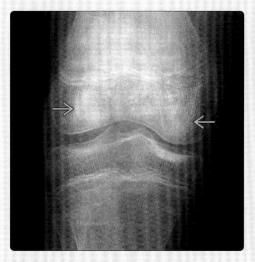

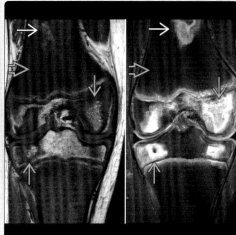

(Left) *AP radiograph of the right knee in a patient with sickle cell disease (SCD) & pain shows patchy sclerosis ⊵ of the femoral condyles, suggesting chronic bone infarcts.* (Right) *Coronal T1 (L) & T2 FS (R) MR images in the same patient show heterogeneous geographic foci with serpiginous margins in the femoral & tibial epiphyses ⊵ & femoral diaphysis ⊳, typical of bone infarcts. The abnormally low T1 & T2 signal intensity of the visualized metadiaphyses ⊵ is due to increased red marrow & iron overload.*

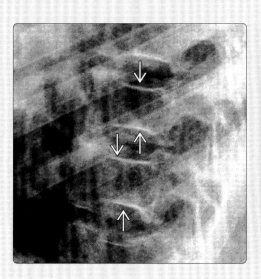

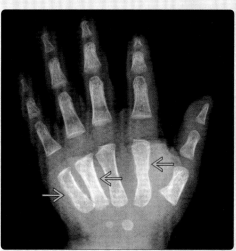

(Left) *Lateral radiograph of the thoracic spine in a patient with SCD shows a classic appearance of H-shaped vertebral bodies with central endplate depressions ⊳ due to infarctions.* (Right) *PA radiograph of the hand in an 11-month-old SCD patient with swelling & pain shows medullary sclerosis & periosteal reaction of the 2nd, 4th, & 5th metacarpals ⊵, typical of dactylitis.*

TERMINOLOGY

- Lateral curvature(s) of spine with Cobb angle of ≥ 10°
- **Curve etiologies** (some diagnoses span categories)
  - Idiopathic: Most common (70-85% of all scoliosis); classified according to age of onset
    - Infantile: < 3 years of age
    - Juvenile: 3-10 years
    - Adolescent idiopathic scoliosis (AIS): > 10 years
      - □ Most common type
      - □ Convex right thoracic curve typical
      - □ M < < F
  - Congenital: 10%
    - Osteogenic: Segmentation anomaly
    - Neuropathic: Tethered cord, split cord malformation
  - Neuromuscular (neuropathic or myopathic)
    - Single long curve
    - Neuropathic: Spina bifida, cerebral palsy, syrinx
    - Myopathic: Muscular dystrophies, spinal muscular atrophy
  - Developmental: Skeletal dysplasias
  - Tumor associated
    - Osteoid osteoma, cord neoplasm, neurofibroma

IMAGING

- Radiographs usually sufficient for AIS
- MR for atypical clinical/radiographic features: Pain, neurologic symptoms, rapid curve progression, unusual curves

CLINICAL ISSUES

- AIS: Usually asymptomatic but may have pain from progressive curvature or degenerative disc & facet disease
  - Young patients presenting with severe curves more likely to progress than older children with lesser curves
    - Most progression occurs during adolescence
  - Typical treatments include bracing for curves of 25-45° or spinal fusion for curves of > 45°

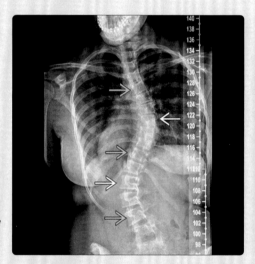
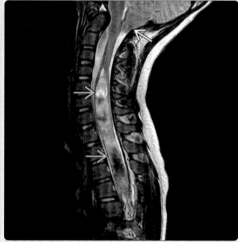

(Left) *PA radiograph of a 13 year old during follow-up for idiopathic scoliosis shows 47° convex right thoracic & 47° convex left thoracolumbar scoliotic curvatures. The terminal ⇨ & apical ➡ vertebrae for each curve are denoted. Note that the image is displayed from the perspective of the examining/operating orthopedist.* **(Right)** *Sagittal T2 MR of the cervical spine in a patient with a rapidly progressive scoliosis shows a large syrinx ⇨ secondary to a Chiari 1 configuration of the cerebellar tonsils ➡.*

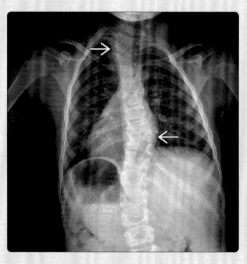
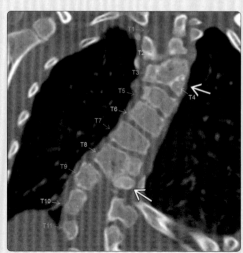

(Left) *Frontal radiograph in a 4 year old with congenital scoliosis shows hemivertebrae ➡ within the thoracic spine.* **(Right)** *Coronal reformatted NECT in a 7 year old with congenital scoliosis shows segmentation anomalies ➡ at T4 & T8. CT can be very helpful in assessing congenital curves due to vertebral anomalies & for planning surgery in cases with complex bony anomalies otherwise.*

Tarsal Coalition

TERMINOLOGY

- Congenital or acquired abnormal fusion of 2 tarsal bones; fusion may be osseous, cartilaginous, or fibrous

IMAGING

- 90% either calcaneonavicular (CN) or talocalcaneal (TC)
  - Up to 50% bilateral
  - Look for > 1 coalition in same foot (rare)
- Uncommon: Talonavicular, calcaneocuboid, cubonavicular
- CN coalition
  - Anteater nose sign: Elongation of anterosuperior calcaneus on lateral radiograph
  - Best tool: 45° oblique foot radiograph (Slomann view)
- TC coalition
  - Most common: Middle facet; less common involvement of anterior or posterior facets
  - Difficult to see radiographically; CT or MR often needed
    - Secondary findings not specific
      - Talar beak: Spur at dorsal head of talus

- C sign: Continuous uninterrupted line formed posteriorly by talar dome & sustentaculum tali on lateral view
  - Ball & socket ankle joint

PATHOLOGY

- Congenital vs. acquired (infection, arthritis, surgery, etc.)

CLINICAL ISSUES

- Presentation: Recurrent sprains, pes planus + heel valgus, flattening of medial arch, midfoot pain, limited subtalar motion, peroneal spastic flatfoot
  - Symptoms ↑ as coalition ossifies
- Treatment conservative initially: Nonsteroidal antiinflammatory medication, arch supports, trial of casting, orthotics, & physical therapy
  - May require surgical or arthroscopic resection

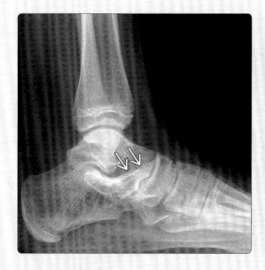
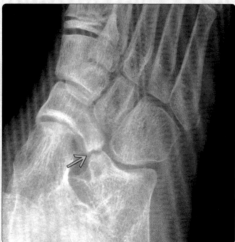

(Left) Lateral radiograph in a 10 year old with foot pain for 1 year shows elongation of the anterior process of the calcaneus (the anteater nose sign) ➡, typical of a calcaneonavicular (CN) coalition. (Right) Oblique foot radiograph in a 10 year old shows narrowing of the CN articulation ➡ with sclerosis & irregularity of the apposed navicular & calcaneus, consistent with a nonosseous CN coalition.

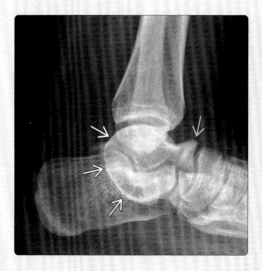
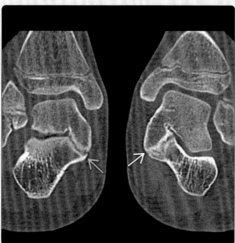

(Left) Lateral radiograph in a teenager who presented with recurrent ankle pain & swelling shows a continuous C sign ➡ of a talocalcaneal (TC) coalition. The C-shaped line is formed superiorly by the medial talar dome with continuity to the sustentaculum talus inferiorly. Note the talar beak ➡. (Right) Coronal bone CT in a 12 year old with bilateral ankle pain shows abnormally oriented & downsloping middle TC facets with partial osseous bridging on the left ➡ & close apposition on the right ➡.

KEY FACTS

TERMINOLOGY

- Brachial plexopathy: Injury to ≥ 1 brachial plexus nerve roots, trunks, or cords → upper extremity contracture
- Glenohumeral dysplasia: Sequelae of brachial plexopathy on developing glenoid & humeral head

IMAGING

- Brachial plexus/cervical spine MR: Shows pseudomeningoceles of root avulsions
- Shoulder imaging: Affected & unaffected sides imaged
  - Ultrasound: Can assess humeral head prior to ossification
    - Allows early detection & dynamic assessment of glenoid dysplasia without radiation or sedation
  - Radiographs: Long-term findings of dysplastic glenoid, winged scapula, hooked coracoid, small humeral head
  - MR: Best overall articular & soft tissue evaluation
    - % humeral head anterior to scapular line (PHHA)
      - ~ 50% normally
    - Angle of glenoid version
      - ↑ retroversion with ↑ glenohumeral dysplasia
      - > 5° difference to unaffected side abnormal

CLINICAL ISSUES

- Shoulder traction at delivery → nerve injury → muscle imbalance → unopposed internal rotation → posterior glenoid/anterior humeral head cartilage loading → glenohumeral dysplasia → posterior subluxation
- Manifestations depend on level of injured nerves (C5-T1)
  - C5 → weak shoulder
  - C5-C6 → weak shoulder & elbow
  - C5-C7 → weak shoulder, elbow, & wrist ("waiter's tip")
  - C5-C8 → weak shoulder, elbow, wrist, & hand
  - C5-T1 → flail hand; ± Horner syndrome
- Most deficits recover by 3 months; 20-30% have permanent deficit; 8-10% develop posterior subluxation
- Conservative treatment: Physical therapy, Botox injections, & closed reduction
- Surgery: Anterior soft tissue release ± tendon transfers

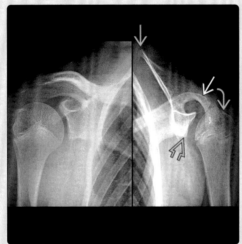
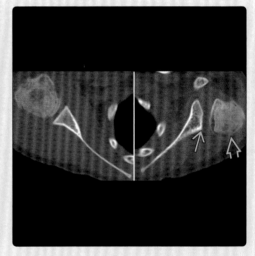

(Left) Frontal radiographs of the normal right shoulder (left image) & abnormal left shoulder (right image) in a 12 year old with glenohumeral dysplasia secondary to a left brachial plexopathy show a small, ovoid left humeral head ➡, winging of the left scapula ➡, a hooked coracoid ➡, & a dysplastic left glenoid ➡. (Right) Axial NECT images of the right (left image) & left (right image) shoulders in the same patient show that the small left humeral head is posteriorly displaced ➡, articulating with a false glenoid ➡.

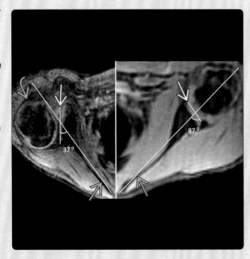
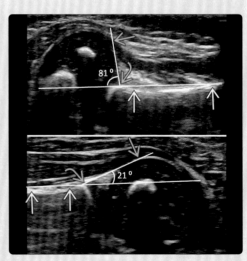

(Left) Axial GRE MR images of abnormal right (left image) & normal left (right image) shoulders show a low right glenoscapular angle (between the scapular ➡ & glenoid ➡ lines) with the humeral head ➡ posterior to the scapular line. (Right) Posterior axial US of the left shoulder (top) in an infant with left brachial plexopathy shows a high α angle (between the posterior scapular margin ➡ & a tangent to the humeral head ➡ from the posterior glenoid ➡), indicating posterior subluxation. The right α angle (bottom) is normal.

Hemophilia

KEY FACTS

TERMINOLOGY

- X-linked recessive (i.e., males only) bleeding disorder resulting from clotting factor deficiencies
  - Hemophilia A (> 80% of cases): Factor VIII deficiency
  - Hemophilia B (< 15% of cases): Factor IX deficiency
- Hemophilic arthropathy: Progressive joint destruction due to recurrent hemarthrosis, synovitis, & erosions

IMAGING

- Location of arthropathy: Knee > elbow > ankle > shoulder
- Radiographs: Distention of joint capsule by effusion & synovitis with eventual joint space narrowing, erosions, & subchondral cysts
- MR: Variable signal intensity & heterogeneity of effusions due to blood products of different ages
  - Chronic hemosiderin deposits line synovium
    - Low signal intensity on all sequences with characteristic blooming of signal loss on T2* GRE
  - Eventual development of osteocartilaginous erosions

- US: Effusion of variable echogenicity/complexity
  - Synovial thickening with hyperemia by Doppler
  - Thinning, irregularity of hypoechoic cartilage

TOP DIFFERENTIAL DIAGNOSES

- Synovial venous malformation
- Pigmented villonodular synovitis
- Juvenile idiopathic arthritis

CLINICAL ISSUES

- Acute hemarthrosis presents with tense, swollen, red, painful joint occurring spontaneously or with minor trauma
  - 1st episode of joint hemorrhage by 2-3 years of age
  - Treat by factor replacement + joint aspiration/irrigation
  - Prevent by aggressive prophylaxis with clotting factors
    - Significantly ↓ joint bleeds & chronic degeneration
    - Some develop antibodies (inhibitors) to factors
- Chronic hemarthrosis treated with synovectomy (surgical or radiosynovectomy) ± arthroplasty

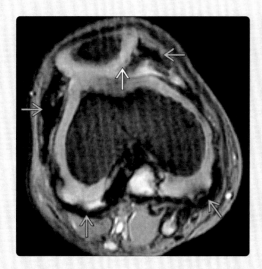

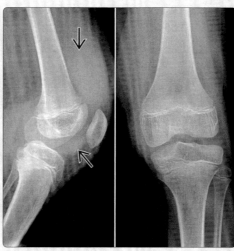

(Left) Axial T2* GRE MR of the knee in a 7 year old with hemophilia A shows extensive blooming (exaggerated signal loss) along the joint capsule ⇒ due to hemosiderin from prior hemarthrosis. Early cartilage damage is seen at the patellar medial facet ➡. (Right) Lateral & AP knee radiographs in the same patient 6 years later at a time of swelling show a large dense joint effusion ➡. The epiphyses are mildly large & irregular due to repeated hemarthroses & synovitis causing local hyperemia & cartilage damage.

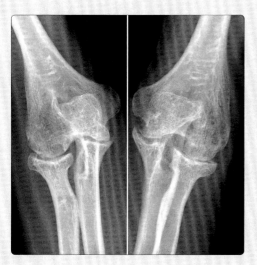

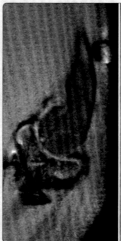
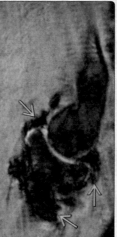

(Left) AP radiographs of the bilateral elbows in the same patient 5 years later show the longstanding effects of recurrent hemarthroses, including irregular, misshapen, & overgrown epiphyses with joint space narrowing. These findings are due to synovitis with hyperemia (particularly during skeletal growth) & osteochondral injury. (Right) Sagittal PD FS (L) & T2* GRE (R) MR images from the same patient show blooming of synovial hemosiderin ⇒. There is irregularity & thinning of the articular cartilage with small erosions.

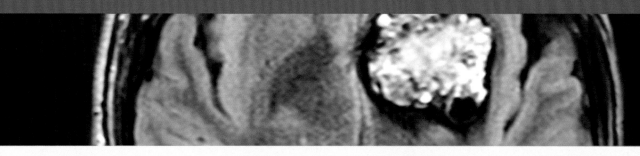

SECTION 7
Brain

Introduction & Normals

Congenital Malformations

Phakomatoses

Cysts and Neoplasms

Traumatic and Vascular Lesions

Metabolic, Infectious, and Inflammatory Disorders

Head/Brain Imaging Modalities

Radiographs

Skull radiographs have limited value in the pediatric patient. They may occasionally be obtained in the setting of trauma, but it should be recognized that they can be falsely reassuring. Pediatric patients can have significant intracranial injuries (including extraaxial hemorrhages & brain parenchymal contusions) without having skull fractures. Additionally, some fractures (particularly of the skull base) will not be readily seen by plain films. In these circumstances, there are typically mechanisms of injury & clinical manifestations that should lead to CT as the modality of choice. Occasionally radiographs of the skull are obtained in the setting of minor trauma for "parental reassurance," yet these patients are the most likely group to have nondisplaced fractures that will be difficult to see on radiographs, particularly regarding the facial bones (other than the nasal bones).

Skull radiographs are regularly employed in certain circumstances, including the evaluation of ventricular shunt catheter continuity (when dysfunction is suspected), the detection of craniosynostosis, the work-up of a palpable bony abnormality or defect, & during skeletal surveys for nonaccidental trauma or multifocal bone lesions (such as Langerhans cell histiocytosis). In the setting of suspected nonaccidental trauma, the patient age & clinical appearance will guide the use of head CT over generalized bone screening in the plain film survey. Some institutions will still obtain radiographs even when a head CT is performed for suspected abusive head trauma, but centers using multiplanar & 3D reconstructions of the CT data may forgo skull plain films.

Computed Tomography

NECT provides a fast & accurate assessment of the skull & intracranial contents. Its main advantages are its wide availability, rapid acquisition (typically just a few seconds of actual scan time, therefore negating a need for sedation in most circumstances), noninvasive nature, & high sensitivity for intracranial hemorrhage, mass effect, hydrocephalus, & skull fractures. Relative to MR, CT is moderately limited in its evaluation of the brain parenchyma, particularly in the detection of acute ischemia or characterization of processes beyond those previously listed. Additionally, CT requires ionizing radiation. While the long-term effects of medical doses of ionizing radiation remain debated, it should be avoided when it is unnecessary. Most centers have taken significant steps in the last 10 years to limit exposure to medical radiation (including implementing dose reduction techniques during scanning & utilizing clinical algorithms to decrease unnecessary exams in the setting of reasonable alternatives).That being said, when there is a true clinical indication & no reasonable alternative for CT in the acute setting, it should not be discouraged.

The use of IV contrast is rarely required for head CT scans in children. In the acute setting, it is most appropriate when a complication of an intracranial infection is suspected (e.g., sinusitis leading to a subdural empyema or brain abscess) or when a vascular abnormality is of concern both clinically & on a preceding NECT (e.g., an atraumatic hemorrhage that suggests an underlying arteriovenous malformation). CECT can also rapidly detect venous thrombosis with sensitivity similar to that of MR venography. Other considerations, such as neoplasm, are best characterized by MR, though NECT will detect any lesions causing mass effect &/or hydrocephalus.

While head CTs have traditionally been viewed in axial planes only (which was at one time the only plane technically achievable), many centers are now reformatting the acquired datasets into additional coronal & sagittal planes. These views greatly increase the accuracy of NECT in the detection of small intracranial lesions & skull fractures, particularly with any abnormality that lies predominantly in the axial plane (such as many linear parietal bone fractures). 3D reformations of bone can also help detect & characterize skull fractures. These tools are generally available without additional charge or radiation, though centers vary on when they are incorporated into imaging protocols.

Ultrasound

The use of ultrasound anywhere in the body is limited by the availability of an "acoustic window" into the region of interest. Specifically, the propagation of sound waves must not be obstructed by bone, gas, or fat. Therefore the use of sonography to evaluate the brain is limited to a timeframe when sufficient calvarial openings exist for the transducer to send & receive sound waves from the brain parenchyma. While several fontanelles may be available in the newborn period, the anterior fontanelle can generally be used up until about 4 months of age.

Because of the location of the anterior fontanelle & the design of the transducer, ultrasound is best at visualizing midline or paramidline structures. Ventriculomegaly, intraventricular hemorrhage, & midline shift are readily detected in the neonatal period. Large parenchymal or extraaxial hemorrhages will also be visualized, though smaller hemorrhages overlying the convexities may not be readily visibile. Ultrasound is much less reliable for early parenchymal injuries, such as lesser degrees of hypoxic ischemic encephalopathy.

A common use of ultrasound beyond the neonatal period is in the infant with macrocephaly. In addition to excluding ventriculomegaly & midline shift, it has excellent visualization of the high extraaxial spaces. A very common but poorly understood underlying disorder is benign macrocrania of infancy, in which the subarachnoid spaces are enlarged (thought to be due to immaturity of the CSF-absorbing arachnoid granulations). However, ultrasound may also visualize more ominous collections incidentally, such as subdural hematomas of child abuse found in an infant with macrocrania.

Another appropriate use of ultrasound during & beyond infancy is in the child with a focal palpable abnormality of the head, particularly when a soft tissue mass is suspected. Vascular anomalies (such as infantile hemangioma), lymph nodes, epidermoids/dermoids, & other lesions may be characterized & sometimes diagnosed by ultrasound. Ultrasound can also detect aggressive bone destruction by some soft tissue lesions, including Langerhans cell histiocytosis, leukemia, & metastatic neuroblastoma. However, if the lesion is very hard on palpation, radiographs should be the 1st imaging evaluation due to the likelihood of heavy calcification &/or bone deformity that will typically not be well characterized by ultrasound.

Magnetic Resonance Imaging

Due to its high contrast & spatial resolution, MR provides much greater detail of the brain parenchyma & intracranial fluid spaces than the previously discussed modalities. This makes it ideal for detecting lesions that do not have much mass effect (& may, therefore, be occult on CT). It also provides much greater characterization of all parenchymal lesions & their effects on the surrounding tissues. For example, a NECT will almost always detect a posterior fossa neoplasm & the resulting obstructive hydrocephalus. It may even provide clues to the tumor type. However, MR will provide the best roadmap for the neurosurgeon to resect the tumor while preserving normal brain tissue; it will also have the greatest chance of detecting metastases elsewhere in the neuraxis. Some MR sequences can also detect ischemic injury hours earlier than CT.

Skull fractures & subarachnoid hemorrhages will not be as well detected by MR as NECT, which adds to the list of reasons that NECT serves the bulk of the need of neuroimaging in the acute patient. Unlike cortical bone, marrow imaging is best performed by MR.

There are many downsides to MR, however. It typically has one of the greatest financial costs of any modality. Additionally, it is one of the lengthiest imaging exams available. While any single imaging sequence ranges from 30 seconds to 5 minutes or more, a full MR exam of the brain is generally comprised of 5-10 different sequence types & anatomical planes, therefore requiring roughly 30-60 minutes for the full study (though this depends on the specific clinical concerns at hand, which generally drive the sequences performed).

Many young patients (particularly under 6 years of age) will not be able to remain still for such a length of time, therefore requiring sedation or general anesthesia. MR compatible video goggles are now used in many centers, making it possible to scan some young patients while awake. Additionally, neonates can often be scanned with a "bundle & feed" technique (by which they often fall asleep during the scan). However, many children will require anesthesia to successfully complete an MR exam. It should be noted that the medical literature has raised increasing concerns about the long-term neurodevelopmental effects of various anesthetic agents on the immature brain. While long-term human data has not yet been established, this has been clearly seen in animal models. It is of particular concern in the patients undergoing a single prolonged anesthetic event or multiple recurrent anesthetic events. Therefore, the risks & benefits of MR must be weighed against those of other modalities, especially CT.

Children with certain preexisting medical problems may have contraindications to being in the magnetic field. This includes most patients with cochlear implants, pacemakers, & vagal nerve stimulators, among other devices, though the exact device must be known to determine its MR compatibility. Patients with retained metallic fragments from prior injuries (such as BBs, other projectiles, & metallic shavings) may also be unable to undergo scanning. Depending on the type of device, the contained metal may be subject to heating or movement. Even surgically implanted metal that is known to be MR safe will result in significant artifacts in that region, which may limit some evaluations. Orthodontic hardware is common source of artifact on brain MR scans, particularly in the inferior frontal lobes & cerebellum; with advanced knowledge, techniques can be adjusted that will largely mitigate these issues.

Due to its length & safety/technical requirements, MR is usually not as readily available as other modalities & may require days to weeks to arrange, depending on a variety of factors.

IV contrast agents for MR are extremely well tolerated & only rarely result in allergic reactions. Unlike CT contrast agents, they are not nephrotoxic, though patients with severe renal failure may be prone to retention & deposition of the gadolinium, leading to the severe long-term cutaneous phenomenon of nephrogenic systemic fibrosis. Recently, concern has been raised about the deposition of dissociated gadolinium in the tissues (especially the brain) of normal patients undergoing numerous repeat exams. The long-term effects of this phenomenon are actively being studied, though it should be noted that certain MR contrast agents (macrocyclics) are much less prone to dissociate than others (linear agents), making such long-term deposition in patients with normal renal function unlikely.

Nuclear Medicine

Nuclear imaging is rarely employed for brain evaluations in children. Most commonly, pediatric nuclear medicine studies are used to search for a seizure focus in patients undergoing advanced epilepsy work-ups (which are usually driven by specialized neurologists). Therefore, nuclear imaging will not be discussed here.

Selected References

1. ACR Appropriateness Criteria: Headache—Child. https://acsearch.acr.org/docs/69439/Narrative/. Published 1999. Reviewed 2012. Accessed March 1, 2017
2. ACR Appropriateness Criteria: Head Trauma—Child. https://acsearch.acr.org/docs/3083021/Narrative/. Published 2014. Accessed March 1, 2017
3. ACR Appropriateness Criteria: Seizures—Child. https://acsearch.acr.org/docs/69441/Narrative/. Published 1995. Reviewed 2012. Accessed March 1, 2017
4. Culotta PA et al: Performance of computed tomography of the head to evaluate for skull fractures in infants with suspected non-accidental trauma. Pediatr Radiol. 47(1):74-81, 2017
5. Radbruch A et al: Pediatric Brain: No Increased Signal Intensity in the Dentate Nucleus on Unenhanced T1-weighted MR Images after Consecutive Exposure to a Macrocyclic Gadolinium-based Contrast Agent. Radiology. 162980, 2017
6. FDA Drug Safety Communication: FDA review results in new warnings about using general anesthetics and sedation drugs in young children and pregnant women
7. Runge VM: Safety of the Gadolinium-Based Contrast Agents for Magnetic Resonance Imaging, Focusing in Part on Their Accumulation in the Brain and Especially the Dentate Nucleus. Invest Radiol. 51(5):273-9, 2016
8. Langford S et al: Multiplanar reconstructed CT images increased depiction of intracranial hemorrhages in pediatric head trauma. Neuroradiology. 57(12):1263-8, 2015
9. Nardone B et al: Pediatric nephrogenic systemic fibrosis is rarely reported: a RADAR report. Pediatr Radiol. 44(2):173-80, 2014
10. Brody AS et al: Radiation risk to children from computed tomography. Pediatrics. 120(3):677-82, 2007

(Left) *Sagittal midline ultrasound of the brain in a term newborn demonstrates normal 3rd ➡️ & 4th ➡️ ventricles & a partially visualized corpus callosum ➡️.* **(Right)** *Coronal head ultrasound of the same newborn shows the corpus callosum ➡️, lateral ventricles ➡️, & cerebellar hemispheres ➡️. The wavy echogenic foci ➡️ in both images represent the normal brain sulcations.*

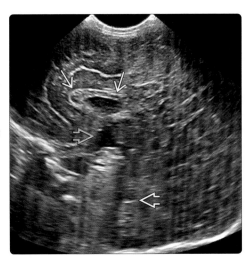
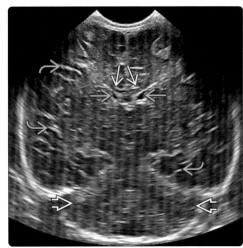

(Left) *Axial NECT in a term 4 day old who is difficult to arouse shows normal differentiation of the gray ➡️ & white ➡️ matter for age. The white matter is quite hypodense at this age due to increased water content. The venous sinuses are hyperdense ➡️ due to hemoconcentration. This overall appearance would not be normal beyond early infancy.* **(Right)** *Axial NECT in a 14 year old shows a normal pattern of gray-white matter differentiation beyond infancy. The venous sinuses ➡️ are also much less dense than in the newborn.*

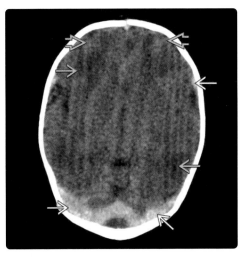
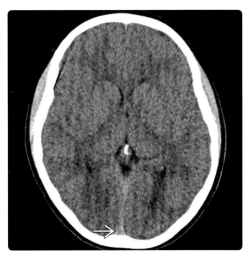

(Left) *Normal MR images from the same 14 year old show several types of sequences able to be obtained with MR, each providing different information. Clockwise from the top left are axial FLAIR, axial diffusion (DWI), coronal T1, & coronal T2.* **(Right)** *Axial perfusion MR image from an arterial spin labeled sequence in a child with left-sided weakness after aortic surgery shows decreased perfusion/blood volume in the right hemisphere ➡️. The DWI was normal, but the follow-up exam confirmed watershed ischemic injury.*

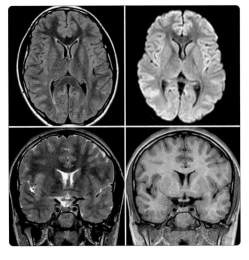
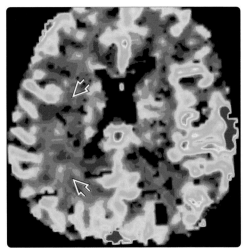

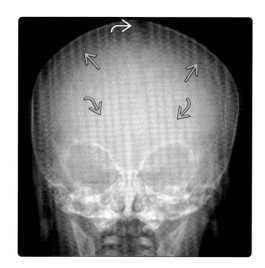

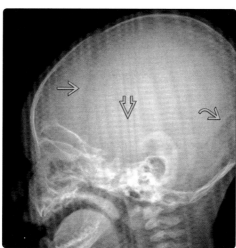

(Left) *AP radiograph in a 4 month old with suspected craniosynostosis shows normal sagittal ➚, coronal ➡, & lambdoid ➘ sutures.* (Right) *Lateral radiograph in the same patient shows normal coronal ➡, lambdoid ➘, & squamosal ➡ sutures.*

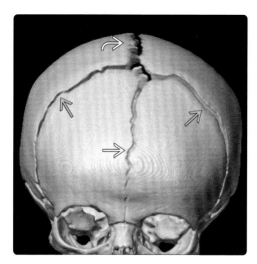

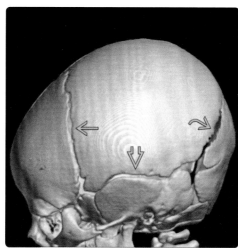

(Left) *Anterior 3D view of a bone CT in a 4 week old with suspected early fontanelle closure shows normal coronal ➡, sagittal ➚, & metopic ➡ sutures, the latter of which typically closes in the 1st few months of life. The anterior fontanelle is normal, as was the underlying brain.* (Right) *Lateral 3D view of a bone CT in the same patient shows normal coronal ➡, lambdoid ➘, & squamosal ➡ sutures. Additional normal sutures are seen near the skull base.*

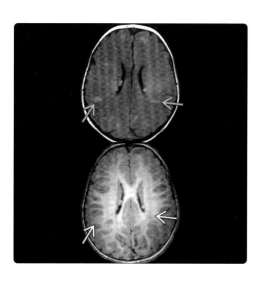

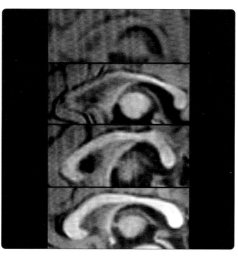

(Left) *Axial T1 MR images in a patient with tuberous sclerosis at 3 months (top) & 10 months (bottom) of age show that, prior to significant myelination, the cortical tubers & radial migration lines are hyperintense ➡. Following myelination, these lesions show varying degrees of hypointensity ➡ compared to the adjacent white matter.* (Right) *Sagittal T1 MR images at 2, 4, 7, & 10 months of age (top to bottom, respectively) show normal progressive myelination & thickening of the corpus callosum during the 1st year of life.*

Enlarged Subarachnoid Spaces

TERMINOLOGY

- Idiopathic enlargement of subarachnoid spaces (SAS) during infancy causing macrocrania [head circumference (HC) > 95%]
  - Likely due to immature CSF drainage pathways
- Synonyms: Benign macrocrania of infancy, benign external hydrocephalus

IMAGING

- Primary imaging modality: US
  - CT/MR used if fontanelle closing or to further investigate atypical clinical/US findings
- Best clue: Enlarged SAS & ↑ HC
  - Symmetric bifrontal & bitemporal SAS
  - Ventricles may be mildly enlarged
- All modalities show veins coursing through SAS
- SAS follow CSF appearance on all modalities
- No inward displacement of arachnoid membrane to suggest subdural collection
- Small nonhemorrhagic subdural collections seen in ~ 4% of patients with enlarged SAS

TOP DIFFERENTIAL DIAGNOSES

- Cerebral atrophy, acquired progressive communicating hydrocephalus, nonaccidental trauma (NAT)

CLINICAL ISSUES

- Family history of macrocephaly > 80%
- Mild developmental delay common & should not prompt further imaging or subspecialty evaluation
  - Further evaluation required only in setting of focal neurologic signs, developmental regression, or rapid deviation of HC from normal curve
  - SAS enlargement & mild developmental delay typically resolve without therapy by 2 years of age
- Consider NAT if enlarged extraaxial spaces atypical
  - Any subdural fluid that is not tiny & simple

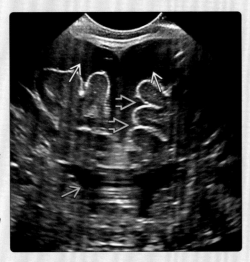

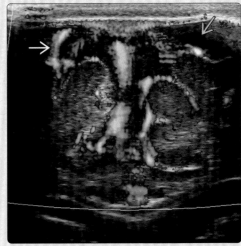

(Left) Coronal US of the head in a 7-month-old boy with macrocrania shows enlarged subarachnoid spaces (SAS) ➡ & normal ventricular size ➡. Note the normal size of the sulci ➡. This is a typical clinical history & imaging appearance for benign enlargement of the SAS. (Right) Coronal color Doppler US in a 4-month-old girl shows vessels ➡ traversing the enlarged SAS ➡. Doppler US can be helpful to exclude subdural collections by demonstrating normal veins in the SAS.

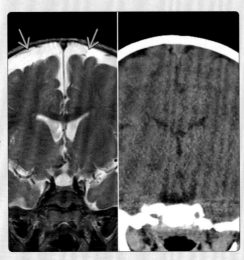

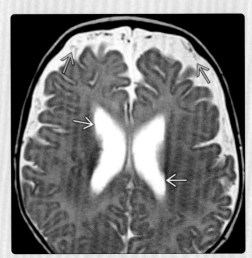

(Left) Coronal T2 MR at 13 months (left) & NECT at 5 years (right) of age show expected resolution of the enlarged SAS ➡ over a 4-year period. Enlarged SAS typically resolve by 24 months of age. (Right) Axial T2 MR in a 6-month-old boy with enlarged SAS shows vessels ➡ coursing through the SAS. Note the lack of mass effect on the underlying brain parenchyma. There is mild enlargement of the lateral ventricles ➡, a common finding in benign enlargement of the SAS.

KEY FACTS

TERMINOLOGY

- Clinically & radiologically heterogeneous group of posterior fossa (PF) malformations: Classic Dandy-Walker malformation (DWM); vermian hypoplasia (VH); Blake pouch cyst (BPC); mega cisterna magna (MCM)
  - Severe to mild: Classic DWM → VH → BPC → MCM

IMAGING

- MR best characterizes severity & associated anomalies
  - DWM: Small or absent cerebellar vermis with 4th ventricle cystic dilation causing enlarged posterior fossa; ± hydrocephalus
  - VH: Degree of hypoplasia variable; ± superior rotation of vermian tissue without PF enlargement
  - BPC: Intact vermis with mild rotation; cyst wall often not seen by imaging
  - MCM: Enlarged CSF cistern posteriorly with intact cerebellum but no rotation

TOP DIFFERENTIAL DIAGNOSES

- PF arachnoid cyst
- Cerebellar hypoplasia

CLINICAL ISSUES

- Age of diagnosis depends on degree of hydrocephalus, supratentorial anomalies, & cerebellar dysfunction
- Marked heterogeneity in clinical findings, even in families with same genetic mutations
  - Motor developmental delay, spastic paraplegia, seizures, variable intellectual disability, hearing &/or visual difficulties, systemic abnormalities
  - Classic DWM: Poor prognosis overall with cognitive abnormalities in 40%-50%
  - ± normal neurodevelopment in isolated VH, BPC, MCM (but may be associated with other anomalies)
- Treatment: CSF diversion (ventriculoperitoneal shunt ± cyst shunt or marsupialization)

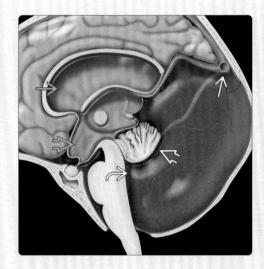

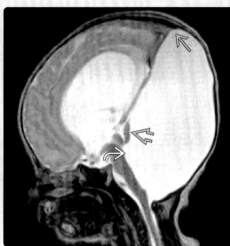

(Left) Graphic of a classic Dandy-Walker malformation (DWM) shows an enlarged posterior fossa, elevated venous sinus confluence ➡, superior rotation of a hypoplastic cerebellar vermis ➡, & posterior expansion of the 4th ventricle ➡. Lateral ➡ & 3rd ➡ ventriculomegaly is shown. (Right) Sagittal T2 MR of a classic DWM in a newborn shows that the venous confluence ➡ is markedly elevated. The vermis ➡ is extremely hypoplastic & rotated. The 4th ventricle ➡ communicates with a large posterior fossa cyst.

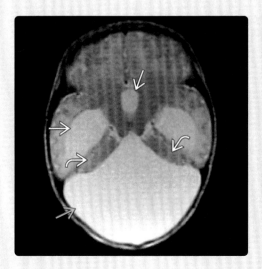

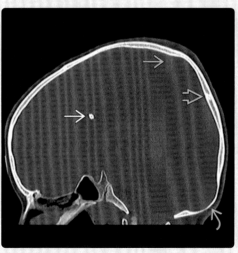

(Left) Axial T2 MR in the same patient with a classic DWM shows hypoplastic cerebellar hemispheres ➡ splayed by the large posterior fossa cyst ➡. The cyst communicates with the 4th ventricle. Note the ventriculomegaly ➡. (Right) Sagittal bone CT of the same patient with a classic DWM at age 7 years (after ventricular shunting ➡) shows that the venous confluence ➡ lies above the lambdoid suture ➡ (torcular-lambdoid inversion). There is remodeling of the occipital bone with scalloping & expansion ➡.

IMAGING

- Pointed cerebellar tonsils extending ≥ 5 mm below foramen magnum with effacement of CSF spaces
- ± syringohydromyelia &/or scoliosis
- Best tool: Head NECT may be performed acutely but MR provides best detail of posterior fossa & cervical spinal cord

TOP DIFFERENTIAL DIAGNOSES

- Normal low-lying cerebellar tonsils
- Chiari 2 malformation
- Tonsillar herniation from increased intracranial pressure
- Intracranial hypotension

PATHOLOGY

- Most common cause believed to be small/underdeveloped posterior fossa; no association with myelomeningocele
- Can be result of premature closure of sutures
  - Causes include shunted infantile hydrocephalus, bone dysplasias, genetic syndromes

CLINICAL ISSUES

- Most common presenting symptom: Occipital headache
  - Induced by cough, Valsalva, or physical exertion
  - Less common: Cranial nerve palsy, ocular disturbances, otoneurologic dysfunction; vertigo, dysphagia, apnea, syncope, rarely sudden death; cord motor/sensory presentations (gait disturbance, neuropathic joint)
  - Up to 30% of patients asymptomatic
    - Degree of tonsillar descent does not always correlate with symptoms: Chiari 1 frequently picked up incidentally
- Goal of surgery in symptomatic patients: Restore normal CSF flow at foramen magnum
  - Posterior fossa (suboccipital) decompression, resection of C1 posterior arch ± duraplasty, cerebellar tonsil cautery
  - Postoperative complications in up to 41% of patients: CSF leak, pseudomeningocele, infection

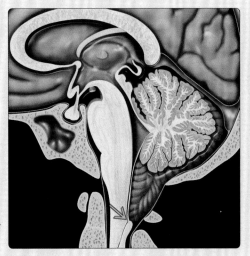
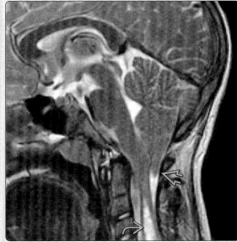

(Left) Sagittal midline graphic demonstrates pointed cerebellar tonsils extending below the foramen magnum to the inferior aspect of the C1 posterior arch. The obex ⊡ is inferiorly displaced as well. (Right) Sagittal T2 MR from a 10-year-old patient demonstrates pointed cerebellar tonsils extending below the foramen magnum to the lower C1 level ⊡, typical of a Chiari 1 malformation. The CSF is largely effaced at the craniocervical junction, & a syrinx ⊡ is seen in the cervical spinal cord.

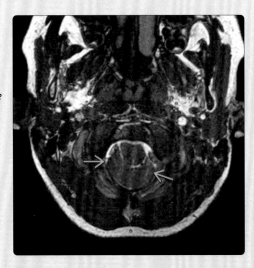
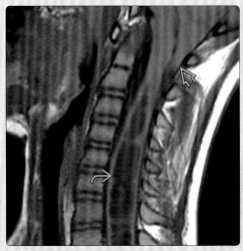

(Left) Axial SSFP MR through the foramen magnum in the same patient shows crowding & effacement of the CSF spaces by the low cerebellar tonsils ⊡. (Right) Sagittal T1 MR of the cervical spine in the same patient further demonstrates the cerebellar tonsillar ectopia ⊡ & large cervicothoracic spinal cord syrinx ⊡.

TERMINOLOGY

Definitions

- Compressed & pointed cerebellar tonsils extending below foramen magnum with effacement of CSF spaces

IMAGING

MR Findings

- T1WI, T2WI, FLAIR
  - Pointed (not rounded) cerebellar tonsils extending ≥ 5 mm below foramen magnum
  - Crowded foramen magnum with small/effaced cisterns ± brainstem compression
  - ± small posterior fossa, elongated 4th ventricle
  - ± syringohydromyelia/syrinx, scoliosis
    - Syrinx reported in 30-70% of cases
    - Patients with syrinx more likely to have scoliotic curve > 20° (~ 70%) than those without syrinx (~ 45%)
- MR cine
  - Restricted CSF flow through foramen magnum ± ↑ brainstem/cerebellar tonsil motion (pistoning)
    - Clinical utility of this sequence debatable

CT Findings

- Crowding of foramen magnum on axial NECT images can mimic cord expansion by tumor
  - Sagittal reconstructions helpful
- Most inferior head CT image may show top of syrinx

Imaging Recommendations

- Best imaging tool
  - Multiplanar brain MR
  - Spine imaging to look for spinal cord syrinx
    - Syrinx makes surgical intervention more likely

DIFFERENTIAL DIAGNOSIS

Normal Variation of Cerebellar Tonsil Position

- Tonsils may normally lie below foramen magnum
  - May be accentuated by certain head positions
- Tonsils retain normal rounded configuration

Chiari 2 Malformation

- Numerous intracranial findings centered around very small posterior fossa with hindbrain herniation
- Almost always occurs in setting of myelomeningocele

Tonsillar Herniation From Increased Intracranial Pressure

- Neoplasm, hemorrhage, hydrocephalus, ischemia

Intracranial Hypotension

- Sagging midbrain + sunken hindbrain with diffuse dural thickening/enhancement, distended veins/dural sinuses, ± subdural hygromas

PATHOLOGY

General Features

- Etiology
  - Primary congenital malformation vs. secondarily acquired morphologic changes

- Primary: Posterior fossa underdevelopment theory most common
    - Not all Chiari 1 patients have small posterior fossa
  - Secondary: Premature closure of cranial sutures &/or generalized abnormal bone formation

CLINICAL ISSUES

Presentation

- Most common signs/symptoms
  - Occipital headache
    - Induced by cough, Valsalva, or physical exertion
  - Less common: Bulbar, cranial nerve, cord motor/sensory presentations
    - Bulbar symptoms: Vertigo, diplopia, dysphagia, apnea, syncope, sudden death (rare)
    - Cranial nerve palsy, ocular disturbances, otoneurologic dysfunction
    - Cord motor or sensory symptoms, gait disturbance, neuropathic joint
  - 15-30% of adults asymptomatic

Demographics

- Epidemiology: 0.5-3.5% of general population
- Age: Evenly distributed in adult & pediatric patients
  - 3% of children & 1% of adults have imaging findings of Chiari 1 malformation, though age of clinical presentation unclear

Natural History & Prognosis

- Natural history not clearly understood
  - Many patients asymptomatic for prolonged periods
  - Increasing ectopia + time → ↑ likelihood of symptoms
- Children respond better to treatment than adults
- Patients selected for nonsurgical management usually have benign course, though spontaneous improvement & worsening have been described

Treatment

- Posterior fossa decompression: Suboccipital craniectomy with C1 laminectomy ± duraplasty, arachnoid opening/dissection, cerebellar tonsil cautery/resection
- Scoliosis may improve from decompression alone but often requires bracing or additional surgery
- Postoperative complications in up to 41% of patients
  - Most common: CSF leak, pseudomeningocele, infection

DIAGNOSTIC CHECKLIST

Consider

- Degree of tonsillar descent does not always correlate with symptoms: Chiari 1 frequently picked up incidentally
  - High likelihood of symptoms if tonsils > 12 mm below foramen magnum

SELECTED REFERENCES

1. Arnautovic A et al: Pediatric and adult Chiari malformation type I surgical series 1965-2013: a review of demographics, operative treatment, and outcomes. J Neurosurg Pediatr. 15(2):161-77, 2015
2. Brockmeyer DL et al: Complex Chiari malformations in children: diagnosis and management. Neurosurg Clin N Am. 26(4):555-60, 2015
3. Leonard JR et al: Chiari I malformation: adult and pediatric considerations. Neurosurg Clin N Am. 26(4):xiii-xiv, 2015

TERMINOLOGY

- Constellation of intracranial findings, mainly hindbrain herniation, due to open spinal dysraphism of myelomeningocele (MMC) or myelocele/myeloschisis

IMAGING

- Prenatal US: Characteristic skull/brain findings (lemon & banana signs) seen as early as 12 weeks
- Postnatal head US: Used to follow change in ventricular size to know if CSF shunt required
- Postnatal MR/CT
  - Small posterior fossa with cerebellum herniating downward through foramen magnum & upward through incisura
    - Elongated, effaced, inferiorly displaced 4th ventricle
    - Cerebellar hemispheres partially wrap around brainstem
  - Caudal brainstem herniation with cervicomedullary kink, corpus callosum dysgenesis, ↓ white matter volume

- ± ventriculomegaly: Occurs in utero or after MMC repair
- ± subependymal gray matter heterotopias, polymicrogyria

PATHOLOGY

- Sequelae of chronic in utero CSF leakage through open spinal dysraphism (4th fetal week)
- Maternal folic acid supplementation during periconceptional period significantly lowers risk

CLINICAL ISSUES

- Lower extremity paresis & spasticity, bowel & bladder dysfunction, symptoms of brainstem compression (swallowing difficulties, stridor, apnea), epilepsy
- MMC classically repaired in first 48 hours after delivery
  - Early intervention required to reduce risk of infection
  - CSF diversion/shunting required in 80-90%
- Prenatal MMC repair in select patients
  - Reduces need for shunting; may improve neurologic outcomes in some patients

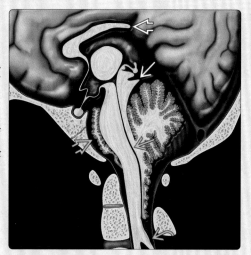

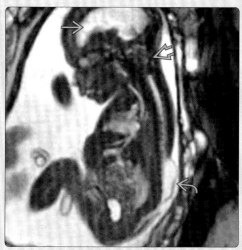

(Left) Sagittal graphic shows characteristic findings of the Chiari 2 malformation (CM2), including caudal displacement of the cerebellum & brainstem, elongation of the 4th ventricle ➡, anterior wrapping of the brainstem by the cerebellum ➡, tectal beaking ➡, cervicomedullary kinking ➡, & callosal dysgenesis ➡. (Right) Sagittal SSFP MR of a 22-week gestation fetus shows a lumbar myelomeningocele (MMC) ➡ with a CM2, including a small posterior fossa with cerebellar herniation ➡ & ventriculomegaly ➡.

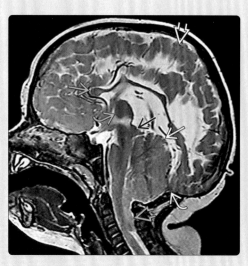

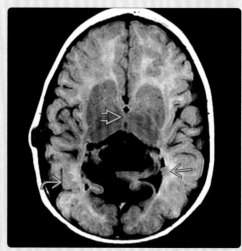

(Left) Sagittal T2 MR in the same patient at 8 months of age after postnatal MMC repair & CSF shunting shows multiple findings of CM2, including cerebellar herniation ➡, a towering cerebellum ➡, tectal beaking ➡, a low torcular Herophili ➡, an enlarged massa intermedia ➡, callosal dysgenesis ➡, & stenogyria (narrow, compacted gyri) ➡. (Right) Axial T1 MR in the same patient demonstrates a thickened massa intermedia ➡, polymicrogyria ➡, & subependymal gray matter heterotopia ➡.

IMAGING

- Nonenhancing T2/FLAIR MR hyperintense lesions
  - 60-85% of children with neurofibromatosis type 1 (NF1)
  - Globus pallidus, cerebellar white matter (WM) typical
  - Little/no mass effect, no enhancement
  - Higher lesion burden may ↓ cognitive functioning
  - ↓ with puberty, resolved by adulthood
- Optic pathway gliomas (OPG)
  - 15-20% of children with NF1
  - Fusiform to lobular in shape, ± contrast enhancement
- Plexiform neurofibromas
  - Lobular infiltrating soft tissue masses
  - Target appearance in cross section on T2/STIR MR
- Vascular dysplasia (moyamoya arteriopathy)
  - 3-7% of children with NF1; ↑ stroke risk
  - Vessel narrowing (especially distal ICA) with collaterals
- Associated tumors: Pheochromocytomas, malignant peripheral nerve sheath tumors

PATHOLOGY

- *NF1* gene locus → long arm of chromosome 17
  - Gene product → neurofibromin (inactivated in NF1)
  - Autosomal dominant; 50% new mutations
  - Variable expression, virtually 100% penetrance

CLINICAL ISSUES

- 1:3,000-5,000 people have NF1
- Phenotype quite variable: Can be dominated by peripheral, paraspinal, or intracranial lesions
  - > 95% have skin lesions (café au lait spots)
  - ~ 50% have macrocephaly → ↑ WM volume
  - ~ 30-60% have learning disability
  - ~ 15% have visual pathway gliomas
  - ~ 15% have scoliosis
- OPG & brainstem gliomas have more indolent behavior in NF1 compared to non-NF1 patients
  - OPG typically not progressive; treatment in ~ 15%

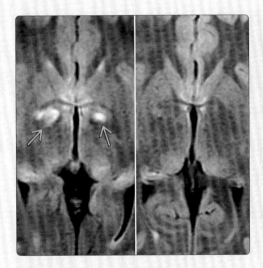

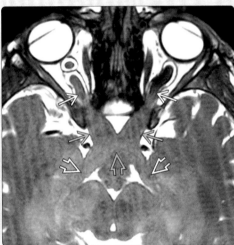

(Left) *Axial FLAIR MR images in a patient with neurofibromatosis type 1 (NF1) at 10 years (left) & 15 years (right) of age show near complete resolution of the characteristic nonenhancing signal abnormalities* ➡ *within the globus pallidus nuclei. It is typical for such lesions to resolve in the late teenage years.* (Right) *Axial MIP of a CISS MR in a 3-year-old girl with NF1 shows enlargement & tortuosity of the orbital* ➡ *& prechiasmatic* ➡ *optic nerves, optic chiasm* ➡, *& optic tracts* ➡, *consistent with an optic pathway glioma.*

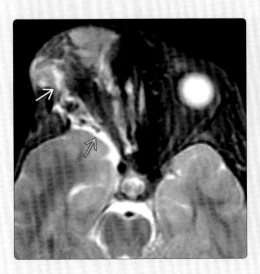

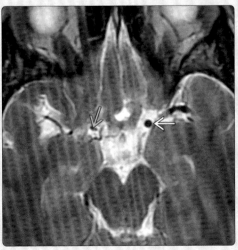

(Left) *Axial T2 FS MR in a 12-year-old girl with NF1 shows a large hyperintense lesion* ➡ *in the right orbit, consistent with a plexiform neurofibroma (PFN). Note the absence of the greater sphenoid wing* ➡, *consistent with sphenoid wing dysplasia. Such osseous changes in the sphenoid occur almost exclusively in the setting of a PFN.* (Right) *Axial T2 MR in a 13-year-old girl with NF1 shows absence of the right carotid terminus* ➡ *(as compared to the left* ➡*) with a few collateral vessels noted, consistent with a moyamoya arteriopathy.*

TERMINOLOGY

- Hamartomas of multiple organs: Central nervous system, skin, kidney, bone

IMAGING

- Cerebral tubers: Cortical/subcortical lesions expanding overlying gyri
- Cerebellar tubers: Wedge-shaped foci of volume loss
  - Often enhance & calcify
- Subependymal nodules (SENs): Elongated nodules in locations of fetal germinal matrix
  - Increasing Ca^{2+} over time
  - 30-80% enhance
- Subependymal giant cell astrocytoma (SEGA): Growing nodule at caudothalamic groove
  - WHO grade I neoplasm

PATHOLOGY

- Criteria: 2 major (definite) or 1 major + 1 minor (probable)

- Major: Tuber, SEN, SEGA, cardiac rhabdomyoma, renal angiomyolipoma, lymphangioleiomyomatosis, adenoma sebaceum, sub-/periungual fibroma, hypomelanotic macules (ash leaf spots), shagreen patch, retinal hamartoma
- Minor: White matter lesions, dental pits, gingival fibromas, rectal polyps, bone cysts, nonrenal hamartoma, retinal achromic patch, confetti skin lesions, multiple renal cysts

CLINICAL ISSUES

- Classic clinical triad: Adenoma sebaceum, seizures, mental retardation; seen in only 30-40%
- Ash leaf spots may be only sign of tuberous sclerosis at birth
- Treatments: Antiseizure medicines, resection of seizure focus; mTOR inhibitors now 1st-line therapy for SEGA
- Prognosis depends on severity of symptoms (seizures, arrhythmias, renal insufficiency) & success of treatment

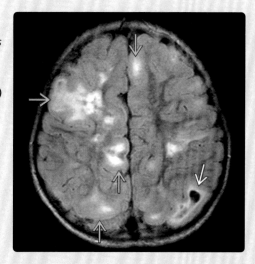
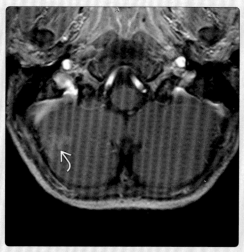

(Left) Axial FLAIR MR of a 3-year-old boy with tuberous sclerosis complex (TSC) shows a moderate to severe burden of cerebral tubers ➡. Cystic change is seen in a left parietal lobe tuber ➡. (Right) Axial T1 C+ MR in the same patient shows a wedge-shaped, enhancing right cerebellar tuber ➡.

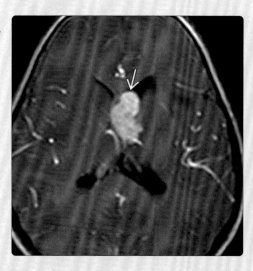
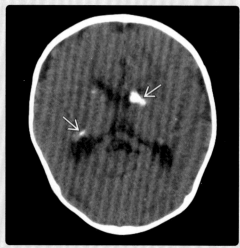

(Left) Axial T1 C+ MR in a 4-year-old girl with TSC shows a lobular, homogeneously enhancing mass ➡ in the left caudothalamic groove, consistent with a subependymal giant cell astrocytoma. (Right) Axial NECT in a 23-month-old girl with TSC shows multiple calcified subependymal nodules ➡. Note that the location of the nodules adheres to the distribution of fetal germinal matrix.

Sturge-Weber Syndrome

KEY FACTS

TERMINOLOGY

- Syndrome of abnormal cortical venous development
- Imaging features result from progressive venous occlusion, recruitment of alternate drainage pathways, & chronic venous ischemia

IMAGING

- NECT: Gyral/subcortical Ca^{2+} (± tram-track appearance)
  - ± calvarial thickening & sinus hyperpneumatization
- MR: Regions of atrophy ± abnormal myelination
  - T2WI: Flow voids in enlarged deep/transcerebral veins
  - FLAIR: Atrophied lobe(s) ± bright sulcal signal of leptomeningeal angiomatosis
  - T1WI C+: Enhancing leptomeningeal angiomatosis
    - Abundant medullary & deep draining veins
    - Choroidal globe enhancement of angioma
  - MRV: Absent normal cortical veins in affected region
- FDG-PET: Progressive ↓ metabolism in affected brain

CLINICAL ISSUES

- Forehead cutaneous capillary malformation (port-wine stain) in ~ 95%: V1 distribution classic
- Seizures (75-90%), hemiparesis (30-66%)
  - Seizures typically develop in 1st year of life
  - Holohemispheric or bilateral angiomatosis (10-20%) worse than focal involvement
- Choroidal angioma in 70% → glaucoma
- Stroke-like episodes, neurological deficit, headaches, & intellectual disability
- Treatment: Aggressive seizure control, resection/hemispherectomy for intractable epilepsy
  - ± aspirin (prior to symptom onset)

DIAGNOSTIC CHECKLIST

- MR in early infancy may be normal: Recommend follow-up if patient at risk for Sturge-Weber syndrome clinically

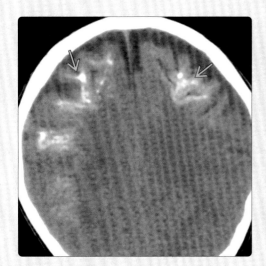

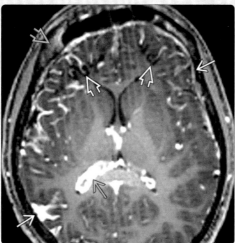

(Left) Axial NECT in an 11-year-old girl with intractable epilepsy shows bilateral (right > left) subcortical Ca^{2+} ➡, characteristic of Sturge-Weber syndrome. (Right) Axial T1 C+ FS MR in the same patient shows bilateral leptomeningeal enhancement ➡ & enlargement of the right choroid plexus ➡. Note the low signal within the subcortical white matter at the depth of sulci ➡, consistent with Ca^{2+}. There is mildly increased right calvarial thickness ➡ secondary to underlying brain parenchymal volume loss.

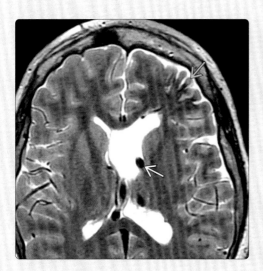

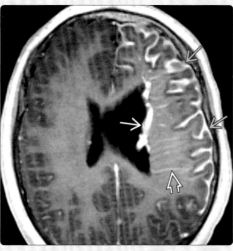

(Left) Axial T2 MR in a 10-year-old boy with right-sided hemiplegia & seizures shows marked parenchymal volume loss & low signal ➡ corresponding to an area of cortical/subcortical Ca^{2+} seen on CT. Also note the ipsilateral enlarged deep draining vein ➡. (Right) Axial T1 C+ MR in the same patient shows extensive left cerebral leptomeningeal enhancement ➡ with multiple prominent medullary veins ➡ & a large subependymal draining vein ➡. Enlargement of the left lateral ventricle is secondary to left cerebral volume loss.

KEY FACTS

TERMINOLOGY

- Arachnoid cyst (AC): Focal extraaxial CSF collection lined by arachnoid; generally lacks free communication with ventricles or subarachnoid space

IMAGING

- Displaces adjacent vessels & nerves
- Typically shows less mass effect than expected
  - Adjacent brain accommodates cyst
- Calvarial remodeling: Thinning/scalloping ± bulging
- US: Anechoic; no internal vascularity; only useful in young infant with open fontanelle
- NECT: Isodense to CSF, unless hemorrhage occurs (rare)
- MR: Follows CSF signal intensity on all sequences
- Locations: Middle cranial fossa (50-70%); retrocerebellar (15-20%); cerebral convexities or interhemispheric fissure (5-10%); cerebellopontine angle (5-10%); quadrigeminal plate (1-5%); suprasellar (1-5%)

TOP DIFFERENTIAL DIAGNOSES

- Epidermoid cyst
- Chronic subdural hematoma
- Subdural hygroma
- Mega cisterna magna

PATHOLOGY

- Wall consists of flattened but normal arachnoid cells
  - No inflammation or neoplastic changes

CLINICAL ISSUES

- Asymptomatic in vast majority (typically found incidentally)
- Symptoms vary with size & location of cyst
  - Headache, dizziness, sensorineural hearing loss, hemifacial spasm/tic
- More likely to grow in younger patients (< 4 years of age)
- Surgery only indicated if symptoms directly attributable to AC & potential benefits outweigh risks

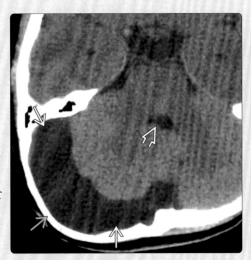
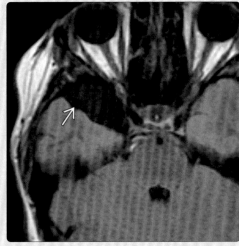

(Left) Axial NECT in a 6-year-old boy shows a right retrocerebellar cystic collection ➡. Note the characteristic imaging features of an arachnoid cyst (AC): Isoattenuating to CSF, bulging & thinning of the overlying calvaria ➡, & relatively mild mass effect on the 4th ventricle ➡. (Right) Axial FLAIR MR in a 14-year-old girl with headaches shows fluid signal suppression within a right middle cranial fossa AC ➡. This is the most common location of ACs.

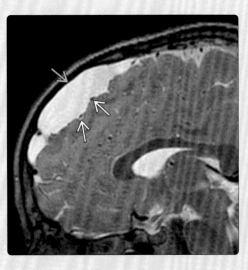
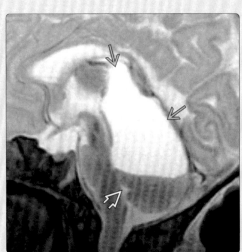

(Left) Sagittal T2 MR in a 9-year-old boy with a right frontal AC shows displacement of vessels ➡ & cortex with scalloping of the calvaria ➡. The relative lack of mass effect despite the size of the lesion is characteristic of an AC. (Right) Sagittal T2 MR in a newborn boy shows a large cyst ➡ in the quadrigeminal cistern with moderate mass effect on the brainstem, 4th ventricle ➡, & cerebellum. While most ACs are incidental, larger cysts in the basilar cisterns can cause significant mass effect & symptoms.

Pilocytic Astrocytoma

KEY FACTS

TERMINOLOGY

- (Juvenile) pilocytic astrocytoma (PA)
  - WHO grade I astrocytic tumor
  - Most common primary brain tumor of children
  - Most common posterior fossa tumor in ages 5-19 years

IMAGING

- Location
  - Without neurofibromatosis type 1 (NF1): Cerebellum (midline or off-midline) > hypothalamus, brainstem, cerebral hemispheres > optic pathway (OP)
  - With NF1: OP most common
- Size: Cerebellar & cerebral lesions often > 5 cm
- > 95% enhance (patterns vary)
  - Nonenhancing cyst with enhancing mural nodule: 50%
  - Heterogeneous enhancement with smaller cysts: 40%
  - Solid, (typically) avid enhancement: 10%
- May show little surrounding vasogenic edema
- Often cause obstructive hydrocephalus

- ↑ diffusivity typical (unlike highly cellular tumors)

TOP DIFFERENTIAL DIAGNOSES

- Posterior fossa: Medulloblastoma, ependymoma
- Hypothalamus/OP: Pilomyxoid astrocytoma, optic neuritis

PATHOLOGY

- Sporadic > syndromic
  - 15% of NF1 patients develop PAs: OP > brainstem
    - 50-60% of patients with OP PAs have NF1

CLINICAL ISSUES

- Location determines presentation, treatment, prognosis
  - ↑ intracranial pressure: Headaches, nausea, vomiting
  - Cerebellar lesions: Ataxia, dysdiadokinesia
  - OP lesions: Visual loss
- Cerebellar & cerebral lesions cured with total resection; OP lesions (especially NF1) may be observed for growth or visual loss prior to chemotherapy or radiation
- 10-year survival > 90%

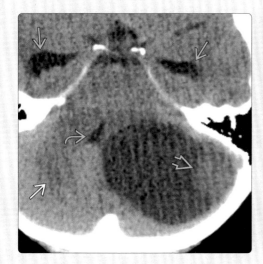

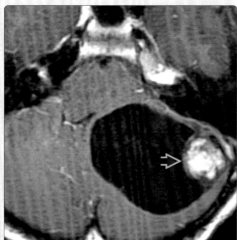

(Left) Axial NECT in a 10-year-old boy with a pilocytic astrocytoma (PA) demonstrates a left cerebellar cystic mass with a solid mural nodule ⇒ that is isoattenuating to the adjacent white matter ➡. Note the mass effect on the 4th ventricle ⇨ with upstream dilation of the lateral ventricle temporal horns ⇨, consistent with obstructive hydrocephalus. (Right) Axial T1 C+ MR in the same patient shows moderate enhancement of the solid nodule ⇨. No cyst wall enhancement is seen.

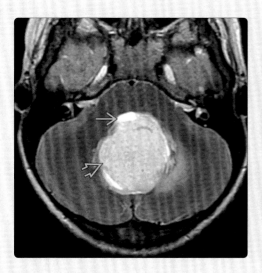

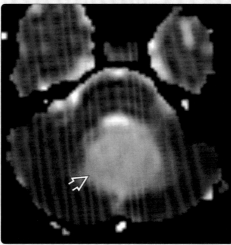

(Left) Axial T2 MR in a 9-year-old girl with headaches shows a solid-appearing midline mass ⇨ with increased signal intensity that is slightly lower than cerebrospinal fluid ⇨, typical for PA. (Right) Axial ADC map MR in the same patient shows signal intensity in the mass ⇨ that is much greater than the adjacent brain parenchyma. This increased diffusivity is typical of a PA. Diffusion characteristics can be helpful in distinguishing PA from medulloblastoma, especially with midline tumors extending into the 4th ventricle.

Medulloblastoma

TERMINOLOGY

- Malignant (WHO grade IV), invasive, highly cellular embryonal tumor

IMAGING

- Round midline 4th ventricular mass
- Obstructive hydrocephalus in 95%
- NECT: 90% hyperattenuating (due to ↑ cellularity)
- NECT: Ca^{2+} in up to 20%; hemorrhage rare
- MR: Restricted diffusion reflects ↑ cellularity
- Contrast & total spine MR to detect spread
  - 33% have subarachnoid metastatic disease at diagnosis
  - 5% develop bone metastases, usually sclerotic

TOP DIFFERENTIAL DIAGNOSES

- Atypical teratoid/rhabdoid tumor
- Ependymoma
- Pilocytic astrocytoma

PATHOLOGY

- Associated with many familial cancer syndromes
- Newly defined molecular subgroups affect prognosis; histology still valuable in treatment decisions

CLINICAL ISSUES

- 15-20% of all pediatric brain tumors
- 75% < 10 years of age
  - Most common posterior fossa tumor in ages 0-4 years
- Presents with ataxia, signs of ↑ intracranial pressure
- Treated with surgical excision, adjuvant chemotherapy
  - Craniospinal irradiation if > 3 years of age
- 5-year survival rate
  - No metastases or gross residual tumor status post resection: 60-100%
  - Presence of gross residual tumor after surgery or metastatic disease: 20%

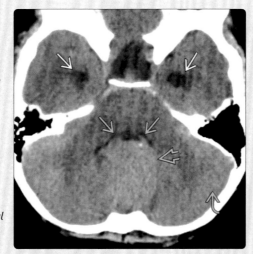

(Left) Axial NECT in a 14 year old with Rubenstein-Taybi syndrome demonstrates a midline posterior fossa mass ⇒ effacing the 4th ventricle ⇒ from posterior to anterior. The mass is similar in attenuation to gray matter ⇒. The enlarged temporal horns ⇒ are due to obstructive hydrocephalus. (Right) Sagittal T1 C+ MR in the same patient shows mild patchy enhancement of the mass ⇒. Note the indistinct interface with the posterior 4th ventricle (roof) ⇒, typical of medulloblastoma.

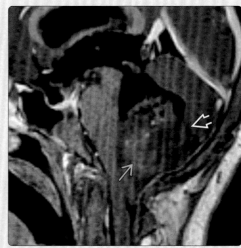

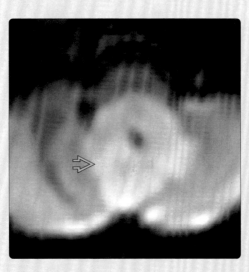

(Left) Axial DWI MR in the same patient shows increased signal intensity of the mass ⇒. The ADC map (not shown) demonstrated decreased signal intensity, consistent with restricted diffusion & reflecting high tumor cellularity. DWI is a key discriminator of posterior fossa tumors. (Right) Axial DWI MR in a 13 year old with medulloblastoma status post gross total resection 3 years ago shows CSF dissemination of recurrent tumor ⇒ along the ependymal lining of the lateral ventricles.

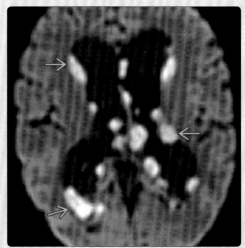

Ependymoma

TERMINOLOGY

- Slow-growing tumor resembling ependymal cells

IMAGING

- 1/3 supratentorial: Periventricular white matter
- 2/3 infratentorial: 4th ventricle/cisterns
- Soft or plastic tumor: Conforms to ventricle & extends through foramina into cisterns
- Variable heterogeneous enhancement
- 3-17% have CSF dissemination
- Requires combination of imaging & clinical findings to distinguish from medulloblastoma

TOP DIFFERENTIAL DIAGNOSES

- Infratentorial: Medulloblastoma, pilocytic astrocytoma, choroid plexus papilloma
- Supratentorial: Numerous glial, neuronal, & mixed neoplasms

PATHOLOGY

- Classic ependymoma: WHO grade II
- Supratentorial, posterior fossa, & spinal ependymomas histologically similar but genetically distinct
- 2 molecular subgroups of posterior fossa ependymoma
  - Group A: Younger children with poorer prognosis
  - Group B: Often older children with better prognosis

CLINICAL ISSUES

- 3rd most common posterior fossa tumor in children (15%)
- Peaks at 1-5 years of age
- Presents with headache, nausea, vomiting, ataxia, hemiparesis, visual disturbances, neck pain, torticollis, dizziness, irritability, lethargy, developmental delay, &/or macrocephaly
- Treatment: Surgical resection ± chemo, radiation therapy
  - Extent of resection strongly correlates with outcome
- Overall 5-year survival for brain lesions: 50-70%
  - 5-year survival after recurrence: 15%

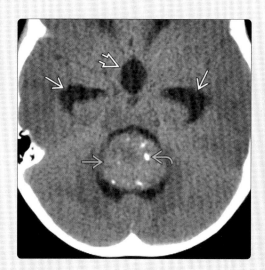
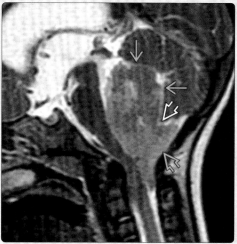

(Left) *Axial NECT in a 2-year-old girl shows a mass* ➡ *in the 4th ventricle containing scattered small Ca²⁺* ➡. *Note the enlargement of the temporal horns* ➡ *& 3rd ventricle* ➡, *consistent with obstructive hydrocephalus.* (Right) *Midline sagittal T2 MR in the same patient demonstrates the mass expanding the 4th ventricle* ➡ *(displacing the cerebellum & brainstem) & extending through the foramen of Magendie* ➡ *into the cisterna magna* ➡.

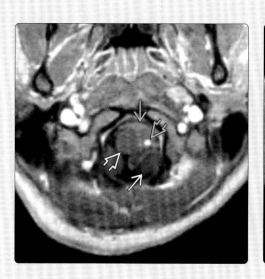
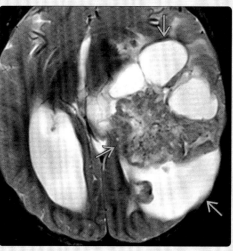

(Left) *Axial T1 C+ MR in a 17-year-old girl demonstrates a lesion* ➡ *in the left cerebellomedullary cistern. The mass encases the enhancing left vertebral artery* ➡ *without narrowing it, further demonstrating its plastic nature as it extends between the left cerebellar tonsil* ➡ *& brainstem* ➡. (Right) *Axial T2 FS MR in a 2-year-old patient demonstrates a large mixed cystic & solid mass* ➡. *The large size, heterogeneous solid component, & cysts are typical of a supratentorial ependymoma.*

TERMINOLOGY

- Brainstem tumors (BST) distinguished by location, imaging appearance, & histology

IMAGING

- Diffuse intrinsic pontine glioma (DIPG): Expansile tumor centered in pons, effacing CSF cisterns & 4th ventricle; often encases basilar artery
- Pilocytic astrocytoma (PA): Exophytic enhancing tumor anywhere in brainstem
- Tectal plate glioma: Nonenhancing lesion in tectum
- Midbrain tumors: Heterogeneous group

TOP DIFFERENTIAL DIAGNOSES

- Brainstem abscess
- Demyelination
- Cavernous malformation

PATHOLOGY

- DIPG: Astrocytomas of varying grade (WHO II-IV)

- o Diagnosis often made solely on imaging
- o ↑ molecular therapy targets will likely ↑ biopsy rates
- Others: PA, PNET, rarely ganglioglioma

CLINICAL ISSUES

- Peak incidence ~ 3-10 years old
- Presentations include cranial nerve palsies, hemiparesis, gait disturbance, ataxia, headache, nausea, vomiting
- Prognosis depends on location & histology
  - o DIPG: Very poor prognosis (unresectable)
    - Radiation therapy if > 3 years old
    - Median survival ~ 1 year; 20% survival at 2 years
  - o PA (dorsally exophytic): Fair to good prognosis
    - ± surgical resection based upon location
  - o Tectum: Good prognosis (only requires CSF diversion)
  - o Medulla or midbrain: Variable prognosis
  - o Better prognosis of BST when associated with neurofibromatosis type I
    - Often asymptomatic, rarely grow

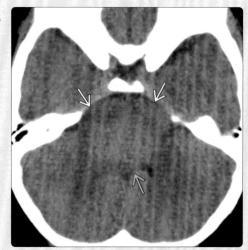

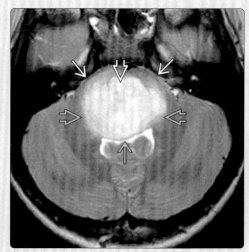

(Left) Axial NECT in a 7-year-old girl shows enlargement of the pons with obliteration of the prepontine cisterns ➡ & near complete effacement of the 4th ventricle ➡. Mass effect on the cisterns & 4th ventricle may be the only clue to a diffuse intrinsic pontine glioma (DIPG) on CT. (Right) Axial T2 MR in the same patient shows a homogeneously hyperintense mass ➡ expanding the pons. The mass shows indistinct margins ➡ with mass effect on the cisterns ➡ & 4th ventricle ➡, typical of DIPG.

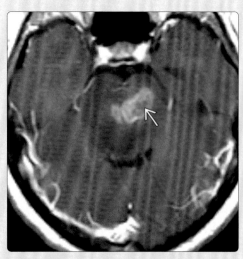

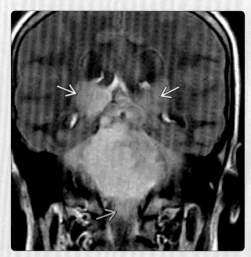

(Left) Axial T1 C+ MR in a 9-year-old girl with DIPG demonstrates focal areas of enhancement with central nonenhancement ➡, suggesting necrosis. Enhancement has been shown to be associated with shorter survival time in DIPG. (Right) Coronal FLAIR MR in a 9-year-old girl with DIPG shows extension of abnormal signal into the bilateral thalami ➡ & medulla ➡. Such distant extension of signal abnormality typically suggests an infiltrative, higher grade tumor.

Craniopharyngioma

TERMINOLOGY

- Benign epithelial tumor arising from squamous rests along involuted hypophyseal-Rathke duct

IMAGING

- Best clue: Complex suprasellar cystic mass with Ca^{2+} & wall enhancement
- Location: Suprasellar 75%; suprasellar & intrasellar 21%
  - Optic chiasm, hypothalamus, & vessels often involved
  - Larger tumors can extend into multiple cranial fossae
  - Retrochiasmatic vs. prechiasmatic configuration key determinant for surgical approach
  - May present with obstructive hydrocephalus from compression on 3rd ventricle & foramen of Monro
- "90% rule"
  - 90% cystic: MR signal intensity highly variable
    - Cystic components frequently T1 hyperintense
  - 90% calcified: SWI/T2* GRE MR helpful to identify Ca^{2+}
  - 90% enhance (wall & solid portions)

TOP DIFFERENTIAL DIAGNOSES

- Rathke cleft cyst, pituitary adenoma, germinoma, hypothalamic-chiasmatic glioma

CLINICAL ISSUES

- Most common nonglial pediatric intracranial tumor
  - Benign tumor with high rate of recurrence
  - 88% overall survival at 20 years
- Peak age of 8-12 years
- Symptoms: Visual changes, endocrine dysfunction, academic decline, headache/vomiting (obstructive hydrocephalus)
  - ~ 1/3 of patients with endocrine symptoms (↓ growth hormone, ↓ thyroid function, diabetes insipidus)
- Poor prognostic factors: Hypothalamic involvement, larger tumor size
- Treatment: Complete resection ideal but must be weighed against high morbidity associated with extensive resection
  - Radiation therapy for incomplete resection

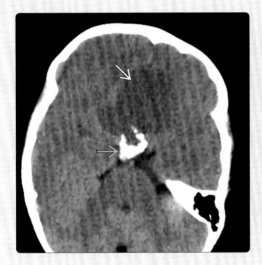
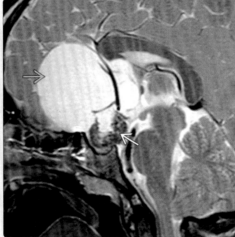

(Left) Axial NECT in a 3-year-old boy with 2 months of headaches & vomiting shows a partially calcified ➡, partially cystic ➡ lesion in the suprasellar region & interhemispheric fissure, characteristic of an adamantinomatous craniopharyngioma. (Right) Sagittal T2 MR in the same 3 year old shows hypointense signal in the posterior components ➡ of the mass, corresponding to Ca^{2+} on the CT. Frontal extension of the large cystic components ➡ is typical of a prechiasmatic location.

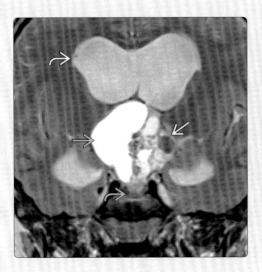
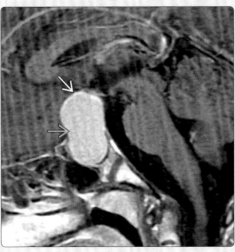

(Left) Coronal T2 MR in an 8-year-old boy with visual changes shows a mixed solid ➡ & cystic ➡ mass with obstructive hydrocephalus ➡. The visual changes are related to mass effect upon the optic chiasm ➡. (Right) Sagittal T1 C+ MR in a 10-year-old boy with increasing headaches shows a predominantly cystic mass with a very thin rim of enhancement ➡. The majority of craniopharyngiomas have some solid components. The cystic contents of these lesions often show intrinsic T1 bright signal ➡ before contrast, as in this case.

TERMINOLOGY

- Nonaccidental trauma, abusive head trauma (AHT)
- Traumatic injury inflicted on infants & children by adults

IMAGING

- Direct impact injury: Direct blow to cranium or impact of skull on object
  - Calvarial (often complex) & skull base fractures
  - Focal brain injury deep to impact
- Shaking injury: Result of violent "to & fro" motion of head
  - Subdural hematomas (SDH) in 90-98%
  - Generalized parenchymal injuries (cytotoxic edema, lacerations, axonal injury)
  - Bridging vein injury & thrombosis common
- CT primary imaging tool in initial evaluation of AHT
  - Multiplanar reconstructions improve detection of
    - Small intracranial hemorrhages
    - Fractures (with bone algorithm & 3D reformats)
- MR best for determining full extent of injury
  - DWI paramount for parenchymal injury
  - PD & SWI/T2* GRE for hemorrhage
  - T1 C+ for chronic SDH membranes

TOP DIFFERENTIAL DIAGNOSES

- Accidental trauma
- Benign macrocrania of infancy
- Mitochondrial encephalopathies
- Bleeding disorders

CLINICAL ISSUES

- Presentation: Poor feeding, vomiting, irritability, seizures, lethargy, coma, apnea, retinal hemorrhages (~ 75%)
  - Discordance between stated history & degree of injury: "Killer couch" (injuries blamed on infant rolling off couch)
- #1 cause of brain injury death in children < 2 years of age
  - 17-25:100,000 annual incidence
  - Risk factors: Developmentally delayed, colicky, premature or low birth weight infants at higher risk

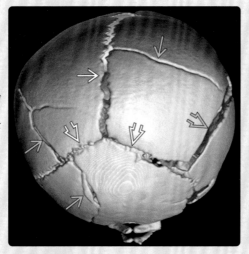
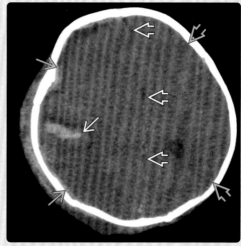

(Left) *Posterior oblique view of a 3D NECT of the head in a 9 week old who "fell off the couch" shows multiple complex skull fractures ➡, including a displaced right parietal fracture ➡. The normal sagittal ➡ & lambdoid ➡ sutures are noted.* (Right) *Axial NECT in the same 9 week old shows a right subdural hematoma (SDH) ➡ & parenchymal laceration ➡ with significant leftward midline shift ➡ & sulcal effacement ➡.*

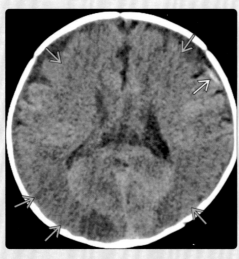
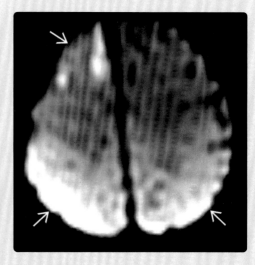

(Left) *Axial NECT in a 4-month-old boy with seizure activity shows multiple bilateral foci of low attenuation with loss of cortical differentiation ➡ as well as a left frontal SDH ➡. There was no fracture, making these findings highly concerning for the shaking type of abusive head trauma (AHT).* (Right) *Axial DWI MR in a 2-month-old boy with AHT shows areas of diffusion restriction ➡ in the right frontal lobe & bilateral parietal lobes, consistent with parenchymal injury. MR is the most sensitive examination for brain parenchymal injury.*

TERMINOLOGY

Abbreviations

- Nonaccidental trauma (NAT), abusive head trauma (AHT), shaken-baby syndrome (SBS)

Definitions

- Traumatic injury inflicted on infants & children by adults

IMAGING

General Features

- 2 major groupings of injuries (but can occur together)
  - Direct impact injury: Result of direct blow to cranium or impact of skull on object
  - Shaking injury: Result of violent "to & fro" head motion
- Direct impact injury typified by skull fractures & injury to subjacent brain
  - Scalp laceration, hematoma, swelling strongly associated
  - High association with injuries to other organs
- Shaking injury typified by subdural hemorrhage (SDH) & generalized brain parenchymal injury
  - Cytotoxic brain injury not conforming to arterial territories
  - May see bridging vein injury ± thrombosis
- Imaging findings may suggest injuries of differing ages

Radiographic Findings

- Sensitive in detection of linear skull fractures
  - CT (with appropriate techniques) better characterizes fractures; often being obtained to evaluate for intracranial hemorrhage
- Some fractures considered more suspicious for NAT
  - Discordance with provided history best indicator

CT Findings

- NECT primary imaging tool for initial evaluation of AHT
- Intracranial hemorrhage (ICH)
  - SDH most common (90-98%)
    - Dominant feature of shaking injury
  - Subarachnoid hemorrhage common (> 50%)
  - Epidural hemorrhage uncommon but may occur
  - Use great caution if attempting to estimate "age" of ICH
- Subdural hygromas may develop after injury
- Bridging vein injury ± thrombosis common (40-50%)
  - Areas of ↑ density in paramedian high convexities
- Parenchymal ischemic injury often seen in shaking injuries
  - Areas of ↓ density (with loss of gray-white differentiation) & sulcal effacement not confined to arterial territories; may be diffuse
- Parenchymal laceration in 10-15%
- Shear injury (axonal injury) in ~ 15%
- Retinal hemorrhages rarely visualized on CT

MR Findings

- DWI: Key for parenchymal injury
- T1WI: Bright foci of hemorrhage or evolving cortical injury
- T2WI: Loss of cortical ribbon & deep nuclei in neonates
- PD/intermediate echo sequences: Very sensitive for detection of small subdural collections
- SWI/T2* GRE: Detects small ICH ± retinal hemorrhages
- T1WI C+: Enhancing membranes best sign of chronic SDH

Imaging Recommendations

- Best imaging tool
  - NECT for acute evaluation
    - Sensitive in detection & characterization of fractures
    - Very sensitive in detection & characterization of ICH
  - MR after 24-48 hours to define extent of brain injury
  - Radiographic skeletal survey to screen for other injuries
- Protocol advice
  - NECT: Multiplanar reconstructions improve detection of
    - Small intracranial hemorrhages
    - Fractures (especially with bone algorithm & 3D)

DIFFERENTIAL DIAGNOSIS

Accidental Trauma

- Appropriate history for degree of injury
- Retinal hemorrhages in only ~ 6%

Benign Macrocrania of Infancy

- Self-limited communicating hydrocephalus
- Prominence of subarachnoid spaces → isodense to CSF

Mitochondrial Encephalopathies

- May cause atrophy with subdural collections
  - Glutaric acidurias (types I & II), Menkes syndrome

Bleeding Disorders

- von Willebrand, thrombocytopenia

CLINICAL ISSUES

Presentation

- Most common signs/symptoms
  - Discordance between stated history & degree of injury
    - "Killer couch": Severe injuries blamed on infant rolling off couch onto floor by perpetrator
  - Unprovoked seizures & apnea raise suspicion for AHT
- Other signs/symptoms
  - Poor feeding, vomiting, irritability, seizures, lethargy, coma, apnea
  - Retinal hemorrhages in ~ 75%
    - Can be missed on cursory exam
    - Can be seen in glutaric acidurias

Demographics

- Most common from 1-6 months of age

Natural History & Prognosis

- Mortality rate: 20-25%
- High rates of impairment for survivors

Treatment

- Notification of local Child Protection Agency
- Multidisciplinary child abuse & neglect team intervention

SELECTED REFERENCES

1. Cramer JA et al: Limitations of T2*-gradient recalled-echo and susceptibility-weighted imaging in characterizing chronic subdural hemorrhage in infant survivors of abusive head trauma. AJNR Am J Neuroradiol. ePub, 2016
2. Cowley LE et al: Validation of a prediction tool for abusive head trauma. Pediatrics. 136(2):290-8, 2015
3. Nadarasa J et al: Update on injury mechanisms in abusive head trauma–shaken baby syndrome. Pediatr Radiol. 44 Suppl 4:S565-70, 2014

Germinal Matrix Hemorrhage

TERMINOLOGY

- Germinal matrix: Transient periventricular regions of fragile thin-walled vessels & migrating neuronal components
  - Involutes by 34 weeks of gestation
- In premature infants, perinatal stresses + poor cerebral autoregulation + germinal matrix → hemorrhage

IMAGING

- US: Globular echogenic focus in caudothalamic groove
  - Acute blood echogenic; later clot retracts & becomes iso- to hypoechoic
  - May appear as abnormally thick choroid plexus but of slightly different echogenicity & lacking vascularity
  - Coronal & sagittal cine clips sweeping though ventricles help differentiate hemorrhage from normal choroid
- MR: Sensitive for detection of germinal matrix hemorrhage (GMH) & intraventricular hemorrhage (IVH)
  - Best imaging modality for detection of associated parenchymal abnormalities

- GMH-IVH grading system
  - Grade I: GMH only
  - Grade II: GMH + IVH, normal ventricle size
  - Grade III: GMH + IVH + ventricular expansion
  - Grade IV: GMH-IVH + intraparenchymal hemorrhage
    - Venous compression leads to venous infarction

CLINICAL ISSUES

- Most common < 32 weeks of gestation & < 1,500 grams
- 1/3-1/2 of all GMHs occur on 1st day of life
  - GMH may occur in utero or after 1st day
- May present with hypotonia, seizures, hyperreflexia, falling hematocrit, irritability, paresis, acidosis, feeding difficulties
- Grade I & II bleeds generally have good prognosis
- Grade III & IV bleeds have variable long-term deficits
  - Spastic diplegia, seizures, developmental delay
- Prenatal steroids, postnatal surfactant, & other treatments have ↓ incidence & poor outcomes of GMH-IVH
- CSF shunting for posthemorrhagic hydrocephalus

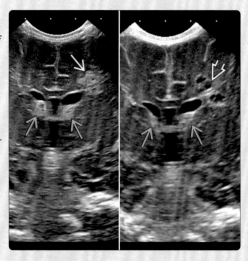
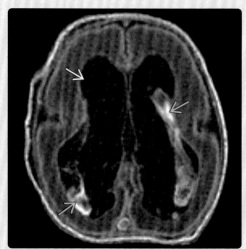

(Left) Coronal head US in a former 29-week gestation newborn shows an asymmetric globular echogenic focus in the right caudothalamic groove ⇨ consistent with a germinal matrix hemorrhage (GMH). The lack of intraventricular hemorrhage (IVH) makes this a grade I hemorrhage. (Right) Axial SWI MR in the same patient at 3 months of age shows a focus of signal loss in the right caudothalamic groove ⇨ consistent with a remote GMH. There is no signal loss in the ventricles otherwise to suggest a component of IVH.

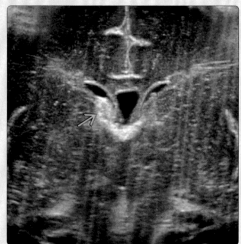
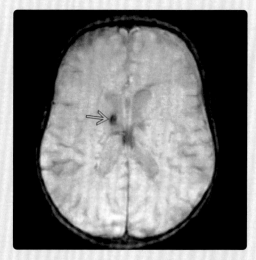

(Left) Coronal head US images in a 29-week premature infant at 3 weeks (L) & 7 weeks (R) of age show echogenic GMHs ⇨ in the caudothalamic grooves. An initially globular echogenic focus in the left frontal periventricular white matter ⇨ shows gradual evolution to cystic encephalomalacia ⇨. (Right) Axial T1 MR in a former 26-week gestation infant 3 weeks after bilateral grade III GMHs shows bright T1 foci from the prior IVHs ⇨. Further ventriculomegaly ⇨ has developed from posthemorrhagic hydrocephalus.

White Matter Injury of Prematurity

TERMINOLOGY

- Definition: Brain injury occurring before 34-week gestation resulting in loss of periventricular white matter (WM)

IMAGING

- Ultrasound: Reliable for more severe or late disease, less reliable for mild/moderate or early disease
  - Acute: Patchy, globular foci of ↑ echogenicity in periventricular/deep WM
  - Subacute/chronic: Clusters of periventricular cysts
- MR: Reliable for entire spectrum of disease
  - Acute: Hyperintense T1, hypointense T2 foci
    - Hypointense SWI/GRE foci with hemorrhage
    - ↓ ADC (may miss if imaging < 24 hours or > 5 days)
    - MRS: Lactate peak or ↑ excitatory neurotransmitters
  - Subacute: Periventricular cysts
  - Chronic: Periventricular/deep WM volume loss
    - Typically minimal associated gliosis

PATHOLOGY

- Preceding inflammation (e.g., chorioamnionitis) + ischemia superimposed on vulnerable premature brain
- Characteristic pattern of injury reflects distribution of immature oligodendrocytes during vulnerable period

CLINICAL ISSUES

- May be clinically silent initially ± EEG findings; spastic diplegia, visual & cognitive impairment
  - ± hydrocephalus (essential to know head size before making diagnosis in order to differentiate "ex vacuo" ventriculomegaly)
- Cerebral palsy: 6.5% in 1990-1993 vs. 2.2% in 2002-2005
  - > 50% with cystic WM injury develop cerebral palsy
  - Motor & visual impairment most common
- Improved outcomes have coincided with increased use of antenatal steroids, antenatal antibiotics, arterial line placement, & surfactant use

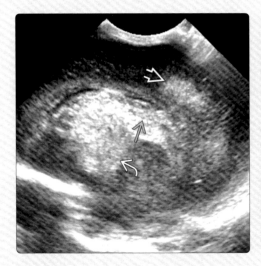

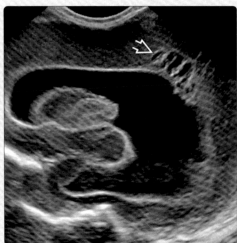

(Left) Sagittal head US of a 5-day-old, former 27-week gestational age infant shows globular increased echogenicity ⇒ in the periventricular white matter, consistent with ischemic injury. Intraventricular hemorrhage ⇒ & deep gray nuclei insult ⇒ are also noted. (Right) Sagittal head US of the same infant 1 month later shows that the previously seen focus of increased echogenicity has now evolved into cystic encephalomalacia ⇒. The new ventriculomegaly may be due to volume loss or obstruction by blood products.

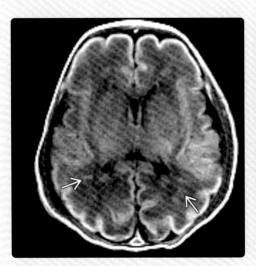

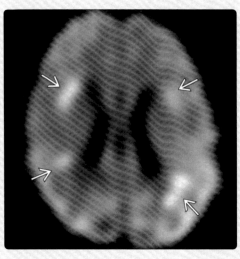

(Left) Axial T1 MR in an 18-day-old, former 33-week gestational age neonate with tricuspid atresia demonstrates patchy foci of hyperintense signal ⇒ in the bilateral parietooccipital periventricular white matter. (Right) Axial DWI MR in the same 18-day-old, former 33-week gestational age neonate with tricuspid atresia shows corresponding foci of restricted diffusion ⇒ (confirmed to have ↓ signal on the ADC map, not shown) in the bilateral periventricular white matter, consistent with ischemic injury.

Hypoxic-Ischemic Encephalopathy

TERMINOLOGY

- Brain injury in neonate caused by hypoxic ischemic insult

IMAGING

- Patterns of injury
  - Deep/central pattern: Basal ganglia, thalamus, ± brainstem
  - Peripheral pattern: Injury to watershed zones of hemispheres
  - Patterns may overlap
- US may be used for screening, particularly in acute setting or with concern for hemorrhage
  - Not sensitive for early parenchymal injury
- MR best imaging test for parenchymal injury
  - T1WI & T2WI MR: Usually normal in 1st few days
  - DWI MR: Best sequence to define extent of injury
    - ↑ DWI, ↓ ADC in affected regions from 2-7 days

PATHOLOGY

- Deep/central pattern due to severe hypoxia of relatively brief (10-25 minutes) duration
- Peripheral pattern due to less severe hypoxia over longer period of time
- Preterm neonates more likely to have associated white matter injury & hemorrhage

CLINICAL ISSUES

- Sarnat stage (based on clinical & EEG findings)
  - I (mild): Hyperalert/irritable, mydriasis, ↑ heart rate
  - II (moderate): Lethargy, hypotonia, miosis, ↓ heart rate
  - III (severe): Stupor, flaccid, reflexes absent, seizures
- Deep/central pattern → dyskinetic cerebral palsy
- Peripheral pattern → spastic cerebral palsy
- Treatment includes resuscitation, correction of fluid & electrolyte imbalances, seizure therapy, hypothermia

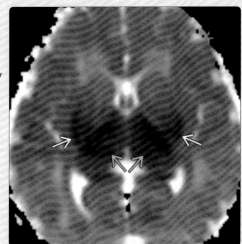

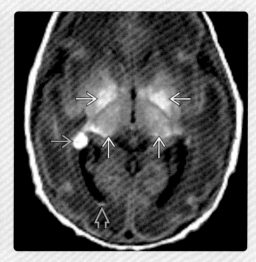

(Left) *Axial ADC MR in 3-day-old term boy (Apgar scores of 1, 1, & 1) shows diffusion restriction in the thalami ➡️ & posterolateral putamina ➡️, consistent with the deep injury pattern of profound hypoxic ischemic encephalopathy (HIE).* (Right) *Axial T1 MR in a 31-week premature infant 11 days following placental abruption shows irregular hyperintense signal ➡️ in the bilateral thalami & nuclei of globus pallidus. Note also the GMH ➡️ & small layering IVH ➡️, findings often seen in premature infants with HIE.*

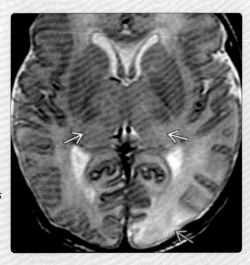

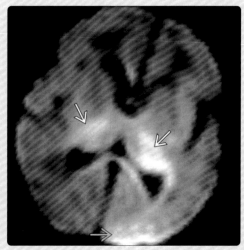

(Left) *Axial T2 MR in a 4-day-old term boy delivered by emergent C-section for fetal bradycardia shows increased signal with loss of cortical differentiation ➡️ in the left occipital lobe + ↑ signal ➡️ in the thalami.* (Right) *Axial DWI MR in the same 4-day-old boy best demonstrates the full extent of injury with definite involvement of the bilateral thalami ➡️ & the left occipital lobe ➡️, suggesting a more severe injury with components of both the central & peripheral patterns.*

Childhood Stroke

TERMINOLOGY

- Acute alteration of neurologic function due to loss of vascular integrity

IMAGING

- NECT: ↓ attenuation of affected gray matter
- NECT: Insular ribbon sign: Loss of distinct insular cortex
- NECT: Hyperdense middle cerebral artery (MCA) sign: Clot in MCA
- MR: ↓ diffusion within ~ 30 minutes of arterial occlusion
- MR: Cytotoxic edema evident in affected territory on FLAIR/T2 by 4-6 hours after arterial occlusion
- MR: Enhancement of infarct typically occurs after 5-7 days
- CTA/MRA: Critical for early evaluation & identification of possible etiology (e.g., dissection, arteriopathy)
- MR perfusion imaging can provide valuable information regarding region at risk in setting of acute stroke

TOP DIFFERENTIAL DIAGNOSES

- Seizure-related injury, acute encephalitis, mitochondrial disorders, posterior reversible encephalopathy

PATHOLOGY

- Major causes: Cardiac disease (~ 25%), moyamoya-type arteriopathy, arterial dissection, CNS vasculitis, hematologic/metabolic
- No underlying cause discovered in ~ 25% of cases

CLINICAL ISSUES

- Incidence: 2-3/100,000 per year in USA
  - Mortality: 0.6/100,000
- Children typically present later than adults (> 24 hours)
- Focal deficit may be masked by lethargy, coma, irritability
- Treatment in pediatric acute stroke usually conservative: Thrombolysis/thrombectomy not well studied in children
- Capacity for recovery in children much > adults

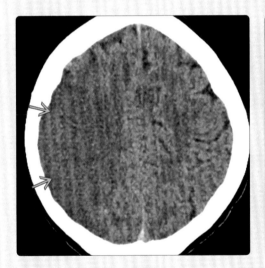
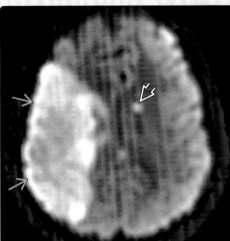

(Left) Axial NECT in a 15-year-old girl with dilated cardiomyopathy shows a large area of low attenuation in the right middle cerebral artery (MCA) territory ➡. Note the sulcal effacement & loss of the gray-white matter differentiation. (Right) Axial DWI MR in the same patient confirms restricted diffusion in the right MCA territory ➡. Also note the focus of restricted diffusion in the left periventricular region ➡. Infarcts in multiple vascular territories should raise suspicion of a proximal embolic source.

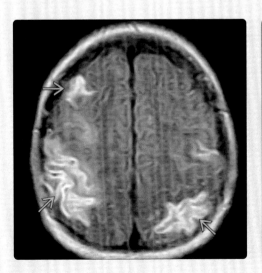
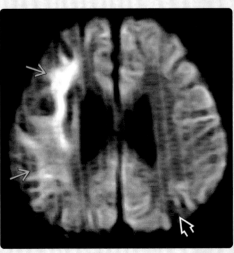

(Left) Axial FLAIR MR in a 2-year-old girl shows multiple areas of cytotoxic edema ➡ in both cerebral hemispheres due to a moyamoya-type vasculopathy (which is predominantly a terminal internal carotid artery occlusion leading to "puff of smoke" collateral vessels). (Right) Axial DWI MR in the same girl shows diffusion restriction in the right frontoparietal hemisphere ➡, suggesting an acute/subacute infarct. However, there is no diffusion restriction in the left parietal region ➡, suggesting this infarct is of an older age.

Arteriovenous Malformation

TERMINOLOGY

- High-flow vascular malformation with AV shunting through nidus of arterioles & venules (without capillary bed)

IMAGING

- Best clue: Parenchymal hemorrhage with extension into ventricle & cluster of adjacent abnormal vessels (nidus) with enlarged draining veins
- NECT: Parenchymal hematoma; small unruptured AVMs often not visible
- CTA: Enhancing feeding arteries, nidus, & draining veins; AVM may be occult if compressed by hematoma
  - Provides rapid diagnosis & adequate detail for therapy
- MR: T1 bright hemorrhage; T2 dark flow voids
- MRA/MRV: Gross depiction of AVM components with flow-related signal in draining veins reflecting AV shunt
- DSA: Gold standard with high temporal & spatial resolution, identifying all components + associated aneurysms & venous stenoses

TOP DIFFERENTIAL DIAGNOSES

- Cavernous malformation
- Hemorrhagic tumor

CLINICAL ISSUES

- Most AVMs sporadic (only 2% syndromic); can develop in previously normal brain
- Presentations: Acute bleed (headache, ↓ consciousness) ~ 50%, ~ seizure 25%, ~ focal neurological changes 15%, ~ incidental 10%
- Annual bleeding risk = 2-4%: ↑ with prior AVM rupture, exclusive deep venous drainage, or deep brain location
- Acute surgical decompression often required for mass effect from hematoma
- Definitive treatment (resection, endovascular embolization, &/or stereotactic radiosurgery) for underlying AVM based on variety of factors

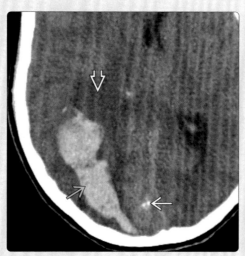
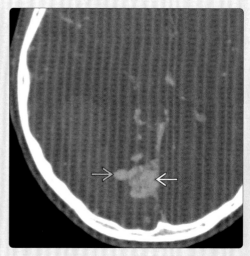

(Left) Axial NECT in a 15-year-old girl who was found unconscious with dilated pupils shows extensive right posterior temporal & occipital intraparenchymal hemorrhage ⬅. Note the surrounding parenchymal edema ➡. A few small calcific foci ➡ in the medial occipital lobe suggest an associated vascular malformation. (Right) Axial CT angiogram in the same patient shows a tightly packed central nidus ➡ with dilated peripheral veins ➡, consistent with an arteriovenous malformation (AVM).

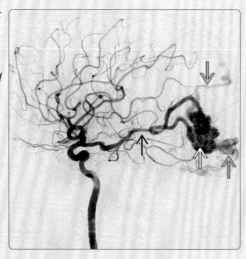
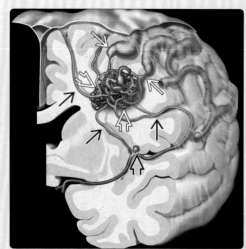

(Left) Lateral DSA image (right ICA injection) in the same 15-year-old girl shows the enlarged arterial feeder ➡ arising from the right ICA via the PComA. The tightly packed nidus ➡ is well defined. Note the 2 separate superficial draining veins that opacify early during the arterial phase ➡, typical of an AVM. (Right) Graphic shows a cerebral AVM with a centrum semiovale nidus ➡ fed from cortical & central arteries ➡ (with a proximal flow-related aneurysm ➡) & drained by enlarged cortical veins ➡.

Cavernous Malformation

TERMINOLOGY

- Benign vascular lesion with dilated sinusoids lined by thin immature walls & containing blood products of various ages

IMAGING

- NECT: Hyperdense lesion ± Ca²⁺; 50% not visible
- CECT: No enhancement of actual lesion
- MR: Heterogeneous core with T2 hypointense rim
  - Popcorn ball appearance with internal fluid-fluid levels
  - Adjacent ↑ FLAIR signal suggests recent hemorrhage
  - SWI/T2* GRE most sensitive for small lesions

TOP DIFFERENTIAL DIAGNOSES

- Diffuse axonal injury
- Venous infarction
- Intracerebral hematoma
- Neoplasm

PATHOLOGY

- Etiology: Initial parenchymal microhemorrhage followed by neoangiogenesis & recurrent hemorrhage
- 70% solitary, 30% multiple (with prior XRT or autosomal dominant familial cavernous malformation syndrome)
- Associated developmental venous anomaly (DVA) in 25%

CLINICAL ISSUES

- 0.6% incidence in children undergoing brain MR
- Symptoms: 1/2 incidental; 1/4 seizures; 1/4 neurologic deficits
- Factors that ↑ annual risk of hemorrhage
  - Zabramski MR classification (I & II > III, IV)
  - Prior hemorrhage
  - Brainstem location
  - Associated DVA
- Treatment: Total surgical excision, sparing DVA
  - DVA removal → venous injury & venous infarct

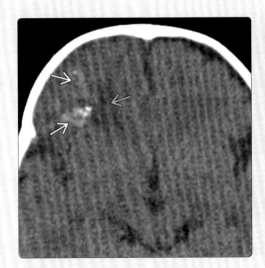

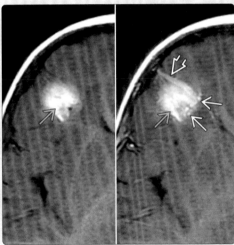

(Left) *Axial NECT in a 1 year old with focal facial seizures shows heterogeneous high attenuation ➡ in the right frontal lobe with low attenuation (edema) ➡ deep to the lesion.* (Right) *Axial T1 (left) & T1 C+ (right) MR images in same 1 year old show intrinsically high signal ➡ (Zabramski type I) in the lesion with multiple small vessels ➡ along the medial margin coalescing into a draining vein ➡, consistent with a developmental venous anomaly (DVA). 25% of cavernous malformations are associated with DVAs.*

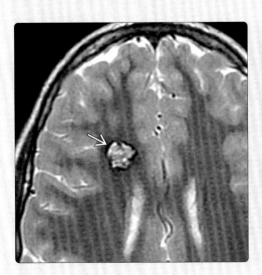

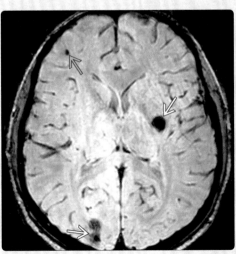

(Left) *Axial T2 MR in a 15 year old with a headache shows the typical popcorn appearance of a Zabramski type II cavernous malformation with a reticulated mixed signal core & hypointense rim ➡.* (Right) *Axial SWI MR in a 15 year old with multiple familial cavernous malformation syndrome shows 2 larger lesions ➡ in the left basal ganglia & right occipital lobe + a smaller lesion ➡ (Zabramski IV) in the right frontal lobe. The 2 larger lesions were visible on T2, but the smaller lesion was only visible on the more sensitive SWI sequence.*

Developmental Venous Anomaly

TERMINOLOGY

- Congenital brain parenchymal vascular malformation composed solely of mature venous elements

IMAGING

- Umbrella-like collection of enlarged medullary (white matter) veins ("Medusa head") converging on single enlarged collecting vein
- Collecting vein drains to deep or superficial venous system
- Usually solitary, of variable size (< 2-3 cm)
- Location: Supratentorial (70%) vs. infratentorial (30%)
- Most commonly visualized by MR; CT less likely
  - Exquisitely depicted on contrast-enhanced MR; may be seen on other sequences without contrast
  - Surrounding parenchymal abnormalities in ~ 11%, of uncertain etiology
    - Gliosis (scarring), edema, hypomyelination
    - Volume loss

PATHOLOGY

- Prevalence of 6.4%, typically isolated
- Associations include
  - Parenchymal cavernous malformations in ~ 6%
  - Other venous malformations: Cervicofacial (especially orbit), blue rubber bleb nevus syndrome
  - Cortical malformations
  - Intracranial neoplasms (rare)

CLINICAL ISSUES

- Hemorrhage: ~ 0.15% per lesion per year; ↑ risk if
  - Stenosis or thrombosis of draining vein
  - Coexisting cavernous malformation
- Usually asymptomatic; rarely associated with headache, seizure (from cortical dysplasia), or neurologic deficit (from hemorrhage of cavernous malformation)
- Treatment of solitary venous anomaly: None (as attempt at removal may cause venous infarction of large territory)

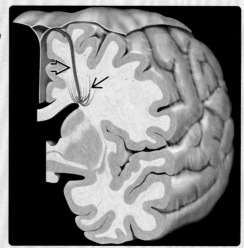
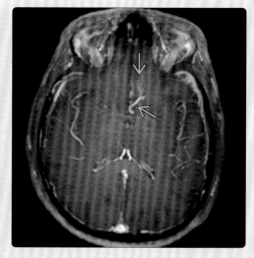

(Left) Coronal oblique graphic shows a classic developmental venous anomaly (DVA) with an umbrella-like "Medusa head" of enlarged medullary (deep white matter) veins ➡ converging on a dilated transcortical "collector" vein ➡. The "collector" vein drains into the superior sagittal sinus in this case but can drain to a variety of normal venous structures (depending on the DVA location). (Right) Axial T1 C+ FS MR MIP image in a 17 year old with possible encephalitis shows an incidental left inferior frontal DVA ➡.

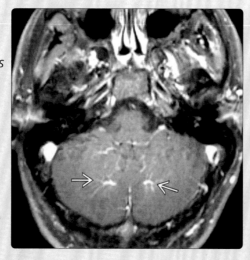
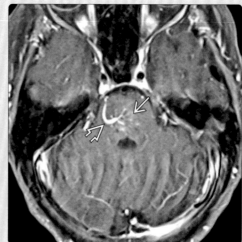

(Left) Axial T1 C+ FS MR in a patient with blue rubber bleb nevus syndrome (BRBNS) shows bilateral cerebellar DVAs ➡. Patients with BRBNS have numerous venous anomalies of the skin & gastrointestinal tract & may have abnormal intracranial venous drainage patterns. (Right) Axial T1 C+ FS MR in the same patient shows the classic "Medusa head" of enlarged veins ➡ draining into a prominent "collector" vein ➡. The brainstem is an uncommon location for a DVA (< 5%).

Metabolic Brain Disease

KEY FACTS

TERMINOLOGY

- Inborn errors of metabolism affecting brain
  - Localized &/or systemic accumulation of metabolites
  - Exclusive of mitochondrial encephalopathies & leukodystrophies
- Mucopolysaccharidoses (MPS)
  - Hunter, Hurler, Sanfilippo, Morquio, Maroteaux-Lamy, Sly, Natowicz syndromes
- Organic & aminoacidopathies
  - Maple syrup urine disease (MSUD)
  - Phenylketonuria
  - Nonketotic hyperglycinemia (NKH)
- Urea cycle disorders
  - Deficiency of enzymes in urea cycle
- Fatty acid oxidation disorders
  - Short, medium, long, or very long chain acyl-CoA dehydrogenase deficiency
  - Carnitine palmitoyl transferase deficiencies (CPT1, CPT2)

IMAGING

- MPS: Enlarged perivascular spaces, often with patchy ↑ white matter signal on T2WI MR
- MSUD: Edema prominently involving brainstem & cerebellar white matter
- NKH: Restricted diffusion & abnormal signal in posterior limb of internal capsule, dorsal midbrain, & cerebellar white matter in neonate
- Urea cycle disorders: Diffuse brain edema, not sparing basal ganglia or thalami
- Medium-chain acyl-CoA dehydrogenase (MCAD) deficiency: Cerebral cortical edema

DIAGNOSTIC CHECKLIST

- Remember to consider metabolic diseases when encountering acutely ill neonate: Characteristic laboratory abnormalities may provide clue
  - Urea cycle disorder → hyperammonemia
  - MCAD deficiency → severe hypoglycemia

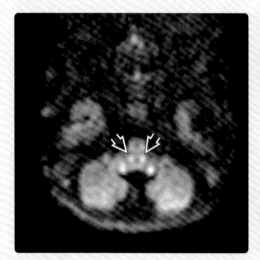

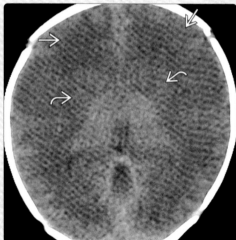

(Left) *Axial DWI MR through the pontomedullary junction in a neonate with nonketotic hyperglycinemia shows characteristic restricted diffusion in the dorsal tegmental tracts* ⇒. (Right) *Axial NECT in a neonate with an inborn deficiency of ornithine transcarbamylase (a urea cycle enzyme) shows diffuse cerebral* ⇒ *& basal ganglia* ⇒ *low attenuation with loss of gray-white matter differentiation from cytotoxic edema brought on by hyperammonemia.*

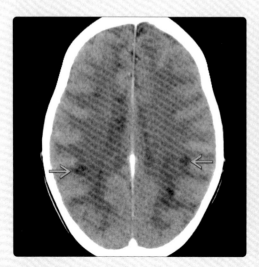

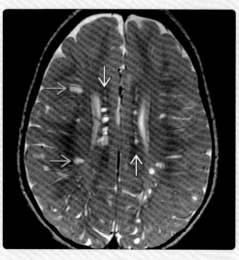

(Left) *CECT in a 14 year old with Hurler syndrome [mucopolysaccharidosis (MPS) I] shows multiple foci of decreased attenuation* ⇒ *in the cerebral white matter reflecting enlarged perivascular spaces.* (Right) *Axial T2 MR in a 2 year old with Hunter syndrome (MPS II) demonstrates markedly enlarged perivascular spaces* ⇒ *throughout the cerebrum to include the body of the corpus callosum* ⇒.

TORCH Infections

TERMINOLOGY

- TORCH/TORCHES: Acronym for congenital infections caused by transplacental transmission of pathogens
  - **T**oxoplasmosis (toxo): *Toxoplasma gondii*
  - **O**ther: Zika virus, etc.
  - **R**ubella virus
  - **C**ytomegalovirus (CMV)
  - **He**rpes: Herpes simplex virus 2 (HSV-2)
  - **H**uman immunodeficiency virus (HIV)
  - **S**yphilis: *Treponema pallidum*

IMAGING

- Toxo, CMV, HIV, Zika, & rubella all cause parenchymal Ca^{2+}
- CMV causes migrational defects, white matter gliosis/hypomyelination, & cystic foci in temporal poles
- Rubella, Zika, & HSV cause lobar destruction/encephalomalacia
- ± microcephaly (not unique to Zika)

CLINICAL ISSUES

- CMV most common TORCH infection in USA
  - Can present at birth (10%) with microcephaly, hepatosplenomegaly, petechial rash
  - 55% with systemic disease have CNS involvement
  - Ganciclovir may benefit CMV-infected infants
- Zika typically apparent at birth due to microcephaly
- Congenital toxo usually inapparent at birth, presenting at 2-3 months; pyrimethamine & sulfadiazine to treat
- Rubella presents with petechial rash, low birth weight, & leukokoria (cataracts)
- HSV acquired during delivery typically presents at 3-15 days with seizures, lethargy; treated with acyclovir as soon as suspected
- HIV: Developmental delay by 6-12 months; antiretroviral treatment in 2nd & 3rd trimesters & during labor can prevent transmission of HIV
- Syphilis → failure to thrive & irritability in newborn, bone pain in infant; treated with penicillin

(Left) Coronal T2 MR in a 1 year old with congenital cytomegalovirus (CMV) & sensorineural hearing loss shows diffusely abnormal white matter signal ➡ & irregularity of gray-white matter junctions, reflecting migrational abnormalities. (Right) Axial T1 MR in 4 year old with congenital CMV shows a large region of abnormal cortical thickening & diminished sulcation in the right hemisphere ➡, reflecting abnormal neuronal migration. More subtle abnormalities can be seen in the left hemisphere ➡.

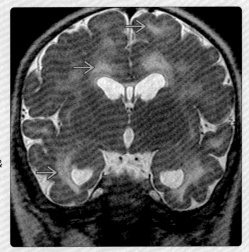
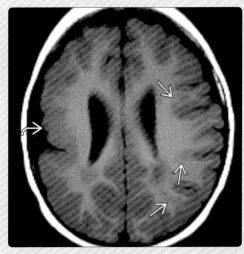

(Left) Axial NECT from an infant with in utero Zika virus infection shows periventricular & subcortical Ca^{2+} ➡ with marked volume loss, resulting in microcephaly (despite the presence of ventriculomegaly). (Courtesy T. Fazecas, MD.) (Right) Axial NECT in a 13 month old with congenital toxoplasmosis infection shows multiple peripheral punctate Ca^{2+} ➡ without superimposed white matter destruction or migration abnormalities.

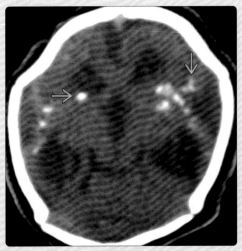
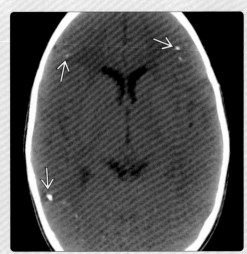

Brain Abscess

KEY FACTS

TERMINOLOGY

- Focal pyogenic infection of brain parenchyma

IMAGING

- Early cerebritis: Ill-defined subcortical lesion with mass effect & patchy enhancement (CT/MR)
- Late cerebritis: T2 hypointense rim (MR) with irregular peripheral rim enhancement (CT/MR)
- Early capsule: T2 hypointense rim (MR) with well-defined, thin enhancing wall (CT/MR)
- Late capsule: Cavity shrinks, edema & mass effect diminish, capsule thickens (CT/MR)

TOP DIFFERENTIAL DIAGNOSES

- Resolving hematoma, pilocytic astrocytoma, demyelination

CLINICAL ISSUES

- 25% occur in patients < 15 years of age
- Headache in up to 90%, fever in only 50%; seizures, altered mental status, focal neurologic deficits less common
  - ↑ ESR in 75%, ↑ WBC count in 50%
- Lumbar puncture can be hazardous
  - Posterior fossa abscess most common cause of herniation after lumbar puncture
- Mortality up to 30%; depends on size & location of abscess, virulence of infecting organism, systemic state of patient
- Treatments
  - Antibiotics (may be adequate in isolation if < 2.5 cm or early cerebritis)
  - Steroids to treat edema & mass effect
  - Surgical drainage or excision may be required
  - Drainage of adjacent source (e.g., infected paranasal sinuses, mastoids)
- Complications of inadequately or untreated abscesses
  - Intraventricular rupture, ventriculitis (may be fatal), meningitis, new daughter lesions
  - Mass effect, herniation

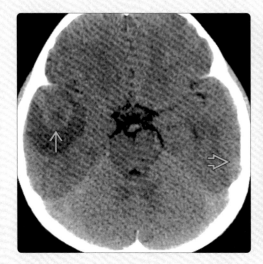

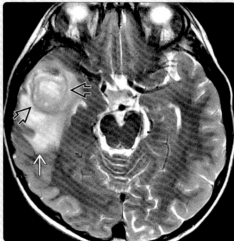

(Left) *Axial NECT in a patient with seizures shows a round temporal lobe lesion with a continuous rim* ⇨ *that is nearly isodense to gray matter* ⇨*. Vasogenic edema is noted in the surrounding temporal lobe.* (Right) *Axial T2 MR in the same patient shows a late cerebritis stage brain abscess with a poorly defined hypointense rim* ⇨ *& extensive surrounding vasogenic edema* ➡*. The characteristic T2 hypointensity of the rim is thought to reflect the presence of collagen, hemorrhage, &/or paramagnetic free radicals.*

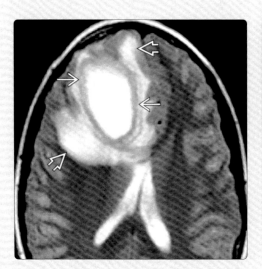

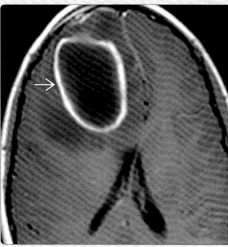

(Left) *Axial T2 MR in a 13 year old with headaches & dizziness shows an ovoid hyperintense lesion with a hypointense wall* ➡ *& moderate surrounding vasogenic edema* ⇨*.* (Right) *Axial T1 C+ MR in the same patient shows a smooth, continuous outer rim of enhancement* ➡ *to the lesion. The constellation of findings is typical for a cerebral abscess. A necrotic tumor would typically show more heterogeneous & irregular enhancement without a T2 hypointense rim.*

Acute Encephalitis

TERMINOLOGY

- Acute brain inflammation caused by infectious agents, most commonly viruses

IMAGING

- Most viral encephalitides have wide-ranging, nonspecific imaging findings that imitate other illnesses
  - Large, poorly delineated parenchymal abnormalities common, ± patchy hemorrhage
    - Variable involvement of gray & white matter, deep gray nuclei, brainstem, & cerebellum
  - Little or no parenchymal enhancement
  - Minimal leptomeningeal enhancement
- Some pathogens (HSV) have characteristic imaging features
  - Temporal & subfrontal hemorrhage classic
  - However, many children with HSV1 do not follow this pattern but have multilobar distribution
- Initial CT negative in vast majority of patients

TOP DIFFERENTIAL DIAGNOSES

- Acute ischemia
- Status epilepticus
- Mitochondrial encephalopathy

PATHOLOGY

- Herpes: Most common sporadic viral encephalitis
  - Include HSV1, HSV2, CMV, EBV, varicella-zoster virus, B virus, HSV6, HSV7
- Marked seasonal variation in USA as arboviruses transmitted by mosquitoes & ticks; travel history useful

CLINICAL ISSUES

- Presentation varies widely from slight meningeal to severe encephalitic symptoms
  - Fever, poor feeding, altered consciousness, seizures, focal neurologic deficits, ± prodrome
- Rapid diagnosis & early treatment with antiviral or antibacterial agents can ↓ mortality, may improve outcome

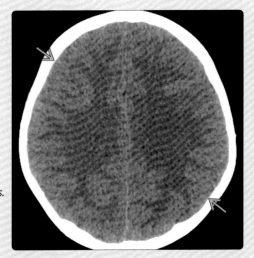

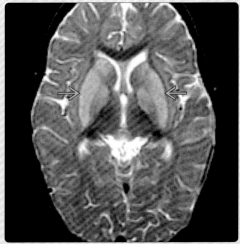

(Left) Axial NECT in a 6 year old with West Nile virus encephalitis shows diffuse effacement of sulci ⮕ with preservation of gray-white matter differentiation. Peripheral sulci should be visible over the convexities at any age; their absence indicates some degree of diffuse cerebral swelling. (Right) Axial T2 MR shows bilateral symmetric lesions in the basal ganglia ⮕ of this 1 year old with EBV encephalitis. EBV is one of many viruses that can cause symmetric basal ganglia or thalamic signal abnormalities.

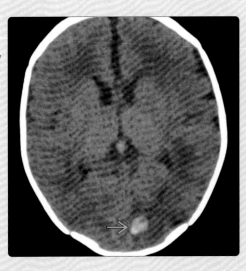

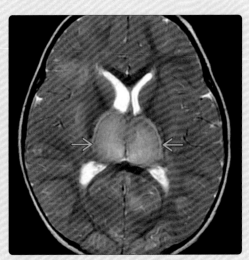

(Left) Axial NECT in a 13 day old with disseminated HSV shows a hemorrhagic lesion in the occipital pole ⮕. Perinatal HSV infection is typically due to HSV2 acquired during passage through an infected birth canal. Older children are more likely to have HSV1 infection. (Right) Axial T2 MR in a 15 month old with acute necrotizing encephalitis complicating an influenza infection shows severe swelling of the thalami ⮕, which is characteristic of this fulminant & frequently fatal complication of viral encephalitis.

Demyelinating Diseases

KEY FACTS

TERMINOLOGY

- Acquired demyelinating processes, often autoimmune & characterized by inflammation: Multiple sclerosis (MS), acute disseminated encephalomyelitis (ADEM), Lyme disease, neuromyelitis optica (NMO) (a.k.a. Devic disease)

IMAGING

- Best tool: MR brain without & with contrast; ± orbits
- MS: Multiple lesions, typically discrete; rarely mass-like
  - Callosal involvement, hemispheric white matter
  - Perpendicular to ventricle margin; often perivenular
- ADEM: Frequent brainstem & thalamic involvement
- Lyme disease: ± cranial nerve inflammation
- NMO: Optic neuritis with spinal cord lesions

PATHOLOGY

- MS: Possibly viral-incited autoimmune reaction in genetically susceptible individuals
- ADEM: Subsequent to infection or vaccination

- Lyme disease: Caused by spirochete *Borrelia burgdorferi*
- NMO: Associated with serum aquaporin-4 immunoglobulin G antibodies; 20-30% of cases are seronegative

CLINICAL ISSUES

- 3-5% of MS diagnosed before age 15
  - ADEM more frequently diagnosed in children
  - 20% of childhood MS initially diagnosed as ADEM
- MS: Initially impaired/double vision of acute optic neuritis, weakness, numbness, tingling, gait disturbances leading to ↓ sphincter control, blindness, paralysis, dementia
  - MS: 45% of patients not severely affected
- ADEM: Cranial nerve palsies, encephalopathy, headache 2 days to 4 weeks after prodrome; seizures in 10-35%; classically monophasic
- Lyme disease: Stereotypical expanding rash around tick bite (erythema chronicum migrans)
- NMO: Rapid vision loss; subsequent spinal cord symptoms

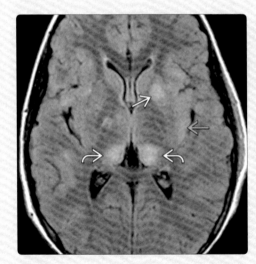

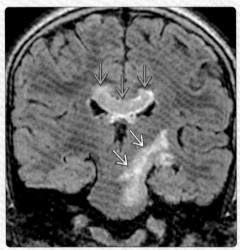

(Left) *Axial FLAIR MR in a 9-year-old patient with altered mental status & hyperreflexia shows ill-defined hyperintense lesions in the thalami ⤢, basal ganglia ⇨, & insula ⇨. Involvement of the deep nuclei is a relatively common feature of acute disseminated encephalomyelitis.* (Right) *Coronal FLAIR MR in a 12-year-old patient with neuromyelitis optica & bladder dysfunction shows large lesions extending across the corpus callosum ⇨ & left cerebral peduncle ⤢.*

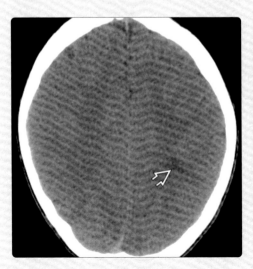

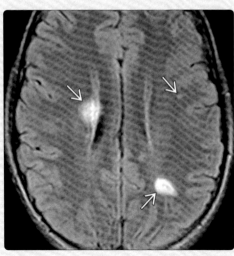

(Left) *Axial NECT in a 14-year-old patient with vomiting shows a nonspecific low-attenuation lesion ⇨ in the left posterior frontal subcortical white matter.* (Right) *Axial FLAIR MR of the same patient acquired the next day shows several ovoid multiple sclerosis plaques ⇨. Active lesions will also demonstrate contrast enhancement & restricted diffusion (not shown here).*

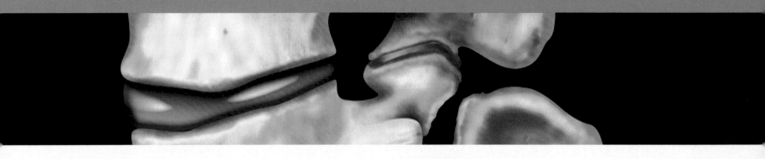

SECTION 8
Spine

Imaging Modalities

Ultrasound

In the newborn, the spine is most commonly imaged when a cutaneous lesion overlies the lumbosacral spine & implies the presence of an underlying spinal abnormality. Common examples requiring deeper imaging investigation include a cutaneous infantile hemangioma, hairy patch, fatty mass, appendage, forked gluteal crease, or atypical dimple (& do not include the common low-lying, shallow midline dimple near the anus). Within the first 4 months of life, ultrasound excels at visualizing the morphologies & spatial relationships of structures within the spinal canal, including the spinal cord, CSF, & nerve roots. This allows for the detection of a low-lying conus medullaris or intraspinal mass that can be associated with tethering & will require release to prevent long-term neurologic damage. After about 4-6 months of age, too much of the pediatric vertebral cartilage has ossified to allow an adequate acoustic window into the spine. Therefore, other methods of interrogation will be required.

Radiographs

Beyond infancy, spine imaging in the child most commonly occurs by plain radiographs, usually in the setting of back pain &/or suspected scoliosis. Two views (frontal & lateral) are typically acquired. In the setting of cervical trauma, a dedicated odontoid/dens view is also obtained in patients who are able to cooperate with positioning (which includes opening of the mouth). It should be noted that the cervicothoracic junction & upper thoracic vertebral elements can be quite difficult to assess on the lateral view & may require additional views (or potentially CT) for adequate visualization.

Flexion & extension views may be used to look for instability (particularly in the cervical spine), but the correlation between radiologic & clinically significant instability has been debated.

With strong suspicion of lumbar spondylolysis (or stress-induced pars interarticularis defects), some clinicians will request oblique views. However, many radiologists recommend conserving this radiation (as such images rarely add valuable information) & choosing another imaging study (such as targeted CT or MR imaging).

When the primary concern is for scoliosis, the obtained long frontal view of the spine is often displayed from the perspective of the examining/operating orthopedist (who is looking at the patient's back) rather than the typical image display that presumes we are face-to-face with the patient.

Computed Tomography

Computed tomography (CT) plays an extremely valuable role in the setting of acute trauma in which concerning mechanisms (such as motor vehicle accidents or falls) &/or symptoms require a rapid assessment for spinal injury. In a patient who is undergoing chest, abdomen, &/or pelvis CT scans due to concern for visceral injuries, the CT data from these scans can usually be reconstructed into spine CT images with no additional scan time or radiation dose. Conversely, patients with mechanisms & presentations specific to 1 region (such as the cervical spine) may only need spine imaging without additional visceral evaluations. In these settings, the mechanism, level of consciousness (i.e., GCS), & other neurologic symptoms will drive the use of CT vs. radiographs. CT is much more sensitive than radiographs at detecting minimally displaced fractures & fractures where critical bone anatomy is poorly visualized by x-rays (usually due to overlap of many structures). It also excels at characterizing complex fractures. However, CT is not typically helpful in the neurologically intact patient with back pain that may have a mild compression-type fracture by radiographs; a follow-up nonemergent MR is most useful in this setting to look for marrow edema (which helps separate a new mild compression fracture from normal developmental wedging that often occurs in the thoracic spine).

Bone CT without contrast has the highest sensitivity & specificity for spondylolysis or osteoid osteoma, & targeted exams (just through the levels of interest) will significantly reduce radiation dose. Bone CT can be combined with nuclear medicine SPECT bone scans to provide physiologic as well as anatomic information in such cases. Bone CT may also be used for assessing the spine preoperatively in complex scoliosis cases, though such cases are typically selected by the orthopedist managing the patient.

IV contrast is rarely useful in spine CT as it is the bones that are well-visualized by CT, not the neural elements or surrounding soft tissues.

Magnetic Resonance

Magnetic resonance (MR) imaging provides the best visualization of the neural elements, intervertebral disks, bone marrow, & surrounding soft tissues. Its ability to detect pathologies that cause increased fluid content (which includes the vast majority of fractures, infections, & tumors) gives it the highest sensitivity & specificity for most abnormalities. It is particularly useful in detecting & characterizing spinal cord pathologies, including congenital anomalies. In the setting of trauma, it will detect nondisplaced fractures (by marrow edema visualization) & ligamentous disruption that cannot be visualized on CT (but may be implied). MR imaging is also the next test performed in infants if ultrasound detects an abnormality.

IV contrast is typically reserved for suspected cases of infection, inflammation, or tumor.

Nuclear Medicine

There are no widely accepted applications of nuclear medicine for evaluating the neural elements of the spine (unlike the brain). However, nuclear studies may help characterize CSF flow (as in patients with complicated ventricular drainage issues) or detect bone pathologies (including infection, spondylolysis, osteoid osteoma, & Langerhans cell histiocytosis, among others), especially when the latter are not clearly localized by symptoms.

Selected References

1. ACR Appropriateness Criteria: Back Pain—Child. https://acsearch.acr.org/docs/3099011/Narrative/. Published 2016. Accessed March 31, 2017
2. ACR Appropriateness Criteria: Suspected Spine Trauma. https://acsearch.acr.org/docs/69359/Narrative/. Published 1999. Reviewed 2012. Accessed March 31. 2017
3. Huisman TA et al: Pediatric spinal trauma. J Neuroimaging. 25(3):337-53, 2015
4. Palasis S et al: Acquired pathology of the pediatric spine and spinal cord. Pediatr Radiol. 45 Suppl 3:S420-32, 2015
5. Rossi A: Pediatric spinal infection and inflammation. Neuroimaging Clin N Am. 25(2):173-91, 2015
6. Malfair D et al: Radiographic evaluation of scoliosis: review. AJR Am J Roentgenol. 194(3 Suppl):S8-22, 2010
7. Grimme JD et al: Congenital anomalies of the spine. Neuroimaging Clin N Am. 17(1):1-16, 2007

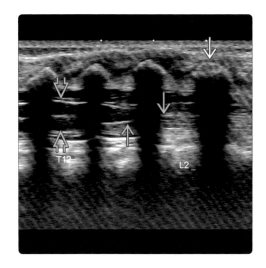

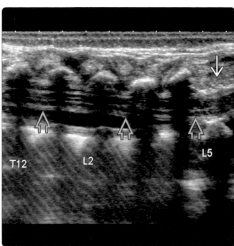

(Left) *Longitudinal US in a 5 week old with a cutaneous lumbar nevus shows a normal spinal cord* ⇨ *tapering to a normal conus medullaris* ⇨ *that ends at the upper L2 level. The partially ossified spinous processes* ➡ *cause posterior acoustic shadowing. Increasing ossification will further obscure the spinal contents over the next few months.* (Right) *Longitudinal US in a 2 day old with an abnormal gluteal cleft shows elongation of the spinal cord* ⇨ *with tethering into a fatty mass* ➡, *consistent with a lipomyelomeningocele.*

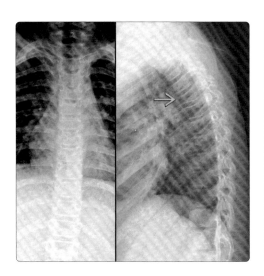

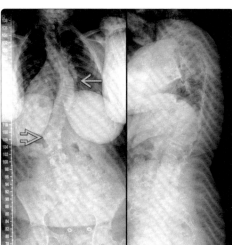

(Left) *AP (left) & lateral (right) radiographs of the thoracic spine in a 7 year old with upper back pain after a fall show mild anterior wedging of the T4 vertebral body* ⇨ *due to a mild compression fracture.* (Right) *PA (left) & lateral (right) radiographs in a 14 year old girl with adolescent idiopathic scoliosis show typical apex right thoracic* ⇨ *& apex left lumbar* ⇨ *curves without significant kyphosis or lordosis. Note that the frontal view is displayed from the perspective of the examining/operating orthopedist.*

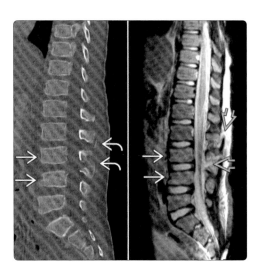

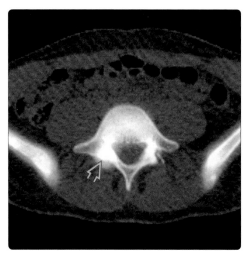

(Left) *Sagittal bone CT (left) & STIR MR (right) images show mixed osseous & soft tissue Chance fractures where the 3 columns of the spine are each involved at 2 different levels. The anterior & middle bony column disruptions* ➡ *are seen on CT & MR. CT shows the posterior bony column disruptions* ➡ *but MR best shows the ligamentous injuries* ⇨. (Right) *Axial fused Tc-99m SPECT-CT through the lumbosacral junction shows increased radiotracer uptake on the right* ⇨ *due to spondylolysis.*

Myelomeningocele

KEY FACTS

IMAGING

- Open neural tube defect leading to Chiari II malformation
- Fetal US/MR: Lumbosacral dysraphism with thin-walled, fluid-filled myelomeningocele sac + intracranial findings of Chiari II (lemon sign, banana sign, ± ventriculomegaly)
- Postnatal spine MR performed after repair
  - Soft tissue now covers defect
  - Neural placode (distal nonneurulated segment of cord) inserts onto dorsal aspect of covered distal thecal sac
  - Elongation of spinal cord (low conus) persists
  - Posterior osseous dysraphic defects persist
- Serial head US to follow ventricular size after spine repair
  - ~ 80-85% have hydrocephalus requiring CSF diversion, though lower incidence reported after fetal repair

PATHOLOGY

- Failure of neural tube closure during 4th gestational week
- Association with maternal folate deficiency or abnormal folate metabolism

CLINICAL ISSUES

- Most common neurologic deficits: Lower extremities, bowel & bladder dysfunction; higher level spine defect correlates with greater motor & somatosensory deficits
- Deficits typically stabilize following repair & CSF diversion
  - Subsequent neurological deterioration prompts imaging evaluation for other findings such as dural ring constriction, cord ischemia, syringohydromyelia, dermoid/epidermoid, arachnoid cyst, brainstem compression, shunt malfunction
- Mortality: 10-30% die before adulthood
- Interventions
  - Folate supplementation to pregnant/conceiving women
  - Myelomeningocele closure < 48 hours after delivery to stabilize neurologic deficits & prevent infection
  - In utero surgical repair: ↓ need for shunting, ↓ Chiari II findings; may improve neurologic function
  - Management of postoperative complications
    - Cord untethering, CSF diversion

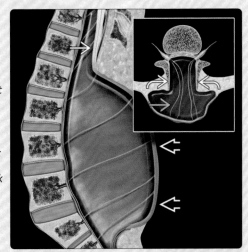
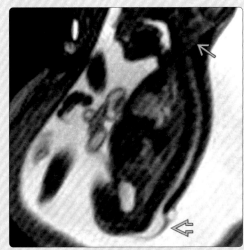

(Left) Sagittal graphic shows ballooning of the meninges & neural placode through a dysraphic spinal defect. The low-lying spinal cord ➡ terminates in the exposed neural placode ➡. Axial insert shows the origin of spinal roots ➡ from the ventral placode as well as the protrusion of the meninges & placode through the dysraphic posterior elements ➡. (Right) Sagittal SSFP MR of a 22-week gestation fetus with a lumbosacral myelomeningocele ➡ also shows posterior fossa findings of a Chiari II malformation ➡.

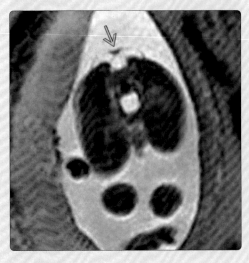
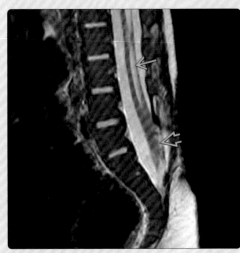

(Left) Axial T2 SSFSE MR from the same 22-week gestation fetus with a lumbosacral myelomeningocele shows the neural placode ➡ (or nonneurulated distal cord) exposed along the dorsal surface of the myelomeningocele sac. (Right) Sagittal T2 MR of the spine in the same patient at 6 months of age shows postoperative changes from the myelomeningocele repair with persistent elongation of the spinal cord (i.e., a low conus) ➡. This patient developed a spinal cord syrinx ➡, which is a common complication.

Dorsal Dermal Sinus

TERMINOLOGY

- Midline/paramidline subcutaneous sinus tract extending from skin surface toward spinal canal
- Located anywhere along neuraxis from cranium to intergluteal cleft; most common location (~ 70%) in lumbosacral region above intergluteal cleft

IMAGING

- US for screening young infant; MR if abnormal or older
- Linear midline/paramidline tract in subcutaneous tissues
- Terminates anywhere from subcutaneous tissues (blind-ending) to spine (epidural, intradural/intrathecal, or even intramedullary)
- ± epidermoid/dermoid cysts along tract (~ 50%)
- ± tethered cord with low-lying conus medullaris, intradural lipoma, split cord malformation

TOP DIFFERENTIAL DIAGNOSES

- Coccygeal pit/simple sacral dimple

- Pilonidal sinus/cyst
- Epidermoid/dermoid without sinus tract
- Lipomyelomeningocele (or other closed dysraphisms)

CLINICAL ISSUES

- Presentations include
  - Asymptomatic with incidentally noted skin dimple above intergluteal cleft ± cutaneous stigmata
    - Hyperpigmentation, capillary malformation/stain, or hypertrichosis
  - Infection (e.g., meningitis, abscess)
  - Neurologic deficits from cord tethering or compression
    - Higher lesions have higher association with tethered cord syndrome or (epi)dermoid with progressive dysfunction of lower limbs & bladder
- Dorsal dermal sinus typically requires excision of entire tract
  - Intraspinal extension may be occult on imaging (necessitating operative exploration of dura)

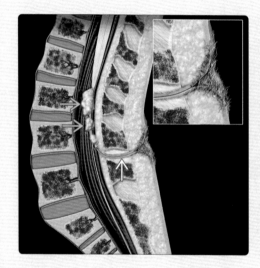
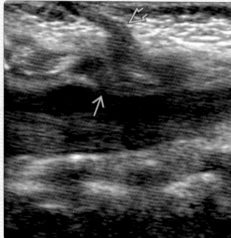

(Left) Sagittal graphic shows a dermal sinus ➡ extending from the skin surface into the spinal canal to terminate with epidermoid cysts ➡ at the conus medullaris. In this case, the sinus opening is marked by a skin dimple with a hairy tuft & capillary stain. (Right) Sagittal ultrasound of the spine in an infant with a cutaneous lumbar dimple demonstrates a hypoechoic dorsal dermal sinus tract ➡ in the subcutaneous tissues. A dural defect ➡ confirms communication of the tract with the thecal sac & subarachnoid space.

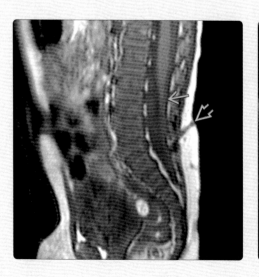
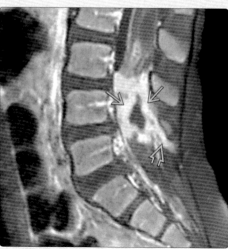

(Left) Sagittal T1 MR in the same patient shows a T1 hypointense dorsal dermal sinus tract ➡ in the subcutaneous tissues. The conus medullaris ➡ is low lying at the L3-4 disc space level. No associated intraspinal mass or cyst was identified. (Right) Sagittal T1 C+ FS MR in the same patient at 3 years of age demonstrates the interval development of a rim-enhancing intraspinal abscess ➡. Note that there is also enhancement along the dorsal dermal sinus tract ➡ entering the spinal canal.

Tethered Spinal Cord

TERMINOLOGY

- Tethered cord syndrome: Clinical diagnosis; imaging in specific screening circumstances or to detect associated anomalies for surgical planning

IMAGING

- Features that may occur with tethering
  - Conus below L2-3 disc level, appearing taut or directly apposed to dorsal thecal sac
    - Lack of conus motion with CSF pulsations
    - Lack of dependent ventral shift of conus when prone
  - Filum > 2-mm thick (at L5-S1 on axial/transverse images)
  - ± echogenic (US) or T1 bright (MR) fatty mass at conus
  - ± bony/soft tissue dysraphism
- Clinical tethering may be present despite normal conus
- Ultrasound to screen infants (< 6 months old) at ↑ risk of spinal anomalies (as suggested by certain cutaneous stigmata or associated systemic anomalies)

- MR to define underlying anomalies for surgical planning in symptomatic older patients

CLINICAL ISSUES

- Cutaneous stigmata in up to 50%
  - Hairy patch, hemangioma, skin tag, atypical dimple
  - Tethering also found in clinically apparent open & closed spinal dysraphism
- Signs & symptoms of tethering: Lower extremity weakness, spasticity, ↓ sensation, ↓ reflexes, bladder dysfunction
- Symptomatic presentation most common during rapid growth (4-8 years of age & adolescent growth spurt)
- Symptomatic patients: Early prophylactic surgery
  - Resect mass (if present), release cord, & repair dura
  - Majority show improvement or stabilization of neurological deficits following surgical untethering
- Asymptomatic patients with radiologic tethering: Management controversial

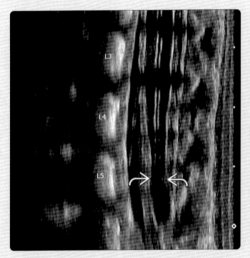

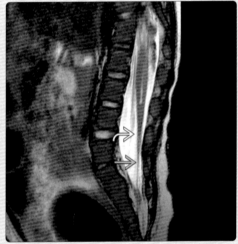

(Left) Sagittal ultrasound of the lumbar spine in an 8-day-old infant with VACTERL association shows that the conus medullaris ➤ extends caudally to the level of L5-S1. The conus remains dorsally positioned despite the patient being prone. (Right) Sagittal T2 MR in the same child again shows the inferior position of the conus ➤ with a thickened filum terminale ➡, findings that suggest tethering. No mass is identified. Up to 40% of children with VACTERL association will be diagnosed with a tethered spinal cord.

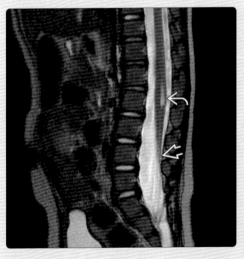

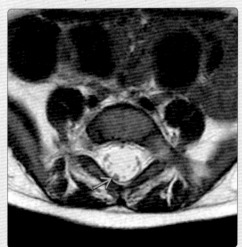

(Left) Sagittal T2 MR in a 5 month old with a cutaneous birthmark over the lower spine shows an abnormally low & dorsal position of the conus medullaris ➤. The mild prominence of the distal spinal cord central canal ➤ is a ventriculus terminalis, a normal finding in infants. (Right) Axial T2 MR at the level of L5-S1 in the same infant further demonstrates the abnormal thickening of the filum terminale ➡, which is directly apposed to the dorsal aspect of the thecal sac. These imaging findings are typical of tethering.

Sacrococcygeal Teratoma

TERMINOLOGY

- Teratomas made up of various parenchymal cell types from > 1 germ layer, usually all 3
- Sacrococcygeal teratoma (SCT) arises from coccyx
- Both benign & malignant (17%) varieties of SCT

IMAGING

- SCT always has presacral components; external/exophytic extension more common than internal growth
- Heterogeneous solid & cystic masses
  - Ca^{2+}, fat, hemorrhage, cysts, various soft tissues in mass
  - ± moderate to high vascularity of solid components
- MR best for identifying intraspinal extension

PATHOLOGY

- American Academy of Pediatrics Surgery Section classification
  - Type I (47%): Primarily external in location

- Type II (34%): Dumbbell shape, equal pelvic & external components
- Type III (9%): Primarily located within abdomen/pelvis
- Type IV (10%): Entirely internal, no external component
- Currarino triad: Presacral mass (SCT or anterior meningocele), anorectal malformation, sacral anomalies

CLINICAL ISSUES

- Presentation varies from large external tumor diagnosed in utero (requiring prenatal intervention or revised delivery plan) to entirely internal mass with delayed diagnosis due to urinary symptoms & constipation
  - Prognosis excellent for benign tumors found at birth
  - Fetal SCT can be quite vascular & grow rapidly → hydrops, intratumoral hemorrhage, rupture → demise
    - Hydrops before 30-week gestation > 90% mortality
  - Malignant characteristics ↑ with age, type IV
- Complete surgical resection must include coccyx
- 5-15% risk of recurrence

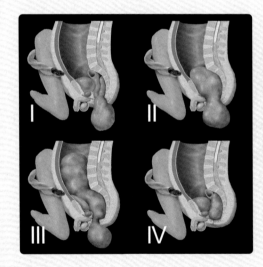
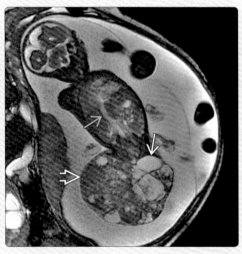

(Left) Graphics show the SCT classification scheme: Type I is primarily exophytic, type II has internal & external masses of similar size, type III has a larger intraabdominal component, & type IV is entirely internal. (Right) Coronal SSFP MR of a twin gestation shows a fetus with a large, predominantly exophytic SCT extending from the perineum. Note the solid ➡ & cystic ➡ foci within the mass. The inferior vena cava ➡ is prominent due to the amount of blood flow coursing through this tumor. However, no hydrops is seen.

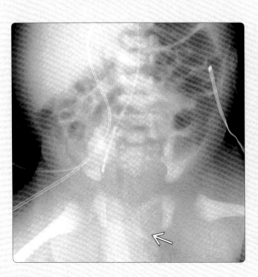
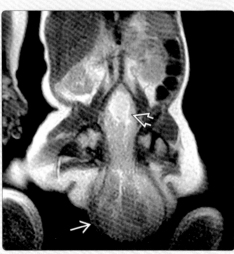

(Left) AP radiograph in a newborn boy with a protruding buttock mass shows soft tissue fullness in the pelvis & perineum with irregular Ca^{2+} ➡ below the pubic bones. (Right) Coronal T2 MR in the same infant shows a heterogeneous solid mass that protrudes externally ➡ & has dumbbell extension internally ➡, splaying the aortic bifurcation in this case of a type II SCT.

TERMINOLOGY

- Bacterial suppurative infection of intervertebral disc & adjacent vertebrae

IMAGING

- Disc-centered process: Disc space narrowing & adjacent endplate irregularity in young children
  - Lumbosacral (75%) > thoracic > cervical spine
- Early: MR imaging most sensitive, specific modality
  - Abnormal disc signal & enhancement
  - Ill-defined abnormal marrow signal & enhancement
  - Paraspinal & epidural phlegmon or abscess
- Subacute
  - Endplate destruction/erosion
- Chronic
  - Increased bone density ± vertebral fusion with healing

TOP DIFFERENTIAL DIAGNOSES

- Langerhans cell histiocytosis
- Spinal metastases
- Chronic recurrent multifocal osteomyelitis (CRMO)
- Degenerative endplate changes

PATHOLOGY

- Hematogenous spread to vascularized disc or subchondral vertebral growth plate in children
- *Staphylococcus aureus* is most common pathogen

CLINICAL ISSUES

- Peak age: 6 months to 4 years
- Variable & nonspecific symptoms (which may delay diagnosis for weeks in children)
  - Difficulty walking, back/hip pain, fever (< 50%)
- Elevated ESR, CRP, WBC
- Treat with empiric IV antibiotics with broad-spectrum coverage until causative pathogen isolated, then organism-specific parenteral antibiotics for 6-8 weeks

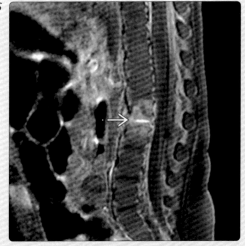

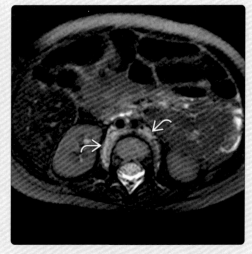

(Left) *Midline sagittal T1 C+ FS MR in a 7 month old shows poor definition & abnormal enhancement of the L2-3 disc space ➡. Patchy abnormal enhancement is also noted in the marrow of the adjoining vertebral bodies. No drainable collection is identified within the adjacent paraspinal soft tissues or epidural space.* (Right) *Axial T2 MR in the same patient shows abnormal thickening & poorly defined fluid signal in the anterior & lateral paraspinal soft tissues ➡ in this patient with spondylodiscitis.*

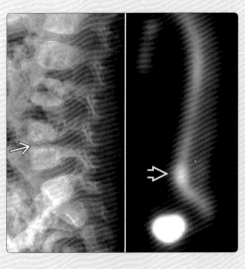

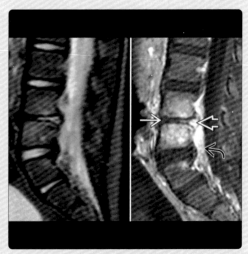

(Left) *Lateral radiograph (left) shows L4-5 disc space narrowing ➡ & endplate irregularity in this 1 year old with back pain. Sagittal SPECT bone scan (right) confirms abnormal uptake ➡ in the vertebral bodies, typical of spondylodiscitis.* (Right) *Sagittal STIR (left) & T1 C+ FS (right) MR images in a 2 year old show disc space narrowing ➡ & enhancement ➡ with abnormal signal/enhancement of the L4-5 vertebral marrow. Enhancing soft tissue in the epidural space ➡ is due to contiguous inflammation.*

TERMINOLOGY

Definitions

- Bacterial suppurative infection of intervertebral disc & adjacent vertebrae

IMAGING

Radiographic Findings

- Radiography
  - Negative up to 2-8 weeks after onset of symptoms
  - Initial endplate & vertebral osteolysis
  - Loss of disc space height
  - Increased bone density ± intervertebral fusion with successful treatment
  - Total vertebral destruction/collapse with treatment delay/failure

MR Findings

- Abnormal disc space
  - Loss of normal disc height, signal, & morphology
  - Diffuse or rim enhancement with contrast
- Vertebral marrow signal abnormality abutting disc
  - Poorly defined increased fluid signal, most conspicuous on FS T2 or STIR images
  - Typically enhances with contrast unless necrotic
- Paraspinal & epidural phlegmon or abscess
  - Poorly defined fluid signal & stranding of fat
  - Diffuse enhancement vs. rim-enhancing collections
- Follow-up: No single MR finding predicts clinical status
  - Abnormal imaging persists for months, does not necessarily equate to residual/recurrent infection

Nuclear Medicine Findings

- Bone scan
  - Increased uptake can localize nonspecific signs & symptoms

Imaging Recommendations

- Best imaging tool
  - MR provides excellent diagnostic detail
  - Nuclear medicine bone scan can localize nonspecific signs & symptoms
- Protocol advice
  - STIR or FS T2 MR for marrow & soft tissue involvement
  - FS T1 C+ MR to evaluate for drainable paraspinal & epidural fluid collections

DIFFERENTIAL DIAGNOSIS

Langerhans Cell Histiocytosis

- Enhancing marrow lesion ± lytic destruction, enhancing soft tissue mass; disc sparing
- Single level vs. noncontiguous multifocal involvement
- Collapse of vertebra → vertebra plana

Chronic Recurrent Multifocal Osteomyelitis

- Autoimmune inflammatory disorder of bone
- Little disc involvement

Spinal Metastases

- Rare in children → neuroblastoma, leukemia
- Marrow abnormalities with disc space preservation

Degenerative Changes

- Rare in children
- Normal marrow ± vertebral endplate preservation

PATHOLOGY

General Features

- Etiology
  - Pathophysiology
    - Intervertebral disc & vertebral growth plates highly vascularized in young children
    - Hematogenous seeding of intervertebral disc/subchondral bone most common source
      □ Lumbosacral (75%) > thoracic > cervical spine
  - Most common pathogen: *Staphylococcus aureus*

CLINICAL ISSUES

Presentation

- Clinical profile
  - Peak age range: 6 months to 4 years
  - Clinical symptoms variable & nonspecific in children
    - Difficulty walking, back/hip pain, fever (< 50%), irritability
  - Elevated ESR, CRP, WBC

Treatment

- Early empiric IV antibiotics, broad-spectrum coverage until causative pathogen isolated
- Organism-specific parenteral antibiotics for 6-8 weeks
- Spinal immobilization with bracing for 6-12 weeks
- CT-guided or open biopsy may be indicated if blood cultures negative & conservative treatment fails
- Surgery rarely indicated except in advanced infection

DIAGNOSTIC CHECKLIST

Image Interpretation Pearls

- Disc-centered process: Abnormal morphology, signal, & enhancement of disc & adjacent marrow is highly suggestive of discitis/osteomyelitis in children

SELECTED REFERENCES

1. Principi N et al: Infectious siscitis and spondylodiscitis in children. Int J Mol Sci. 17(4):539, 2016
2. Fucs PM et al: Spinal infections in children: a review. Int Orthop. 36(2):387-95, 2012
3. Spencer SJ et al: Childhood discitis in a regional children's hospital. J Pediatr Orthop B. 21(3):264-8, 2012
4. Treglia G et al: The role of nuclear medicine in the diagnosis of spondylodiscitis. Eur Rev Med Pharmacol Sci. 16 Suppl 2:20-5, 2012
5. Chandrasenan J et al: Spondylodiscitis in children: a retrospective series. J Bone Joint Surg Br. 93(8):1122-5, 2011
6. Dunbar JA et al: The MRI appearances of early vertebral osteomyelitis and discitis. Clin Radiol. 65(12):974-81, 2010
7. de Lucas EM et al: CT-guided fine-needle aspiration in vertebral osteomyelitis: true usefulness of a common practice. Clin Rheumatol. 28(3):315-20, 2009
8. Kowalski TJ et al: Follow-up MR imaging in patients with pyogenic spine infections: lack of correlation with clinical features. AJNR Am J Neuroradiol. 28(4):693-9, 2007
9. Ledermann HP et al: MR imaging findings in spinal infections: rules or myths? Radiology. 228(2):506-14, 2003

Guillain-Barré Syndrome

TERMINOLOGY

- Group of disorders characterized by acute onset of weakness & diminished reflexes secondary to inflammatory polyradiculopathy; diagnosis primarily clinical

IMAGING

- Smooth pial enhancement of cauda equina & conus medullaris: Ventral roots > dorsal roots
  - May be slightly thickened but not nodular
- May see cranial nerve enhancement

PATHOLOGY

- Inflammatory immune-mediated demyelination
- Antecedent event or "trigger" in 70% of Guillain-Barré syndrome cases
  - *Campylobacter jejuni* or CMV infection
  - Temporal link has been suggested with vaccines but no correlation has been shown
- Many variants/subtypes, including
  - Acute inflammatory demyelinating polyradiculoneuropathy: Most common form in USA
  - Acute motor axonal neuropathy: Pure motor form
  - Miller-Fisher variant (~ 5%): Ophthalmoplegia, ataxia, areflexia, normal extremity strength

CLINICAL ISSUES

- Acute flaccid paralysis or distal paraesthesias rapidly followed by ascending paralysis
  - Ascent up to brainstem may involve cranial nerves
    - Uncommon descending pattern mimics botulism
  - Autonomic disturbances & absence of reflexes common
  - Sensory loss common but less severe
- Treated medically with plasma exchange or intravenous immunoglobulin (IVIg)
  - Prolonged respiratory support in severe cases
- Most patients somewhat better by 2-3 months; 30-50% have persistent symptoms at 1 year; relapse in 2-10%

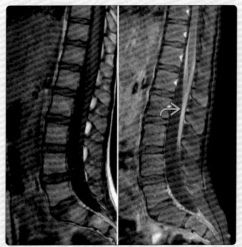
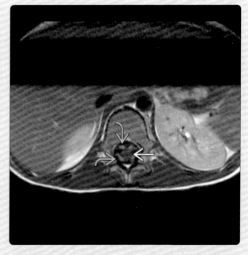

(Left) *Sagittal T1 (left) & T1 C+ FS (right) MR images show marked enhancement of the cauda equina nerve roots ⮕ in this 10-year-old patient with Guillain-Barré syndrome (GBS).* (Right) *Axial T1 C+ MR in the same patient shows a striking degree of enhancement of the nerves ⮕ relative to the conus medullaris ⮕. Some nerve root enhancement can be normal, but this degree is not physiologic.*

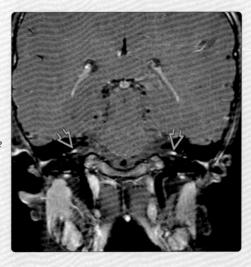
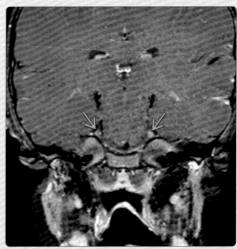

(Left) *Coronal T1 C+ FS MR through the internal auditory canals in a 3-year-old patient with the Miller-Fisher variant of GBS shows abnormal enhancement of the facial nerve on each side ⮕.* (Right) *Coronal T1 C+ FS MR more anteriorly in the same patient shows bilateral & symmetric abnormal enhancement of the trigeminal nerves ⮕.*

Transverse Myelitis

TERMINOLOGY

- Poorly understood inflammatory disorder of spinal cord resulting in bilateral motor, sensory, & autonomic dysfunction
- Requires exclusion of other definable causes of spinal cord inflammation: Neuromyelitis optica, multiple sclerosis (MS), acute disseminated encephalomyelitis, Lyme disease

IMAGING

- Normal imaging in up to 40%
- Thoracic more common than cervical cord
- > 2 vertebral segments in length (often much longer)
- Smooth cord expansion with CSF effacement
- Bright cord signal on T2 MR
  - Involves > 2/3 of cross-sectional area of cord
  - Centrally located with peripheral cord sparing
- No enhancement in up to 1/2 of cases
- Affected cord may atrophy over time

PATHOLOGY

- Clinical syndrome that can be idiopathic or associated with systemic disease or prodrome; no etiology in 1/3

CLINICAL ISSUES

- 2 age peaks: 10-19 & 30-39 years old
- Prodrome of viral-like illness with rapid progression to maximal neurologic deficits in days
- Signs & symptoms bilateral with well-defined sensory level, band-like dysesthesia, loss of pain & temperature sensation, paraplegia or quadriplegia, bladder & bowel dysfunction; hypotonia → spasticity & hyperreflexia over time
  - Cord inflammation confirmed by CSF pleocytosis, elevated IgG index, or gadolinium enhancement
- Treated with high-dose intravenous steroid pulse therapy; plasmapheresis for cases that fail to respond
  - Recovery variable: 1/3 good, 1/3 fair, 1/3 poor
- Typically monophasic; recurrence rate between 24-40%
  - Must consider MS with recurrence

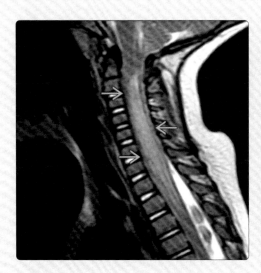

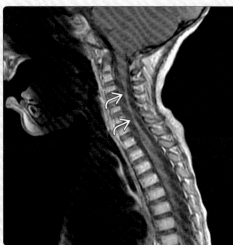

(Left) Sagittal T2 MR in a 2 year old who developed quadriparesis 6 days after receiving an influenza vaccine shows swelling & hyperintense signal of the cervical & upper thoracic cord with effacement of the subarachnoid CSF spaces at the cervical levels ➡. (Right) Sagittal T1 C+ MR in the same patient 7 months after presentation shows marked atrophy of the cervical cord ➡. Up to 1/3 of patients with transverse myelitis will have persistent fixed neurological deficits, usually accompanied by imaging abnormalities.

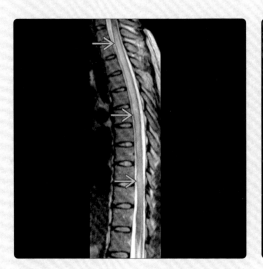

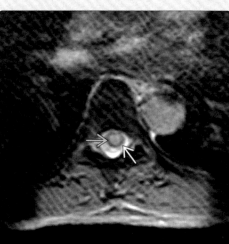

(Left) Sagittal T2 MR shows a long segment of abnormal hyperintensity & expansion ➡ of the visualized spinal cord, characteristic of transverse myelitis. (Right) Axial T2* GRE MR in the same patient shows diffuse hyperintensity ➡ within the central cord. Note the peripheral sparing ➡ of the cord, a typical appearance of transverse myelitis.

TERMINOLOGY

- Traumatic injury to upper cervical region: Occiput to C2

IMAGING

- Normal cervical spine measurements in adults may not translate to children due to dynamic skeletal changes in early life
- Radiography: Initial screening test of choice
  - \> 20% of cervical fractures missed by radiography alone
  - 10% of craniocervical junction (CCJ) fractures shown by CT, not radiography
  - Remember entity of Spinal Cord Injury WithOut Radiographic Abnormality (SCIWORA)
- CT: Asymmetry & ↑ joint space measurements; ± retroclival hematoma & perimedullary hemorrhage
- MR: Ligament disruption; edema/hemorrhage of spinal cord, bone marrow, & soft tissues
- MRA: ± vertebral artery injury (often clinically occult)

CLINICAL ISSUES

- Injury at CCJ most common in 1st decade
  - Disproportionate head size, ligamentous laxity, & immature muscles may contribute
- Neurological status at presentation predicts outcome
- Atlantooccipital dissociation: Many die prior to reaching medical care; 25-30% neurologically intact at presentation
- Jefferson (C1) fracture: Axial loading injury (e.g., diving)
- Odontoid & hangman fractures: Flexion or extension with distraction (usually motor vehicle accident)
- Rotational injuries: Present with painful torticollis; may have little or no trauma antecedent
- Treatment
  - Temporary stabilization to prevent further injury
    - Correct stabilization prevents iatrogenic injury
  - Emergent decompression of spinal cord impingement
  - Internal or external surgical stabilization
  - Steroids for acute cord injury no longer recommended

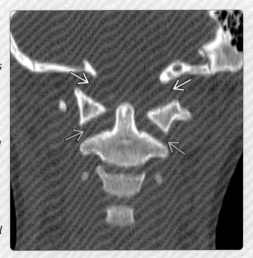
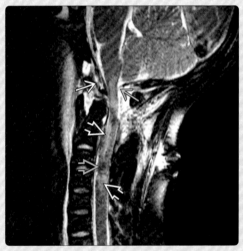

(Left) *Coronal NECT in a 9-year-old girl after a motor vehicle accident shows an increase of the condyle-C1 intervals* ➡ *& the lateral mass intervals* ➡, *consistent with severe atlantooccipital dissociation (AOD) & atlantoaxial dissociation.* (Right) *Sagittal STIR MR in the same patient shows disruption of the tectorial membrane* ➡ *& complete transection of the posterior atlantooccipital ligament* ➡. *The spinal cord shows areas of hyperintense signal (likely contusion)* ➡ *as well as a few foci of low signal (possibly hemorrhage)* ➡.

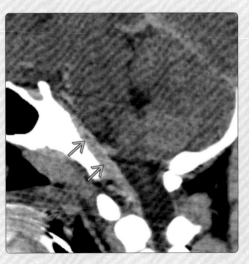
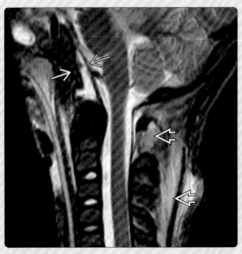

(Left) *Sagittal NECT in a 7-year-old girl involved in a motor vehicle accident shows a hyperintense collection (hemorrhage)* ➡ *between the clivus & the tectorial membrane. A retroclival hematoma indicates AOD until proven otherwise.* (Right) *Sagittal STIR MR in the same patient shows that the linear hypointense tectorial membrane* ➡ *has been lifted off the clivus* ➡. *Also note the extensive abnormal signal in the posterior neck soft tissues* ➡, *suggestive of a severe flexion-related injury. The spinal cord appears normal.*

Chance Fracture

TERMINOLOGY

- Synonyms: Flexion-distraction injury, seat belt fracture
- Definition: Compression injury of anterior column of spine with distraction of middle & posterior columns
  - Anterior column: Anterior longitudinal ligament, anterior 1/2 of vertebral body, anterior annulus fibrosis
  - Middle column: Posterior longitudinal ligament, posterior 1/2 of vertebral body, posterior annulus fibrosis
  - Posterior column: Posterior neural arch, facet joint capsular ligaments, ligamentum flavum, inter- & supraspinous ligaments
- May be completely osseous, ligamentous (rare "Chance equivalent"), or mixed (most frequent)
- 3-column extension may invoke adjacent levels

IMAGING

- 78% occur between T12-L2
- Wedging of anterior vertebral body

- Posterior bony & ligamentous distraction injuries result in
  - Focal kyphosis
  - Wide "splitting" of pedicles & laminae on AP view
  - Separation of facet joints with ↑ interspinous distance
  - Artifactual ↑ in radiolucency of vertebral body on AP radiograph secondary to splayed spinous processes

CLINICAL ISSUES

- Traumatic back pain ± neurologic injury
- Classic history: Motor vehicle collision with lap belt restraint & cutaneous seat belt sign over abdomen
  - Up to 40% have 3-point restraint (not just lap belt)
- Up to 80% have significant abdominal injuries
  - Bowel/mesentery (most common), aorta
- Osseous injury acutely unstable
  - Bracing vs. fixation if reduction not maintained
- Osteoligamentous or purely ligamentous injuries
  - Poor prognosis for healing unless fusion performed

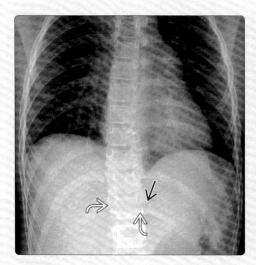

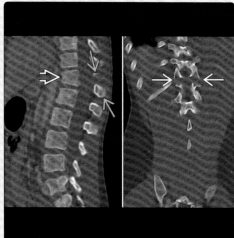

(Left) AP chest radiograph of a teenager injured in a motor vehicle collision while wearing a seat belt shows a horizontal lucency splitting the T12 pedicles ➡ with widening of the costovertebral joints ➡, indicative of a Chance fracture. (Right) Sagittal (left) & coronal (right) bone windowed CECT images in the same patient show anterior wedging of the T12 vertebral body ➡ with a horizontal fracture plane "splitting" the posterior elements ➡. Note the splaying/distraction of the T12 spinous process fragments ➡.

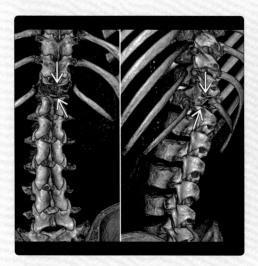

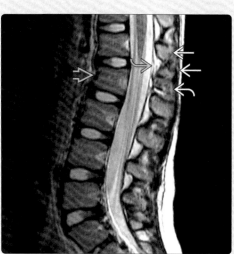

(Left) 3D posterior oblique CT images in the same patient clearly show the horizontal "splitting" & distraction of the T12 posterior elements ➡, characteristic of the posterior column injury in a Chance fracture. (Right) Sagittal T2 MR in a 7 year old shows mild anterior wedging of the L2 vertebra ➡ with disruption of the ligamentum flavum ➡, interspinous ligaments ➡, & L1 posterior elements ➡.

Spondylolysis and Spondylolisthesis

TERMINOLOGY

- Spondylolysis: Defect/break in pars interarticularis
- Spondylolisthesis: Spondylolysis + anterior slippage of vertebra in relation to vertebra below

IMAGING

- Radiographs (insensitive): Break in neck of "Scotty dog" (pars interarticularis defect on oblique standing views of lumbar spine)
- Bone CT
  - Linear lucency or defect in pars interarticularis
    - Sagittal or oblique sagittal reformatted imaging vital in assessment
  - Incomplete ring sign on axial imaging ± distraction
  - Spondylolisthesis & foraminal narrowing on sagittal reformatted images
  - Secondary finding of sclerosis &/or hypertrophy of contralateral pedicle & lamina
- SPECT bone scan imaging helpful for diagnosis
  - Intense focal uptake in posterior elements, unilateral or bilateral
  - Remote or healed may be occult (normal)
- SPECT/CT: Confirms diagnosis with anatomy & physiology
- MR: ↑ conspicuity of marrow & soft tissue edema with fat suppressed fluid-sensitive techniques

PATHOLOGY

- Repetitive microtrauma results in stress fracture
  - Participation in gymnastics, weightlifting, wrestling, cricket, & American football at young age
  - L5 affected in 85%, L4 in 5-15%

CLINICAL ISSUES

- Asymptomatic (80%); back pain (exacerbated by rigorous activities), back spasms, &/or radiating pain
- 40% incidence in children with lower back pain
- Therapy mainly conservative; surgical if conservative treatment fails or subluxation progresses

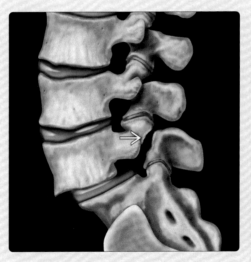
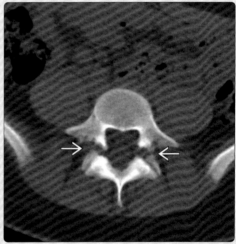

(Left) Lateral graphic shows a defect within the pars interarticularis (spondylolysis) at L5 ➡. Notice the resultant anterior slippage (spondylolisthesis) of L5 on S1. (Right) Axial NECT in a 14-year-old girl who presents with severe left flank pain for a renal stone evaluation shows an incomplete ring with bilateral distracted pars interarticularis defects ➡ (spondylolysis) at L5.

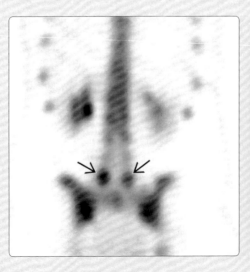
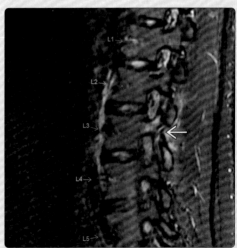

(Left) Coronal SPECT bone scan in a 15 year old who presents with lower back pain shows asymmetric uptake ➡ in the posterior elements of L5, right > left. NECT images (not shown) demonstrated right L5 spondylolysis with reactive stress changes at the left L5 pars interarticularis. (Right) Sagittal STIR MR in 14 year old with back pain shows a pars defect ➡ with edema in the marrow of the posterior elements & adjacent soft tissues. STIR images can be helpful in detecting marrow edema associated with spondylolysis.

IMAGING

General Features

- Location
  - L5: 85%; L4: 5-15%
  - Cervical spine usually congenital
  - 10-15% unilateral

Radiographic Findings

- Classic: Break in neck of "Scotty dog" (pars interarticularis defect on oblique views of standing lumbar spine)
  - ± anterolisthesis
  - Positive predictive value of 57%

CT Findings

- Bone CT: Linear lucency or defect in pars interarticularis
  - Sagittal or oblique sagittal reformatted imaging vital in assessment
  - Incomplete ring sign on axial imaging ± distraction

MR Findings

- T2WI: ↓ signal in pars interarticularis (reactive sclerosis), ↑ signal in pars interarticularis (marrow edema)
- STIR/T2 FS: ↑ conspicuity of surrounding marrow & soft tissue edema, suggesting spondylolysis at classic location even if fracture not seen
- MR for lysis: Sensitivity: 57-86%; specificity: 81-82%

Nuclear Medicine Findings

- ↑ uptake best seen on SPECT bone scan

Imaging Recommendations

- Best imaging tool
  - If suspicious for this diagnosis
    - Targeted helical/volumetric bone CT with multiplanar reformats
    - Bone scan SPECT/CT better than SPECT alone
      - □ Anatomic & physiologic confirmation
  - If source of back pain not clear, MR may be more beneficial
    - Include STIR or T2 FS for marrow & soft tissue edema

DIFFERENTIAL DIAGNOSIS

Spectrum of Radiologic Findings in Back Pain

- Musculoskeletal
  - Normal (muscular)
  - Scoliosis, vertebral or sacral fracture, spinous process avulsion, Baastrup disease, facet degeneration, Bertolotti syndrome, degenerative disc disease, ring apophyseal injury, Scheuermann disease
- Infection
  - Discitis, osteomyelitis, sacroiliitis, paraspinal inflammation/abscess, pyelonephritis, pelvic inflammatory disease
- Tumor
  - Osteoid osteoma, osteoblastoma, Langerhans cell histiocytosis, leukemia, lymphoma, metastatic disease, neurofibroma
- Inflammatory
  - Ankylosing spondylitis, psoriatic arthritis, inflammatory bowel disease

PATHOLOGY

General Features

- Etiology
  - Believed to be caused by repetitive microtrauma, resulting in stress fracture
  - Participation in gymnastics, weightlifting, wrestling, cricket, & football at young age
- Associated abnormalities
  - Spondylolisthesis (50%), scoliosis, Scheuermann disease, spina bifida occulta

CLINICAL ISSUES

Presentation

- Most common signs/symptoms
  - Asymptomatic (80%)
  - 40% incidence in children with lower back pain
- Other signs/symptoms
  - Tight hamstring muscles
    - Waddling gait secondary to tight hamstring muscles
  - Back spasms or radiating pain
  - Back pain exacerbated by rigorous activities
  - Radiculopathy & cauda equina syndrome with high-grade spondylolisthesis

Demographics

- Gender
  - M:F = 2-4:1
- Epidemiology
  - Incidence: 3-6% of Caucasian population
  - Higher incidence in competitive athletes, especially male patients

Treatment

- Mainly conservative 1st; surgical if conservative treatment fails or subluxation progresses

DIAGNOSTIC CHECKLIST

Image Interpretation Pearls

- Sagittal or oblique sagittal bone CT reformats & sagittal STIR/T2 FS MR images are most important for diagnosis
- Identify complete ring at each lumbar level on axial bone CT or MR
- Typical bone scan findings with normal radiographs or bone CT suggest stress reaction or early spondylolysis

SELECTED REFERENCES

1. Nitta A et al: Prevalence of symptomatic lumbar spondylolysis in pediatric patients. Orthopedics. 39(3):E434-7, 2016
2. Bouras T et al: Management of spondylolysis and low-grade spondylolisthesis in fine athletes. a comprehensive review. Eur J Orthop Surg Traumatol. 25 Suppl 1:S167-75, 2015
3. Gum JL et al: Characteristics associated with active defects in juvenile spondylolysis. Am J Orthop (Belle Mead NJ). 44(10):E379-83, 2015
4. Leonidou A et al: Treatment for spondylolysis and spondylolisthesis in children. J Orthop Surg (Hong Kong). 23(3):379-82, 2015
5. Trout AT et al: Spondylolysis and beyond: value of SPECT/CT in evaluation of low back pain in children and young adults. Radiographics. 35(3):819-34, 2015

SECTION 9
Head and Neck

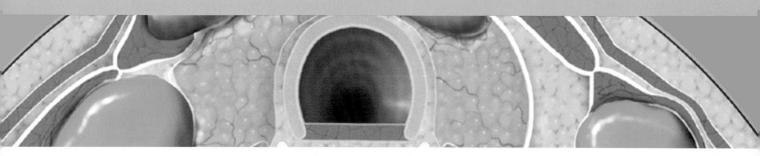

Imaging Modalities

Note that the airway, spine, & skull are largely discussed in other sections.

Radiography

Plain films of the face have limited indications in children. They are often used as a quick screening tool for sinus disease or facial trauma. However, their sensitivity & specificity are low, particularly when the clinical suspicion is low (which is often when such studies are ordered, unfortunately).

Regarding the neck, radiographs are most useful in the initial assessments of the airway & cervical spine (both of which are discussed in separate chapters). It should be remembered that radiographs can be a useful tool in looking for lodged foreign bodies, though many ingested items (such as toys & food) will not be radiopaque.

Fluoroscopy

Contrast studies of the upper digestive tract may be of benefit with penetrating trauma of the oropharynx or in the setting of suspected swallowing dysfunction/aspiration.

Ultrasound

As with other regions of the body, sonography proves to be an excellent tool for the initial investigation of a palpable mass of the pediatric head or neck, be it cystic or solid. Common masses of the infant neck, including infantile hemangioma, lymphatic malformation (sometimes referred to as cystic hygroma), & fibromatosis colli, are readily diagnosed by radiologists experienced with pediatric ultrasound. However, large masses with deeper extension, or those with an unclear diagnosis by ultrasound, often require additional cross-sectional imaging with CECT or MR to determine the exact relationship of the lesion to the airway or spine.

In the setting of cervical adenitis, ultrasound can help distinguish enlarged hyperemic nodes vs. necrotic but not liquefied conglomerations vs. drainable abscesses. However, some locations of inflammatory collections (such as the peritonsillar & retropharyngeal regions) are better assessed by CECT.

Ultrasound provides an excellent visualization of the pediatric thyroid gland & should serve as the primary imaging modality for palpable abnormalities or thyroid dysfunction.

Doppler ultrasound provides an excellent assessment of the jugular veins & carotid arteries, though visualization will be limited approaching the skull base. Doppler is typically adequate to exclude thrombus in the vessels of the neck or upper chest (including the brachiocephalic & subclavian vessels), though the superior vena cava may not be fully visualized due to the sternum. In the setting of traumatic vascular injury, however, these time-consuming studies should be bypassed for a more rapid & sensitive assessment of the vessel (as performed with CT angiography)

Ultrasound has some role in evaluating the globes & orbits, but that is typically the domain of the ophthalmologist & will not be discussed here.

Computed Tomography

In the acute setting, when deeper infectious collections are suspected, CECT is the modality of choice as it clearly determines the relationship of the collection to the airway & demonstrates associated vascular complications. However, it can rarely have difficulty distinguishing a necrotic phlegmonous collection from drainable fluid.

In the setting of blunt trauma that causes concern for a vascular injury (such as a seat belt injury to the neck), CT angiography is the modality of choice. Depending on the clinical stability of the patient, penetrating trauma may also benefit from CT angiography, though mucosal injuries will not be well-demonstrated by any cross-sectional imaging study.

Bone CT has 3 important uses in the head & neck region. In the setting of significant orbital/facial/skull base trauma, it remains the gold standard imaging exam for detecting fractures. It also provides exquisite evaluation of the paranasal sinuses, which is useful in the difficult to diagnose patient, the patient with suspected sinusitis complications (where CECT may be necessary for orbital or intracranial processes), & the patient with chronic or recurrent sinus disease requiring operative management. Additionally, temporal bone imaging by CT remains critical to the evaluation of hearing loss by otolaryngologists.

CECT is now used less commonly in the evaluation of primary neck masses due to 2 concerns: 1st is the use of unnecessary radiation (when US &/or MR will often suffice prior to biopsy), & 2nd is the interference of iodinated contrast with thyroid cancer therapy. Regarding the latter, it is generally recommended that any neck mass that could be thyroid cancer not undergo CECT as the administered iodinated contrast will interfere with iodine uptake by the mass during subsequent nuclear medicine imaging & therapy, thus delaying treatment for weeks. CECT is still used in the evaluation of lymphoma of the neck as chest CT remains better than MR for detecting lung involvement.

Magnetic Resonance

Soft tissue masses not fully characterized by ultrasound should undergo evaluation by MR as MR will provide the best tissue characterization & assessment of extent compared to other modalities. Lesions that involve bone may require combination imaging with CT & MR due to their different strengths.

Nuclear Medicine

Nuclear studies of the neck are most commonly employed to evaluate the thyroid, either in the characterization of a thyroid nodule or the treatment of a known thyroid malignancy. PET studies are also used to stage & follow-up lymphoma, typically as part of a whole-body scan; the physiologic information provided by PET in these cases has substantial implications regarding therapy.

Selected References

1. ACR Appropriateness Criteria: Penetrating Neck Injury. https://acsearch.acr.org/docs/3099165/Narrative/. Published 2017. Accessed April 4, 2017
2. ACR Appropriateness Criteria: Sinusitis—Child. https://acsearch.acr.org/docs/69442/Narrative/. Published 1995. Reviewed 2012. Accessed April 4, 2017
3. Ho ML et al: The ABCs (airway, blood vessels, and compartments) of pediatric neck infections and masses. AJR Am J Roentgenol. 1-10, 2016
4. Friedman ER et al: Imaging of pediatric neck masses. Radiol Clin North Am. 49(4):617-32, v, 2011
5. Ludwig BJ et al: Diagnostic imaging in nontraumatic pediatric head and neck emergencies. Radiographics. 30(3):781-99, 2010

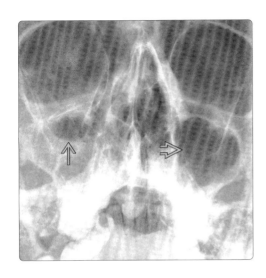

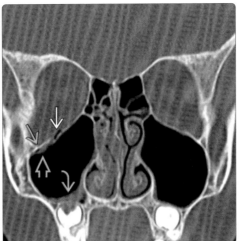

(Left) AP Waters view of the sinuses in a 17 year old shows an air-fluid level in the right maxillary sinus ⮑, consistent with acute sinusitis. The left maxillary sinus is clear ⮑. (Right) Coronal bone CT in an 8 year old after being hit by a baseball shows a bony lucency ⮑, herniated fat ⮑, intraorbital gas ➡, & maxillary sinus fluid ⮑ from a nondisplaced orbital floor fracture. These findings would likely not be seen on radiographs.

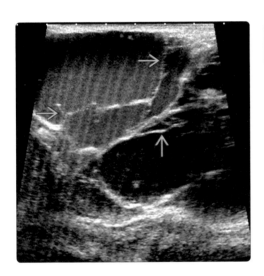

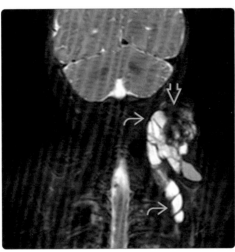

(Left) Transverse ultrasound through a compressible posterior neck mass in a newborn shows a large cystic mass with numerous thin septations ⮑ & no solid component, typical of a lymphatic malformation. The internal echogenicity of the fluid content varies in different compartments due to hemorrhagic debris. (Right) Coronal STIR MR of the same infant defines the craniocaudal & deep extent of the lesion ⮑. Thicker, lower signal components ⮑ in this case were due to internal hemorrhage.

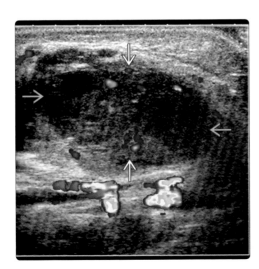

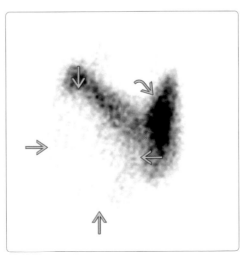

(Left) Longitudinal color Doppler ultrasound of the lateral neck in a 2 year old with fever shows partially necrotic lymph nodes with vascular flow ➡ still visible between the hypoechoic pockets ⮑. No swirling debris was seen upon compression to suggest drainable fluid. (Right) Anterior neck image from a radioiodine thyroid study in a 17 year old shows a large, "cold" nodule ⮑ (with no uptake) in the right lobe with normal uptake in the left lobe ⮑. This lesion was solid on ultrasound, & biopsy showed papillary carcinoma.

Acute Rhinosinusitis

TERMINOLOGY

- Acute inflammatory sinonasal process lasting ≤ 4 weeks
- Related terms: Acute bacterial sinusitis (ABS), viral upper respiratory infection (URI)

IMAGING

- Clinical diagnosis; imaging rarely necessary & does not distinguish bacterial from viral
- NECT: Confirms diagnosis, evaluates when medical therapy has failed, delineates anatomic variants (especially presurgical)
  - Best sign: Air-fluid level ± aerosolized secretions with mucosal thickening
    - Most common in ethmoid & maxillary sinuses
    - Often asymmetric sinus involvement
- CECT vs. MR: If complications suspected
- Radiography: Inaccurate, should be supplanted by CT

PATHOLOGY

- Most cases of ABS follow viral URI

CLINICAL ISSUES

- Signs/symptoms of sinusitis in children: Nasal drainage (± purulence), facial pain, fever, & cough
  - Viral URI: Signs/symptoms last < 10 days, do not progress; usually self-limited
  - ABS: Signs/symptoms for > 10 days (but < 4 weeks) without improvement; symptoms may worsen after initial improvement or be severe at onset
    - Imaging only with concern for complication (rare)
      - Orbital cellulitis, subperiosteal abscess, meningitis, epidural or subdural empyema, brain abscess, venous sinus thrombosis, subgaleal abscess (Pott puffy tumor)
- Treatment: ABS course may be shortened by saline irrigation & medical therapy (antibiotics); surgical drainage rarely required

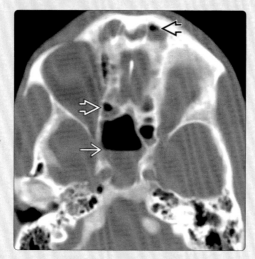
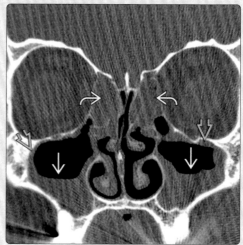

(Left) Axial NECT shows "pansinusitis" with air-fluid levels in the frontal ➡, ethmoid ➡, & sphenoid ➡ sinuses. (Right) Coronal bone CT shows acute bilateral maxillary & ethmoid sinusitis. Note the air-fluid levels ➡ & mucosal thickening ➡ in the maxillary sinuses with complete opacification of the ethmoid sinuses ➡.

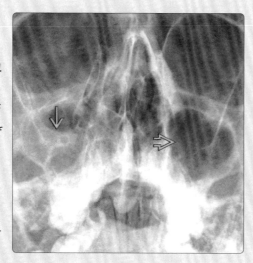
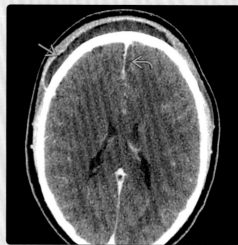

(Left) AP radiograph in a teenager with acute sinusitis shows an air-fluid level ➡ in the right maxillary sinus. The left maxillary sinus is clear ➡. (Right) Axial CECT in a teenager with altered mental status & facial swelling shows a large subgaleal abscess ➡. There is diffuse effacement of cerebral sulci (due to edema) plus a left frontal parafalcine subdural collection ➡. The frontal sinuses (not shown) contained air-fluid levels. The subdural empyema was emergently evacuated in this patient with Pott puffy tumor of complicated sinusitis.

TERMINOLOGY

Abbreviations

- Acute bacterial sinusitis (ABS)
- Viral upper respiratory infection (URI)

Definitions

- Acute inflammation of sinonasal mucosa lasting ≤ 4 weeks
  - Viral URI vs. ABS distinguished by clinical presentation
- Generally clinical diagnosis; imaging only needed if complications suspected

IMAGING

Radiographic Findings

- Mucosal thickening or sinus opacification ± air-fluid level
- Inaccurate & should be supplanted by CT

CT Findings

- NECT
  - Air-fluid level, bubbly or frothy-appearing secretions
  - Moderate mucosal thickening, generally > 1 cm in sinus cavity, ostium, or nasal cavity
    - Lesser thickening often present without sinusitis
    - Difficult to separate fluid from mucosal thickening on NECT if sinus completely opacified
  - May see polypoid inflammatory tissue obstructing drainage pathways
- CECT
  - Indicated when orbital or intracranial complications suspected clinically
  - Inflamed sinus mucosa enhances but thin, linear soft tissue deep to mucosa does not
  - Central secretions do not enhance
- Bone CT
  - Bone destruction not typical for acute infection
    - If present, suspect aggressive invasive sinus infection or neoplasm
  - Osteoneogenesis (sinus wall sclerosis & thickening) usually indicates chronic inflammation

Imaging Recommendations

- Best imaging tool
  - Sinusitis, whether ABS or viral URI, is clinical diagnosis
  - Radiographs inaccurate with little role in clinical practice
  - CT: Consider only if evaluating for complications, failed medical therapy, alternative diagnoses, or surgery
    - NECT delineates anatomic variants prior to functional endoscopic sinus surgery
  - CECT or MR for orbital or intracranial complications; MR for invasive fungal disease or possible neoplasm

PATHOLOGY

General Features

- Etiology
  - 80% of ABS follows viral URI; however, only 6-8% of viral URI cases develop ABS
    - URI → mucosal swelling → sinus outflow obstruction → static secretions in sinus → bacterial infection
    - Viral symptoms usually improve in 7-10 days

- Symptoms > 10 days or worsening after 5-7 days suggest bacterial superinfection
  - Common organisms: *Streptococcus pneumonia, Haemophilus influenzae, Moraxella catarrhalis*
- Associated abnormalities
  - Structural abnormalities may narrow drainage pathways
    - Anatomic variants of septum, uncinate process, middle turbinate, frontal recess, ethmoid sinuses
    - Polyps, either isolated or associated with allergic sinusitis with diffuse polyposis
    - Benign or malignant neoplasms
  - Predisposing systemic disorders: Allergies, immunoglobulin deficiency, immotile cilia syndrome, cystic fibrosis, vitamin D deficiency

CLINICAL ISSUES

Presentation

- Most common signs/symptoms
  - Nasal drainage (± purulence), facial pain, fever, & cough
    - Viral URI: Signs/symptoms last < 10 days, do not progress
    - ABS: Signs/symptoms fail to improve within 10 days or worsen within 10 days after initial improvement
  - Irritability common in children
- Other signs/symptoms
  - Malaise, hyposmia, anosmia, ear pressure/fullness

Natural History & Prognosis

- Viral URI usually self-limited
- ABS may resolve without antibiotics
- ABS course may be shortened by medical therapy, surgical drainage, & possibly saline irrigation
- If ABS untreated, rarely complications may ensue
  - Orbital cellulitis, subperiosteal or subgaleal abscess (Pott puffy tumor), meningitis, epidural or subdural empyema, brain abscess, venous sinus thrombosis

Treatment

- Medical therapy
  - Saline nasal sprays & irrigants
  - Antibiotics
  - ± nasal steroids
- Surgical therapy
  - More often performed for chronic rhinosinusitis
  - Drainage procedures may be performed in acute disease with complications

SELECTED REFERENCES

1. ACR Appropriateness Criteria: Sinusitis—Child. https://acsearch.acr.org/docs/69442/Narrative/. Published 1995. Reviewed 2012. Accessed Feb. 2017
2. Joshi VM et al: Imaging in sinonasal inflammatory disease. Neuroimaging Clin N Am. 25(4):549-68, 2015
3. Magit A: Pediatric rhinosinusitis. Otolaryngol Clin North Am. 47(5):733-46, 2014
4. Nocon CC et al: Acute rhinosinusitis in children. Curr Allergy Asthma Rep. 14(6):443, 2014
5. DeMuri GP et al: Clinical practice. Acute bacterial sinusitis in children. N Engl J Med. 367(12):1128-34, 2012

Orbital Cellulitis

KEY FACTS

TERMINOLOGY

- Preseptal cellulitis: Infection anterior to orbital septum
- Postseptal cellulitis: Infection posterior to orbital septum
- Orbital septum: Periosteal reflection from bony orbit to tarsal plates

IMAGING

- Thickening & edema of orbital/periorbital soft tissues
- Preseptal cellulitis: Limited to anterior tissues
- Postseptal cellulitis
  - Low-attenuation, rim-enhancing collection
    - Drainable subperiosteal abscess (SPA) in majority
    - 20% without drainable abscess (phlegmon)
  - Associated myositis common with swollen extraocular muscles, ± abnormal enhancement
  - ± thrombosed superior ophthalmic vein
- ± extraorbital complications of sinusitis
  - Frontal osteomyelitis, meningitis, subdural/epidural effusion or empyema, cerebritis, parenchymal abscess

TOP DIFFERENTIAL DIAGNOSES

- Idiopathic orbital inflammatory pseudotumor
- Orbital soft tissue or osseous neoplasm: Rhabdomyosarcoma, metastatic neuroblastoma
- Orbital vascular anomaly: Infantile hemangioma, venous malformation

CLINICAL ISSUES

- Sinusitis most common cause of pediatric orbital cellulitis
  - Other causes: Trauma, foreign body, skin infection, nasolacrimal duct mucocele; rarely retinoblastoma
- Presentation: Fever, eyelid swelling, erythema, tenderness, chemosis, proptosis, ophthalmoplegia with diplopia, ↓ visual acuity, intracranial complications → seizures, mental status changes
- Treatment: Intravenous antibiotics ± sinus drainage procedures, SPA drainage with postseptal cellulitis
  - Chandler classification + imaging characteristics ↑ ability to predict surgical need

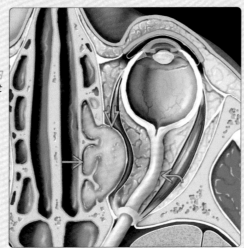
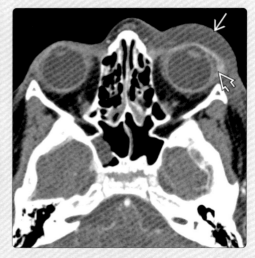

(Left) Axial graphic shows the spread of infection from the ethmoid sinuses ➡ through the lamina papyracea into the medial orbit, resulting in a subperiosteal abscess (SPA) ➡ & putting the optic nerve ➡ at risk. (Right) Axial CECT in a 7 year old with neutropenia & eyelid swelling shows left preseptal periorbital soft tissue edema ➡. There is a low-attenuation crescent marginating the anterolateral globe ➡, consistent with chemosis in this patient with preseptal cellulitis.

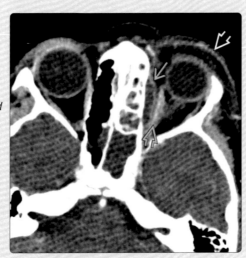
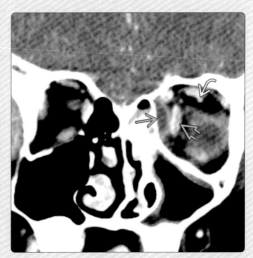

(Left) Axial CECT in a 7 year old demonstrates extensive, primarily left-sided ethmoid & sphenoid sinus disease with a medial rim-enhancing SPA ➡. This collection causes lateral deviation of the left medial rectus muscle ➡. There is mild associated preseptal cellulitis ➡. (Right) Coronal CECT in the same patient shows the left medial SPA ➡ & better defines the thickening of the deviated medial rectus muscle ➡. The left superior ophthalmic vein remains patent ➡.

TERMINOLOGY

Definitions

- Preseptal cellulitis: Inflammation anterior to orbital septum
- Postseptal cellulitis: Inflammation posterior to septum
- Orbital septum: Periosteal reflection from bony orbit to tarsal plates of eyelids

IMAGING

CT Findings

- CECT
  - Infiltrative edema & mild enhancement of periorbital &/or intraorbital fat
  - ± focal elongated lentiform rim-enhancing subperiosteal abscess (SPA) or intraorbital abscess
    - Medial > > superior orbit
    - ± foci of gas in abscess
  - ± extraocular muscle (EOM) enlargement due to myositis; EOM deviation by inflammatory collections
  - ± enlarged, centrally nonenhancing superior ophthalmic vein due to thrombosis
  - Careful review of anterior & middle cranial fossae for fluid collection or findings of parenchymal edema

Imaging Recommendations

- Best imaging tool
  - CECT: Obtain acutely in most cases of suspected postseptal cellulitis
    - Impairment in visual acuity or ophthalmoplegia
    - Severe eyelid edema prohibiting evaluation of vision & EOM motility
    - No improvement or worsening of symptoms on appropriate antibiotics
  - MR C+: Evaluate intracranial complications of sinusitis
    - Clinical & CT findings may dictate operative intervention before MR

DIFFERENTIAL DIAGNOSIS

Idiopathic Orbital Inflammatory Pseudotumor

- Subacute onset of poorly marginated, mass-like enhancing soft tissue involving any region of orbit

Langerhans Cell Histiocytosis

- Classic punched-out round or geographic lytic bone lesion, often filled with homogeneously enhancing soft tissue

Orbital Neoplasm

- Malignant bone lesions show permeative destruction & periosteal reaction, particularly in superolateral orbit

Orbital Vascular Anomaly

- Infantile hemangioma: Characteristic cutaneous features (red "strawberry mark") if superficial
- Venous malformation: ± bluish skin discoloration that bulges with Valsalva

PATHOLOGY

General Features

- Etiology
  - Most common cause in children: Sinusitis
    - Up to 3% develop cellulitis
  - Other causes: Trauma, foreign body, skin infection, nasolacrimal duct mucocele
- Associated abnormalities
  - Superior ophthalmic vein &/or cavernous sinus thrombosis
  - Frontal osteomyelitis (Pott puffy tumor)
  - Meningitis, epidural or subdural effusions or empyema, cerebritis or parenchymal abscess

Staging, Grading, & Classification

- Chandler classification: Orbital complications of sinusitis
  - Preseptal cellulitis: Inflammation anterior to orbital septum with eyelid edema; no tenderness, visual loss, or impaired EOM motility (ophthalmoplegia)
  - Orbital cellulitis without abscess: Diffuse postseptal edema of orbital fat
  - Orbital cellulitis with SPA: ± proptosis, impaired vision, or limited EOM motility
  - Orbital cellulitis with abscess in orbital fat: Usually severe proptosis, ↓ vision, & limited EOM motility
  - Cavernous sinus thrombosis secondary to orbital phlebitis: Unilateral or bilateral

CLINICAL ISSUES

Presentation

- Most common signs/symptoms
  - Fever, eyelid swelling, erythema, tenderness, chemosis, proptosis, ophthalmoplegia with diplopia, ↓ visual acuity
- Other signs/symptoms
  - Cranial nerve palsies (III-VI) with cavernous sinus thrombosis
  - Seizures, mental status changes with intracranial complications

Demographics

- 50% of affected children < 4 years of age

Treatment

- Medical management: Intravenous antibiotics
- Surgical management: Chandler classification + imaging characteristics ↑ ability to predict surgical need
  - SPA: Not absolute surgical indication
    - Younger children may only require antibiotics with more aggressive surgical drainage in older children
    - Emergent surgery if visual disturbance from optic nerve or retinal compromise
  - Sinus drainage procedures
  - Intracranial empyema classically considered surgical emergency, particularly with neurologic signs/symptoms

SELECTED REFERENCES

1. Sharma A et al: Pediatric orbital cellulitis in the Haemophilus influenzae vaccine era. J AAPOS. 19(3):206-10, 2015
2. Le TD et al: The effect of adding orbital computed tomography findings to the Chandler criteria for classifying pediatric orbital cellulitis in predicting which patients will require surgical intervention. J AAPOS. 18(3):271-7, 2014
3. Bedwell J et al: Management of pediatric orbital cellulitis and abscess. Curr Opin Otolaryngol Head Neck Surg. 19(6):467-73, 2011

Retinoblastoma

TERMINOLOGY

- Retinoblastoma (RB): Malignant primary retinal neoplasm

IMAGING

- Unilateral in 60%, bilateral in 40%
- Trilateral/quadrilateral RB (bilateral ocular RB + pineal tumor ± suprasellar tumor) rare
- Extraocular extension in < 10%: Poor prognosis
  - < 10% 5-year disease-free survival
- CT: Ca^{2+} in > 90%
- MR: Assess extent of intraocular tumor + presence of optic nerve, orbital, &/or intracranial involvement
  - T1: Mild hyperintensity
  - T2: Moderate to marked hypointensity
  - T1 C+: Moderate to marked heterogeneous enhancement

TOP DIFFERENTIAL DIAGNOSES

- Persistent hyperplastic primary vitreous

- Coats disease
- Retinopathy of prematurity
- Orbital toxocariasis

PATHOLOGY

- Primitive neuroectodermal tumor
- Sporadic (nongermline) *RB1* mutation: Most unilateral
- Inherited (germline) *RB1* mutation: Multilateral > unilateral
  - ↑ risk of 2nd remote malignancy: Sarcoma, etc.

CLINICAL ISSUES

- Most common intraocular tumor of childhood
  - 90-95% diagnosed by age 5 years
- Leukocoria in 50-60%; inflammatory signs in 10%
  - Strabismus if macular involvement, retinal detachment
  - Proptosis with significant orbital disease
  - Severe vision loss
- > 95% of children with RB in United States cured with modern techniques; retaining eye & vision still problematic

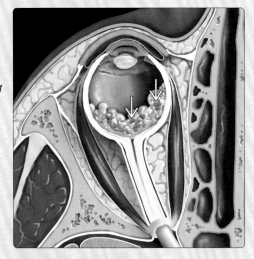

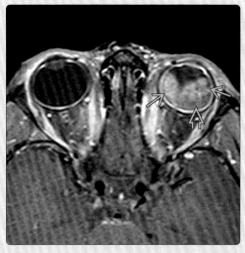

(Left) *Axial graphic depicts a retinoblastoma (RB) with lobulated tumor extending through the limiting membrane into the vitreous. Characteristic punctate Ca^{2+} ➡ are shown.* (Right) *Axial T1 C+ FS MR in a 3 year old with leukocoria demonstrates a large, moderately enhancing, bilobed left RB ➡. Mild decreased signal intensity posteriorly ➡ represents subretinal fluid secondary to retinal detachment.*

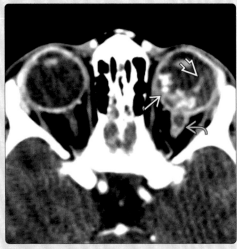

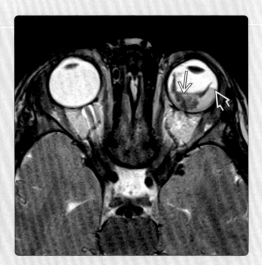

(Left) *Axial CECT in a 3 year old with leukocoria shows a partially calcified RB in the left globe ➡ with a focus of retinal detachment &/or noncalcified subretinal tumor at the temporal aspect of the globe ➡. There is also optic nerve sheath invasion ➡, an uncommon finding on CT imaging.* (Right) *Axial T2 MR in the same child shows hypointensity ➡ in the calcified portions of the ocular mass with a lateral subretinal fluid level ➡ secondary to ocular detachment.*

Congenital Cholesteatoma

TERMINOLOGY

- Congenital cholesteatoma (CCh): Benign mass secondary to epithelial rests of embryonal origin
- CCh most commonly occurs in middle ear (ME) behind intact tympanic membrane (TM) in patient without history of surgery, chronic otitis media, or otorrhea

IMAGING

- Majority in ME
  - Anterosuperior tympanic cavity near eustachian tube or stapes most common
- Temporal bone CT findings
  - Small well-circumscribed ME lesion medial to ossicles
  - Large mass may erode ossicles, ME wall, lateral semicircular canal, or tegmen tympani
- MR findings: Peripherally enhancing ME mass with diffusion restriction in larger lesions

TOP DIFFERENTIAL DIAGNOSES

- Acquired cholesteatoma
- Rhabdomyosarcoma
- Langerhans cell histiocytosis
- Glomus tympanicum paraganglioma

CLINICAL ISSUES

- Avascular pearly white ME mass behind intact TM without prior history of inflammation or trauma
- Unilateral conductive hearing loss in 30%
- May be discovered surgically after chronic ME effusion unresponsive to tympanostomy tubes
- Rarely external auditory canal mass with bone destruction
- Complete surgical extirpation = treatment of choice
- If untreated, keratin debris accumulates over time → enlarging mass → rupture throughout ME cavity
  - Large ME lesions can obstruct eustachian tube → ME effusion & infection

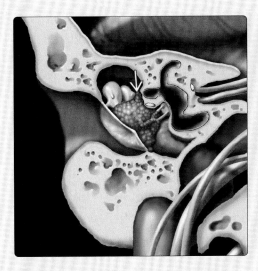

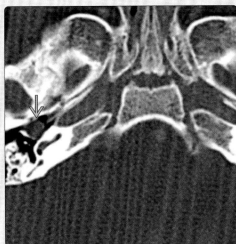

(Left) Coronal graphic shows a congenital cholesteatoma (CCh) involving the middle ear (ME) cavity. Notice that the lesion has extended medial to the ossicles ➡ as it engulfs the entire ossicular chain. The tympanic membrane (TM) is intact, a typical finding in congenital lesions, as opposed to acquired cholesteatomas (which are associated with TM perforation). (Right) Axial bone CT in a 3-year-old child without a history of chronic otitis media shows a typical CCh ➡ anteromedial to the malleus manubrium.

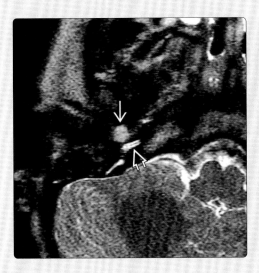

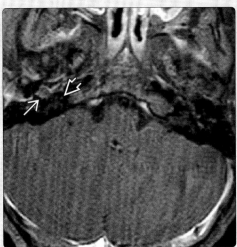

(Left) Axial T2 MR in the same patient shows the CCh as a high signal intensity well-defined ME mass ➡ anterolateral to the basal turn ➡ of the right cochlea. (Right) Axial T1 C+ FS MR in the same patient shows the centrally nonenhancing CCh with a thin rim of peripheral enhancement ➡ adjacent to the cochlea ➡. This is a typical appearance & location for a CCh.

Acquired Cholesteatoma

TERMINOLOGY

- Secondary or acquired cholesteatoma: Tympanic membrane (TM) retraction or perforation → accumulation of stratified squamous epithelial cells in middle ear (ME) → mass-like keratin ball
- Progressive ↑ in size → destruction of surrounding structures (ossicles, semicircular canals, tegmen tympani, facial nerve canal, transverse sinus invasion)

IMAGING

- Nonenhancing ME soft tissue mass + ossicular erosion
  - Noncontrast bone CT: Axial & coronal
    - Ossicular & adjacent bone evaluation
  - Coronal T1 C+ FS MR
    - Suspected intracranial extension/infection
- Associated granulation tissue or scar may enhance

TOP DIFFERENTIAL DIAGNOSES

- Chronic otitis media with ossicular erosion

- Acute coalescent otomastoiditis with abscess
- Congenital cholesteatoma
- Langerhans cell histiocytosis
- Rhabdomyosarcoma

CLINICAL ISSUES

- Recurrent or chronic ME infections with TM perforation or retraction pocket on otoscopy
  - ± conductive hearing loss, painless otorrhea, vertigo, otalgia, facial nerve paralysis
- Unusual in children < 4 years of age
- If untreated, complications include: CNVII involvement, venous sinus thrombosis, intracranial extension
- Excellent prognosis with complete removal of small lesions
- Mastoidectomy & ossicular chain reconstruction for more extensive involvement

(Left) Coronal graphic shows a large acquired cholesteatoma of the pars flaccida (PF) portion of the tympanic membrane. Complications include erosion of the ossicles & lateral semicircular canal (SCC) ⇨ & thinning of the tegmen tympani ⇨. (Right) Axial bone CT in a 5 year old with chronic otitis media & conductive hearing loss shows complete opacification of the right middle ear cavity & mastoid air cells. There is truncation of the incus ⇨ without a definable long process.

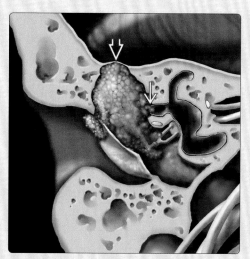
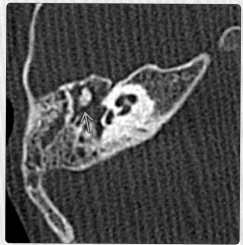

(Left) Coronal bone CT in a 10 year old with chronic right otitis media & otorrhea shows a large PF cholesteatoma ⇨ nearly filling the mesotympanum & epitympanum. The partially eroded ossicles ⇨ are deviated inferiorly & medially. (Right) Axial bone CT in the same child shows focal dehiscence of the right lateral SCC ⇨ compared to the normal covering on the left ⇨. Also note the underdevelopment of the right mastoid air cells ⇨ relative to the left ⇨, a common finding with chronic inflammation.

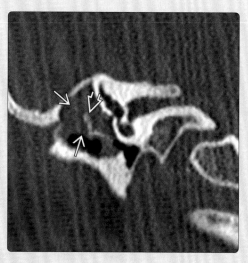
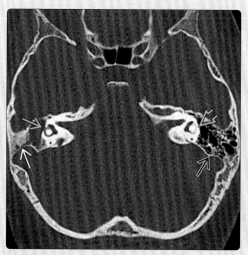

Acute Mastoiditis With Abscess

IMAGING

- CECT for acute evaluation will define most mastoiditis complications & provide excellent bone detail
  - Opacified mastoid cells
  - Rim-enhancing fluid collection (abscess) adjacent to opacified mastoid cells with eroded bone cortex
    - Subperiosteal: Periauricular fluid collection
    - Middle or posterior fossa: Epidural or parenchymal
  - Dural sinus thrombosis: Adjacent venous filling defect
- MR provides better intracranial detail (meningitis, subdural empyema, parenchymal abscess)

TOP DIFFERENTIAL DIAGNOSES

- Acquired cholesteatoma, Langerhans cell histiocytosis, rhabdomyosarcoma

PATHOLOGY

- 46% of children have > 2 episodes of acute otitis media (AOM) by 3 years of age

- 0.24% of patients with AOM develop mastoiditis
  - *Streptococcus* species, polymicrobial aerobes & anaerobes
- 70-100% of mastoiditis patients have concurrent AOM

CLINICAL ISSUES

- Presentation: Young child with 1-day to 1-week history of intense otalgia, fever, & otorrhea (overlaps AOM)
  - Findings favoring mastoiditis
    - Retroauricular pain, swelling, & redness
    - Pinna protrusion/lateralized auricle
  - Imaging reserved for suspected mastoiditis complications
- Treatments: IV antibiotics ± tympanocentesis with myringotomy tube placement, I&D of extracranial subperiosteal abscess
  - Mastoidectomy typically reserved for patients that fail initial conservative management

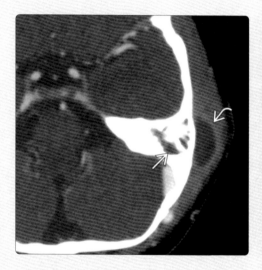
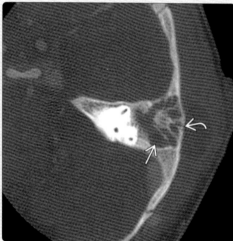

(Left) Axial CECT in an 8-month-old girl shows a rim-enhancing fluid collection ➡ superficial to opacified left mastoid air cells ➡, consistent with a subperiosteal abscess. There is edema of the surrounding soft tissues. (Right) Axial bone CT in the same patient shows opacification of the mastoid air cells ➡ without septal destruction. Subtle bony dehiscence ➡ is suggested deep to the abscess. However, bone destruction need not be present to establish a diagnosis of acute mastoiditis.

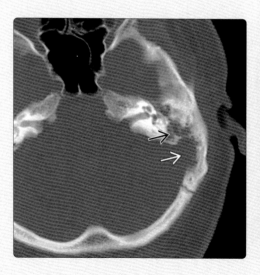
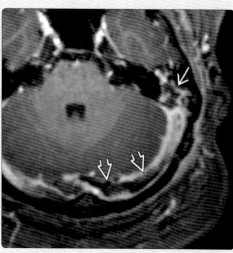

(Left) Axial bone CT in a 17-year-old boy shows complete opacification of the left mastoid air cells ➡ & middle ear cavity with extensive destruction of the mastoid septa & medial wall ➡, consistent with acute coalescent otomastoiditis. (Right) Axial T1 C+ FS MR in the same patient shows extensive intramastoid enhancement ➡ & a large, hypointense filling defect in the left transverse sinus ➡, consistent with secondary venous thrombosis.

TERMINOLOGY

- Thyroglossal duct cyst (TGDC): Cystic remnant of embryologic thyroglossal duct

IMAGING

- Best diagnostic clue: Round or ovoid midline/paramidline cystic neck mass about hyoid bone
  - Suprahyoid neck: ~ 20-25%, typically midline
  - At hyoid bone: ~ 50%
  - Infrahyoid neck: ~ 25%, midline or paramidline
- Typically well-defined, simple-appearing cyst
- ± wall enhancement, soft tissue stranding if infected

TOP DIFFERENTIAL DIAGNOSES

- Dermoid or epidermoid cyst
- Lingual thyroid
- Lymphatic malformation
- 4th branchial apparatus anomaly
- Thymic cyst

CLINICAL ISSUES

- Most common congenital neck lesion
  - Associated anomalies: Thyroid agenesis, ectopia, or pyramidal lobe
- Midline or paramidline doughy, compressible, painless neck mass; < 10 years of age at presentation (up to 90%)
  - Cyst elevates when tongue protrudes if TGDC located around hyoid bone
- May present intermittently with midline neck mass upon upper respiratory tract infections or trauma
  - Rapidly enlarging mass suggests either infection or thyroid carcinoma (< 1%, typically papillary)
  - Rarely, lingual TGDC may lead to infantile airway obstruction
- Treatment: Sistrunk procedure (excision of cyst, tract, & midline hyoid bone) → ↓ recurrences from 50% to < 4%
  - Confirm normal thyroid present by US prior to TGDC or lingual thyroid resection
  - Isolated lingual TGDC may be treated endoscopically

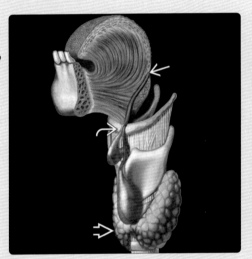
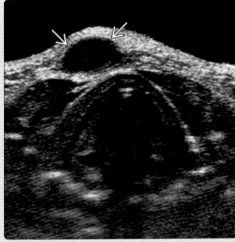

(Left) Sagittal oblique graphic shows the potential sites of a thyroglossal duct cyst (TGDC) from the foramen cecum ➡ to the thyroid bed ⇨. Note the close relationship of the midportion of the hyoid bone ➡ to this pathway. A cyst can occur anywhere along this tract. (Right) Transverse ultrasound of the anterior neck shows a well-defined, subcutaneous, right paramidline hypoechoic mass ➡ ventral to the strap muscles. This was surgically removed & confirmed to be a TGDC.

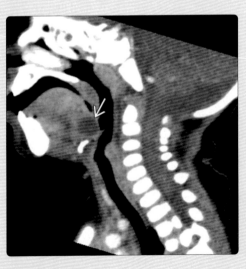
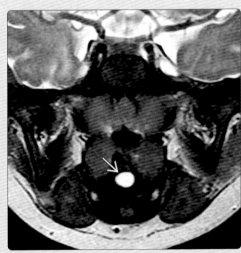

(Left) Sagittal CECT shows a well-defined, cystic-appearing mass ➡ at the midline base of the tongue. This mass was incidentally found on a CT performed to evaluate the extent of a deep neck infection (not shown). The mass was subsequently proven to be a TGDC. (Right) Coronal T2 MR shows a well-defined, hyperintense base of tongue TGDC ➡ found incidentally in a 1 year old undergoing a brain MR for developmental delay.

TERMINOLOGY

- Synonyms: Branchial cleft cyst, branchial apparatus cyst (BAC), branchial apparatus anomaly (BAA)
  - May be cyst, fistula, or sinus tract

IMAGING

- Best clue: Well-defined, smooth-walled unilocular cyst of face/neck
  - ± wall thickening, enhancement, & septation with surrounding edema if infected
- Locations
  - 1st BAC: Periauricular, in or adjacent to parotid
  - 2nd BAC (most common): Anterior to sternocleidomastoid muscle, posterior to submandibular gland, lateral to carotid sheath
  - 3rd BAC: Posterior triangle in upper neck or anterior triangle in lower neck
  - Cervical thymic cyst: Anywhere from lateral hypopharynx to normal thymus in superior mediastinum

- 4th BAA: Typically sinus tract or fistula extending from apex of pyriform sinus to anterior lower neck, usually in or adjacent to left thyroid lobe
- Ultrasound useful for initially assessing palpable lesions; MR or CT often needed to establish deep extent & relationship to vital structures

TOP DIFFERENTIAL DIAGNOSES

- Suppurative lymph node or abscess
- Thyroglossal duct cyst
- Lymphatic malformation
- Dermoid & epidermoid cysts

CLINICAL ISSUES

- Typical presentations include soft, painless mass vs. recurrent infections or drainage
  - 1st BAC: ± otorrhea or recurrent parotid abscess
  - 4th BAA: ± left thyroid lobe abscess
- Treatment requires complete surgical excision of cyst & associated fistula or sinus tract, if present

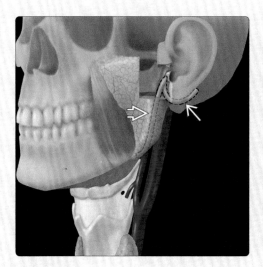

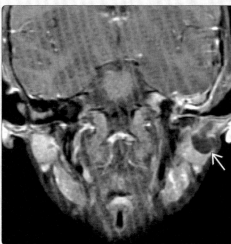

(Left) Oblique graphic shows the 2 forms of a 1st branchial apparatus cyst (BAC). Type I ➡ courses from the medial bony external auditory canal (EAC) toward the retroauricular area. The tract of a type II BAC ➡ connects the EAC to the angle of the mandible. (Right) Coronal T1 C+ FS MR in a 3-year-old patient with a 1st BAC shows a lobulated, nonenhancing periparotid cyst ➡ extending towards the junction of the cartilaginous & bony EAC.

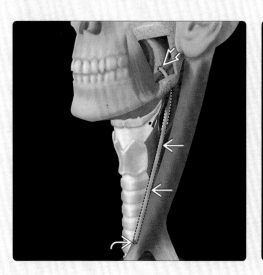

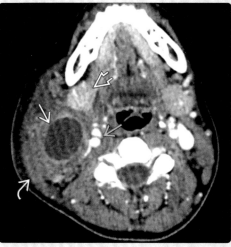

(Left) Oblique graphic of the tract of a 2nd BAC ➡ shows a proximal opening ➡ in the faucial tonsil & a distal opening in the anterior supraclavicular neck ➡. (Right) Axial CECT in teenager with enlarging mass shows a cystic-appearing lesion ➡ in typical location of a 2nd BAC (dorsal to the submandibular gland ➡, anterior to the sternocleidomastoid ➡, & lateral to the carotid sheath vessels ➡). Note the thick, irregular rim & overlying edema, consistent with superimposed infection plus cellulitis/myositis.

Lymphatic Malformation, Cervical

TERMINOLOGY

- Lymphatic malformation (LM): Subtype of slow/low flow congenital vascular malformation composed of embryonic lymphatic sacs; not neoplastic
- Composed of macrocysts > 1 cm &/or microcysts < 1 cm

IMAGING

- Macrocystic LM: Multiloculated cystic neck mass with imperceptible wall, thin septations, & fluid-fluid levels
- Microcystic LM: More ill-defined, infiltrative, &/or solid appearing
- Transspatial, often crossing midline extensively
  - Insinuates between vessels & other normal structures
  - May infiltrate upper airway or cause extrinsic compression
- US: Cysts can show varying degrees of ↑ echogenicity; Doppler shows no significant internal vascularity
- T2 FS/STIR MR: Hyperintense; frequent fluid-fluid levels
  - Best defines extent + relationship to airway & vessels

- T1 FS C+ MR: No significant or minimal rim enhancement
  - Must compare with precontrast T1 as hemorrhage & protein often show hyperintensity before contrast

TOP DIFFERENTIAL DIAGNOSES

- 2nd branchial cleft anomaly
- Abscess
- Teratoma
- Neuroblastoma
- Soft tissue sarcoma

CLINICAL ISSUES

- Nontender, compressible mass
  - Present since birth, grows commensurate with patient
  - May not be clinically apparent until hemorrhage, infection, or hormonal stimulation → rapid ↑ in size
- Depending on size & extent, treatment options include resection, sclerotherapy (for macrocysts), & sirolimus
  - Combination therapy, often staged, may be required

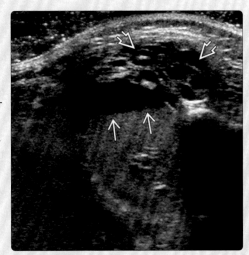
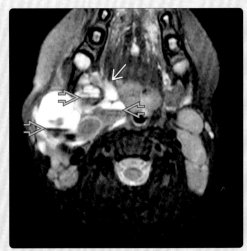

(Left) Transverse US in a 2-year-old boy who presented with the sudden onset of neck swelling shows a multiloculated transspatial lymphatic malformation (LM) with a fluid-debris level ➡ in the largest macrocyst. Smaller microcysts ➡ are seen anteriorly. (Right) Axial T2 FS MR in the same patient better shows the deep extent of the lesion ➡. Multiple fluid-fluid levels ➡ (secondary to layering blood products) are scattered throughout the cysts, a common feature of LMs.

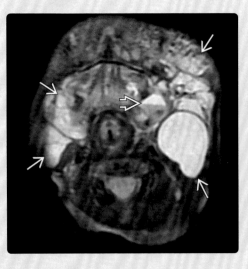
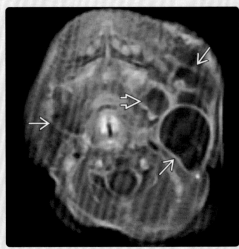

(Left) Axial T2 FS MR in a 1-week-old infant demonstrates a multiloculated, mixed micro- & macrocystic transspatial LM ➡ involving the left anterior neck more than the right. Layering blood products are seen in a single left-sided submandibular macrocyst ➡. (Right) Axial T1 C+ FS MR in the same child shows a typical appearance of an extensive LM. The macrocysts show only mild peripheral enhancement ➡, & the fluid-fluid level ➡ is much more difficult to discern.

Acute Parotitis

TERMINOLOGY

- Acute inflammation of parotid gland

IMAGING

- US/CECT/MR: ↑ size & enhancement of parotid ± stranding of surrounding fat; parotid retains shape
  - CECT best for stone or rim-enhancing abscess
  - Viral rarely requires imaging
- Bacterial parotitis: Typically unilateral; ± abscess
- Calculus-induced parotitis: Typically unilateral with calcified stone + dilated parotid duct
- Viral parotitis: 75% bilateral; ± submandibular &/or sublingual gland involvement; clinical diagnosis
- Autoimmune: Usually bilateral
- Juvenile recurrent (JRP): Unilateral or asymmetric clinical presentations with bilateral imaging findings
- Reimage if mass persists after resolution of infection (to exclude underlying branchial cyst or malignancy)

TOP DIFFERENTIAL DIAGNOSES

- Infected 1st branchial cleft anomaly
- Salivary gland neoplasms

CLINICAL ISSUES

- Bacterial: Indurated, erythematous, tender gland; purulent ostial discharge; ± abscess
  - Responds well to antibiotics: *Staphylococcus aureus* > *Streptococcus*, *Haemophilus*, *Escherichia coli*, anaerobes
- Viral: Parotid swollen but not erythematous or warm; usually from systemic self-limited viral infection with headache & malaise followed by parotid pain, earache, trismus; may also experience orchitis, meningoencephalitis, pancreatitis, thyroiditis, depending on virus
  - Mumps paramyxovirus most common
  - Swelling ≤ 2 weeks with supportive treatment
- Calculus induced: Swollen, painful gland, often related to eating due to ductal obstruction by sialolith
- JRP: 1-10 episodes per year, resolving in 2nd decade

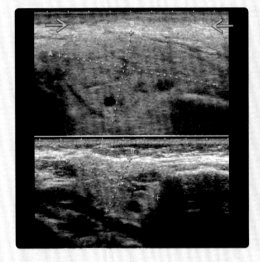
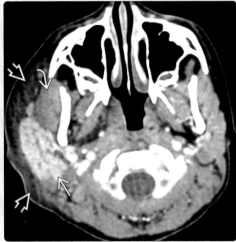

(Left) *Longitudinal US of the right (upper) & left (lower) parotid glands (denoted by calipers) in a toddler with right facial swelling shows a normal size & echogenicity of the left parotid gland & overlying soft tissues. The right parotid gland is enlarged & mildly heterogeneous with induration of the overlying soft tissues* →, *typical of parotitis.* **(Right)** *Axial CECT shows diffuse asymmetric enlargement & enhancement of the right parotid gland* → *with associated facial cellulitis* → *& myositis* → *due to acute bacterial parotitis.*

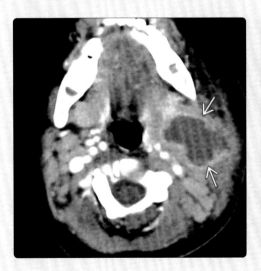
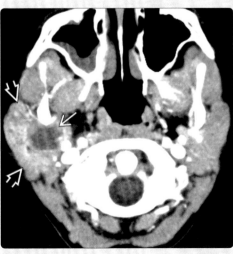

(Left) *Axial CECT shows a low-density, rim-enhancing collection* → *replacing the left parotid gland. There is substantial surrounding fat stranding. These findings are consistent with an abscess complicating acute bacterial parotitis.* **(Right)** *Axial CECT shows an irregular collection* → *deep within the enlarged, asymmetrically enhancing right parotid gland* →. *This collection, which could represent phlegmon or abscess, was treated as the former & resolved without drainage on IV antibiotics.*

Suppurative Adenitis

TERMINOLOGY

- Pus formation within nodes from bacterial infection
- Synonyms: Adenitis, lymphadenitis, intranodal abscess

IMAGING

- Enlarged node(s) with internal fluid & surrounding inflammation (cellulitis)
  - Most often jugulodigastric, submandibular, or retropharyngeal
- Loss of normal nodal architecture & internal vascularity/enhancement
- Conglomeration of necrotic nodes progressing to abscess shows marked heterogeneity of irregular collection
  - Well-defined enhancing/hyperemic wall
  - Complex hypoechoic/nonenhancing center
- US useful to confirm true liquefaction with drainable pus
  - Swirling internal debris upon compression
- CECT best defines deep extent & complications

- Lemierre syndrome (venous thrombophlebitis), internal carotid artery spasm or pseudoaneurysm, airway compression, mediastinal extension

TOP DIFFERENTIAL DIAGNOSES

- Nontuberculous *Mycobacterium* adenopathy, tuberculous adenopathy, 2nd branchial cleft anomaly, rhabdomyosarcoma, lymphoma, lymphatic malformation

PATHOLOGY

- *Staphylococcus* & *Streptococcus* most frequent organisms

CLINICAL ISSUES

- Painful neck mass, fever, poor oral intake; symptoms referable to primary infection
- Treatment: Antibiotics
  - Incision & drainage for large suppurative nodes, abscesses, or poor response to antibiotics

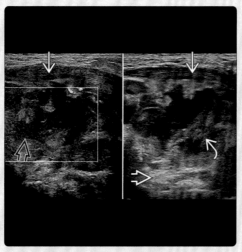
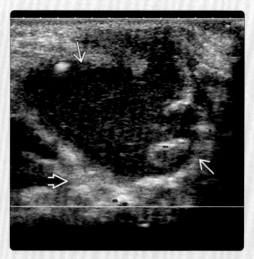

(Left) Transverse (left) & longitudinal (right) color Doppler & grayscale US images of an infant with suppurative adenopathy show an enlarged, heterogeneous conglomeration of cervical nodes ⇒ with internal debris ⇒, posterior acoustic enhancement ⇒, & peripheral hyperemia ⇒. (Right) Transverse color Doppler US in a 6 year old with fever & a tender neck mass shows an irregular hypoechoic abscess ⇒ with posterior acoustic enhancement ⇒, internal echoes, & no internal vascularity.

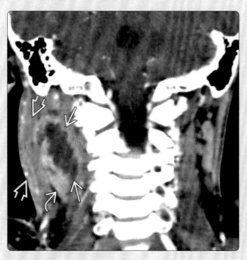
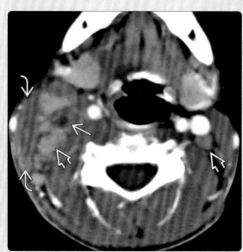

(Left) Coronal CECT in a 6 year old with fever & a fluctuant neck mass shows an irregular, rim-enhancing abscess ⇒ with overlying myositis/cellulitis ⇒ & an adjacent nonsuppurative lymph node ⇒. (Right) More inferior image from an axial CECT in the same child shows a round focus of nonenhancement representing segmental clot ⇒ in the right internal jugular vein, consistent with Lemierre syndrome. Note the right-greater-than-left nonsuppurative nodes ⇒ as well as the overlying myositis/cellulitis ⇒.

TERMINOLOGY

Definitions

- Pus formation within nodes from bacterial infection

IMAGING

General Features

- Location: Any nodal groups of head/neck, unilateral or bilateral
- Size: Enlarged single node or conglomeration of nodes; often in 1-4 cm range
- Morphology: Ovoid to round large node with central necrosis; margins may be poorly defined; additional abnormal nodes typically present

Ultrasonographic Findings

- Early adenitis may show enlarged ovoid foci with retained nodal architecture & hyperemia
- Loss of architecture & internal vascularity with necrosis
  o Central ↓ echogenicity with ↑ through transmission
- Conglomeration of necrotic nodes progressing to abscess shows marked heterogeneity of irregular collection
  o Liquefied pus: Swirling internal debris with compression
  o ↑ peripheral vascularity
- Thickening of overlying subcutaneous fat ± serpentine foci of poorly defined fluid (cellulitis)

CT Findings

- CECT
  o Enhancing nodal wall with central hypoattenuation/lack of enhancement
  o Stranding/edema of surrounding tissues
  o With progression to abscess: Irregular, ill-defined, peripherally enhancing, low-attenuation collection
    – Represents nondrainable phlegmon in ~ 20% rather than drainable pus → consider US
  o ± myositis, Lemierre syndrome (venous thrombophlebitis), deviation of carotid sheath vessels, internal carotid artery spasm or pseudoaneurysm, retropharyngeal soft tissue edema, mass effect on airway, mediastinal extension

Imaging Recommendations

- Best imaging tool
  o US to determine phlegmon vs. abscess & guide aspiration
    – May be difficult to determine deep extent
  o CECT best for deep neck infections
    – Defines total extent for aspiration or surgical planning

DIFFERENTIAL DIAGNOSIS

Nontuberculous *Mycobacterium* Adenopathy

- Asymmetric enlarged nodes with necrotic ring-enhancing masses
- Minimal or absent subcutaneous fat stranding
- Purified protein derivative (PPD) weakly reactive in 55%
- Usually ≤ 5 years of age

Tuberculous Adenopathy

- Painless, low jugular & posterior cervical low-density nodes
- Strongly reactive PPD
- Systemically unwell if active pulmonary infection

2nd Branchial Cleft Anomaly

- Solitary unilocular cyst, posterior to submandibular gland

Rhabdomyosarcoma

- Solid firm soft tissue neoplasm of children (typically beyond infancy) occurring in many head/neck locations

Lymphoma

- Multifocal solid enhancing nodes, often of bilateral neck & chest; ± enlargement of tonsillar tissue

Lymphatic Malformation

- Congenital multicystic mass with thin rim & septations
- Variable internal echogenicity due to internal hemorrhage
- No significant internal vascularity
- Often infiltrative & transspatial

PATHOLOGY

General Features

- Primary head/neck infection (e.g., pharyngitis)
  o Adjacent lymph nodes enlarge 2° to pathogen: Reactive
  o Intranodal exudate forms, containing protein-rich fluid with dead neutrophils (pus): Suppurative
  o If untreated or incorrectly treated, suppurative nodes rupture → interstitial pus walled-off by immune system → extranodal abscess in soft tissues
- Pediatric infections show clustering of organisms by age
  o Infants < 1 year: *S. aureus*, group B *Streptococcus*
  o Children 1-4 years: *S. aureus,* group A β-hemolytic *Streptococcus*, atypical mycobacteria
  o 5-15 years: Anaerobic bacteria, toxoplasmosis, cat scratch disease, tuberculosis

CLINICAL ISSUES

Presentation

- Most common signs/symptoms
  o Painful neck mass
    – Overlying skin often warm, erythematous
  o Fever, poor oral intake
  o Elevated WBC & ESR
- Other signs/symptoms
  o Symptoms referable to primary infection
    – Pharyngeal/laryngeal: Drooling, respiratory distress
    – Peritonsillar: Trismus
    – Retropharyngeal: Neck stiffness

Treatment

- Mainstay of therapy: Antibiotics
- Incision & drainage for large suppurative nodes, abscesses, or poor response to antibiotics
  o ± CT & US-guided aspiration
- Nodes from atypical mycobacteria should be excised to prevent recurrence or fistula/sinus tract

SELECTED REFERENCES

1. Worley ML et al: Suppurative cervical lymphadenitis in infancy: microbiology and sociology. Clin Pediatr (Phila). 54(7):629-34, 2015
2. Rosenberg TL et al: Pediatric cervical lymphadenopathy. Otolaryngol Clin North Am. 47(5):721-31, 2014
3. Sauer MW et al: Acute neck infections in children: who is likely to undergo surgical drainage? Am J Emerg Med. 31(6):906-9, 2013

TERMINOLOGY

- Benign fibrosis of sternocleidomastoid (SCM) muscle
- Most common cervical "mass" of infancy: Postulated to be muscular response to birth trauma or peripartum injury

IMAGING

- Often diagnosed clinically without imaging
- Ultrasound modality of choice when imaging required
- Process entirely intramuscular (contained within SCM), without local invasion or inflammatory changes
- Fusiform expansion of central SCM muscle
  - Thick & short compared to contralateral SCM
- Variable heterogeneity of lesion with loss of normal muscle architecture
  - Ranges from nearly homogeneous to markedly heterogeneous on US/CECT/MR
- Variable internal vascularity within/about mass
- Fascial planes surrounding SCM preserved
- No associated adenopathy or fluid collection

TOP DIFFERENTIAL DIAGNOSES

- Cervical lymphadenopathy
- Infantile hemangioma
- Cervical teratoma
- Congenital neuroblastoma
- Rhabdomyosarcoma
- Branchial cleft anomalies
- Lymphatic malformation

CLINICAL ISSUES

- Peak presentation at 24 days old
  - Painless palpable mass with torticollis
  - Contralateral occipital flattening (plagiocephaly)
- Treatment: Self-limited, usually resolves by 6 months of age
  - 90% fully recover with conservative treatment & physiotherapy
  - Surgery only in unusual cases when craniofacial asymmetry or refractory torticollis persists after 1 year

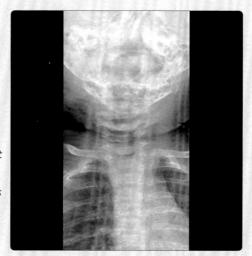
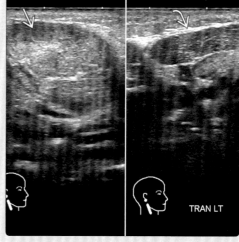

(Left) AP radiograph of the neck shows mild torticollis with the left ear closer to the left shoulder & the chin slightly turned away. No bony anomalies are seen to explain this neck positioning in this infant with fibromatosis colli. (Right) Split screen transverse US images in a 3-week-old girl with torticollis show a homogeneously enlarged right sternocleidomastoid (SCM) muscle ➡ as compared to the left ➡, typical of fibromatosis colli.

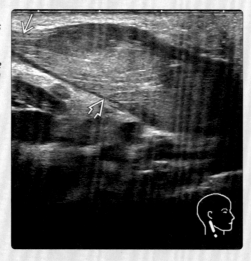
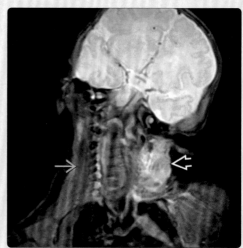

(Left) Orienting the US transducer along the long axis of the SCM optimally shows the mildly heterogeneous enlargement/expansion of the muscle belly with normal SCM tapering ends ➡ & sharp, distinct borders ➡. (Right) Coronal STIR MR in an infant with obvious torticollis shows heterogeneously increased signal intensity & thickness of the left SCM ➡ in a patient with fibromatosis colli. Note the normal right SCM ➡.

TERMINOLOGY

Synonyms

- Sternocleidomastoid (SCM) pseudotumor, SCM tumor of infancy, congenital muscular torticollis, neonatal torticollis

Definitions

- Most common cervical "mass" of infancy
- Represents benign fibrosis of SCM muscle, typically in response to birth trauma or peripartum injury

IMAGING

General Features

- Best diagnostic clue
  - Focal thickening & fibrosis of SCM muscle
  - Process entirely intramuscular without local invasion or inflammatory changes
- Location
  - Middle or lower 1/3 of SCM muscle belly
- Morphology
  - Focal heterogeneous to homogeneous expansion of SCM muscle, distorting normal muscle architecture
  - SCM tapers to normal proximal & distal to lesion
  - Affected SCM mildly shorter than contralateral side
  - No surrounding inflammatory changes or adenopathy

Radiographic Findings

- Cervical spine films may be obtained to exclude bony abnormality causing torticollis
- May see nonspecific unilateral soft tissue fullness or "mass"
- Virtually never calcifies

Ultrasonographic Findings

- Grayscale ultrasound
  - Focal mass mildly or moderately expanding SCM muscle belly
  - Loss of normal muscle architecture
  - Variable echogenicity of mass; may be homogeneous or heterogeneous
  - Affected SCM shorter & thicker than contralateral side
    - Comparison with asymptomatic side useful
  - No associated adenopathy, edema, or fluid collection
  - Lack of extramuscular involvement excludes other differential diagnoses
- Color Doppler
  - Variable hyperemia in acute phase

CT Findings

- Focal thickening/expansion of unilateral SCM muscle
  - Variable enhancement & heterogeneity

MR Findings

- Variable enhancement & heterogeneity
  - Marked muscle edema of SCM surrounding mass

Imaging Recommendations

- Best imaging tool
  - Often diagnosed clinically without imaging
  - Ultrasound modality of choice when imaging required
    - No ionizing radiation or sedation
    - Clearly localizes mass within SCM muscle
- Protocol advice

- Regardless of modality, fibromatosis colli does not show
  - Involvement of tissues outside SCM
  - Lymphadenopathy
  - Airway compression
  - Vascular encasement
  - Bone involvement
  - Intracranial/intraspinal extension

DIFFERENTIAL DIAGNOSIS

Cervical Lymphadenopathy

- Nodes discrete & easily recognizable, though may appear mass-like when enlarged & confluent

Infantile Hemangioma

- Rapidly growing highly vascular benign neoplasm presenting weeks to months after birth, ultimately regressing over years

Cervical Teratoma

- Congenital mixed solid & cystic mass, often large

Congenital Neuroblastoma

- Look for Ca^{2+}, intraspinal extension, & bony erosion

Rhabdomyosarcoma

- Solid mass outside SCM, typically in older children

Branchial Cleft Anomalies

- Unilocular cyst adjacent to SCM

Lymphatic Malformation

- Compressible multicystic congenital mass

CLINICAL ISSUES

Presentation

- Most common signs/symptoms
  - Painless palpable mass with torticollis
  - Contralateral occipital flattening (plagiocephaly)
  - History of breech presentation & "difficult" vaginal birth common but not mandatory

Demographics

- Age
  - Classically noticed < 8 weeks of age but may worsen in first 2-3 months of life

Treatment

- Self-limited, usually resolves by 6 months of age
- 90% fully recover with conservative treatment & physiotherapy
- Surgery only indicated in unusual cases when craniofacial asymmetry or refractory torticollis persists after 1 year

SELECTED REFERENCES

1. Lowry KC et al: The presentation and management of fibromatosis colli. Ear Nose Throat J. 89(9):E4-8, 2010
2. Murphey MD et al: From the archives of the AFIP: musculoskeletal fibromatoses: radiologic-pathologic correlation. Radiographics. 29(7):2143-73, 2009
3. Parikh SN et al: Magnetic resonance imaging in the evaluation of infantile torticollis. Orthopedics. 27(5):509-15, 2004
4. Ablin DS et al: Ultrasound and MR imaging of fibromatosis colli (sternomastoid tumor of infancy). Pediatr Radiol. 28(4):230-3, 1998

Radiology Abbreviation Index

A

ACL: anterior cruciate ligament

ADC: apparent diffusion coefficient

ALCAPA: anomalous left coronary artery origin from pulmonary artery

AP: anteroposterior

ARDS: acute respiratory distress syndrome

ASD: atrial septal defect

ASL: arterial spin labeling

AV: atrioventricular

AVM: arteriovenous malformation

B

BP: brachial plexus

BPD: bronchopulmonary dysplasia

C

CBD: common bile duct

CCAM: congenital cystic adenomatoid malformation

CECT: contrast-enhanced computed tomography

C+: with contrast

CISS: constructive interference in steady state

CT: computed tomography

CTA: computed tomography angiography

CTV: computed tomography venography

D

DORV: double outlet right ventricle

DSA: digital subtraction angiography

DTI: diffusion tensor imaging

DWI: diffusion-weighted imaging

E

ERCP: endoscopic retrograde cholangiopancreatography

F

F-18 FDG: F-18 fluorodeoxyglucose

FIESTA: fast imaging employing steady-state acquisition

FLAIR: fluid-attenuated inversion recovery

fMRI: functional magnetic resonance imaging

FNH: focal nodular hyperplasia

FS: fat suppression or fat saturation

G

GMH: germinal matrix hemorrhage

GRE: gradient echo

H

HSV: herpes simplex virus

HU: Hounsfield unit

I

IVC: inferior vena cava

IVH: intraventricular hemorrhage

IVP: intravenous pyelogram

L

LAD: left anterior descending

LUQ: left upper quadrant

LVOT: left ventricular outflow tract

M

MCL: medial cruciate ligament

MDCT: multidetector computed tomography

MIP: maximum intensity projection

MR: magnetic resonance

MRA: magnetic resonance angiography

MRCP: magnetic resonance cholangiopancreatography

MRP: magnetic resonance perfusion

MRS: magnetic resonance spectroscopy

MRU: MR urogram

MRV: magnetic resonance venography

N

NECT: nonenhanced computed tomography

P

PA: posteroanterior

PA: pulmonary artery

PACS: picture archiving and communications system

PC: phase contrast

PD: proton density

PDA: patent ductus arteriosus

PET: positron emission tomography

PFO: patent foramen ovale

PIE: pulmonary interstitial emphysema

PNET: primitive neuroectodermal tumor

Radiology Abbreviation Index

R

RA: right atrium

RF: radiofrequency

RHD: rheumatic heart disease

RI: resistive index

RUQ: right upper quadrant

RV: right ventricle

S

SBFT: small bowel follow-through

SCFE: slipped capital femoral epiphysis

SPECT: single photon emission computed tomography

SSFP: steady-state free precession

SSFSE: single shot fast spin-echo

STIR: short tau inversion recovery

SVC: superior vena cava

SWI: susceptibility weighted imaging

T

T1: T1 relaxation time or T1-weighted

T2: T2 relaxation time or T2-weighted

T2*: T2 star relaxation time or T2 star-weighted

T2* GRE: T2 star gradient-echo

TOF: tetralogy of Fallot

TOF: time of flight

U

UGI: upper gastrointestinal tract

US: ultrasound

V

VCUG: voiding cystourethrography

VSD: ventricular septal defect

VUR: vesicoureteral reflux

W

WI: weighted imaging

WSCE: water-soluble contrast enema

Numbers

99mTC: technetium-99m

INDEX

INDEX

INDEX

INDEX

INDEX

INDEX

INDEX

INDEX

INDEX

INDEX

U